Basics of Functional Outcome and Measurements Scales

Basics of Functional Outcome and Measurements Scales

Dr Nikhil Mathur
BPT, MPH (Epidemiology) (Honours)
Senior Physiotherapist, NPCDCS (NCD)
Government District Hospital Mandore, Jodhpur (Raj)

ACMERI

SCIENTIFIC PUBLISHERS

Published by
SCIENTIFIC PUBLISHERS (INDIA)
5 A, New Pali Road, P.O. Box 91
Jodhpur 342 001 (INDIA)
E-mail: info@scientificpub.com
Website: http://www.scientificpubonline.com

Print 2026

ISBN: 978-93-94645-88-2 (HB)
eISBN: 978-93-94645-89-9 (E/B)

Printed in India

Dedication

To My Parents
Smt. Manju Mathur
Sh. Suresh Mathur
for raising me to believe that
anything is possible

And to My Guru Ji
Dr Harish Agarwal Sir M.D (Medicine)
Faculty, Regional Geriatric Centre
Dr S N Medical College, Jodhpur, Rajasthan
for making everything possible

Foreword

For more than four decades as a practising physician, particularly in geriatrics, I have realized the necessity of functional assessment in clinical practice.

As a medical teacher, I have been impressed by the talent of Dr Nikhil Mathur, whom I have known as a bright student, a sensitive practitioner and a keen research collaborator.

It's a pleasure to present his book "Basics of Functional Outcome and Measurement Scales". The book is a comprehensive collection of Medical Functional Outcomes and Measurement Scales frequently used in clinical practice and medical research. Dr Nikhil Mathur has gone deep into the subject and presented it in an easily understandable manner.

Besides clinical practitioners, the book will be helpful for physiotherapy students on the subject of Functional Outcome Measures (FOM).

The book is a valuable addition to the subject for undergraduate and postgraduate students, healthcare professionals and medical researchers.

Dr Arvind Mathur
Editor, Journal of the Indian Academy of Geriatrics
Director, Asian Centre for Medical Education, Research & Innovation
Chairperson, Caregivers Asha Society
Ex-Principal and Controller, Professor of Medicine,
Dr S. N. Medical College, Jodhpur

Message

Felicitations and Blessings to Dr Nikhil Mathur that he had collaborated all medical functional outcome and measurement scales on a platform. Functional outcome and scales play important role in diagnosing patient at every aspect level. This book provides theoretical information about intended population on which scales has to be applied, reliability, validity, and responsiveness of all scales which is the main key point and feature of book.

Best Wishes for success of book.

Dr Harish Agarwal
M.D (Medicine), Associate Professor
Regional Geriatrics Centre, Mathura Das Mathur Hospital
Dr S N Medical College, Jodhpur (Raj.)

Foreword

The health care delivery system in present times believes in evidence-based approach. To establish a fact into a true clinical science we rely on functional assessment, data collection and statistical analysis. The Functional Outcome Assessments are extremely important for planning the interventions in clinical research.

This book on functional assessment contains daily regular basic assessments and measurements, which are clinically used by professional therapists and students at their regular college, clinic, hospitals and during research studies.

This book "Basics of Functional Outcome and Measurement Scale" is the basic collection of all the scales and outcome measure, which helps the therapists and medicos to evaluate the current situation of patient and plan effectively with clinical reasoning.

The Book covers all the pattern of problems of patients coming to our regular OPD. It would be best for students enrolled for Bachelor of Physiotherapy course covering Functional and Outcome subject.

I would congratulate the author Dr Nikhil Mathur, who had been my student and a sincere professional for his persistent efforts. I also congratulate him and his team for gathering all the basic functional and outcome measurement scales at one platform.

Best wishes for success of this book.

Prof. Umasankar Mohanty
B.P.T(Hons), MPT(Manual Therapy),
MIASP, MISEP, FAGE, PhD.
The Founder President of
Manual Therapy Foundation of India (MTFI)

Foreword

Functional outcome assessment, the innovative premier book written exclusively for the Physiotherapy for students and clinicians, provides a detailed information important for understanding of the outcome measures. Measures of the successful intervention is key in deciding. managing and changing the strategies of intervention for betterment of patient. The intervention program has to be planned and implemented appropriately as per changing status and needs of the patient. The referral to Physiotherapy treatments for variety of the disorders, diseases are increasing day by day. This book has taken care of growing public demands and inclination towards Physiotherapy. There was need of such content rich, focused book on the outcome measures specially dedicated towards needs of Physiotherapy students, clinicians and researchers.

The evidence-based practice (EBP) is the need of the current time. The outcome measurement is one of the critical areas in achieving the EBP. The book is rich resource for the Physiotherapy fraternity and will also help other health care professionals. With rapid advancement in health care and evolvement of newer techniques, such books becomes essential.

The technology of information sector is rapidly changing and plenty of information is easily available on various platform however the clarity and wisdom seems as rare as authentic information. This book will be welcomed by everyone in our speciality from novice to experienced one.

I appreciate the efforts of Dr. Nikhil Mathur & Dr. Harish Agrawal for their efforts to address this area. I have great pleasure in writing forward for the book.

Dr. Sudeep Kale
Professor, Terna Physiotherapy College, Navi Mumbai
President, Maharashtra Physiotherapy Council

Prologue

"Necessity is the mother of innovation." For me the lack of Functional Outcomes and Measurements Scales during my stint as a Physical Therapist lead me to ponder over compiling a book on this line. The result – Was pouring over thousands of papers, scouring various journal and surfing umpteen hours on net. The final product – a glossary where a Physical Therapy student or medical research fellow will find a needy reference for his needs. I am thankful to PhysioPedia for providing essentials.

As with all major works, I too was blessed by a number of individuals without whose guidance, the book wouldn't have seen the light of day. Foremost my sincere gratitude to Dr Harish Agarwal Sir (MD, Medicine) , a mentor, a friend, the backbone of this book. His guidance was akin to what Krishna's was for Arjun.

The blessings of my parents, the love and patience of my wife and encouragement by my soul (my younger brother) and his wife, children made my enduring task simple. A big thank you to them.

Currently there is no any specific book covering the basic functional scales at one platform. We had compiled these functional outcomes scales at one. The functional outcome measurement scales contains their theoretical part which include objective of scale, material and methodology to applying scale, Responsibility, Validity and Reliability of that specific scale on to the patient.

The functional outcome measures are essential component of assessment, planning and monitoring in research and treatment aspects. The chapters of book can further be included according to categories wise segments like: -

- Cardiopulmonary and Cardiovascular Functional Outcome Scales like: 2 Minute Walk Test, Borg Rating of Perceived Exertion, 6 Minute Walk Test, 10 Meter Walk Test, Glasgow Coma Scale etc.
- Mental Health Outcome Measures like: - Fever Avoidance Belief Questionnaire, Mental Health Outcome Measure for Physiotherapist in Clinical Practice, Nottingham Health Profile etc.
- Neurological Outcome Measures like – 10 Meter Walk Test, 2 Minute Walk Test, Action Research Arm Test, Arm Mobility Ability Test, Balance Evaluation System Test, Berg Balance Test, Box and Block Test, Coma Recovery Scale (Revised), Community Balance and Mobility Scale, Edinburgh Handedness Inventory, Falls Efficacy Scale – International, Functional Ambulation Category, Functional Gait Assessment, Functional Reach Test, Galveston Orientation Amnesia Test, Glasgow Coma Scale, Mass Attention Rating Scale, NIH Stroke Scale, Nine Hole Peg Test, Oswestry Disability Index, Parkinson's Disease Questionnaire, Progressive Supra Nuclear Palsy Rating Scale etc.
- Geriatric Outcome Measure – 10 Meter Walk Test, @ minute Walk Test, 30 Second Sit to Stand Test, 4 Item Dynamic Gait Index, Barthel Index, Berg Balance Scale, Community Balance and Mobility Scale, DASH Outcome Measure, Elderly Mobility Scale, Falls Efficacy Scale- International, Fear Avoidance Belief Questionnaire, Functional Gait Assessment, Functional Independence Measure, Functional Reach Test, Harris Hip Score, Hip Disability and Osteoarthritis Outcome Score, Katz ADL, Mental Health and Outcome Measure for Physiotherapist in Clinical Practice, Mini – Mental State Examination, Neck Disability Index, Oswestry

Disability Index, Oxford Hip Score, Oxford Knee Score, Physical Activity Scale for the Elderly, Sarc – F : A Simple Questionnaire to Rapidly Dispose Sarcopenia, Short Form McGill Pain Questionnaire, Time Up and Go Test , Tinetti Test, Tragus to Wall Test, VAS Scale, WOMAC – Osteoarthritis Index etc.

- Pediatric Measures – 2 Minute Walk Test, Bangla Club Foot Tool, Functional Ability Description ool, Gait and Lower Limb Observation of Pediatrics, Gross Motor Function Measure, Knee Injury and Osteoarthritis Outcome Score – Child, Pediatrics Balance Scale, Pirani Score, Revised Hammersmith Scale for Spinal Muscular Atrophy, Roye Score etc.
- Orthopedic Measurement Outcome Scales like: Neck Disability Index, Tragus to Wall Test, DASH Outcome Measure, Upper Extremity Functional Index, Lower Extremity Functional Index, 8-Item Sports Sub Scale, Foot and Ankle Ability Measure, Foot Function Index, Manchester Oxford Foot Questionnaire, Pirani Score, Roye Score, Harris Hip Score, Hip Disability and Osteoarthritis Outcome Score, Ibadan Knee / Hip Osteoarthritis Outcome Score, Knee Injury and Osteoarthritis Outcome Score – Adult, Knee Injury and Osteoarthritis Outcome Score – Child, 36 – Short form Survey etc.

Lastly, I would like to acknowledge the book designer Scientific Publisher – Sh. Tanay Sharma who give the final touches to my book.

Loads of heartfelt thanks to developers of these scales. I hereby confirm that the scales used are of the developers and they have the sole authority of copyright and that these scales would be used for students and researchers' awareness and updating their knowledge.

Dr Nikhil Mathur

BPT, MPH (Epidemiology) (Honours)

Senior Physiotherapist, NPCDCS (NCD)

Government District Hospital Mandore, Jodhpur (Raj)

Visiting Faculty:

a. **Physiotherapy**
K S Memorial College of Physiotherapy, Jodhpur
(Affiliated: Rajasthan University of Health Science, Jaipur)

b. **Public Health**
Jodhpur School of Public Health, Jodhpur
(Affiliated: Maulana Azad University, Jodhpur)

c. **Public Health**
Lachoo Memorial College of Science & Technology, Jodhpur
(Affiliated: Jai Narain Vyas University, Jodhpur)

Contents

PART A Basics

PART B Outcome Scales

Part A

BASICS

1 Outcome Measures

Introduction

An outcome measure is a tool used to assess a patient's current status[1]. Outcome measures may provide a score, an interpretation of results and at times a risk categorization of the patient. Prior to providing any intervention, an outcome measure provides baseline data. The initial results may help determine the course of treatment intervention. Once treatment has commenced, the same tool may be used in serial assessments to determine whether the patient has demonstrated change. With the move towards Evidence Based Practice (EBP) in health care, outcome measures provide credible and reliable justification for treatment on an individual patient level. The results from outcome measures may also be grouped for aggregated analysis focused on determining quality of care. When outcome measures are used in an aggregated data situation to compare results, a risk adjustment process is required to fairly compare results.[2][3]

Outcome measures that we use in clinical practice are divided into four categories:

1. Self-report measures
2. Performance-based measures
3. Observer-reported measures
4. Clinician-reported measures

Self-report measures are typically captured in the form of a questionnaire. The questionnaires are scored by applying a predetermined point system to the patient's responses. Although self-report measures seem subjective in nature, self-report measures objectify a patient's perception. Historically, the questionnaires required that either a therapist interviewed the patient or the patient independently completed the questionnaire. Self-report outcome measures that use paper and pencil for completion are considered a fixed-form questionnaire. Computer based or electronic self-report measures are available. Electronic measures may be fixed-form or adaptive. Computerized adaptive testing is a method of testing that determines the questions for a response based on the patient's previous responses.[4] The questionnaires where the patient reports on health or physical function are known as patient-reported outcomes (PRO).[5] PROs can be categorized as disease specific or generic. PROs have been defined as "any report of the status of a patient's health condition that comes directly from the patient, without interpretation of the patient's response by a clinician or anyone else."[6]

Performance-based measures require the patient to perform a set of movements or tasks. Scores for performance-based measures can be based on either an objective measurement (e.g., time to complete a task) or a qualitative assessment that is assigned a score (e.g., normal or abnormal mechanics for a given task).

Performance-based measures and patient reported measures both capture a current status. These measures do not typically equate with each other. Performance-based measures tend to bring to light physiologic factors. Patient reported outcome measures may capture a patient's perception, beliefs, social factors and/or health factors. [7]

Observer-reported measures are measurements completed by a parent, caregiver or someone who regularly observes the patient on a daily basis.

Clinician-reported measures are measurements that are completed by a health care professional. The professional uses clinical judgement and reports on patient behaviors or signs that are observed by the professional.

Statistical Analysis

Important features of an outcome measure that need to be taken into account when using an outcome measure are its psychometric properties. Psychometric properties are the intrinsic properties of an outcome measure. Ideally, the psychometric properties of an outcome measure used in practice should have been developed and tested through a series of research studies. These properties include validity, inter-rater reliability, intra-rater reliability, responsiveness, ceiling effects, floor effects and minimal clinically important difference. Validity refers to the how accurately the test actually measures what it is supposed to measure. High validity means the measure is consistently stable in its ability to measure its intended focus. Inter-rater reliability takes into consideration the consistency of the results of the measure when two different people are evaluating the results of a common subject. With performance-based measures, if two physiotherapists scored the performance, high inter-rater reliability would mean that both determined similar scores on the performance evaluated. For patient reported outcome measures, a high intra-rater reliability indicates that the patient consistently responds to attain the same results. (This would be more relevant with serial testing and no intervention or change in status. Intra-rater reliability falls under test-retest reliability.) Responsiveness refers to the ability for the measure to be able to capture change in status. Ceiling effect occurs when the majority of patients are able to complete the measure and score within the highest range of the measurement. (The test is too easy and is not capturing their full capability.) Floor effect occurs when the majority of the patients score within the lowest range of the measurement. (The test is too hard and does not have enough easier items to distinguish varying levels of status.) When determining if change is relevant, the p-value has no value. For outcome measures, the clinician needs to know the minimal important difference. Minimal important difference refers to the amount of change that is relevant from the patient's perspective. (clinical meaningfulness).

Clinical Utility of an Outcome Measure

Choosing appropriate outcome measures for your patients is critical to understanding their status and progress over time.[8]

References

1. Fetters L, Tilson J. Evidence based physical therapy. FA Davis; 2012 May 5.
2. Gvozdyev BV, Carreon LY, Graves CM, Riley SA, McGraw KE, Head RJ, Dimar JR, Glassman SD. Patient-reported outcome scores underestimate the impact of major complications in patients undergoing spine surgery for degenerative conditions. Journal of Neurosurgery: Spine. 2017 Oct 1;27(4):397-402.
3. Deutscher D, Werneke MW, Hayes D, Mioduski JE, Cook KF, Fritz JM, Woodhouse LJ, Stratford PW. Impact of risk adjustment on provider ranking for patients with low back pain receiving physical therapy. Journal of Orthopaedic & Sports Physical Therapy. 2018 Aug;48(8):637-48.
4. McCabe E, Gross DP, Bulut O. Procedures to develop a computerized adaptive test to assess patient-reported physical functioning. Quality of Life Research. 2018 Sep 1;27(9):2393-402.
5. Kyte DG, Calvert M, Van der Wees PJ, Ten Hove R, Tolan S, Hill JC. An introduction to patient-reported outcome measures (PROMs) in physiotherapy. Physiotherapy. 2015 Jun 1;101(2):119-25.
5. Black N. Patient reported outcome measures could help transform healthcare. BMJ: British Medical Journal. 2013;346.
6. Bean JF, Ölveczky DD, Kiely DK, LaRose SI, Jette AM. Performance-based versus patient-reported physical function: what are the underlying predictors? Physical Therapy. 2011 Dec 1;91(12):1804-11.
7. Hefford C, Abbott JH, Baxter GD Arnold R. Outcome measurement in clinical practice: practical and theoretical issues for health related quality of life (HRQOL) questionnaires. Physical Therapy Reviews. 2011;16(3):155-167.

2 Guide to Selecting Outcome Measures

Why Am I Using the Outcome Measure?

- Identifying the impact of a disorder on an individual?
- Establishing a baseline measure from which to monitor changes over time?
- Evaluating the impact of an intervention?
- Evaluating the needs of those attending a service?

What Am I Aiming to Measure?

- Impairments of body structure and function?
- Activity limitations?
- Participation restrictions?
- Quality of life?

Have the Clinimetric Properties of this Tool Been Measured in a Population Similar to Mine? Consider:

- Do the study samples have the same condition?
- Is the study sample similar in disease severity?
- Is the study sample similar in disease-specific factors?

Is the Outcome Measure Reliable?

- Do I know the rate of error detected with scores?
- Do I know the minimum detectable change?

Is the Outcome Measure Valid?

- Does it measure what I want it to measure?

Is the Outcome Measure Responsive to Change?

- Is there a known minimum clinically important difference?

Financial Considerations

- What is the cost of this test?
- Is a licence required?
- Is equipment required?

Therapist Implementation

- Is the measure easy for a clinician to conduct?
- Is special training required/available?
- Are there clear standardised instructions on how to carry out and score the measure?
- How long does it take to carry out the measure?
- How long does it take to record results?

Resources

- Is special equipment or are special forms required?
- Is space sufficient for this measure to be carried out?

Client

- How much time does it take for the person to complete?
- Is the task difficult?
- Is privacy required?

Patient-Reported Outcome Measures (PROM)

- Is face-to-face contact required or can this measure be completed in the waiting room?
- Does the questionnaire cover sensitive personal issues?
- Is there a specific reading level required?
- Is the measure available in other languages?

References

1. Iansek R, & Morris ME (Eds.) (2013). Rehabilitation in movement disorders. Cambridge University Press.

❑❑❑

3 Wheelchair Related Outcome Measures

Introduction

An outcome measure is any characteristic or quality measured to assess a patient's status[1]. An outcome measure is the result of a test that is used to objectively determine the baseline function of a patient at the beginning of treatment. Once treatment has commenced, the same instrument can be used to determine progress and treatment efficacy. With the move towards Evidence Based Practice (EBP) in the Health Sciences, objective measures of outcome are important to provide credible and reliable justification for treatment. The instrument should also be convenient to use for the wheelchair service personnel and comfortable for the wheelchair user. An integral part of evaluating clinical practice is to objectively assess the intervention and measure it against a set of outcomes to determine its efficacy. [2] This means the wheelchair service personnel can ensure they are providing the most appropriate intervention that meets the goals and expectations of the wheelchair user, their family member/caregiver and the wheelchair service provision team.

Considerations before Choosing an Outcome Measure

If you are considering using an outcome measure for a wheelchair user it is worth considering the questions posed on the Guide to Selecting Outcome Measures Physiopedia Page. At the very least you should consider these questions with your wheelchair user in mind.

Why Am I Using an Outcome Measure?

- Am I trying to establish a baseline measure from which I can monitor changes over time for an individual user?
- Am I trying to predict how the wheelchair is going to perform?
- Am I trying to evaluate the impact of a wheelchair, a wheelchair component or treatment programme on an individual or a group?
- Am I trying to evaluate the needs of the wheelchair user attending my service?
- Am I trying to evaluate how my service is responding to needs of the wheelchair user?

What Am I Aiming to Measure?

- Impairments of Body Structure and Function?
- Activity Limitations?
- Participation Restrictions?
- Quality of Life?
- Something Else?

Have the Clinimetric Properties been Measured in a Population Similar to Mine?

1. Is the Outcome Measure Reliable?
    - Do I know the rate of error detected with scores?
    - Do I know the minimum detectable change?
2. Is the Outcome Measure Valid?
    - Does it measure what I want it to measure?
3. Is the Outcome Measure Responsive to Change?
    - Is there a known minimum clinically important difference?

Other Considerations

Other considerations (Outcome Measures) may come into play when deciding which outcome measure to use:

Financial Considerations:

- What is the cost of this test?
- Is a licence required?
- Is equipment required?

Therapist Implementation

- Is the measure easy for a clinician to conduct?
- Is special training required/available?
- Are there clear standardised instructions on how to carry out and score the measure?
- How long does it take to carry out the measure?
- How long does it take to record results?

Resources

- Is special equipment or are special forms required?
- Is space sufficient for this measure to be carried out?

Wheelchair User

- How much time does it take for the person to complete?
- Is the task difficult?
- Is privacy required?

Patient-Reported Outcome Measures (PROQ)

- Is face-to-face contact required or can this measure be completed in the waiting room?
- Does the questionnaire cover sensitive personal issues?
- Is there a specific reading level required?
- Is the measure available in other languages?

References

1. Fetters L, Tilson J. Evidence based physical therapy. FA Davis; 2012 May 5.
2. Debuse D, Brace H. Outcome Measures of Activity for Children with Cerebral Palsy: A Systematic Review. Pediatr Phys Ther. 2011 Fall;23(3):221-31

❑❑❑

4 Outcome Measures for Patients with Lower Limb Amputations

General Introduction

Outcome measures can be used for many different purposes. A predictive measure should be able to classify individuals according to a set of pre-defined categories either concurrently or prospectively e.g. whether an amputee will use a prosthesis successfully [1] [2]. Detecting differences between people or groups demonstrates the discriminative value of an outcome measure e.g. being able to determine the different abilities of a trans-tibial or trans-femoral amputee or differences between prosthetic components from scores or times recorded [3].

Whereas an evaluative measure should be able to detect changes, usually over a period of time in an individual or group. An evaluative outcome measure may also detect changes occurring following some kind of intervention, e.g a therapy programme[4] or provision of a prosthetic component. Some outcome measures are designed to do only one of the above, while others may do a combination, though some of the requirements of these different types of outcome measures are competing [5]. Whichever purpose it is designed for, the psychometric properties of the outcome measure need to be reported to satisfy the user that it is fit for purpose with the population they wish to use it [6].

The psychometric properties of an outcome measure are the characteristics that express its adequacy in terms of reliability, validity and responsiveness. Another term often used is clinimetric properties. While being developed from similar origins as psychometrics, clinimetrics has been described as the practice of assessing or describing symptoms, signs, and laboratory findings by means of scales, indices, and other quantitative instruments, all of which should have adequate psychometric properties [7] [8].

It is important in the initial stages of rehabilitation to use outcome measures that help predict the ability a patient will have to walk with a prosthesis and to determine which prosthetic components would be best for the patient[9].

Considerations Before Choosing an Outcome Measure

If you are considering using an outcome measure with an amputee it is worth asking yourself the questions posed on the Outcome Measures page here in Physiopedia (Guide to Selecting Outcome Measures). At the very least you should consider these questions with your amputee patient or group in mind.

Why am I using an outcome measure?

- Am I trying to establish a baseline measure from which I can monitor changes over time for an individual patient?
- Am I trying to predict how my patient is going to perform?
- Am I trying to evaluate the impact of a treatment programme or prosthetic component on an individual or a group?
- Am I trying to evaluate the needs of the amputee attending my service?
- Am I trying to evaluate how my service is responding to the needs of the amputee?

What am I aiming to measure?

- Impairments of body structure and function?
- Activity limitations?
- Participation restrictions?
- Quality of life?
- Something else?

When you think you may have an outcome measure in mind you should also consider these questions.

Have the clinimetric properties of the outcome measure I am considering been measured in a population similar to mine?

- Is the outcome measure reliable?
- Do I know the rate of error detected with scores?
- Do I know the minimum detectable change?
- Is the outcome measure valid?
- Does it measure what I want it to measure?
- Is the outcome measure responsive to change?
- Is there a known minimum clinically important difference?

Here are some examples of studies where the clinimetric, sometimes called psychometric, properties have been reported in an amputee population and what the results may tell you.

Reliability

Reliability is usually measured by Intra-class correlation coefficients (ICC) and is presented as a number between 0 (no consistency) to 1 (complete consistency) [10] Intra-rater Reliability: This indicates how consistently a rater administers and scores an outcome measure. Inter-raterReliability:Thisindicateshowwelltworatersagree in the way they administer and score an outcome measure. Test-retest reliability: If an individual completes a self-report survey and then repeats the survey on a second occasion when no change is expected, the results should be similar.

- Brooks, Hunter et al (2002) examined the reliability of the 2 minute walk test (2MWT) [11]. Participants completed 2 successive timed walks measured by 2 different raters on 2 consecutive days. Intra class correlations (ICC) were >0 .98 showing excellent intra- and inter-rater reliability.

Measurement error: This is the degree to which scores or ratings are identical irrespective of who performs or scores the test and can be reported using the standard error of measurement (SEM) or minimal detectable change (MDC), which is the same as smallest detectable change (SDC) [12].

- Deathe & Miller (2005) reported the SEM in absolute values, which was 3 sec for the L-Test [13].
- Resnik & Borgia (2011) also reported MDC in absolute values for all the measures they studied: 2MWT (34.3m), 6 minute walk test (6MWT) (45m), timed up and go (TUG) (3.6s) and amputee mobility predictor (AMP) (3.4pts) [14]

Internal Consistency: This reliability property is reserved for outcome measures that are designed to test only one concept. Internal consistency assesses the extent to which all items or questions in an outcome measure address the same underlying concept, e.g. in a mobility scale, all the items should deal with mobility [5]. There are two main methods used to report internal consistency. The Classical Test theory uses Cronbachs alpha (α) to indicate the reliability of an outcome measure as a whole. And the Item Response Theory uses Rasch Analysis to assess internal consistency by looking at each item within the outcome measure [15].

- The internal consistency of the ABC scale was considered excellent as measured by Cronbachs alpha (0.93) in a study by Milleret al (2003) [16].
- Rasch analysis was used to examine all the items in the Berg Balance Scale which confirmed that it was able to test a range of difficulty and identify four levels of ability [17].

Validity

Content /Face validity: This is the degree to which the content of an outcome measure is an adequate reflection of the construct or concept to be measured (5). It is usually considered and agreed by consensus of an expert group of clinicians and can and should include patient representatives. For example an instrument measuring activity limitation in young athletic individuals should include not only walking but also running, jumping, and climbing.

Structural validity: This refers to the degree to which the scores of an outcome measure are an adequate reflection of the dimension or factor of the construct being measured [5]. It can be measured by performing factor analysis where the result demonstrate that if >50% of data refer to one factor this confirms that the outcome measure is measuring one factor / dimension. Anything less indicates more than one factor is being assessed. Rasch Analysis may also be used where the outcome measures unidimensionality, i.e. whether it is measuring one or more factors or dimensions.

- Wong et al (2013) reported results from factor analysis performed on the Berg Balance Score (BBS). The results showed that 70% of the data were explained in the model related to one dimension, i.e. balance capability [17].
- Franchignoni et al (2007) used Rasch modelling on a modified Locomotor Capability Index to confirm good structural validity when level 1 and 2 category responses were combined and 4 items

were deleted due to either over or under-fitting [18]. The resultant modified index is known as LCI-5 which many clinicians now use.

Construct Validity: This is the degree to which the scores of an outcome measure are consistent with pre-defined (apriori) hypotheses that outline relationships to the scores of other instruments, or differences between groups. If > 75% of hypotheses are proved this is an indication of good validity [19]. It can also be referred to as: Concurrent validity – showing the ability to distinguish between groups (e.g. older and younger lower limb amputees (LLAs)) which is often measured by testing hypotheses, or; Convergent validity – showing that measures that should be related are related, which can also be measured using intraclass correlation coefficient (ICC) with high values indicating good validity.

- Major et al (2013) hypothesised positive relationships between the Berg Balance scale (BBS) scores and the Activities specific Balance Confidence (ABC) scale, the mobility scale of the Prosthetic Evaluation Questionnaire (PEQ (ms), the Frenchay Activities Index (FAI) and the 2MWT and a negative relationship with the L-test score [20]. These were all proved.
- To assess concurrent and convergent validity of the L-test Deathe & Miller (2005) asked subjects to complete walks test; TUG,10-Meter Walk Test, and 2MWT, followed by self-reported measures; ABC scale, FAI, PEQ (ms). Concurrent validity was high (ICC = 0.86-0.97) between the L-Test data and the other walk tests and fair-to-moderate (ICC = 0.22 – 0.54) for self-report measures. Higher mean times were observed for those subjects who:

1. were older
2. used a walking aid
3. had to concentrate on each step they took
4. had a vascular amputation and
5. had a TF amputation.

Therefore it was demonstrated that the L Test was able to discriminate between all groups as hypothesized [13].

Criterion validity: This is the degree to which the scores of an outcome measure are an adequate reflection of a 'gold standard'. However there are very few situations in rehabilitation where such a gold standard test exists. If no gold standard is available then it may be appropriate to test hypothetical relationships with comparator measures. The estimation of criterion validity depends on the type of data. Intra-class correlations are used if both instruments (outcome instrument and comparator) have continuous scores (e.g. time, distance etc) and the results should preferably be above 0.70. If the outcome instrument has a continuous score but the comparator has a dichotomous score (e.g. Yes / No) then area under the receiver operated characteristic (ROC) is the preferred method. Again, a criterion of 0.70 is suggested [19].

- Gremeauxet al (2012) presented ROC curves for the 2MWT. The modified Houghton Scale was used to stratify the patients into two groups; those with no mobility problems (scored 20/20) and those who scored less than 20 indicating a functional limitation. According to the ROC analysis cut off values of 130m or 150m were highly associated with the existence of functional limitations [21].

Responsiveness

Internal responsiveness is the ability of a measure to change over a specified time frame. It will depend on the particular population being studied, the treatment or intervention which occurs during the time frame and the outcome measure used to determine any changes [5]. Standard effect size is the difference between the mean baseline scores and the follow-up scores, divided by the baseline standard deviation (SD). If there is a high variability in baseline scores in relation to the mean change scores the effect size will be small and the ability of the outcome measure to detect meaningful changes is also small. A small effect will be 0.2 representing a change of approx 1/5 that of the baseline SD, 0.5 is considered moderate and anything over 0.8, or a change of at least 4/5 of the baseline SD is considered large [22]. The paired-t-test is a statistical test that can be used to detect the change in the average scores at two time points, but is dependent on the sample size and variability / reliability of the outcome measure used[15]. In a study by Devlinet al (2004) the effect size calculated for the change in mean scores for the Houghton Scale, from discharge to follow-up, was 0.60, indicating a moderate difference[23].

- Findings by Brooks et al (2001) indicated that the 2MWT was "responsive to change during rehabilitation". Significant improvements were seen in means and SDs of the distances walked between baseline and discharge and follow-up [24]. However, effect sizes were not calculated.

Other Considerations

Other considerations (Outcome Measures) may come into play when deciding which outcome measure to use: Financial Considerations:

- What is the cost of this test?
- Is a licence required?
- Is equipment required?

Therapist Implementation

- Is the measure easy for a clinician to conduct?
- Is special training required/available?
- Are there clear standardised instructions on how to carry out and score the measure?
- How long does it take to carry out the measure?
- How long does it take to record results?

Resources

- Is special equipment or are special forms required?
- Is space sufficient for this measure to be carried out?

Client

- How much time does it take for the person to complete?
- Is the task difficult?
- Is privacy required?

Patient-Reported Outcome Measures (PROQ)

- Is face-to-face contact required or can this measure be completed in the waiting room?
- Does the questionnaire cover sensitive personal issues?
- Is there a specific reading level required?
- Is the measure available in other languages?

List of Outcome Measures Validated for Use With Lower Limb Amputees

Before using an outcome measure remember to consider the questions stated above.

Post-amputation

- Amputee Mobility Predictor without a Prosthesis (AMPnoPRO)
- Basic Amputee Mobility Score (BAMS) - this is a newly developed outcome measure that evaluates four basic mobility activities of individuals who underwent major lower limb amputations.

Prosthetic Rehabilitation

The following outcome measures are included in the most recent version (2014) of the British Association of Chartered Physiotherapists in Amputee Rehabilitation (BACPAR) Outcome Measures Toolbox

- Activities-specific Balance Confidence (ABC) Scale-UK
- Amputee Mobility Predictor (www.oandp.org/olc/lessons/html/SSC_06/Gailey_AMP_Arch_of_Phys_Med_Rehab_2002.pdf) Amputee Mobility Predictor without prosthesis (AMPnoPRO) - has the best statistical predictor for motor ability/outcome [9]
- Houghton Scale (www.archives-pmr.org/article/S0003-9993%2803%2901223-1/fulltext)
- Locomotor Capabilities Index-5
- Trinity Amputation and Prosthesis Experiences Scales (www.archives-pmr.org/article/S0003-9993%2803%2900978-X/fulltext)
- Timed Up and Go Test (TUG)
- L-Test (ptjournal.apta.org/content/85/7/626.long)
- 2 min timed walk test (www.archives-pmr.org/article/S0003-9993%2802%2900252-6/fulltext)
- 6 min timed walk test
- Berg Balance Scale

High-level Activity Amputees

The outcome measures listed above can be used use with high level activity amputees but it should be noted that ceiling effects may be seen, i.e. the amputee will achieve maximum scores when using ordinal scales, whether observed or self reported.

A Comprehensive High-Level Activity Mobility Predictor (CHAMP) was developed to asses patients with limb loss that need to return to high-level activity. This outcome measure was found to be safe and reliable with wounded army servicemen at Walter Reed Medical Center with high-level mobility and traumatic lower limb amputations. [25]

Pre-prosthetic and/or Immediate Post-operative Period

A narrative review undertaken by the BACPAR Outcome Measures project group, looking into the evidence for the use of outcome measures for lower limb amputees (LLAs) in the acute or pre-prosthetic phase. The review was presented in the Spring 2014 BACPAR Journal bacpar.csp.org.uk/. A search of MEDLINE, CINAHL and PsychINFO in May 2013 using such search terms as 'Acute Care' and 'Outcome Measures' with 'Lower-limb Amputees' OR 'Lower-limb Amputation' resulted in a total of 26 articles which, after screening, produced two articles that merited further reading. From these articles only the Functional Independence Measure (FIM) was identified as of potential interest and a further search was conducted adding the specific FIM title. While there is evidence that the FIM is used in the acute and / or early rehabilitation phase with LLAs and can demonstrate an improvement between admission and discharge, the evidence was weak. There was no evidence that the total FIM score was effective as a predictor tool, but there was good correlation in one study for the motor subscale with prosthetic outcome.

When the Toolbox was updated in October 2014 it was decided that not to include the FIM or any other specific outcome measure into the Toolbox for this population as the current evidence was not strong enough. The other outcome measures included in the Toolbox all had good evidence with larger sample sizes. In addition the FIM requirés training before using it and is recommended as an MDT tool so does not fit the "easy to use" criteria.

References

1. Condie ME, McFadyen AK, Treweek S, Whitehead L. The trans-femoral fitting predictor: a functional measure to predict prosthetic fitting in transfemoral amputees--validity and reliability. Arch Phys Med Rehabil 2011 08;92(8):1293-1297.
2. Raya M, A., Gailey R, S., Gaunaurd I, A., Ganyard H, Knapp-Wood J, McDonough K, et al. Amputee Mobility Predictor-Bilateral: A performance-based measure of mobility for people with bilateral lower-limb loss. J Rehabil Res Dev 2013 11;50(7):961-968.
3. Hafner BJ, Willingham LL, Buell NC, Allyn KJ, Smith DG. Evaluation of function, performance, and preference as transfemoral amputees transition from mechanical to microprocessor control of the prosthetic knee. Archives of Physical Medicine & Rehabilitation 2007 02;88(2):207-217.
4. Rau B, Bonvin F, de Bie R. Short-term effect of physiotherapy rehabilitation on functional performance of lower limb amputees. Prosthet Orthot Int 2007;31(3):258-270.
5. Mokkink LB, Terwee CB, Patrick DL, Alonso J, Stratford PW, Knol DL, et al. The COSMIN study reached international consensus on taxonomy, terminology, and definitions of measurement properties for health-related patient-reported outcomes. J Clin Epidemiol 2010;63(7):737-745.
6. Kirshner B, Guyatt G. A methodological framework for assessing health indices. J Chronic Dis 1985;38(1):27-36.
7. Streiner DL. Clinimetrics vs. psychometrics: an unnecessary distinction. J Clin Epidemiol 2003 12;56(12):1142-1145.
8. Galea M. Introducing Clinimetrics. Australian Journal of Physiotherapy 2005;51(3):139-140.
9. Spaan MH, Vrieling AH, van de Berg P, Dijkstra PU, van Keeken HG. Predicting mobility outcome in lower limb amputees with motor ability tests used in early rehabilitation. Prosthetics and orthotics international. 2017 Apr;41(2):171-7.
10. Shrout PE(1), Fleiss JL. Intraclass correlations: Uses in assessing rater reliability. Psychol Bull 1979 / 03 / 01 /;86(2):420-428.
11. Brooks D, Hunter JP, Parsons J, Livsey E, Quirt J, Devlin M. Reliability of the two-minute walk test in individuals with transtibial amputation. Arch Phys Med Rehabil 2002 11;83(11):1562-1565
12. Stratford P, W., Riddle D, L. When Minimal Detectable Change Exceeds a Diagnostic Test-Based Threshold Change Value for an Outcome Measure: Resolving the Conflict. Phys Ther 2012 10;92(10):1338-1347.
13. Deathe AB, Miller WC. The L test of functional mobility: measurement properties of a modified version of the timed "up & go" test designed for people with lower-limb amputations. Phys Ther 2005 07;85(7):626-635
14. Resnik L, Borgia M. Reliability of outcome measures for people with lower-limb amputations: distinguishing true change from statistical error. Phys Ther 2011 04;91(4):555-565.
15. Streiner DL, Norman GR. Health measurement scales : a practical guide to their development and use / David L. Streiner and Geoffrey R. Norman. : Oxford : Oxford University Press, 2003; 3rd ed; 2003.
16. Miller WC, Deathe AB, Speechley M. Psychometric properties of the Activities-Specific Balance Confidence Scale among individuals with

a lower-limb amputation. Arch Phys Med Rehabil 2003 05;84(5):656-661.

17. Wong C, Kevin, Chen C, C., Welsh J. Preliminary Assessment of Balance With the Berg Balance Scale in Adults Who Have a Leg Amputation and Dwell in the Community: Rasch Rating Scale Analysis. Phys Ther 2013 11;93(11):1520-1529.
18. Franchignoni F, Giordano A, Ferriero G, Muñoz S, Orlandini D, Amoresano A. Rasch analysis of the Locomotor Capabilities Index-5 in people with lower limb amputation. Prosthet Orthot Int 2007 12;31(4):394-404.
19. Terwee CB, Bot SDM, de Boer M,R., van der Windt D,A.W.M., Knol DL, Dekker J, et al. Quality criteria were proposed for measurement properties of health status questionnaires. J Clin Epidemiol 2007 01;60(1):34-42.
20. Major MJ, Fatone S, Roth EJ. Validity and reliability of the berg balance scale for community-dwelling persons with lower-limb amputation. Arch Phys Med Rehabil 2013 11;94(11):2194-2202.
21. Gremeaux V, Damak S, Troisgros O, Feki A, Laroche D, Perennou D, et al. Selecting a test for the clinical assessment of balance and walking capacity at the definitive fitting state after unilateral amputation: a comparative study. Prosthet Orthot Int 2012 12;36(4):415-422.
22. Kazis LE, Anderson JJ, Meenan RF. Effect sizes for interpreting changes in health status. Med Care 1989 / 03 / 01 /;27(3):S178-189.
23. Devlin M, Pauley T, Head K, Garfinkel S. Houghton Scale of prosthetic use in people with lower-extremity amputations: reliability, validity, and responsiveness to change. Arch Phys Med Rehabil 2004 08;85(8):1339-1344.
24. Brooks D, Parsons J, Hunter JP, Devlin M, Walker J. The 2-minute walk test as a measure of functional improvement in persons with lower limb amputation. Arch Phys Med Rehabil 2001 10;82(10):1478-1483.
25. Gailey RS, Gaunaurd IA, Raya MA, Roach KE, Linberg AA, Campbell SM, Jayne DM, Scoville C. Development and reliability testing of the Comprehensive High-Level Activity Mobility Predictor (CHAMP) in male servicemembers with traumatic lower-limb loss. WALTER REED ARMY MEDICAL CENTER WASHINGTON DC; 2013 Jan.

❑❑❑

5 Physical Activity and Outcome Measures

Introduction

For clinical and research purposes, measuring physical activity is vital for studying and evaluating its health benefits. Being a variable with many dimensions (frequency, intensity, mode, duration, volume, context), there is no standardised outcome measure for physical activity, hence, the choice of assessment/proxy measure of physical activity is dependent on which dimension is being studied.

Measures

Physical activity can be measured across all age groups and health spectrum, with choice of tool dependent on the type of activity being examined:

- Preschool children (2-5 years)
- Children (6-12 years)
- Adolescents (13-17 years)
- Adults (18-64 years)
- Older adults (65+)

Physical activity can be measured using different techniques[1] such as:

Method of measurement	Unit of measurement
Self-report	Bouts of physical actvity
Activity monitors/motion sensors	Movement counts
Heart rate	Beats per minute
Pedometers	Step counts
Direct observation	Activity rating
Indirect calorimetry	Oxygen consumption
Doubly labelled water	Carbon dioxide production

Self-report Techniques

The self-report approach to measuring physical activity is one that is commonly used because of its affordability, low respondent burden and ability to capture large population in a shorter time frame[2]. It relies on the ability of participants to recall their physical activity in retrospect, and can be documented by use of a questionnaire, either self-administered or interview-administered[3] or by daily logs and diaries[4].

Self-report physical activity instruments can be further classified into:

Physical Activity Records & Diaries

While logs involve the participants documenting the amount of time spent in broad categories of activity (sitting, standing, walking), records/diary require the participant to record the individual sessions of activity as they occur prospectively[5]. Examples include: Physical activity log book[6] and Bouchard's activity diary[7].

Gobal Self-report

When the objective of the researcher or clinician is to stratify an individual's level of physical activity as either high or low using generic terms, self-report assessments are usually used[8]. This involves using an instrument that contains one to four items to identify the physical activity pattern of the individual, in a specific domain over a specific period of time[9].

Recall Questionnaires

In surveillance studies, the physical activity patterns of participants are quantified using short and easy instruments that contain less than 15 items[3]. Data from these questions can further be described and individuals classified into broad categories.

Quantitive History Questionnaire

When the objective of the researcher is to capture the physical activity patterns of participants over multiple domains, a more detailed approach of assessment such as the quantitative history questionnaire is used. This usually entails more questions over multiple segments designed to provide comprehensive information on the physical activity patterns over a period of time such as a day, week, month or year[6] [5].

Objective Monitors

The use of monitoring devices such as accelerometers, pedometers and heart rate monitors in measuring physical activity have been made possible through recent advances in technology[10]. When worn, intensity of body acceleration is measured using an electronic component embedded within the device[11], which usually has the capacity to store and record these data over a period of time.

The different types of objective monitors are further discussed below:

Pedometers

Since walking has been shown to provide substantial health benefits[12] and is a known form of physical activity commonly employed by people, measuring walking-based activity is made possible by the use of pedometers which are usually worn on the waist, or the wrist, ankle, shoe, and counts the number of steps taken by the individual over a period of time.[13] A 2017 study found that accuracy of waist pedometers was higher than those worn on the wrist.[14] Pedometers are fairly inexpensive, but more advanced versions with added features may cost higher. Available types include Kenz Lifecorder, New-Lifestyles NL-2000 (piezoelectric), and Yamax Digi-Walkers SW-200 and SW-70.

Accelerometers

Accelerometers are often used in research to obtain more detailed information about physical activity and to help to address the limitations of self-report methods.[15] Uniaxial and multi axial measurements across one to three orthogonal planes of movement can be obtained by the use of accelerometers[16][10], which is a more advanced and slightly more expensive electronic device than the pedometer[16] with an added advantage of being able to distinguish between walking and running by the wearer (PARC-PH). Information on the amount, frequency and duration of physical activity can be obtained with the aid of accelerometers. Accelerometers are portable, noninvasive and provide quality information on human movement[17]. Available types include GT3x Actigraph and Activpal monitor.

Heart Rate Monitor

Heat rate monitors, usually worn on the chest or wrist, have an electrocardiogram (ECG) transmitter that sends signals to the receiver which calculates average heart rate within 5 to 15 seconds intervals and displays it as beats per minute[1]. Although more expensive than pedometers and accelerometers, data obtained from heart rate monitors can be transferred to a computer, are useful in calculating energy expenditure and physical activity for observational and intervention studies[18]. Available types include Fitbit Surge fitness superwatch, Timex personal trainer, Polar FT7, Garmin vivofit.

Direct Observation

Obtaining accurate information on the frequency, duration, intensity and type of physical activity carried out by an individual is only possible through systematic observation[10]. In direct observation, the physical activity levels are assessed in specific settings[19] such as playground, classes etc. and can be done by a trained observer or videotaping[1]. Several instruments such as System for Observing Fitness Instruction Time (SOFIT), Fargo Activity Timesampling Survey (FATS) and Children's Activity Rating Scale (CARS) have been specifically designed to capture different dimensions of interest depending on the behavioural category of interest[20]. The results obtained can be useful in assessing and designing intervention programs for a target group[21].

Evidence

Reliability

Self-report measure[22]	ICC 0.67 (95% CI 0.54-0.77) ICC 0.70 (95% CI 0.66-0.83) ICC 0.52 (95% CI 0.33-0.66)
Accelerometry-based activity monitors[17]	0.62 – 0.80
Heart rate monitor[23]	0,993
Pedometer[24]	ICC 0.71 (95% CI 0.47-0.86)

Validity

Self-report instruments[25]	(0.50-0.60)
Accelerometry- based activity monitors[26]	0.9
Heart rate monitor[27]	0.81
Pedometer[28]	0.60

Responsiveness

The ability of physical activity outcome measures to respond to changes in physical activity intensity is important when selecting the appropriate tool for the intended objective. From several studies, accelerometers have been shown to have high responsiveness e.g. Actical (1.2-4.7) and Actigraph (1.1-3.3)[29].

References

1. Welk, G. J. (2002). Introduction to physical activity research. In G. J. Welk (Ed.), Physical Activity Assessments in Health Related Research (pp. 3–18). Champaign IL: Human Kinetics.
2. Siegel, D. (2005). A Self-Report Measure of Physical Activity. Journal of Physical Education, Recreation & Dance (JOPERD), 76(7), 11.
3. Matthews, C. (2002). Use of self-report instruments to assess physical activity. In G. J. Welk (Ed.), Physical activity assessments for health-related research (2002nd ed., pp. 107–23). Champaign, IL: Human Kinetics.
4. Sylvia, L. G., Bernstein, E. E., Hubbard, J. L., Keating, L., & Anderson, E. J. (2014). Practical guide to measuring physical activity. Journal of the Academy of Nutrition and Dietetics, 114(2), 199–208.
5. · Strath, S. J., Kaminsky, L. A., Ainsworth, B. E., Ekelund, U., Freedson, P. S., Gary, R. A., Swartz, A. M. (2013). Guide to the assessment of physical activity: Clinical and research applications: A scientific statement from the American Heart association. Circulation, 128(20), 2259–2279
6. Ainsworth, B. E., Haskell, W. I. L., Whitt, M. C., Irwin, M. L., Swartz, A. M., Strath, S. J., Leon, A. S. (2000). Compendium of physical activities: an update of activity codes and MET intensities. Medicine and Science in Sports and Exercise, 32(9 Suppl), S498–S504
7. Wickel, E. E., Welk, G. J., & Eisenmann, J. C. (2006). Concurrent validation of the Bouchard diary with an accelerometry-based monitor. Medicine and Science in Sports and Exercise, 38(2), 373–379
8. Biddle, S. J. H., Gorely, T., Pearson, N., & Bull, F. C. (2011). An assessment of self-reported physical activity instruments in young people for population surveillance: Project ALPHA. The International Journal of Behavioral Nutrition and Physical Activity, 8(1), 1
9. Steene-Johannessen, J., Anderssen, S. A., Van Der Ploeg, H. P., Hendriksen, I. J. M., Donnelly, A. E., Brage, S., & Ekelund, U. (2016). Are self-report measures able to define individuals as physically active or inactive? Medicine and Science in Sports and Exercise, 48(2)
10. Taylor, N. (2014). Available methods for measuring physical activity. In A. Clow & S. Edmunds (Eds.), Physical Activity and Mental Health (pp. 35–40). Champaign, IL: Human Kinetics.
11. Graham, D. J., & Hipp, J. A. (2014). Emerging technologies to promote and evaluate physical activity: cutting-edge research and future directions. Frontiers in Public Health, 2, 66
12. Lee, I. M., & Buchner, D. M. (2008). The importance of walking to public health. Medicine and Science in Sports and Exercise, 40(7 SUPPL.1), 512–518
13. Bassett Jr, D., & Tudor-Locke, C. (2004). How many steps / day are enough ? Preliminary pedometer indices for public health . PubMed Commons. Sports Medicine, 34(1), 1–8
14. Husted HM, Llewellyn TL. The Accuracy of Pedometers in Measuring Walking Steps on a Treadmill in College Students. Int J Exerc Sci. 2017;10(1):146-53.
15. Arvidsson D, Fridolfsson J, Börjesson M. Measurement of physical activity in clinical practice using accelerometers. J Intern Med. 2019;286 (2):137-53.
16. Corder, K., Brage, S., & Ekelund, U. (2007). Accelerometers and pedometers: methodology and clinical application. Current Opinion in Clinical Nutrition & Metabolic Care, 10(5), 597–60
17. Welk, G. J. (2002b). Use of Accelerometry-Based Activity Monitors to Assess Physical Activity. In G. J. Welk (Ed.), Physical Activity Assessments in Health Related Research (pp. 125–140). Champaign, IL: Human Kinetics
18. Janz, K. F. (2002). Use of Heart Rate Monitors to Assess Physical Activity. In G. J. Welk (Ed.), Physical Activity Assessments in Health Related Research (pp. 143–158). Champaign, IL: Human Kinetics
19. Dugdill, L., & Stratton, G. (2007). Evaluating sport and physical activity interventions: A guide for practitioners. Salford University, 44(0), 9–10
20. Mckenzie, T. L. (2002). Use of Direct Observation to Assess Physical Activity. In G. J. Welk (Ed.), Physical Activity Assessments in Health Related Research (pp. 179–191). Champaign, IL: Human Kinetics

21. Bird, M. E., Datta, G. D., van Hulst, A., Kestens, Y., & Barnett, T. A. (2015). A reliability assessment of a direct-observation park evaluation tool: the Parks, activity and recreation among kids (PARK) tool. BMC Public Health, 15(1), 906

22. Murphy, J. J., Murphy, M. H., MacDonncha, C., Murphy, N., Nevill, A. M., & Woods, C. B. (2017). Validity and Reliability of Three Self-Report Instruments for Assessing Attainment of Physical Activity Guidelines in University Students. Measurement in Physical Education and Exercise Science, 0(0), 1–8

23. Brage, S., Brage, N., Franks, P. W., Ekelund, U., & Wareham, N. J. (2005). Reliability and validity of the combined heart rate and movement sensor Actiheart. European Journal of Clinical Nutrition, 59(4), 561–570

24. Kooiman, T. J. M., Dontje, M. L., Sprenger, S. R., Krijnen, W. P., van der Schans, C. P., & de Groot, M. (2015). Reliability and validity of ten consumer activity trackers. BMC Sports Science, Medicine and Rehabilitation, 7, 24

25. Sallis, J. F., & Saelens, B. E. (2000). Assessment of physical activity by self-report: status, limitations, and future directions. Res Q Exercise Sport, 71(2), 1–14

26. Leenders, N. Y. J. M., Nelson, T. E., & Sherman, W. M. (2003). Ability of different physical activity monitors to detect movement during treadmill walking. International Journal of Sports Medicine, 24(1), 43–50

27. Barreira, T., Kang, M., & Caputo, J. (2009). Validation of the Actiheart monitor for the measurement of physical activity. International Journal of Exercise Science, 2, 60–71

28. Jago, R., Watson, K., Baranowski, T., Zakeri, I., Yoo, S., Baranowski, J., & Conry, K. (2006). Pedometer reliability, validity and daily activity targets among 10- to 15-year-old boys. Journal of Sports Sciences, 24, 241–251

29. Montoye, A. H., & Pfeiffer, K. A. (2014). Change in Physical Activity. Measurement in Physical Education and Exercise Science, 18(4), 273–285

❑❑❑

6 Evaluating Physical Activity

Introduction

There are many reasons that, as physiotherapists we might want to measure physical activity (PA) levels. If we are devoting clinical time to promoting PA then we need to be able to demonstrate effectiveness and show that we are making a difference, this might be with individual patients or with populations so measurement of some form is necessary. Before you think about how to measure, think about why you want to measure and who the information is for. For example you might want to measure for any of the following reasons;

1. To understand baseline levels in the population of interest?
2. To see whether a certain intervention is having an impact on PA levels?
3. To motivate patients by showing progress?

Each of the above reasons might require a different type of data, for a different audience with a different objective.

There are also different components of PA that can be measured, for example you could measure the frequency with which someone is physically active, the intensity of their activity, the type of activity they engage in and the duration of that activity. In some situations it's more appropriate to measure one of these aspects of activity but frequently it's more practical to try to get an overall measurement of someones activity (their total physical activity over a given period of time). It's really important to keep in mind that none of these measures are perfect and they all have advantages and disadvantages, it's a case of weighting up the pros and cons of a selection of measures in a given context.

Program evaluations using quality physical activity measures can contribute to achieving the goal of improved health. At a community level good evaluations can lead to program improvements, documenting positive results can attract funding to continue and expand programs, and communicating results can persuade other communities to adopt effective approaches[1].

Ways of gathering physical activity data

Existing Records

This might include using information that is routinely collected, for example census information, surveys, polls, government data. There is more information available than ever before and a quick literature search may reveal the information you need. Sometimes the existing data doesn't quite meet our needs, this could be for many reasons including; it may be too broad and not focus on our population of interest, it may be in a format that doesn't suit us, it may have been gathered in a way that we don't feel is sufficiently detailed or it may be out of date.

Indirect Measures

These rely on self-report i.e. they ask the patient to estimate how much activity they have done in a given period. They are useful because they are cheap and easy to complete. There are obvious issues with relying on recall though, they may not be appropriate for some older populations and people with dementia for example. There are also other issues such as trying to give a favourable result to please the assessor.

There are lots of questionnaires and surveys available, in 2011 the UK National Obesity Observatory produced a report which reviewed the available tools and suggested the following shortlist are the most robust measurement tools (this doesn't mean that they are user friendly though!).

Shortlist of selected questionnaires

Physical activity: children and young people

1. The Physical Activity Questionnaire for Older Children/Adolescents (PAQC/PAQ-A)
2. Youth Risk Behaviour Surveillance Survey (YRBSS)
3. The Teen Health Survey

Physical activity: adults

1. Stanford 7-day recall (7-DR)
2. International Physical Activity Questionnaire Long version (IPAQ-Long)
3. New Zealand Physical Activity Questionnaire (Short Form) (NZPAQ-Short)
4. 7-day Physical Activity Diary

Direct Measures

Direct measures use technology to measure activity levels, this is usually in the form of a device that will measure and record movement. This might be a simple pedometer, an app on a smart phone or a sophisticated movement tracker.

Direct measures are considered to be more accurate than self-report measures but they are costly and may not be appealing to some patients. They also have limitations including;

- Variable ability to detect very slow walking speeds; obvious implications for clinical populations.
- Variable ability to measure movement in abnormal gait patterns.
- Variable ability to gather data on certain types of activity. Walking is usually fine but if the monitor is worn on the lower limb, upper limb activity is unlikely to be detected. This has implications for wheelchair users or anyone who engages in chair-based exercise.

Evaluating PA is challenging and often hindered by the challenge of employing a valid, reliable measure that also adequately satisfies the research question or design[2] and literature suggests that there is little agreement between indirect and direct measures[3] However because of the barriers to accessing technology indirect measures are still frequently used. In their systematic review Skender et al [3] explored the correlation between self-reported PA and accelerometer data and found that accelerometers appear to provide slightly more consistent results in relation to self-reported physical activity but due to overall limited consistency both questionnaires and accelerometers should be used to gain the most complete physical activity information Kowalski[4] performed a systematic review of studies that had used direct and indirect tools to measure PA in older adults and found lack of a clear trend regarding the agreement between PA measures in older adults.

Challenges

The more robust and reliable these are the more detailed and time consuming they become. Trying to find something that it valid, reliable AND user-friendly in clinical practice is a really difficult! It's important to remember;

- Health and PA behaviours are complex.
- Changes may take a long time to become apparent.
- Different stakeholders are interested in different things.
- You simply can't measure everything.

References

1. Sallis JF. Measuring physical activity: practical approaches for program evaluation in Native American communities. Journal of public health management and practice: JPHMP. 2010 Sep;16(5):404.
2. · Sylvia LG, Bernstein EE, Hubbard JL, Keating L, Anderson EJ. A Practical Guide to Measuring Physical Activity. Journal of the Academy of Nutrition and Dietetics. 2014 Feb;114(2):199.
3. · Skender S, Ose J, Chang-Claude J, Paskow M, Brühmann B, Siegel EM, Steindorf K, Ulrich CM. Accelerometry and physical activity questionnaires-a systematic review. BMC Public Health. 2016 Jun 16;16(1):1.
4. Kowalski K, Rhodes R, Naylor PJ, Tuokko H, MacDonald S. Direct and indirect measurement of physical activity in older adults: a systematic review of the literature. International Journal of Behavioral Nutrition and Physical Activity. 2012 Dec 18;9(1):1.

❑❑❑

7

Clinical Reasoning

Introduction

Clinical Reasoning is the process by which a therapist interacts with a patient, collecting information, generating and testing hypotheses, and determining optimal diagnosis and treatment based on the information obtained. It has been defined as "an inferential process used by practitioners to collect and evaluate data and to make judgments about the diagnosis and management of patient problems"[1]

Clinical reasoning is "the sum of the thinking and decision-making processes associated with clinical practice"[2][1]. During this process, the therapist analyses multiple variables contributing to the patient's limited physical capacity (the ability to execute a task or action in a standard environment) and performance (what the patient can do in his or her own current environment). The key elements of the process include generation of hypotheses of factors assumed to underlie the limitations of physical capacity and performance and postulation of the magnitude of those factors. The therapist interacts with the patient and other persons involved in the patient's care (family, other health care professionals) and guides the patient in finding meaningful goals and health management strategies[3]. All decisions and actions need to be made in line with professional ethics and community expectations[3].

Clinical Reasoning

Clinical Reasoning is integral to physiotherapy practice. As a concept, clinical reasoning is quite a simple one; however in practice, it is difficult and fraught with errors. The aim of clinical reasoning is to prevent misdirection [5] A robust clinical reasoning process is vital so the threshold of suspicion of serious pathology is at an appropriate level[6]. The way a therapist clinically reasons their findings can strongly influence how the case is interpreted. This has implications as to how the clinician views the red flags and gives weight to any red herrings presented therein [7].

The most common form of clinical reasoning within the physiotherapy profession is hypothetico-deductive reasoning[8]. Within hypothetico-deductive reasoning, the clinician gains initial clues in regards to the patient's problem (from the subjective assessment), which forms the initial hypotheses in the therapists mind. Further data is collected in the objective assessment, which may confirm or negate the hypotheses. Continual hypothesis generation may occur during management and reassessment[2].

Reflection after the initial assessment and also after the subsequent sessions will help the therapist to recognise patterns and their clinical reasoning process will improve[5][6].

Process of Clinical Reasoning

Clinical reasoning should begin as soon as the therapist meets the patient, as their behaviour can inform the therapist's clinical reasoning[6]. There should be ongoing data collection which should not stop at the end of the assessment to aid this process. A hypothetico-deductive model of clinical reasoning can be seen in Figure 1.

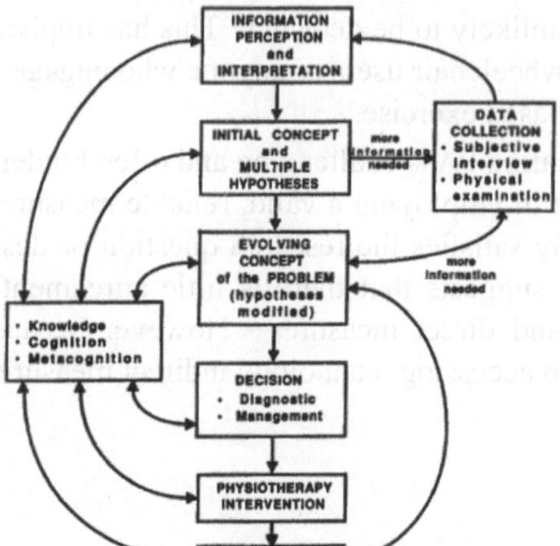

Figure 1: A Hypothetico-deductive model of Clinical Reasoning[5]

The therapist may be able to ascertain quickly that something is wrong with the patient due to the subjective and objective assessment along wither their subsequent clinical reasoning. The data gathered over sessions should be collated to best inform the therapist. This will contribute to the therapist's evolving concept of the patient's problem[6][5].

Pattern Recognition

Pattern recognition is an important part of clinical reasoning however, this will be limited in students and newly qualified physiotherapists[5][8].

Knowledge is also an important consideration. The newly qualified therapist is expected to have many more potential hypotheses in comparison to a experienced therapist[5]. There is suggested to be differences in novice and expert therapists in the process of clinical reasoning[8]. Although largely similar, novice physiotherapists have to go through a longer process of clinical reasoning compared to expert therapists due to lack of knowledge in comparison and less experience in pattern recognition. Figure 2 demonstrates the clinical reasoning process of expert therapists (with at least 3 years of experience) and novice therapists (with under three years' experience or students)[8].

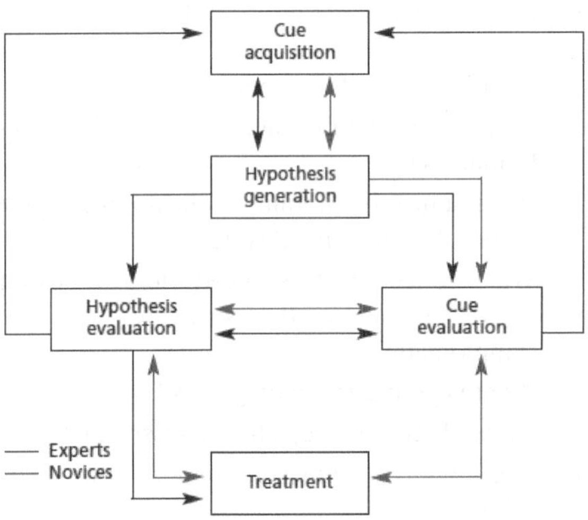

Figure 2: Difference in clinical reasoning between expert and novice therapists[8].

Patient Involvement in the Clinical Reasoning Process

The patient should be an integral part of the clinical reasoning process, as this can help the clinician to form hypotheses and lead towards the review of the outcome post physiotherapy intervention[5](See Figure 3).

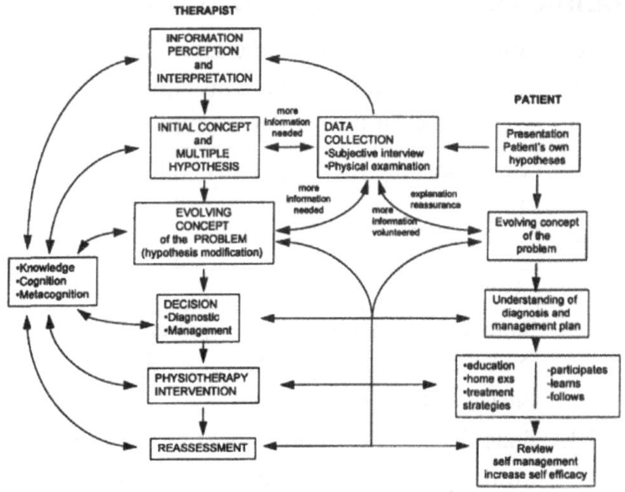

Figure 3: Patient involvement in the clinical reasoning process[5].

References

1. Higgs J, Jones M. Clinical decision making and multiple problem spaces. In: Higgs J, Jones MA, Loftus S, Christensen N. Clinical reasoning in health professions. Amsterdam: Elsevier;2008. p. 4-19.
2. Edwards I, Jones M, Carr J, Braunack-Mayer A, Jensen GM. Clinical reasoning strategies in physical therapy. Physical therapy. 2004;84(4):312-30.
3. Atkinson HL, Nixon-Cave K. A tool for clinical reasoning and reflection using the International Classification of Functioning, Disability and Health (ICF) framework and patient management model. Physical therapy. 2011;91(3):416-30.
4. Rahul Patwari Clinical reasoning Available from:https://www.youtube.com/watch?v=6DzeF8hCNb8&app=desktop (last accessed 3.3.2020)
5. Jones, M. Clinical reasoning and pain. Manual Therapy. 1995; 1:17-24.
6. Greenhalgh, S. Red Flags, and clinical Presentation Mapping. Available from: https://macpweb.org/home/index.php?m=file&f=873. (accessed 21 October 2008)
7. Greenhalgh, S. and Selfe, J. Margaret: a tragic case of spinal Red Flags and Red Herrings. Physiotherapy. 2004; 90:73-76.
8. Doody C, McAteer M. Clinical reasoning of expert and novice physiotherapists in an outpatient orthopaedic setting. Physiotherapy. 2002;88 (5): 258-268.

❑❑❑

CLINICAL REASONING – POST SUBJECTIVE

To be completed after the subjective assessment:

1. Which structure(s) do you think could be responsible for the patient's symptoms?

Structures in order of priority	Reasons
1.	
2.	
3.	

2. State the irritability of the patient's condition:
   Not Mild Moderate Severe
   Please justify your answer:
3. State the severity of the patient's condition:
   Mild Moderate Severe
   Please justify your answer:
4. State the pain mechanisms involved:
5. Is the nociceptive component predominantly inflammatory or mechanical? List the factors that support and negate your decision.
6. At what stage of the healing/inflammatory process is the patient at?
7. State the nature of the condition (% for each component)
   Discogenic Arthrogenic Myogenic
   Neurogenic Soft tissue Osteogenic
   Vascular Psychogenic Sociogenic
   Visceral
8. Are there any contributing factors associated with the patient's symptoms?
   Physical
   Environmental/biomechanical
   Cognitive/affective
9. Is there any indication for caution? Yes No
   If yes, please justify (irritability, severity, red flags, yellow flags)
10. Do you think you would need to be gentle, moderate or vigorous with your examination movements? Why?
11. Do you expect a comparable sign to be easy or hard to find? Why?
12. What relationship will there be between pain and resistance?
    P R P>R R>P R=P
    Explain?
13. Is neurological examination necessary...why?
14. What must you test on day 1?
15. What should you test after day 1?
16. From the S/E, what are your O/E findings likely to be?
17. State your working **hypothesis?**

CLINICAL REASONING – OBJECTIVE PLANNING

To be completed after the subjective prior to the objective assessment

1. Name all the possible structures which could be a source of the symptoms:
   Symptomatic Area –
   Structure Under Area –
   Structures which can refer to the area –
2. What needs to be examined today and why?
3. Will a neurological examination be required and why?
4. Behaviour of symptoms
   (a) Is the condition severe? Explain why.
   (b) Is the condition irritable? Explain why.
   (c) Are there any precautions or contraindications?
5. How is the severity, irritability or nature of the condition going to affect your physical examination and treatment?
6. Will the comparable sign be easy or hard to find? Explain why.
7. What subjective findings indicate likely physical findings? Subjective Physical
8. What other factors need to be examined as reasons why the structure has become symptomatic?
9. What is your clinical diagnosis?

To be completed after the objective assessment:

1. Were your hypotheses supported or negated? Why?
2. What is you main hypothesis now with regard to the primary disorder and the dominant pain mechanism?
3. Is there anything about your physical exam that would indicate caution in your management?
4. How will you manage this patient?
5. What comparable signs will you check on return?

6. Indicate your treatment progression over time.
7. What is the patients prognosis? Justify:
8. What goals do you expect to achieve?
9. Would you expect the patient to have residual signs and symptoms at the end of the course of treatment?
10. How many treatments would be required?

CLINICAL REASONING – POST OBJECTIVE

To be completed after the objective assessment:

1. Were your hypotheses supported or negated? Why?
2. What is your hypothesis now with regard to the primary disorder and the dominant pain mechanism?
3. Is there anything about your physical exam that would indicate caution in your management? Why?
4. How will you manage this patient? Justify your choice.
5. What comparable signs will you check on return?
6. Indicate your treatment progression over time? (Include ergonomics, posture, electrotherapy...)
7. What is the patient's prognosis? Justify:
8. What goals do you expect to achieve (function/ VAS)?
9. Would you expect the patient to have residual signs and symptoms at the end of the course of treatment?
10. How many treatments would be required?

❑❑❑

8 Clinical Decision Making in Physiotherapy Practice

Introduction

The majority of time spent working in clinical practice involves thinking and decision making.[1][2][3] Because decisions are so commonly made, it is easy to assume that anyone can make effective decisions.[1] Effectiveness in clinical practice depends on the decisions made which stresses the importance of learning how to optimally make decisions.[4][5]Clinical or diagnostic reasoning has been proposed to be the most important core skill of any health care practitioner.[6] The dynamic and ever-changing realm of health care demands that practitioners provide meaningful improvements in patients and the clinical decision process is the only path to achieving it.[5][7] The rate at which practitioners fail at this critical skill is alarmingly high. Not only have large discrepancies (20-40%) been reported between ante and postmortem diagnoses but many of these postmortem examinations would not have been necessary if the correct diagnosis was made.[8][9]. It has been estimated that nearly 18% ($2.7 trillion) of the United States' GDP is spent on healthcare, yet more than 30% is wasted on inappropriate care.[10] Up to 80 000 deaths occur annually in hospitalised patients in the United States due to incorrect diagnoses and in the outpatient setting, around 5% of adults (12 million US adults annually) are incorrectly diagnosed. [11]

The majority of these failures are not attributed to system problems or knowledge failure, but to how practitioners think - how they solve problems, reason and ultimately make decisions[5]. To improve healthcare it is of great importance to improve clinical reasoning and hence clinical decision making.

What is Clinical Decision Making?

Clinical decision making (CDM) has been defined as a contextual, continuous and evolving process where data is gathered, interpreted and evaluated in order to select an evidence-based choice of action. [12] "The CDM process is a highly complex, multi-faceted skill that is developmental in nature and requires a substantial amount of practice with realistic patients to develop." i.e. learnt behaviour. [7][13] The understanding of CDM is still evolving and largely based on research in psychology, medicine and nursing.[7][14] It involves multiple different types of reasoning [7] and is therefore wrapped up in the "Great Rationality Debate" about the most optimal course of our reasoning, decision-making and actions. [15] Rationality is proposed to be the foremost characteristic of the accomplished decision-maker.[5]

What is the great rationality debate all about?

There are multiple major theories of rationality that could in part be relevant to the medical field.[15] "Rationality is often defined as acting in a way that helps us achieve our goals, which in the clinical setting typically means a desire to improve our health."[15] Most major theories of consequence agree that in order to achieve our goals we need to take into account both the benefits (gains) and harms (losses) of alternative courses of action. [15] Djulbegovic & Elqayam[15] developed a list of "core ingredients" of rationality and its relevance to the medical field (Table 1).

Table 1: Core ingredients/ Principles of rationality commonly identified across theoretical models (highlighted in bold) (Adapted from Djulbegovic & a Elqayam)[15]

Principle	Description
Principle 1	Rational decision-making requires the integration of • Benefits (gains) • Harms (losses) in order to accomplish our goals like improved health
Principle 2	It generally happens under conditions of uncertainty. • The rational approach requires the use of reliable evidence to deal with the intrinsic uncertainties. • It depends upon cognitive processes that permit the integration of probabilities/uncertainties.
Principle 3	"Rational thinking should be informed by human cognitive architecture." • Made up of type 1 "old mind" reasoning processes (affect-based, intuitive, fast, resource-frugal) and type 2 "new mind" processes ("analytic and deliberative, consequential driven, and effortful")
Principle 4	Rationality is context dependant and should be aware of environmental, and computational constraints of human brains
Principle 5	Rationality (in medicine) is closely related to ethics and morality of our actions • requires consideration of utilitarian (society-oriented), duty-bound (individual-oriented), and right-based (autonomy, "no decision about me, without me") ethics

Despite this ongoing debate about defining rationality, there is consensus that it should conform to a normative standard - how the decision "ought" to be made[5]. The dominant paradigm seems to be that "Decision-making should be logical, evidence-based, follow the laws of science and probability and lead to decisions that are consistent with the rational choice theory"[5]

How Do We Make Decisions?

There are two main frameworks (mental models) described in medical literature that clinicians employ in clinical decision making:

- Fast and frugal heuristics[16]
- Dual system theory[17] - which can also be described as a two system mind

Fast and frugal heuristics (FFH) is based on the theory that "people do not rely on a single cognitive strategy but rather select an adequate heuristic from what has been dubbed an adaptive toolbox. Each of the heuristics (decision making tools) in this cognitive "toolbox" is suitable for a different class of environments. By relying on a heuristic that fits a particular environment, people can make efficient decisions in little time and based on little information (hence 'fast -and-frugal')".[18]

Heuristics can be defined as:

- "...mental shortcuts developed by a clinician over time and include recognizing patterns of disease, case experience, intuitive judgment and the "rule of thumb" applications" [13]
- "...short-cuts, abbreviated ways of thinking, maxims, 'seen this many times before' ways of thinking" [19]
- "...cognitive strategies or mental shortcuts that are automatically and unconsciously employed - are particularly important for decision making. Heuristics can facilitate decision making but can also lead to errors. When a heuristic fails, it is referred to as a cognitive bias" [20]

Heuristics are our "gut decisions" and rely on our intuition - our recognition based on our past experiences. Heuristics utilizes the capacities developed through extended practice.[21] The aim of heuristics is not to "optimise" (find the best solution) but rather to "satisfice" (find a good enough solution).[21]

FFH is therefore used when there is a need to make quick and accurate decisions and the information is limited to only what is absolutely necessary at that specific time.[22][23] This is commonly seen in the field of medicine with triage or emergency medicine. In emergency situations there is no need for a wide spectrum of information, the clinician only needs the immediate information necessary to know what to do at that specific moment, whether to resuscitate, intubate, apply a tourniquet or identify if the patient had a stroke. In these life-or-death situations, FFH strategies are important and the algorithmic decision making trees come into play. The clinician now only considers a series of "yes/no" questions until an answer is reached.[24] These fast-and-frugal decision-making trees and tools can be even more accurate than multiple regression.[21]

This approach cannot be applied to every situation and in healthcare, it is only applicable in two instances, where:

- Rapid decisions need to be made, the amount of information is therefore limited and simple decision making tools/trees are used
- The decision maker has intuition - a substantial amount of experience in similar enough situations to draw upon.[24]

FFH is not universal in Physiotherapy[24], because

- Not everybody has intuition, for example, newly qualified clinician don't have an experience bank yet to draw upon
- Most of the situations in physiotherapy are non-urgent, therefore fast decisions are not always needed and physiotherapists can spend the time to gather more information.
- The decision making trees used are largely dependent on the biomedical model which is essential in triage-type situations where patient-oriented factors like goal setting are not needed. Physiotherapy has been moving away from the biomedical model, rather utilising the biopsychosocial approach to healthcare.

The second, and more commonly used approach to CDM, is the Dual-Process theory, developed by Kahneman & Tversky.[17] Dual-process theory incorporates the use of intuitive (System 1) and analytical (System 2) processes toward thinking, reasoning and deciding.[6][17][20][25] See Table 2.

Intuitive/System 1 reasoning

- Similar to FFH and most commonly used in clinical practice.
- Heavily reliant on the experience of the clinician making the decision[6]
- It is fast, automatic and uses thin-slicing - relying on our instinctive first impressions to form an unconscious diagnosis [2][6]
- These decisions use heuristics [6]
- It is an adaptive mechanism that saves us time and effort when making decisions. We spend the majority of our time in this "automatic zone" - where few events are deliberate and most events automatically trigger the next.[19]
- These unconscious processes may control our behaviour without us being aware of them.[25]
- Heuristics are most effective but they are also prone to error/biases.[19]

Analytical/System 2 processes

- A slower and more deliberate process.[2][6]
- Methodical and analytical and involves critical thinking and hypothesis testing[2][6][25]
- More reliable, safe and effective but also slower and more resource-intensive.[6][26]

Table 2: Comparison of Intuitive and Analytical Approaches to Decision Making[5][6][15][25]

Intuitive decision making (System 1/"old mind")	Analytical decision making (System 2/"new mind")
• Depends on experiential-inductive logic	• Uses hypothetico-deductive processes
• Fast	• Slow
• Unconscious thinking	• Deliberate conscious thought
• Automatic, little effort	• Effortful and controlled
• Pattern recognition/gestalt effect	• Hypothesis generation
• High capacity	• Low capacity
• Associative cognition	• Rule-based cognition
• Evolutionary/hardwired	• Acquired through critical thought
• Heuristic	• Normative reasoning
• Default process	• Inhibitory
• Reflexive	• Reflective
• More prone to error - based on our own personal biases	• Less prone to error as a high level of attention is present in cognitive load

The Decision Making Process

The decision making process starts with the presentation of the patient's signs and symptoms.

- If the clinician recognizes the signs and symptoms - the visual presentation (swelling, posture, area of symptoms, biomechanics) or the combination of symptoms/findings (behaviour of symptoms, history, imaging reports) - the Intuitive process (System 1) is immediately and automatically activated. This process is reflexive and unconscious and does not involve any deliberate thinking.[6] Besides the pattern recognition, other System 1 responses may be simultaneously triggered for example, the clinician's feelings, experiences and perceptions or the ambient environment. [6][19]
- If the clinician does not recognize the presented signs and symptoms or there is uncertainty, Analytical/System 2 processes are triggered instead. The clinician now incorporates analytical thinking to systematically analyse the presented data to reach multiple hypotheses. This process is slow, effortful and requires conscious thought. [6][13][26]

Even though there seems to be a complete distinction between the Intuitive and Analytical approaches, it seems more probable that the two approaches would interact and clinicians would integrate both approaches.[6][28]

Dual Process Theory Model

The relationship between these two systems (intuitive and analytical) is informed by a model developed by Croskerry[6][19] in the context of diagnostic reasoning. It recognizes that a continuous fluctuation may exist between both approaches within a clinical setting (Figure 1).

He proposes eight major features of this model[19] :

1. System 1 processing is fast, automatic and most prevalent. It is usually effective but leans heavily on heuristics and because it is unchecked, it is more prone to biases
2. System 2 is slower, but deliberate and conscious, which may limit mistakes.
3. Errors in reasoning occur more often in System 1 reasoning
4. Repetitive use of Analytical/System 2 processing as well as the repeated presentation of the same problem to System 2, will lead to System 1 processing as learning occurs and skills are acquired.[4]. Following this concept, skilled clinicians are more prone to automatically use System 1 processing whereas novices initially rely more on System 2 processing.[28]
5. Heuristics/biases can be overridden by the deliberate use of clinical reasoning, which means System 2 processes can override System 1 processes.
6. Conversely, over-reliance on System 1 processes can also override System 2 processes leading to unchecked decisions. This is evident when clinicians ignore well-developed clinical decision rules or habitually persist with clinical practices with no substantial evidence.[4]
7. The clinician can toggle/fluctuate between both systems
8. In its continuous effort for cognitive ease, the brain will generally default to System 1 processing when possible.

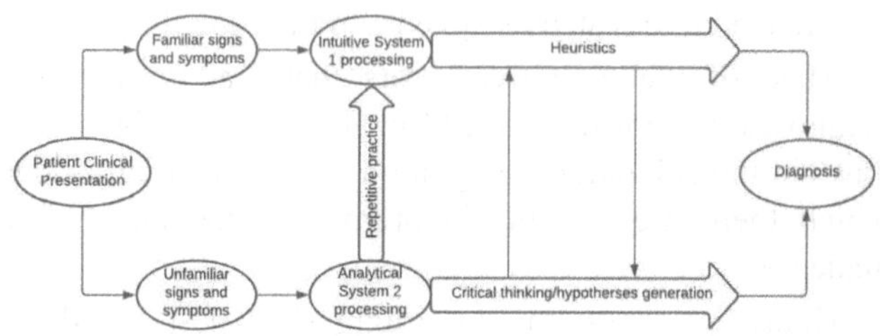

Figure 1. Model for diagnostic reasoning (Adapted from Croskerry [6])

What Influences our Clinical Decision Making?

Clinical decision making is influenced by a complex interaction between the following: [3][5][6][19][26]

- **Intrinsic factors**
    - o professional experience, skills and training
    - o context-specific knowledge - mindware gaps (lack of knowledge acquirement or forgetting of knowledge)
    - o Mindware contamination by bias and incorrect thinking
    - o Personal factors like general fatigue, affective state, sleep deprivation, cognitive overload, decision fatigue
    - o Individual factors like gender, personality, intelligence
    - o Self-reflection
    - o Communication

- o Metacognition (thinking about what we are thinking) during the process of gaining experience (on a cognitive level)

- **Extrinsic factors**
  - o Patient characteristics (appearance, demeanour, communication issues, past experiences with the patient)
  - o The unique presentation of the patient (their condition - severity, previous experience with the presenting complaints)
  - o Organisational factors in the medical environment (workload, other patients' needs, interruptions, time restraints, ergonomic factors, cost)
  - o Resource limitations (availability of specific tests, procedures, consultants etc)

Biases can occur in both approaches but the majority of biases are related to the failure of heuristics (cognitive biases) and are therefore seated in System 1 processing.[5][6] [13]

Most of the cognitive errors that lead to incorrect diagnoses are not due to a lack of knowledge but rather flaws in the collection, integration and verification of data which then often results in premature diagnoses being made.[13]

Heuristics (system 1) might be best used by experienced clinicians who are able to also recognise patterns more efficiently. Therapists using heuristic style decisions should be aware of the increased chance for bias and the consequences of error and use their analytical system 2 processes to check their decisions. As was discussed previously, errors in decision making have a great impact on patient safety and satisfaction and it is imperative to increase our understanding of the approaches to decision making and their potential biases in order to improve our clinical decision making through increased awareness of our biases/heuristics and limitations.

References

1. Croskerry P, Nimmo GR. Better clinical decision making and reducing diagnostic error. The journal of the Royal College of Physicians of Edinburgh. 2011 Jun1;41(2):155-62.
2. Smyth O, McCabe C. Think and think again! Clinical decision making by advanced nurse practitioners in the Emergency Department. Int Emerg Nurs. 2017 Mar 1;31:72-4.
3. Whelehan DF, Conlon KC, Ridgway PF. Medicine and heuristics: cognitive biases and medical decision-making. Irish journal of medical science. 2020 May 14;189:1477-1484.
4. Croskerry P. Context is everything or how could I have been that stupid. Healthc q. 2009 Aug 15;12(Spec No Patient):e171-176.
5. Croskerry P. A model for clinical decision-making in medicine. Medical Science Educator. 2017 Dec 1;27(1):9-13.
6. Croskerry P. A universal model of diagnostic reasoning. Academic medicine. 2009 Aug 1;84(8): 1022-8.
7. Huhn K, Black L, Christensen N, Furze J, Vendrely A, Wainwright S. Clinical reasoning: survey of teaching methods and assessment in entry-level physical therapist clinical education. Journal of Physical Therapy Education. 2018 Sep 1;32(3):241-7.
8. Gawande A. Final cut. In: Complications: A Surgeon's Notes on an Imperfect Science. New York: Henry Holt and Company; 2002;197-198
9. Graber M. Diagnostic errors in medicine: a case of neglect. The Joint Commission Journal on Quality and Patient Safety. 2005 Feb 1;31(2):106-13.
10. Berwick DM, Hackbarth AD. Eliminating waste in US health care. Jama. 2012 Apr 11;307(14):1513-6.
11. Singh H, Meyer AN, Thomas EJ. The frequency of diagnostic errors in outpatient care: estimations from three large observational studies involving US adult populations. BMJ quality & safety. 2014 Sep 1;23(9):727-31.
12. Tiffen J, Corbridge SJ, Slimmer L. Enhancing clinical decision making: development of a contiguous definition and conceptual framework. Journal of professional nursing. 2014 Sep 1;30(5):399-405.
13. Hussain A, Oestreicher J. Clinical decision-making: heuristics and cognitive biases for the ophthalmologist. Survey of Ophthalmology. 2018 Jan 1;63(1):119-24.
14. Chowdhury A, Bjorbækmo WS. Clinical reasoning—embodied meaning-making in physiotherapy. Physiotherapy theory and Practice. 2017 Jul 3;33(7): 550-9.
15. Djulbegovic B, Elqayam S. Many faces of rationality: implications of the great rationality debate for clinical decision-making. Journal of Evaluation in Clinical Practice. 2017 Oct;23(5):915-22.
16. Gigerenzer G, Todd PM. Simple heuristics that make us smart. Oxford University Press, USA; 1999.

17. Tversky A, Kahneman D. Judgment under uncertainty: Heuristics and biases. science. 1974 Sep 27;185(4157):1124-31.
18. Hafenbrädl S, Waeger D, Marewski JN, Gigerenzer G. Applied decision making with fast-and-frugal heuristics. Journal of Applied Research in Memory and Cognition. 2016 Jun 1;5(2):215-31.
19. Croskerry P, Singhal G, Mamede S. Cognitive debiasing 1: origins of bias and theory of debiasing. BMJ quality & safety. 2013 Oct 1;22(Suppl 2):ii58-64.
20. Norman GR, Monteiro SD, Sherbino J, Ilgen JS, Schmidt HG, Mamede S. The causes of errors in clinical reasoning: cognitive biases, knowledge deficits, and dual process thinking. Academic Medicine. 2017 Jan 1;92(1):23-30.
21. Gigerenzer G. Why heuristics work. Perspectives on psychological science. 2008 Jan;3(1):20-9.
22. Gigerenzer G. Moral intuition= fast and frugal heuristics? In:Moral psychology 2008 (pp. 1-26). MIT Press.
23. Gigerenzer G, Kurzenhaeuser S. Fast and frugal heuristics in medical decision making. Science and medicine in dialogue: Thinking through particulars and universals. 2005 Jan 30:3-15.
24. Walston Z. How do we make clinical decisions? [Accessed on 22 January 2021]
25. Evans JS. Dual-processing accounts of reasoning, judgment, and social cognition. Annu. Rev. Psychol.. 2008 Jan 10;59:255-78.
26. Trimble M, Hamilton P. The thinking doctor: clinical decision making in contemporary medicine. Clinical Medicine. 2016 Aug;16(4):343.
27. Learn Liberty. Heuristics, Explained. Published 25 Sep 2017. Available from https://youtu.be/ReFqFPJHLhA. [last accessed 9 Jan 2021]
28. Price A, Zulkosky K, White K, Pretz J. Accuracy of intuition in clinical decision-making among novice clinicians. Journal of advanced nursing. 2017 May;73(5):1147-57.
29. ACAPT. Clinical reasoning in Physical Therapy: Fast & slow thinking. Published on 27 Aug 2020. Available from https://youtu.be/LekUj7dlxlw. [last accessed 9 Jan 2021]
30. EmPROinsurance. PRI Interviews Dr. Pat Croskerry about How Physicians Make Decisions. Published on 18 Dec 2018. Available from https://youtu.be/hgGlrzKaoqI. [last accessed on 9 Jan 2021]

❑❑❑

9 Hypothesis-Oriented Algorithm for Clinicians II (HOAC II)

Introduction

The Hypothesis Orientated Algorithm for Clinicians (HOAC) – a method for evaluation and treatment planning - was first published in 1986[1]. In 2003 the algorithm was updated to be compatible with the contemporary physical therapy practice[2]. The update was termed the Hypothesis Orientated Algorithm for Clinicians II (HOAC II). The HOAC II offers a conceptual, patient-centred framework for physical therapists to use in the management of any type of patient[3]. It addresses the five elements of patient management: examination, evaluation, diagnosis, prognosis and intervention. Important for contemporary physical therapy, the HOAC II provides a means to engage in evidence-based practice and to differentiate between the types of evidence and science used[4]

Clinical Reasoning Using the HOAC

Much of the clinical reasoning language utilized below has been modified from the Hypothesis-Oriented Algorithm for Clinicians 2nd Edition (HOAC II)[5]

Evaluation

Pathobiological Mechanisms

- mechanisms relating to tissues - tissues injured, nature of injury, stage of healingmechanisms relating to pain - input (nociceptive, neurogenic), processing (central, cognitive), output (motor, sympathetic).

Dysfunction/Impairment

Clinical manifestations of the pathobiological processes, these are the patients main problems at that time.

- dysfunction - general physical dysfunction as describedbythepatientsuchaslimitationsinactivity restriction in participation
- impairment - specific impairments in body functions and structures identified on examination.

Patho-Anatomic Hypothesis

The actual anatomical location of the pathobiological mechanisms. What discrete anatomical structure is generating the primary complaint.

Contributing Factors

Any factor relating to the predisposition, development and maintenance of the problem

- physical - previous injury, nerve root involvement, pain provoked by multiple trunk movemements, reduced muscle control, reduced physical fitness
- Biomechanical
- Psychosocial - yellow flags determine a patients potential to proceed to chronicity.
- Environmental - Ergonomics, Stress,
- Emotional
- Behavioural
- Nutritional
- Cultural

Biomechanical Contributions

There are 3 primary forces the human body must dissipate. The biomechanical nature of the condition helps the clinician to determine which of these forces may be the primary contributor to a patient's symptoms. For example: tension overload may be the primary biomechanical nature of a patient who is experiencing patellar tendonitis.

- Compression
- Tension
- Shear

Mechanism of Injury (physical)

Biomechanically mediated injuries should be categorized according to the cause of their symtpoms in the following way:

1. Microtraumatic
2. Macrotraumatic
3. Microtraumatic and Microtraumatic

Centrally Mediated (Central Nervous System) Contributions

- Central symptoms or dysfunction is a complex cause of symptoms, impairments, funcitonal limitations and/or disability.

Problem List

Patient Identified Problems (PIP)

These are the patient identified problem(s), either in a symptom AND/OR functional limitation/disability level.

Non Patient Identified Problems (NPIP)

This is essentially a problem list generated by the clinician. This is an ongoing process of evaluation as the subjective examination and physical examination is taking place.

Anticipated Problems

These are problems that if they are not addressed, will lead to PIPs or NPIPs in the future. This is based on the clinicians utilization of best practice as well as there own prognostic skills. For example, research has shown that those wiht a BMI ?25 kg/m^2 have an increased likliehood of disc degeneration, notably if this develops at an early age.[6]

Precautions

- red flags - need referral on for appropriate medical intervention.
- yellow flags - highlight the need for a more detailed psychosocial assessment.
- SIN factor - severity, irritability, nature.

Stage of the Condition

The stage of the condition should closely follow the phases of healing. There is not a consistent language used across physical therapy literature on how to stage a condition. Some refer to symptoms lasting >6 weeks as chronic.

- **Acute:** Early onset of symptoms. This patient is in the inflammatory phase of healing.
- **Subacute:** The inflammatory phase of healing is subsiding and the patient should be in the reparative/proliferative phase of healing.
- **Chronic:** This patient should have completed the maturation stage of healing; however, there may be intrinsic or extrinisc factors limiting the complete recovery of this patient
- **Acute on Chronic:** This patient has reinitiated the inflammatority phase of healing, on a previous chronic condition that may or may not have completed the maturation phase of healing.

Irritability

The irritiability also helps determine the vigorousness of your examination, the examination sequence and strategy, as well as the dosage of your intervention. The VAS (or audible pain scale of 0-10) is very helpful when determining the irritability. The average 24 hour VAS must be used in context. The presence or absence of pain at rest is helpful and over the course of the day. However, how easily pain is exacerbated and relieved may have just as much relevance.

Severity

This helps determine the vigorousness of the examination and the tactics of your intervention, notably the exact positions to avoid and dosage to control. Functional forms are primarily used to will help determine the severity of the condition. Pain scales (such as the VAS) may also be helpful in determining the severity, but these can be misleading at times as pain is a relative experience for each person. Therefore, how the symptoms affect function is a very helpful way to identify how severely this problem is affecting a persons function.

Positive Patient Behaviors

These are behaviors that may improve a patient's prognosis. Example: active participant in plan of care, internal locus of control, trusts therapists judgement/ rapport, compliant, respects therapists schedule.

Negative Patient Behaviors

These are behaviors that may negatively affect a patient's prognosis. Example: fear avoider, kinesiophobia, passive participant in POC, non-compliant with recommendations, disrepect for therapists time, external locus of control

Phase of Healing

The phase of tissue healing is closely related to the prognosis of the patient.

Primary phases of healing include:

1. Inflammatory phase
2. Fibroblastic (Reparative or Proliferative) phase
3. Maturation (Remodeling) phase
4. Degenerative phase

Management and Intervention

Optimal management with a dynamic clinical working diagnosis should follow if all the above categories have been considered.

Strategy Traditional Physiotherapy Interventions for Pain Conditions (of intervention)

There are basic strategies of physical therapy intervention that may be employed.

1. Stretch
2. Soft Tissue Mobilization (STM)
3. Joint Mobilization (JM)
4. Strengthening/Stabilization
5. Re-training/Re-education
6. Education
7. Offloading
8. Pain inhibition
9. Modalities/Physical Agents

Tactics

- These are the detailed and specific elements of an intervention. Tactics specify the frequency, duration, and intensity of interventions.
- In a direct access environment, the therapist decides the stategy and tactic(s) of the treatment, not the physician. In a non-direct access environment, the physician may at times request a specific strategy; however, they rarely dictate the tactics employed. Therefore, it is the therapists responsibility to prescribe and modify the tactics implemented. The strategy may be to strengthen, but the tactics will specificy: quadriceps eccentric load on single leg to maximum tissue failure for 3 sets, 30 second rest between sets. 3 times per week.
- The strategy to use ultrasound will need specific tactics to highlight the dosage. Example: 50% pulsed ultrasound, 1.0mhz, .5 w/cm^2, 8minutes, to insertion of extensor carpi radialis brevis, 1.5 ERA (effective radiating area).

Post Test (Testing Criteria)

- These represent critical values that if attained, would suggest the hypothesis is correct and the associated problem/impairment are improving or has resolved.
- Establishing valid post-test criteria is an important component of clinical reasoning as it helps to determine if the interventions are moving towards the goals.
- This is different than goal setting as this is the specific testing employed to prove that your goals have been met, or that your goals are moving in a positive direction.
- Example: You have a long term goal for a patient to have symmetrical quadriceps strength. Your post-test could look quite different. EXAMPLE: hand-held maximum isometric strength in the 90 degree position of the knee VS. isokinetic strength throughout the entire range at a specific angular velocity to measure endurance over a 60 second period.

Slope of Recovery

It is key to monitor the patients slope of recovery. Understanding the patients slope of symptoms and functions assists with case management, prognosis, as well as the dosage of interventions. These slopes can be categorized below.

1. Static
2. Positive
3. Negative
4. Oscillating

Prognosis and Outcomes

To predict potential improvement identify positive and negative prognostic indicators. Consider age, occupation, hobbies, previous treatment response, stage and stability od condition, general health, past medical history, pain mechanisms.

Discharge Criteria

When is the patient ready for discharge? When does optimal care end to address all key NPIP and PIP. You must also consider anticipated problems and the need for re-admittance to physical therapy secondary to inadequate rehabilitation. All patients must of course be discharged. There are some patients that will be discharged prior to the recommended time frame secondary to monetary constraints. Please assume that there are no significant monetary restraints (but be reasonable) and focus on what criteria is in the best interest of the patient as you complete this section. Someone with severe degeneration will be discharged with different criteria than an acute injury. Often, the patient will be ready for discharge because they are back to functioning normally but you are not pleased with their protective mechanisms and HEP intensity. To prevent reinjury, your D/C criteria may be very specific. For instance, normalized core ratios with McGill testing. [7] Tolerating Core IV/V level exercises. Normal cervical ROM for a young neck. 110% of external rotation strength (per hand-held dynamometer) relative to the non-dominant throwing shoulder for a college pitcher. You may officially discharge this college pitcher 6—9 months after surgery. Consider the discharge criteria your absolute last patient encounter before they re-enter the general populace without limitations OR once they have reached their MMI (maximum medical improvement).

References

1. Rothstein JM, Echternach JL. Hypothesis-Oriented Algorithm for Clinicians: a method for evaluation and treatment planning. 1986;66(9):1388-94
2. Rothstein JM, Echternach JL, Riddle DL. The Hypothesis-Oriented Algorithm for Clinicians II (HOAC II): a guide for patient management. Phys Ther. 2003;83(5):455-70.
3. Riddle DL, Rothstein JM, Echternach JL. Application of the HOAC II: an episode of care for a patient with low back pain. Phys Ther. 2003;83:471-85.
4. Thoomes EJ, Schmitt MS. Practical use of the HOAC II for clinical decision making and subsequent therapeutic interventions in an elite athlete with low back pain. J Orthop Sports Phys Ther. 2011;41(2):108-17.
5. Rothstein JM, Echternach JL, Riddle DL. The Hypothesis-Oriented Algorithm for Clinicians II (HOAC II): a guide for patient management. Physical Therapy. 2003;83(5):455. Available at: http://www.ncbi.nlm.nih.gov/pubmed/12718711
6. Liuke M, Solovieva S, Lamminen A, et al. Disc degeneration of the lumbar spine in relation to overweight. International Journal of Obesity (2005). 2005;29(8):903-908. Available at: http://www.ncbi.nlm.nih.gov/pubmed/15917859.
7. McGill SM, Childs a, Liebenson C. Endurance times for low back stabilization exercises: clinical targets for testing and training from a normal database. Archives of physical medicine and rehabilitation. 1999;80(8):941-4. Available at: http://www.ncbi.nlm.nih.gov/pubmed/10453772.

❑❑❑

10 Clinical Outcome Assessment

Introduction

A clinical outcome assessment (COA) is a measure that describes or reflects how a patient feels, functions, or survives. Types of COAs include[1]:

1. Patient-reported outcome (PRO) measures
2. Observer-reported outcome (ObsRO) measures
3. Clinician-reported outcome (ClinRO) measures
4. Performance outcome (PerfO) measures.[2]

Types of Clinical Outcome Assessments

Patient-Reported Outcomes (PRO)

- Outcome where the patient is the rater
- Rely on a patient's direct responses to questions
- Responses may be recorded by the patient in a variety of ways such as on paper, via computerized questionnaire forms, or via interviews where the patient's observations or reports are recorded exactly as spoken, without any interpretation (judgment) on the part of the interviewer.
- Patient's direct report can capture a wide range of feelings and functions, as well as provide a direct measurement of how a patient feels, e.g., pain or low mood

Increasing interest in developing PRO COAs. FDA guidance on the topic [3] has highlighted the regulatory agency's interest in these instruments[2]

Clinician-Reported Outcomes (ClinRo)

- Reflects the evaluation of a patient's condition by a healthcare professional
- Based on the report that comes from a trained health care professional after observation of a patient's condition. a good example of this is the pain rating scale

Observer-Reported Outcomes (ObsRo)

- Measurement based on an observation by someone other than the patient or a health professional.
- Usually done by patient's non-clinical care giver, family or anyone living around patient and observes the patient in daily life. A good example is the assessment of a patient's cognition.

Performance Outcome (PerfO)

- The patient is assessed, but no rater judgment impacts the measurement, categorized as COAs because a patient's motivation or volition is involved in the task performance.
- Based on the patient's performance of a defined task that is quantified in a specified way that does not rely on judgment to determine the rating.
- Include instruments such eg distance walked in 6 minutes and Timed up and go (TUG)
- Clinician or observer is administering and monitoring performance of the PerfO assessment task, this individual does not apply judgment to quantifying the performance..[2]

The Context of Use of the COA

The context of use typically includes the following elements;

- Disease, injury, impairment or condition being treated
- Patient population demographics (age, disease severity, language, culture, education)
- Clinical treatment objectives and plan of treatment

Conclusion

- An outcome assessment, the patient assessment used in an endpoint, is the measuring instrument that provides a rating or score (categorical or continuous) that is intended to represent some aspect of the patient's health status.
- Outcome assessments are used to define efficacy endpoints when developing a therapy for a disease or condition.
- Most efficacy endpoints are based on specified clinical assessments of patients.
- When clinical assessments are used as clinical trial outcomes, they are called clinical outcome assessments (COAs).[2].

References

1. FDA COA Available from:https://www.fda.gov/about-fda/clinical-outcome-assessment-coa-frequently-asked-questions#COADefinition (last accessed 14.5.2020)
2. Walton MK, Powers III JH, Hobart J, Patrick D, Marquis P, Vamvakas S, Isaac M, Molsen E, Cano S, Burke LB. Clinical outcome assessments: conceptual Foundation—Report of the ISPOR clinical outcomes assessment–emerging good practices for outcomes research Task force. Value in Health. 2015 Sep 1;18(6):741-52. Available from:https://www.ncbi.nlm.nih.gov/pmc/articles/PMC4610138/ (last accessed 14.5.2020)
3. US Food and Drug Administration. Patient-Reported Outcome Measures: Use in Medical Product Development to Support Labeling Claims. [Accessed July 20, 2014];2009 Available from :http://www.fda.gov/Drugs/GuidanceCompliance RegulatoryInformation/Guidances/ucm064981.htm.

❑❑❑

11 Health Insurance

Health insurance is a type of insurance that covers medical expenses that arise due to an illness. These expenses could be related to hospitalisation costs, cost of medicines or doctor consultation fees.

Why is Health Insurance important?

- **Savings:** The best part about health insurance is it helps to keep your savings intact in case there is a medical emergency. The insurer will take care of all the expenses such as hospitalization, drugs/ medicines, etc. A health insurance plan is a trusted way to ensure a healthy and financially stable future.
- **Security of Family's health:** Protecting the health of self and your family members or parents is necessary. You can protect your family members by investing regularly in the family floater plan wherein you can also get health cover for your parents. This type of health insurance ensures that all types of medical treatments are covered.
- **High Medical Costs:** Due to the high healthcare services cost, you may not be able to afford treatment. But when you have a health insurance cover, you can avail quality treatment at the best network hospitals. Network hospitals are those wherein insurers have a tie-up with hospitals that helps you get cashless treatment. With this facility, the insurance company directly settles the bills with the hospital.
- **Lifestyle changes:** Our fast-paced lives have influenced our lifestyle choices. Work stress, indulgence in junk food, smoking, environmental changes, etc., affect our overall health, and this could lead to life-threatening diseases such as cancer, liver problem, kidney failure and so on. In such situations, health insurance will cover the medical and surgical expenses incurred during an illness. It is an established way to provide for health-related or medical emergencies.

Benefits of a Health Insurance Plan

1. **Financial Security:** With the passing of time, the medical costs are rising and lifestyle-related diseases such as diabetes, cancer, stroke, etc. are also surging. In such a case, having health insurance in the present time is of utmost importance as it can financially protect you against the unavoidable expenses. This way, your savings also remain protected.
2. **Domiciliary treatment:** Some health insurance companies provide cover for domiciliary treatment, wherein the treatment for certain diseases is provided at home under medical supervision. Note that there is a limitation on the amount and the number of days when availing insurance cover for domiciliary treatment.
3. **Free health check-up:** Health insurance understands that health is wealth; therefore, it needs consistent health monitoring. As a policyholder, you are eligible for a free preventive health check-up after an every 4 to 5 claim-free year. Some insurers also offer cashless treatments at their network hospital.
4. **Tax benefits:** You can avail tax benefits under Section 80D of the Income Tax Act. As part of the law, you can avail tax benefit for the expenses incurred on the preventive health check-up of parents above 60 years. Below is the table which shows the tax deductions for various health cover:

Scenario	Tax exemptions	Total Tax Exemption
Individual and parents are below 60 years	Rs.25,00 + Rs.25,000	Rs.50,000
Individual below 60 years and parents above 60 years	Rs.25,000 + Rs.50,000	Rs.75,000
Individual and parents both are above 60 years	Rs.50,000 + Rs. 50,000	Rs.1,00,000

5. **Coverage against critical illness:** To treat life-threatening diseases, the sum assured of a basic health insurance cover would not be enough; therefore, insurers provide critical illness cover as an add-on or rider option. When you seek critical illness add-on cover under your existing health insurance policy, you are entitled to receive lumpsum on detection of diseases like cancer, heart stroke, kidney failure, bone marrow transplant, etc.

Features of Health Insurance

The most notable features of a modern health insurance plan are-

1. **Coverage:** Insurance plans offer comprehensive coverage for all expenses that can be occurred during any health-related emergency. It includes hospitalization charges, post-hospitalization charges, ambulance expenses all under a single policy. Critical illnesses like cancer, kidney failure, and stroke are also covered for in a health insurance plan.
2. **Renewal discounts:** A No Claim Bonus is provided to the person insured in the following year if no claim has been made against the policy in the previous year. This bonus can be in the form of a high discount of the premium or the sum assured can be increased. Some insurers also provide a free check-up if there is a good record of no-claim bonuses.
3. **Co-payment:** Co-payment is an option provided by most insurers that helps to decrease the yearly premium. A percentage of the total expenses is paid by the insured while the insurance company pays the balance.
4. **Tax benefits:** Among the lesser-known health insurance benefits, is that under section 80D of the Income Tax Act, 1961, health insurance policies entitle you to receive tax benefits. The premium paid for a health insurance policy is tax-deductible, both for your own policy or for your family members.
5. **Flexibility:** An insurance plan provides high flexibility to the insured person. Insurance buyers can reduce their premium after a certain period or can change their policy duration entirely. Health insurance providers are also willing to also adjust the terms of your insurance plan in accordance with a change in your lifestyle, like change in your marital status.

Types of Health Insurance in India

1. **Individual Health Insurance:** An individual health insurance policy, like its name suggests covers the treatment cost of a single individual. This cover can be availed for yourself, parents including your spouse and children. Under this plan, every family member gets an individual sum insured. For example, if your plan sum insured is Rs 10 lakhs, each family member gets to use up to 10 lakhs each for that policy period, i.e. if you're buying an individual plan for three members, the collective sum insured for the three would be Rs 30 lakhs. It means that if something were to happen to all/more than one of your family members at the same time, this health insurance policy will be enough to cover them all due to the separate sum insured amount.
2. **Family Floater Health Insurance:** Under such plans, a single sum insured is available for all individuals under one policy. This entire sum can be disbursed for treatment of one person respectively, in which case no subsequent claims are covered in the event of another medical emergency. Senior citizens are not eligible under family floater plans, as their medical needs tend to be more complicated.
3. **Senior Citizen Health Insurance:** These types of plans can only be obtained by people above the age of 60 years. Comprehensive coverage for different types of illnesses which might develop due to old age is extended.
4. **Group Health Insurance:** Companies extend such plans to their employees. Premium is paid by the employer itself and has provisions which

ensure refill of the sum insured. Such group health insurance policies are cost-effective and are undertaken disbursed as an employee retention tactic.

However, you should remember that this insurance cover can only be availed as long as you are employed at the company. The benefits of the cover cannot be availed if you are terminated or have left your job at the company.

5. **Health Insurance with Maternity Insurance:** All pre and postnatal care expenses incurred during pregnancy are covered under maternity insurance cover. Medical bills of a new-born are included for the first three months as well. However, such policies come with a waiting period of two years.
6. **Critical Illness:** As life-threatening diseases are accompanied by extensive medical bills generated for adequate treatment. A critical illness insurance policy provides coverage against such specific conditions, providing financial protection for optima treatment and recovery of a patient.

   However, you should remember that the fixed sum insured offered under this cover can only be availed under the condition of the insured person remaining alive for 30 days post-diagnosis.
7. **Top-Up Health Insurance:** Oftentimes, the treatment costs you estimate while availing a health insurance cover can increase over time even though your sum insured remains unchanged.

   Under such circumstances, you can choose to avail a top-up for your existing cover, instead of purchasing a separate policy. This top-up policy helps to increase the overall sum insured which you can use in case of any emergency.

But to avail the top-up, you will first need to choose a deductible amount. For example, if you go for top-up plan of Rs. 3 Lakhs with a deductible of Rs. 50,000. Then, at the time of claim, you will first have to bear this Rs. 50,000 from your pocket. Once the deductible amount is exhausted, the insurance provider will come into the picture and will borne the remaining expenses up to 3 Lakhs. These health insurance plans are obtained to meet all healthcare expenditures a person might incur in their lifetime. It is significantly different from life insurance plans, as the latter provides financial coverage based on the life or death of an insured individual.

Difference between Health Insurance and Medical Insurance

Before purchasing health insurance or medical insurance plans, analyse the thin line between the two.

1. Medical insurance will provide you coverage only for hospitalization, pre-specified ailments and accidents that too for a pre-specified amount while health insurance will provide you with comprehensive coverage against hospitalization expenses, pre-hospitalization and post hospitalization expenses and ambulance charges.
2. Medical insurance will not provide you with any add-on coverage while health insurance, on the other hand, offers add-on coverage such as critical illness, accidental disability, etc.
3. Medical insurance doesn't offer any flexibility in terms of coverage whereas health insurance policyholders can reduce their policy duration, health insurance premium amount after a certain period, etc.
4. Medical insurance doesn't provide the insured with the critical illness cover while health insurance provides the insured with critical illness cover for diseases like cancer, heart attack, etc.
5. In medical insurance, the pre-assured sum cannot exceed INR 5 Lakhs while in health insurance the limit is INR 6 Crores.

What Should You Look for While Availing a Health Insurance Policy?

People should carefully factor in the following parameters before choosing a plan:

1. **Benefits and Sum Insured:** An insurance plan should be selected depending upon the age and medical history of an individual. Also, look into the coverage benefits extended by an insurance provider, as well as the waiting period before which any claims can be made.
2. **Market Reputation of the Insurance Company:** This is a significant factor to be analysed carefully, as it reflects the method and time taken for disbursement of the claim amount.

   To ensure hassle-free distribution, ensure your insurance provider satisfies the following conditions –

   - **High claim settlement ratio:** This reflects the percentage of insured individuals who applied for claims successfully received the requested amount to meet all medical bills generated.

- **Assets under management:** This reflects the total number of people opting for an insurance policy from the specified company, through total funds available. Cumulative premium amounts collected from all policyholders are categorised as assets under management. A high AUM value implies a larger proportion of individuals are opting for plans from the stipulated company, hence reflecting its reputation in the market.
- **Solvency ratio:** This indicates the ability of a company to meet its short term and long-term liabilities in the event of multiple claims simultaneously. A higher solvency ratio indicates sound management of a company, as the assets managed is substantially higher than total claims which have been or might be made.
- **The number of years in business:** Experience of an insurance company speaks volumes regarding the manner in which all claims are settled, as well as a mannerism of fund disbursal.

3. **Network hospitals:** A higher number of network hospitals ensure cashless claim transfer required for treatment. The hassles of third-party involvement are diminished by facilitating the treatment process.
4. **Routine Medical check ups:** Major insurance companies have provisions for free annual check-ups of policyholders, allowing them to keep track of their health conditions.
5. **Renewability:** Choose insurance providers who have lifetime renewability clause in their policies. Such a facility allows individuals to remain financially secured in any unpredicted situations causing deterioration in their health conditions at constant premiums.

You can choose an ideal health insurance policy suited to meet all your medical requirements by keeping the following pointers. Nominal premium charges can go a long way into easing the financial burden significantly in your lifetime through a health insurance policy.

Reference

1. ICICI Prudential's - https://www.iciciprulife.com/health-insurance/what-is-health-insurance.html
2. Health Care.gov - https://www.healthcare.gov/why-coverage-is-important/coverage-protects-you/
3. Aditya Birla Capital – ABS of Money - https://www.adityabirlacapital.com/abc-of-money/what-is-health-insurance
4. GoDigit : https://www.godigit.com/health-insurance/what-is-health-insurance
5. Jagaran Josh - https://www.jagranjosh.com/general-knowledge/difference-between-health-insurance-and-medical-insurance-1584521528-1
6. Max Life Insurance - https://www.maxlifeinsurance.com/blog/life-insurance/difference-between-life-insurance-and-health-insurance

Part B

OUTCOME SCALES

1 The Mohanty Flat Palpation Grades

(Prof. Dr Umashankar Mohanty, 2010)

The Mohanty Flat Palpation Grades is used to identify the extent of Trapezius muscle involvement with respect to the surrounding soft tissues.

- Layer 1 = Skin
- Layer 2 = Subcutaneous Tissue
- Layer 3 = Superficial Muscles
- Layer 4 = Deep Muscles

These Grades are described as follows:

- **Grade 1** = Adherence of 1,2,3 & 4
- **Grade 2** = Adherence of 2,3 & 4
- **Grade 3** = Adherence of 3 & 4
- **Grade 4** = Toughness in deep fascia
- **Grade 5** = Normal

(**Note:** The patient / subject should be in prone lying and the palpation done by circular movements with graded pressure)

Reference

1. Prof. Dr Umashankar Mohanty – Clinical presentation and examination of trapezius: Manual therapy and taping techniques for trapezius pain: Ch. 04: Clinical Symposia in Manual Therapy: Vol. 01- Edition 01

2

10 Meter Walk Test

Objective

The 10 Metre Walk Test is a performance measure used to assess walking speed in meters per second over a short distance. It can be employed to determine functional mobility, gait, and vestibular function.

Normative Values

Age (Men and Women)	Average Walking Speed (m/s)
20-29	1.36-1.34 m/s
30-39	1.43-1.34 m/s
40-49	1.43-1.39 m/s
50-59	1.43-1.31 m/s
60-69	1.34-1.24 m/s
70-79	1.26-1.13 m/s
80-990	0.97-0.94 m/s

Walking Speed m/s - Household Ambulator <0.40 m/s; Limited Community Ambulator 0.40 to <0.80 m/s; Community Ambulator ≥0.80 m/s[1]

Calculating Gait Speed - total distance/time. For example: if you did a 10-meter gait speed test and it took you 7 seconds, the equation would like: 10 meters / 7 seconds = 1.4 meters per second.[2]

Intended Population

Preschool children (2-5 years), children (6-12 years), adolescents (13-17 years), adults (18-64 years), elderly adults (65+) with a range of diagnoses including:

- Acquired Brain Injury
- Cerebral Palsy
- Geriatrics
- Hip Fracture
- Lower Limb Amputation
- Movement Disorders
- Multiple Sclerosis
- Parkinson's Disease
- Spinal Cord Injury
- Stroke
- Traumatic Brain Injury

Method of Use

Equipment Required

- Stopwatch
- A clear pathway with set distance (6, 8, 10 meters in length depending on distance tested)

Set-Up

- Measure and mark a 10-meter walkway
- Add a mark at 2-metres
- Add a mark at 8-metres

Instructions

- The individual walks without assistance for 10 meters, with the time measured for the intermediate 6 meters to allow for acceleration and deceleration
- Assistive devices may be used, but must be kept consistent and documented for each test
- Start timing when the toes pass the 2-meter mark
- Stop timing when the toes pass the 8-metre mark
- Can be tested at either preferred walking speed or maximum walking speed (ensure to document which was tested)
- Perform three trials and calculate the average of three trials

Patient Instructions

- Normal comfortable speed: "I will say ready, set, go. When I say go, walk at your normal comfortable speed until I say stop"
- Maximum speed trials: "I will say ready, set, go. When I say go, walk as fast as you safely can until I say stop"

Evidence

Reliability

The 10-meter walk test has demonstrated excellent reliability in many conditions including healthy adults, children with neuromuscular disease, Parkinson's disease, hip fracture, Spinal cord injury, Stroke, and Traumatic brain injury.

Test-Retest Reliability

Children with Neuromuscular Disease: (n = 29; mean age = 11.5 (3.5) years (6-16), Children with Neuromuscular Disease)

- Excellent test-retest reliability (ICC = 0.91) [4]

Healthy Adults

- Excellent test-retest reliability for comfortable gait speed (r = 0.75 - 0.90) [5]
- Excellent test-retest reliability for comfortable and fastest gait speeds (ICC = 0.93 - 0.91) [6]

Hip Fracture

- Excellent test-retest reliability (ICC = 0.823 with 95% CI = 0.565 to 0.934) [7]

Parkinson's Disease or Parkinsonism:

- Excellent test-retest reliability for comfortable gait speed (ICC = 0.96)
- Excellent test-retest reliability for maximum gait speed (ICC = 0.97) [8]

SCI:

- Excellent test-retest reliability (ICC = 0.97) [9]
- Excellent test-retest reliability (r = 0.983) [10]

Stroke: (n = 25; mean age = 72 years;
stroke onset = 2 to 6 years, Chronic Stroke)
Test-retest assessed three times within a single session:

- Excellent test-retest reliability (ICC = 0.95 to 0.99) [11]
- Excellent reliability for comfortable (ICC = 0.94) and fast (ICC = 0.97) gait speeds [12]

TBI (Traumatic brain injury):

- Excellent between day reliability at comfortable (ICC = 0.95) and fast speeds (ICC = 0.96) [13]
- Excellent test-retest reliability (r = 0.97 - 0.99) [5]

Interrater/Intrarater Reliability

Healthy Adults: (n = 28 healthy adults; mean age = 56.43 (+/- 13.82) years)

- Excellent interrater reliability (ICC = 0.980) [14]

SCI (Spinal cord injury):

- Excellent intrarater reliability (r = 0.983, p < 0.001)
- Excellent interrater reliability (r = 0.974, p < 0.001)
- Bland-Altman plots indicate reliability as being excellent when completed in under 40 seconds, but reliability decreases with marginal walkers requiring > 40 seconds to complete [15]
- Scivoletto et al 2011 (n = 37; median age = 58.5 (range 19 - 77) years; median time from onset = 24 (range 6 - 109) months; AIS D = 35, C = 2; Median WISCI = 16) utilized 2 methods in chronic SCI (measured 10 m with a static start and measured middle 10 m of 14 m walkway to include acceleration and deceleration), both showing:
    - o Excellent interrater reliability (ICC > 0.95)
    - o Excellent intrarater reliability (ICC > 0.98) [16]

Stroke: (Wolf et al, 1999; n = 28 with history of stroke; mean age = 56.04 (12.80) years; mean time since lesion = 13.59 (12.30) months, Chronic Stroke)

- Excellent intrarater reliability; ICC = 0.87 to 0.88 [11]
- Excellent interrater reliability; (ICC = 0.998) [14]

TBI (Traumatic brain injury): (Tyson & Connell, 2009; review of seventeen measures; n = 12 mobile TBI patients, TBI)

- Excellent interrater reliability (ICC = 0.99) [17]

Validity

Criterion Validity

Multiple Sclerosis: (*Paltamaa et al, 2007; n = 120; mean age = 45.0 (10.8) years; mean duration since symptom onset 12.3 (8.8) years, MS) Predictive Validity* [18]:

- Excellent correlation with dependence in self-care (r = 0.60 - 0.87) at comfortable speed
- Adequate to Excellent correlation with dependence in mobility (r = 0.34 - 0.74) at comfortable speed
- Adequate to excellent correlation with dependence in domestic life (r = 0.34 - 0.81) at comfortable speed

Stroke: (*Tyson & Connell, 2009; n = 40, review article of 17 measures, Stroke)*

Predictive Validity [17]:

- Excellent correlation with dependence in instrumental activities of daily living (r = 0.76)
- Excellent correlation with Barthel Index (r = 0.78

Construct Validity

Healthy Adults:

- Poor correlation with BBT (r = 0.052)
- Adequate correlation with FRT (r = 0.307) [14]

Hip Fracture:

- Excellent correlation with 6MWT (correlation coefficient = 0.82)
- Adequate correlation with LE strength (r = 0.51)
- Adequate correlation with LE power (r = 0.58)
- Poor correlation with hip pain (r = -0.23)
- Poor correlation with bodily pain (r = 0.30)
- Poor correlation with vitality (r = 0.26)
- Adequate correlation with physical role (r = 0.54)
- Adequate correlation with social role (r = 0.42) [19]

Convergent Validity

SCI (Spinal cord injury):

- Excellent correlation between the TUG and 10MWT (r = 0.89, n = 70)
- Excellent correlation between 10MWT and 6MWT (ρ = -0.95, n = 62)
- Subgroup comparisons of WISCI II and 10MWT
- Excellent correlation between WISCI II and 10MWT when testing individuals with WISCI II scores 11 - 20 (p = -0.68, n = 47)
- Poor correlation between the WISCI II and 10MWT when testing individuals with WISCI II scores 0 - 10 (r = -0.24, n = 20)
- Adequate but not significant correlation between WISCI II (0-8,10,11,14,17), dependent walkers (r = -0.35, n = 15)
- Adequate correlation between WISCI II (9,12,13,15,16,18-20) independent walkers (r = -0.48, n = 43)
- Overall, improved validity in individuals who are less impaired, higher walking ability, and do not require assistance [20]

Stroke:

- Excellent correlation between comfortable gait speed and TUG (ICC = -0.84), FGS (ICC = 0.92), Stair climbing ascend (SCas) (ICC = -0.81), Stair climbing descend (SCde) (ICC = -0.82), 6MWT (ICC = 0.89)
- Excellent correlation between fast gait speed and TUG (ICC = -0.91), CGS (ICC = 0.88), SCas (ICC = -0.84), SCde (ICC = -0.87) and 6MWT (ICC = 0.95) [12]

Responsiveness

Geriatrics:

- Small meaningful change = 0.05 m/s
- Substantial meaningful change = 0.10 m/s [21]

SCI (Spinal cord injury):

- Smallest real difference = 0.13 m/s
- Mean change between 1 and 3 months post-injury, effect size = 0.92
- Mean change between 3 and 6 months post-injury, effect size = 0.47 [10]

Stroke:

- Small meaningful change = 0.05 m/s
- Substantial meaningful change = 0.10 m/s [21]

References

1. Walk Guide Online Resources 14. Quick Look-Up Sheet: Reference Values for 10mWT & 6MWT © University of Toronto, Toronto, Canada 1 Quick Look-Up Sheet: Reference Values for 10-metre Walk Test and 6-Minute Walk Test Available

from:https://www.physicaltherapy.utoronto.ca/wp-content/uploads/2018/03/14_Quick-Look-Up-Sheet-Reference-Values-for-10mWT-6MWT-FINAL-.pdf (last accessed 5.2.2020)

2. wikiHow How to Measure Your Gait Speed Available from:https://www.wikihow.fitness/Measure-Your-Gait-Speed (last accessed 5.2.2020)
3. SCIREWebVideo. SCIREproject.com - 10 Meter Walk Test. Available from: http://www.youtube.com/watch?v=vKhgHOFCamU [last accessed 09/09/16]
4. Pirpiris, M., Wilkinson, A., et al. "Walking speed in children and young adults with neuromuscular disease: comparison between two assessment methods." Journal of Pediatric Orthopaedics 2003 23(3): 302
5. Watson, M. J. "Refining the ten-metre walking test for use with neurologically impaired people." Physiotherapy 2002 88(7): 386-397
6. Bohannon, R. W. "Comfortable and maximum walking speed of adults aged 20-79 years: reference values and determinants." Age Ageing 1997 26(1): 15-19
7. Hollman, J. H., Beckman, B. A., et al. "Minimum detectable change in gait velocity during acute rehabilitation following hip fracture." J Geriatr Phys There 2008 31(2): 53-56
8. Steffen, T. and Seney, M. "Test-retest reliability and minimal detectable change on balance and ambulation tests, the 36-item short-form health survey, and the unified Parkinson disease rating scale in people with parkinsonism." Physical Therapy 2008 88(6): 733-746
9. Bowden, M. G. and Behrman, A. L. "Step Activity Monitor: accuracy and test-retest reliability in persons with incomplete spinal cord injury." J Rehabil Res Dev 2007 44(3): 355-362
10. Lam, T., Noonan, V., et al. "A systematic review of functional ambulation outcome measures in spinal cord injury." Spinal Cord 2007 46(4): 246-254
11. Collen, F., Wade, D., et al. "Mobility after stroke: reliability of measures of impairment and disability." Disability and Rehabilitation 1990 12(1): 6-9
12. Flansbjer, U.B., Holmback, A. M., et al. "Reliability of gait performance tests in men and women with hemiparesis after stroke." J Rehabil Med 2005 37(2): 75-82
13. van Loo, M. A., Moseley, A. M., et al. "Test-re-test reliability of walking speed, step length and step width measurement after traumatic brain injury: a pilot study." Brain Inj 2004 18(10): 1041-1048
14. Wolf, S. L., Catlin, P. A., et al. "Establishing the reliability and validity of measurements of walking time using the Emory Functional Ambulation Profile." Phys There 1999 79(12): 1122-1133
15. van Hedel, H. J., Wirz, M., et al. "Assessing walking ability in subjects with spinal cord injury: validity and reliability of 3 walking tests." Archives of Physical Medicine and Rehabilitation 2005 86(2): 190-196
16. Scivoletto, G., Tamburella, F., et al. "Validity and reliability of the 10-m walk test and the 6-min walk test in spinal cord injury patients." Spinal Cord 2011 49(6): 736-740.
17. Tyson, S. and Connell, L. "The psychometric properties and clinical utility of measures of walking and mobility in neurological conditions: a systematic review." Clin Rehabil 2009 23(11): 1018-1033
18. Paltamaa, J., Sarasoja, T., et al. "Measures of physical functioning predict self-reported performance in self-care, mobility, and domestic life in ambulatory persons with multiple sclerosis." Archives of physical medicine and rehabilitation 2007 88(12): 1649-1657
19. Latham, N., Mehta, V., et al. "Performance-based or self-report measures of physical function: which should be used in clinical trials of hip fracture patients?" Archives of physical medicine and rehabilitation 2008 89(11): 2146-2155
20. van Hedel, H. J., Wirz, M., et al. "Assessing walking ability in subjects with spinal cord injury: validity and reliability of 3 walking tests." Archives of Physical Medicine and Rehabilitation 2005 86(2): 190-196
21. Perera, S., Mody, S., et al. "Meaningful change and responsiveness in common physical performance measures in older adults." Journal of the American Geriatrics Society 2006 54(5): 743-749

□□□

3 Arm Motor Ability Test

Objective

- Assess the functional capacity of the upper extremity in Activities of Daily Living (ADL) using both qualitative and quantitative method [1]
- Was developed in 1988 by McCulloch to supplement the WMFT as it was unable to detect the improvements in ADL activities of people with stroke receiving constraint-induced movement therapy.[2] The AMAT focuses mainly on activity limitation rather than impairment. [3]

Intended Population

- Mostly Stroke patient[1][4]
- People with a neurological problem like vestibular dysfunction, multiple sclerosis, spinal cord injury, traumatic brain injury [4]

Method of Use

The Arm Motor Ability Test(AMAT) has different versions and the components vary accordingly. Originally, AMAT consisted of 17 components. The AMAT version 13 has 13 components, the AMAT version 10 has 10 components, and the AMAT version 9 consists of 9 components.[2][5]The tasks in the tool are further divided into 1-3 subtasks or movements and the tasks may involve different contributions from the bilateral arm or distal and proximal part of the affected arm.[5]

Although the subtasks are timed individually, the patient is allowed to perform the task continuously and fluently. The time limit for each task is usually 1-2 minutes.[5] The task is evaluated in two scales: the Functional Ability scale (ability to perform the task) and the Quality of Movement (how the task is performed). [2][5] Each component is scored on 6 points Likert scale from 0 (no hand use) to 5(normal hand use). The Functional Ability: 0 = no use, 1 = very slight use, 2 = slight use,3 = moderate use, 4 = almost normal use, 5 = normal use and the Quality of Movement: 0 = no use, 1 = very poor, 2 = poor, 3= fair, 4 = almost normal, 5 = normal. [5]The more score means the fewer activity limitations and the less score means more activity limitations. [2][5]

The examiner/evaluator should read the instructions for each task carefully and the task is demonstrated to the patient three times using same arm/arms as the patient would use. The patient is not allowed to practice the task from both affected and unaffected arms because of the possibility of inter manual transfer of motor learning effects. If a subject could not complete a task component within the given time limit(1-2 minutes), the time limit is arbitrarily assigned as the score and timing of the remaining task components are resumed. The median is taken for all the time taken while performing and the mean for Functional Ability and Quality of Movement.[5][2]

The equipment needed to perform tasks are:

- Silverware and plate
- Play-doh
- Mug
- Comb
- Foam sandwich
- Towel
- Jar
- 2 shirts (different styles)
- Light switch
- Door
- Dried beans
- Shoe and Shoelaces
- Telephone

Evidence

Minimal Detectable Change (MDC):

The minimal detectable change in AMAT based on therapists' perception of change(Global Rating of Change (GROC)=5)[6]

- Grasp: 0.44
- Release: 0.42
- Ability to move affected arm and hand: 0.42
- Ability to perform Canadian Occupational Performance Measure activity: 0.42
- Overall arm and hand function: 0.42

The minimal detectable change in AMAT based on participants' perception of change (GROC=5)[6]

- Grasp: 0.44
- Release: 0.42
- Ability to move affected arm and hand: 0.40
- Ability to perform Canadian Occupational Performance Measure activity: 0.40
- Overall arm and hand function: 0.40

Minimally Clinically Important Difference (MCID):

The Minimally Clinically Important Difference in AMAT based on therapists' perception of change (GROC=5)[6]

- Grasp:0.34
- Release: 0.42
- Ability to move affected arm and hand: 0.40
- Ability to perform Canadian Occupational Performance Measure activity: 0.35
- Overall arm and hand function: 0.42

The minimal detectable change in AMAT based on participants' perception of change (GROC=5)[6]

- Grasp: 0.29
- Release: 0.31
- Ability to move affected arm and hand: 0.29
- Ability to perform Canadian Occupational Performance Measure activity: 0.30
- Overall arm and hand function: 0.40

Reliability

Test/retest reliability

- Excellent (ICC=0.93-0.99)[5]

Interrater/Intrarater reliability

- Excellent (ICC=0.95-0.99)[5]

Internal consistency

- Excellent with Cronbach's alpha 0.93[3]
- Excellent with inclusion of extreme scores using Pearson Separation Index (0.86)[3]
- Excellent with exclusion of extreme scores using Pearson Separation Index (0.88)[3]

Validity

Concurrent Validity

- Adequate to excellent with Motricity Index Arm (correlation coefficent=0.45-0.61)[5]
- ExcellentwithFugylMeyerAssessment(correlation coefficient= 0.92-0.94)[1]

Construct Validity

- Excellent Correlation with Wolf Motor Function Test (WMFT), Fugl-Meyer Assessment (FMA) and Action Research ArmTest (ARAT) (0.78-0.79)[3]
- Excellent Correlation with FMA wrist/hand subscore(0.74) [3]
- Excellent Correlation with FMA shoulder/elbow subscore (0.66) [3]
- Adequate Correlation with Stroke Impact Scale (SIS) hand subscore (0.40)[3]
- Poor Correlation with SIS communication subscore (-0.16)[3]

Content Validity

- Consistencies between the AMAT-9 and the Rash model expectations [3]

Floor/ceiling effect

- The AMAT time of performance exhibited significant ceiling and floor effects with respect to FMA[1]

Responsiveness

Sensitivity in AMAT based on Therapists' perception of change [6]

- Grasp: 0.64
- Release: 0.60
- Ability to move affected arm and hand: 0.58
- Ability to perform COPM tasks: 0.62
- Overall arm and hand function: 0.62

Sensitivity in AMAT based on Participants' perception of change [6]

- Grasp: 0.67
- Release: 0.64
- Ability to move affected arm and hand: 0.53
- Ability to perform COPM tasks:0.56
- Overall arm and hand function: 0.50

References

1. Chae J, Labatia I, Yang G. Upper limb motor function in hemiparesis: concurrent validity of the Arm Motor Ability test. American journal of physical medicine & rehabilitation. 2003 Jan 1; 82 (1): 1-8.
2. Scale Library. Finding a clinical assessment scale-Physical medicine and rehabilitation.Arm Motor Ability Test. accessed on 2021/3/19. Available from:http://scale-library.com/assessment_scale_result.php?echelle=Wolf%20Motor%20Function%20Test%20(WMFT)&theme=&type=&scalage=adulte&retour=liste&cle=&echelle_box=Arm%20Motor%20Ability%20Test%20(AMAT)
3. O'Dell MW, Kim G, Rivera L, Fieo R, Christos P, Polistena C, Fitzgerald K, Gorga D. A psychometric evaluation of the Arm Motor Ability Test. Journal of rehabilitation medicine. 2013 Jun 5;45(6):519-27.
4. Shirley Ryan Ability lab.Rehabilitation measures database.Arm Motor Ability Test.Accessed on 2021/03/13.Available from:https://www.sralab.org/rehabilitation-measures/arm-motor-ability-test
5. Kopp B, Kunkel A, Flor H, Platz T, Rose U, Mauritz KH, Gresser K, McCulloch KL, Taub E. The Arm Motor Ability Test: reliability, validity, and sensitivity to change of an instrument for assessing disabilities in activities of daily living. Archives of physical medicine and rehabilitation. 1997 Jun 1;78(6):615-20.
6. Fulk G, Martin R, Page SJ. Clinically important difference of the arm motor ability test in Stroke survivors. Neurorehabilitation and neural repair. 2017 Mar;31(3):272-9.

□□□

4 Balance Evaluation Systems Test (BESTest)

Objective

BESTest is the quantitative assessment tool that aims to identify the disordered systems underlying the postural control responsible for poor functional balance. It was first developed by Dr. Horak in 2009 for clinicians to differentiate balance problems into six underlying systems that may constrain balance. It was developed from the theoretical understanding of balance control systems based on Bernstein's concept that postural control results from a set of interacting systems. It has 36 items that evaluate performance of 6 balance systems: bio-mechanical constraints, stability limits/verticality, anticipatory responses, postural responses, sensory orientation, and stability in gait.[1]

Strength of BESTest

- It incorporates different balance systems which help in postural control.
- It helps clinicians to determine the type of balance problems so as to direct the specific treatments for their patients.[2]
- It will help to improve third party reimbursement by identifying the specific system affected and change with therapy.[1]

Constraints of Postural Control Systems Addresses Following

- **Bio-mechanical Systems:** Ankle strategy or compensatory steps for postural recovery (eg: flexed posture in frial elderly and Person's with Parkinson diseases).
- Limits of Stability (how far the body's center of mass can be moved over it's base of support) and Verticality (represent gravitational upright).
- **Anticipatory Postural Adjustments:** Readiness prior to the voluntary movements which depend on interaction of supplementary motor areas with basal ganglia and brain stem areas.
- **Automatic Postural Responses:** Impulses carried by short, medium and long proprioceptive feedback loops.
- **Sensory Orientation:** Spatial orientation maintain by pathways involving vestibular system and sensory integrative areas of the temporo-parietal cortex.
- **Stability in Gait:** Co-ordination between spinal locomotor and brain stem postural sensorimotor programs.[1]

Intended Population

It can be used in varied age and severity of ambulator patients with neurological conditions (Parkinson'ss, Stroke,Cerebellar Ataxia, Neuropathies, Head injury, Mulitiple Scelerosis, Cerebral palsy, etc.), Vestibular disorders, Cognitive Deficits and Elderly.

Method

Time to Administer

20-30 minutes.[1]

Examiner Instructions for BESTest

1. Subjects should be tested with flat heeled shoes or with shoes and socks off.
2. If subject must use an assistive device for an item, score that item one category lower.[1]

Equipment Required

- Stop watch
- Measuring tape mounted on wall for Functional Reach test

- Approximately 60 cm x 60 cm (2 X 2 ft) block of 4-inch, medium-density, Tempur® foam
- 10 degree incline ramp (at least 2 x 2 ft) to stand on
- Stair step, 15 cm (6 inches) in height for alternate stair tap
- 2 stacked shoe boxes for obstacle during gait § 2.5 Kg (5-lb) free weight for rapid arm raise
- Firm chair with arms with 3 meters in front marked with tape for Get Up and Go test
- Masking tape to mark 3 m and 6 m lengths on the floor for Get Up and Go.[1]

Scoring

It consist of 27 tasks, with 36 items in total. Each items is scored based on ordinal scale scoring from 0- 3 where 3 representing best performances and 0 representing worst performances. Scores for the total test is provided as a percentage of total points i.e. 108. In addition, 6 sub-systems scores can be generated separately in percentage of total score each representing a specific balance system.[1]

Required Training

Reading Original Article/Manual.

Psychometric Properties

For Non- Specific Patient Population

Reliability

The excellent inter-reliability of the total score with inter-class correlation (ICC) of 0.91 and subsection ICC ranged from 0.79 to 0.95:

- Bio-mechanical constraints: 0.80
- Stability limits/verticality: 0.79
- Anticipatory Postural Adjustments: 0.92
- Postural Reactions: 0.92
- Sensory Orientation: 0.96
- Stability of Gait: 0.88[1]

Criterion Validity (Concurrent/ Predictive)

- With Activities- Specific Balance Confidence (ABC) scale, it shows moderate correlation (r=.41–.78) where Stability Limits/Verticality scores had the best correlation (r=.78) and Anticipatory Postural Adjustments scores had the worst correlation (r=.41).[1]
- BBS, BESTest, Mini-BESTest, and Brief-BESTest were significantly correlated with each other with Spearman correlation coefficients (ρ=.83-.96) and with the ABC Scale (ρ=.46-.61).[4]

Construct Validity

- Control subjects scored significantly higher (better) than the subjects with balance problems (P=.036) via Mann-Whitney U test.[1]
- Discriminated between people with different balance deficits: subjects with unilateral vestibular loss scored the worst in Sensory Orientation (60%), whereas the subjects with Parkinson's scored the worst in Postural Responses (50%) and subjects with neuropathies in Anticipatory Postural Adjustment.

Minimal Detectable Change (MDC)

MDC at 95% confidence level= 9[4]

Cut-off score

82% differentiate from fallers to non- fallers.[4]

For Parkinson's

Reliability

Excellent inter-rater reliability of total BESTest with ICC 0.96 and subsection ICC ranging from 0.79-0.96.

- Bio-mechanical constraints:0.81
- Stability Limits/verticality: 0.79
- Anticipatory Postural Adjustments: 0.91
- Postural Responses: 0.91
- Sensory Orientation: 0.96
- Stability in Gait: 0.86[5]

Excellent to Adequate Test- retest reliabilty for total score with ICC (0.88) and for subsection mentioned below:

- Bio-mechanical constraints:0.69
- Stability Limits/verticality: 0.63
- Anticipatory Postural Adjustments: 0.83
- Postural Responses: 0.87
- Sensory Orientation: 0.72
- Stability in Gait: 0.72[5]

Cut-off Score:

- To identify individual as fallers and non-fallers 69% cut-off score with sensitivity=0.84, specificity = 0.76, LR+ = 3.49, LR-=0.21AND AUC=0.85. [5]

- With 69% of cut off score to detect fallers.
  - with sensitivity of 0.84, specificity= 0.76, LR+=3.49, LR-= 0.21 and AUC= 0.84, adequate for detecting retrospective fallers.
  - with sensitivity of 0.93, specificity= 0.84, LR+=5.81, LR-= 0.08 and AUC= 0.89, adequate for detecting prospective fallers.
  - with sensitivity of 0.46 specificity= 0.74, LR+=1.77, LR-= 0.73 and AUC= 0.68, poor for detecting 12 months prospective fallers.[2]

Criterion Validity:

- Excellent Correlation between Mini-BESTest and BESTest total score (r=0.955).[5]
- Adequate Correlation with ABC (r=0.757).
- Excellent Correlation with berg balance scale (r= 0.87)
- Excellent Correlation with Functional Gait Assessment (r=0.882)[2]

Limitations

- The limitation of the BESTest is the time required to complete the assessment (35 minutes) [6]. Time to complete the assessment is longer with even longer depending upon the severity of conditions. A short form of the BESTest, the Mini-BESTest, and Brief-BESTest was developed to reduce the assessment time. Mini-BESTest has 14 tasks and needs only 10 to 15 minutes.
- Equipment required is too many which may not be practical for regular use in all clinical settings.[7]

References

1. Horak FB, Wrisley DM, Frank J. The balance evaluation systems test (BESTest) to differentiate balance deficits. Physical therapy. 2009 May 1;89(5):484-98.
2. Duncan RP, Leddy AL, Cavanaugh JT, Dibble LE, Ellis TD, Ford MP, Foreman KB, Earhart GM. Comparative utility of the BESTest, mini-BESTest, and brief-BESTest for predicting falls in individuals with Parkinson disease: a cohort study. Physical therapy. 2013 Apr 1;93(4):542-50.
3. dcscott325. Mini BESTest Demonstration. Available from: https://www.youtube.com/watch?v =jK43dcXrhWM [last assessed 3/2/2019]
4. Marques A, Almeida S, Carvalho J, Cruz J, Oliveira A, Jácome C. Reliability, validity, and ability to identify fall status of the balance evaluation systems test, Mini–balance evaluation systems test, and Brief–balance evaluation systems test in older people living in the community. Archives of physical medicine and rehabilitation. 2016 Dec 1;97(12):2166-73.
5. Leddy AL, Crowner BE, Earhart GM. Utility of the Mini-BESTest, BESTest, and BESTest sections for balance assessments in individuals with Parkinson disease. Journal of neurologic physical therapy: JNPT. 2011 Jun;35(2):90.
6. Yingyongyudha A, Saengsirisuwan V, Panichaporn W, Boonsinsukh R. The Mini-Balance Evaluation Systems Test (Mini-BESTest) demonstrates higher accuracy in identifying older adult participants with history of falls than do the BESTest, Berg Balance Scale, or Timed Up and Go Test. Journal of geriatric physical therapy. 2016 Apr 1;39(2):64-70.
7. Di Carlo S, Bravini E, Vercelli S, Massazza G, Ferriero G. The Mini-BESTest: a review of psychometric properties. International journal of rehabilitation research. 2016 Jun 1;39(2):97-105.
8. Huang M, Pang MY. Psychometric properties of Brief-Balance Evaluation Systems Test (Brief-BEST est) in evaluating balance performance in individuals with chronic stroke. Brain and behavior. 2017 Mar; 7(3): e00649.

❑❑❑

5 Balance Error Scoring System

Objective

The Balance Error Scoring System is an objective measure of assessing static postural stability (designed for the mild head injury population, to assist in return to sports play decisions).

Intended Population

Those diagnosed with concussion, mild traumatic brain injury, vestibular disorders

Method of Use

Equipment Required:

- Foam pad
- Stopwatch
- An assistant to act as a spotter
- BESS testing protocol (instructions to be read to subject during testing)
- BESS score card

Description:

- 6 conditions each tested barefoot, eyes closed for 20 seconds each:
    - o Double leg stance (feet together) – firm / foam surfaces Single leg stance (non-dominant foot) – firm / foam surfaces
    - o Tandem stance (non-dominant foot in back) – firm / foam
- Score of 0-60 (lower scores indicate better balance and less errors).
- Each trial is scored by counting errors (deviations from the proper stance). If multiple errors occur at the same time, only one is counted. The maximum number of errors for a single condition is 10.
- Errors include moving hands off of iliac crests, opening eyes, step stumble or fall, abduction or flexion of the hip beyond 30 degrees, lifting forefoot or heel off testing surface, remaining out of the proper testing position for > 5 seconds.
- Number of errors in each trial are added together to obtain a total score (out of 60).
- Read instructions to subject as they are written in the testing protocol.

Evidence

Reliability

Test-retest Reliability

- Athletes: (Bell et al, 2011) [2]
- Adequate test retest reliability in youth participants aged 9-14 (ICC = 0.70)

Interrater/Intrarater Reliability

- Athletes (without neurological / orthopedic injury): (Susco et al, 2004; n = 34 subset of subjects) [3]
    - o Adequate to Excellent intrarater reliability (ICC from 0.62-0.82)
    - o Excellent: Double support / firm surface (ICC = 0.82)
    - o Adequate: Double support / firm surface (ICC = 0.63)
- Athletes: (Bell et al, 2011; n = 18 college athletes)[2]
    - o Excellent interrater reliability (ICC = 0.78-0.96)
    - o Adequate-excellent interrater reliability (ICC=0.57-0.85 for total score (systematic review looking at 8 studies)

- o Adequate-excellent intrarater reliability for total score (ICC = 0.60-0.92)

Validity

Criterion Validity (Predictive/Concurrent)

- Athletes: (Bell et al, 2011) [2]
  - o Adequate-excellent correlations with target sway in male athletes
  - o Significant correlations for 5 of the 6 stances ($r = 0.31$-0.79, $p < 0.01$)
- Concussion: (Barlow et al, 2011 retrospective chart review of middle and high school students; n = 106; mean age = 15.38(1.7) years; mean days between testing = 15.5(14.1) days) [4]
  - o Adequate correlation with ImPACT (Immediate Post-Concussion Assessment and Cognitive Testing)Impulse control (r = -0.31)
  - o Adequate correlation with ImPACT verbal score (r = 0.37)
  - o Poor correlation with ImPACT visual motor speed change (r = -0.33)
  - o Poor correlation with ImPACT reaction time (r = -0.02)
  - o Poor correlation with PCSS (r = 0.15)
- Athletes (controls without neurological/orthopedic injury): (Susco et al, 2004) [3]
  - o Positive correlation with RPW score (r = 0.542)

Construct Validity (Convergent/Discriminant)

- Athletes: (Bell et al, 2011) [2]
  - o Convergent validity: BESS and sensory organization test (SOT), validated in a concussed population. More errors seen at day 1 post injury compared to healthy individuals, but returned to baseline at 3 and 5 days post injury. Average errors 9(4) for control, 15(8) for concussed, effect size 1.0.
  - o Discriminant: BESS does not discriminate between concussed athletes with and without a headache (p = 0.87)
  - o BESS performance worsens after 50 years of age ($p < 0.01$), r = 0.36
  - o Increase in total BESS score (poorer performance) after whole-body or central fatigue ($p < 0.01$)
  - o Barefoot BESS performance better than braced BESS (p = 0.04), before walking, better than braced (p=.03 or taped (p = 0.04) after walking. Differences not seen in SOT between conditions.
- Healthy adults: (Iverson et al, 2008) [5]
  - o Adequate correlation between BESS and age(r = 0.36)
  - o Poor correlation between BESS and height (r = -0.03)
  - o Poor correlation between BESS and weight (r = 0.16)
  - o Poor correlation between BESS and waist circumference (r = 0.26)
  - o Poor correlation between BESS and BMI (r = 0.23)

Responsiveness

Not established

References

1. Duke Neurology. Sports Concussion Exam (3 of 9): Balanced Error Scoring System (BESS). Available from: https://www.youtube.com/watch?v=fA392PbM3-A
2. Bell, D. R., Guskiewicz, K. M., et al. "Systematic review of the balance error scoring system." Sports Health 2011 3(3): 287-295
3. Susco, T. M., Valovich McLeod, T. C., et al. "Balance Recovers Within 20 Minutes After Exertion as Measured by the Balance Error Scoring System." J Athl Train 2004 39(3): 241-246
4. Barlow, M., Schlabach, D., et al. "Differences in change scores and the predictive validity of three commonly used measures following concussion in the middle school and high school aged population." Int J Sports Phys Ther 2011 6(3): 150-157
5. Iverson, G. L., Kaarto, M. L., et al. "Normative data for the balance error scoring system: implications for brain injury evaluations." Brain Inj 2008 22(2): 147-152

❑❑❑

6

Four Square Step Test

Objective

The Four Square Step Test (FSST) is used to assess dynamic stability and the ability of the subject to step over low objects forward, sideways, and backward.[1]

Intended Population

- Older adults/geriatrics
- Stroke
- Parkinson's
- Vestibular Disorders
- Limb Loss/Amputation

Method of Use

Test Description:

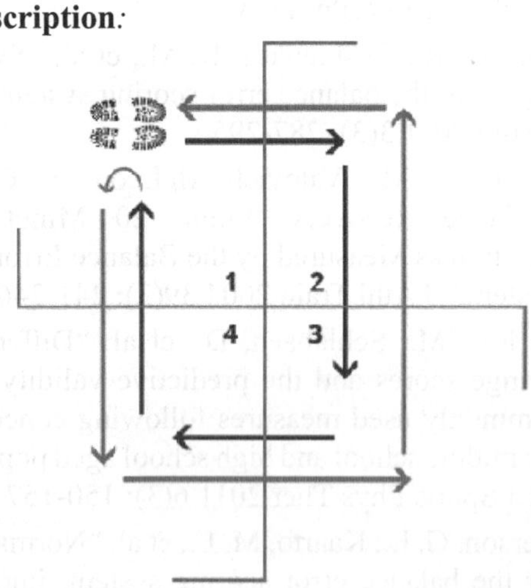

- The subject is required to sequentially step over four canes set-up in a cross configuration on the ground.
- At the start of the test, the subject stands in Square 1 facing Square 2.
- The aim is to step as fast as possible into each square with both feet in the following sequence: Square 2, 3, 4, 1, 4, 3, 2, 1 (clockwise to counter-clockwise)
- Test procedure may be demonstrated, one practice trial is allowed prior to administering the test.
- Two trials are then performed, and the better time (in seconds) is taken as the score.
- Timing starts when the first foot contacts the floor in Square 2 and finishes when the last foot comes back to touch the floor in Square 1.
- Instructions: "Try to complete the sequence as fast and as safely as possible without touching the sticks. Both feet must make contact with the floor in each square. If possible, face forward during the entire sequence."[2][3]
- Repeat a trial if the subject:
    - o Fails to complete the sequence successfully
    - o Loses balance
    - o Makes contact with the cane
- Subjects who are unable to face forward during the entire sequence may turn before stepping into the next square and are timed accordingly.
- Any assistive device used during the test are noted down accordingly.

Equipment

- Stopwatch
- 4 canes/ rods (approximately 100cm in length and 2.5cm in diameter[4])

Time to Administer

Less than five minutes

Evidence

The FSST may be an effective and valid tool for measuring dynamic balance and the subject's fall risk. It has been shown to have strong correlations with other measures of balance and mobility with good reliability shown in a number of populations.[5] A recent study showed a stronger relationship between gait and balance disorder and TIA/minor stroke, which was measured by logistic regression analysis of six measurements (Four Square Step [OR, 24.07; 95% CI 5.90–98.13; p<0.001], Tandem, Functional Reach, Gait and Pivot Turn, Timed "Up and Go", and Single Leg Balance tests).[6]

Reliability

Older adults/geriatrics

(Dite & Temple, 2002)

- Excellent test-retest reliability (ICC = 0.98)
- Excellent inter-rater reliability (ICC = 0.99)

Parkinson's

(Duncan & Earhart et al, 2013)[7]

- Excellent reliability on medication (ICC = 0.78)
- Excellent reliability off medication (ICC = 0.90)
- Excellent inter rater reliability (ICC = 0.99)

Vestibular Disorders

(Whitney et al, 2007)[8]

- Excellent test retest reliability (ICC = 0.93)

Cut-off scores

Older adults/geriatrics

- > 15 seconds = increased risk of falls

Stroke

- > 15 seconds or failed attempt = increased risk of falls

Parkinson's

- > 9.68 seconds = increased risk of falls

Vestibular Disorders

- > 12 seconds = increased risk of falls

Limb Loss/Amputation

- > 24 seconds = at risk for fall

References

1. Shirley Ryan Ability Lab. Rehabilitation measure: four square step test. www.sralab.org/rehabilitation-measures/four-step-square-test (accessed 12 March 2018).
2. Dite W, Temple VA. A clinical test of stepping and change of direction to identify multiple falling older adults. Archives of physical medicine and rehabilitation. 2002 Nov 1;83(11):1566-71.
3. Blennerhassett JM, Jayalath VM. The Four Square Step Test is a feasible and valid clinical test of dynamic standing balance for use in ambulant people poststroke. Archives of physical medicine and rehabilitation. 2008 Nov 1;89(11):2156-61.
4. McKee KE, Hackney ME. The Four Square Step Test in individuals with Parkinson's: Association with executive function and comparison with older adults. NeuroRehabilitation. 2014 Jan 1;35(2):279-89.
5. Moore M, Barker K. The validity and reliability of the four square step test in different adult populations: a systematic review. Systematic reviews. 2017 Dec;6(1):187. https://systematicreviewsjournal.biomedcentral.com/articles/10.1186/s13643-017-0577-5 (accessed 12 March 2018).
6. Li N, Li J, Gao T, Wang D, Du Y, Zhao X. Gait and balance disorder in patients with transient ischemic attack or minor stroke. Neuropsychiatric disease and treatment. 2021;17:305.
7. Duncan RP, Earhart GM. Four square step test performance in people with Parkinson disease. Journal of Neurologic Physical Therapy. 2013 Mar 1;37(1):2-8.
8. Whitney SL, Marchetti GF, Morris LO, Sparto PJ. The reliability and validity of the Four Square Step Test for people with balance deficits secondary to a vestibular disorder. Archives of physical medicine and rehabilitation. 2007 Jan 1;88(1):99-104.

❑❑❑

7 Motor Assessment Scale

Objective

The Motor Assessment Scale (MAS) is a performance-based scale used to assess everyday motor function in patients with stroke[1].

Intended Population

Used widely in assessing functional ability for patients with stroke by Physical therapists and Occupational therapists.

Method of Use

Description:

- 8 items assess 8 areas of motor function. Takes 15 mins to complete.
- Patients perform each task 3 times, only the best performance is recorded.
- Items (with the exception of the general tonus item*) are assessed using a 7-point scale (0 to 6)
- A score of 6 indicates optimal motor behavior.

*For the general tonus item, the score is based on continuous observations throughout the assessment. A score of 4 on this item indicates a consistently normal response, a score > 4 indicates persistent hypertonus, and a score < 4 indicates various degrees of hypotonus[2].

Equipment Required:

- Stopwatch
- 8 Jellybeans
- Polystyrene cup
- Rubber ball
- Stool
- Comb
- Spoon
- Pen
- 2 Tea cups
- Water
- Prepared sheet for drawing lines
- Cylindrical shaped object like a jar
- Table

Items Assessed:

- Supine to side lying
- Supine to sitting over the edge of a bed
- Balanced sitting
- Sitting to standing
- Walking
- Upper-arm function
- Hand movements
- Advanced hand activities

Scoring:

- Item scores (with the exception of the general tonus item) are summed to provide an overall score (out of 48 points)
- Completing a higher-level item suggests successful performance on lower-level items and thus lower-items can be skipped.

Evidence

Reliability

Test-retest Reliability:

Chronic Stroke:

(Carr et al, 1985; n = 15; mean age = 70 years, range = 42 to 85)[2]

- Excellent test-retest reliability: r ranged from 0.87 to 1.00 (mean r = 0.98)

Interrater/Intrarater Reliability:

Chronic & Acute Stroke:

(Carr et al, 1985; 20 clinical raters; n = 5; mean age = 65 years, range = 55 to 78; mean time since stroke onset = 14 (range = 6 to 40) weeks)[2]

- Excellent Interrater Reliability; 87% overall agreement between raters (mean correlation r = 0.95; most agreement = balanced sitting (r = 0.99); least agreement = sitting to standing (r = 0.89).

Validity

Criterion Validity:

Acute Stroke:

(Malouin et al, 1994, n = 32, mean age = 60 years, mean time since stroke = 64.5 days)[3]

- Excellent Concurrent Validity with Fugl-Meyer (FMA) total scores (r = 0.96, not including general tonus items)
- Adequate to Excellent item level Concurrent Validity between MAS items and similar FMA items (r = 0.65 to 0.93)
- Poor Concurrent Validity with MAS and FMA sitting balance (r = -0.10)

Construct Validity:

Acute Stroke:

(Tyson & DeSouza, 2004; n = 48; mean age = 66.7 (12.5) years; median time since stroke = 11 weeks)[4]

MAS and functional balance test:

- Adequate Convergent Validity: Sitting arm raise (no. of raises; r = 0.33*)
- Adequate Convergent Validity: Sitting forward reach (cm, r = 0.54**)

*$p < 0.05$

**$p < 0.01$

Content Validity:

The MAS was developed by Carr and Shepherd (1985) based on many years of experience with similar measures[2]

Responsiveness

Chronic & Acute Stroke:

MAS sensitivity[5]:

Item	Dimension	Effect	Effect Size (d)	% Change
1	Rolling	Large	1.03	31.1
2	Lie to sit	Moderate	0.74	44.3
3	Balanced Sitting	Moderate	0.61	60.7
4	Sit to Stand	Large	0.85	18
5	Walking	Large	1.02	19.7
6	Upper arm function	Small	0.36	44.3
7	Hand movements	Small	0.43	55.7
8	Advanced hand activities	Moderate	0.50	63.9

References

1. Dean, C. M., Mackey, F. M. Motor assessment scale scores as a measure of rehabilitation outcome following stroke. Aust J Physiother. 1992; 38, 31-35.
2. Carr, J. H., Shepherd, R. B., Nordholm, L., Lynne, D. Investigation of a new motor assessment scale for stroke patients. Phys Ther 1985 65: 175-180
3. Malouin, F., Pichard, L., Bonneau, C., Durand, A., Corriveau, D . Evaluating motor recovery early after stroke: comparison of the Fugl-Meyer Assessment and the Motor Assessment Scale. Arch Phys Med Rehabil 1994; 75: 1206-1212
4. Tyson, S. F. and DeSouza, L. H. Reliability and validity of functional balance tests post stroke. Clin Rehabil 2004; 18(8): 916-923
5. English, C. K., Hillier, S. L. The sensitivity of three commonly used outcome measures to detect change among patients receiving inpatient rehabilitation following stroke. Clin Rehabil, 2006; 20(1): 52-55

❑❑❑

8 12-Item Short Form Survey (SF-12)

Objective

The SF-12 is a self-reported outcome measure assessing the impact of health on an individual's everyday life. It is often used as a quality of life measure.

The SF-12 is a shortened version of it's predecessor, the SF-36, which itself evolved from the Medical Outcomes Study[1]. The SF-12 was created to reduce the burden of response[2].

The SF-12 uses the same eight domains as the SF-36:

1. Limitations in physical activities because of health problems.
2. Limitations in social activities because of physical or emotional problems
3. Limitations in usual role activities because of physical health problems
4. Bodily pain
5. General mental health (psychological distress and well-being)
6. Limitations in usual role activities because of emotional problems
7. Vitality (energy and fatigue)
8. General health perceptions

Intended Population

Like the SF-36, the SF-12 is designed as a general measure of health so can be used with the general population.

Method of Use

Patients fill out a 12 question survey which is then scored by a clinician or researcher.

Unlike the SF-36, the SF-12 is not available for free by its authors, due to a scoring programme. However, there is an online calculator here that uses the first version.

There is a scoring guide for both versions available here.

Evidence

Like the SF-12 has been tested in a range of disease populations, including mental health, stroke, and myocardial infarction.

Validity

When compared to the SF-36 in various patient groups varying in age, physical and mental health, the SF-12 scores were similar to the SF-36 but almost always had bigger standard errors[3].

A separate study[4] compared the SF-12 to the SF-36 in treatments for congestive heart failure, sleep apnoea and inguinal hernia. The authors found that the SF-12 agreed with the MCS and PCS of the SF-36, noting that the scores recorded the same level of health and change over time.

A third study of responses from nine European countries also confirmed correlation between SF-12 and SF-36 component summaries and recommended the SF-12 to be useful for assessment of large populations[5].

Responsiveness

The SF-12 has been shown to reflect change over time like the SF-36[4].

Miscellaneous

There are two versions of the SF-12 which have some differences in scoring so it is recommended that users document which version they are using.

References

1. Ware J. SF-36 Health Survey Update. Spine. 2000. 25; 24: 3130-3139.
2. Rand Health Care. 12-Item Short Form Survey (SF-12). Available from: https://www.rand.org/health-care/surveys_tools/mos/12-item-short-form.html. (Accessed 29 February 2020).
3. Ware J, Kosinski M, Keller SD. A 12-Item Short-Form Health Survey: construction of scales and preliminary tests of reliability and validity. Med Care. 1996. 34; 3:220-33.
4. Jenkinson C, Layte R, Jenkinson D, Lawrence K, Petersen S, Paice C, Stradling J. A shorter form health survey: can the SF-12 replicate results from the SF-36 in longitudinal studies? Journal of Public Health. 1997. 19; 2: 179-186. Accessed 29 February 2020.
5. Gandek B, Ware J, Aaronson N, Apolone G, Bjorner J, Brazier J, Bullinger M, Kaasa S, Leplege A, Prieto L, Sullivan M.. "Cross-validation of item selection and scoring for the SF-12 Health Survey in nine countries: results from the IQOLA Project." Journal of clinical epidemiology. 1998. 51;11: 1171-1178.

❑❑❑

S F – 12 Patient Questionnaire

This information will help your doctors keep track of how you feel and how well you are able to do your usual activities. Answer every question by placing a check mark on the line in front of the appropriate answer. It is not specific for arthritis. If you are unsure about how to answer a question, please give the best answer you can and make a written comment beside your answer.

1. In general, would you say your health is:
   Excellent (1) Very Good (2)
   Good (3) Fair (4)
   Poor (5)

   The following two questions are about activities you might do during a typical day. Does YOUR HEALTH NOW LIMIT YOU in these activities? If so, how much?
2. MODERATE ACTIVITIES, such as moving a table, pushing a vacuum cleaner, bowling, or playing golf:
   Yes, Limited A Lot (1)
   Yes, Limited A Little (2)
   No, Not Limited At All (3)
3. Climbing SEVERAL flights of stairs:
   Yes, Limited A Lot (1)
   Yes, Limited A Little (2)
   No, Not Limited At All (3)

   During the PAST 4 WEEKS have you had any of the following problems with your work or other regular activities AS A RESULT OF YOUR PHYSICAL HEALTH?
4. ACCOMPLISHED LESS than you would like:
   Yes (1) No (2)
5. Were limited in the KIND of work or other activities:
   Yes (1) No (2)

   During the PAST 4 WEEKS, were you limited in the kind of work you do or other regular activities AS A RESULT OF ANY EMOTIONAL PROBLEMS (such as feeling depressed or anxious)?
6. ACCOMPLISHED LESS than you would like:
   Yes (1) No (2)
7. Didn't do work or other activities as CAREFULLY as usual:
   Yes (1) No (2)
8. During the PAST 4 WEEKS, how much did PAIN interfere with your normal work (including both work outside the home and housework)?
   Not At All (1) A Little Bit (2)
   Moderately (3) Quite A Bit (4)
   Extremely (5)

   The next three questions are about how you feel and how things have been DURING THE PAST 4 WEEKS. For each question, please give the one answer that comes closest to the way you have been feeling. How much of the time during the PAST 4 WEEKS –
9. Have you felt calm and peaceful?
   All of the Time (1)
   Most of the Time (2)
   A Good Bit of the Time (3)
   Some of the Time (4)
   A Little of the Time (5)
   None of the Time (6)
10. Did you have a lot of energy?
    All of the Time (1)
    Most of the Time (2)
    A Good Bit of the Time (3)
    Some of the Time (4)
    A Little of the Time (5)
    None of the Time (6)
11. Have you felt downhearted and blue?
    All of the Time (1)
    Most of the Time (2)
    A Good Bit of the Time (3)
    Some of the Time (4)
    A Little of the Time (5)
    None of the Time (6)
12. During the PAST 4 WEEKS, how much of the time has your PHYSICAL HEALTH OR EMOTIONAL PROBLEMS interfered with your social activities (like visiting with friends, relatives, etc.)?
    All of the Time (1)
    Most of the Time (2)
    A Good Bit of the Time (3)
    Some of the Time (4)
    A Little of the Time (5)
    None of the Time (6)

9

2 Minute Walk Test

Objective

The Two/2 Minute Walk Test (2MWT) is a measure of self-paced walking ability and functional capacity[1], particularly for those who cannot manage the longer Six Minute Walk Test (6MWT) or 12 Minute Walk Test.

Intended Population

The 2MWT has been used as an outcome measure in a variety of health conditions including COPD[1][2], lower limb amputation[3], neuromuscular disease[4] in adults as well as pediatric population[5], cardiac disease[6], functionally restrictive conditions like cystic fibrosis[7] and the elderly[8], including those in long term care[9].

Method of Use

PROCEDURE:

The 2MWT is a simple measure of the distance a person can walk in two minutes. Rest breaks are allowed if needed. The person is encouraged to walk as fast as they can, safely, for two minutes.

Walking aids can be used as needed e.g. for elderly people with a record made of walking aid used.

If Assistive devices are used , they should be kept consistent and documented from test to test.

EQUIPMENT: A clear course such as a hallway with cones or similar to mark an approximately 15m "out and back" course[10], stopwatch, pen and paper or a device to record distance walked and any other observations e.g BORG scale.

INSTRUCTIONS: Commands given are based on those of the 6MWT: before the participant starts walking the observer advises them to "Cover as much ground as possible without running" or "Walk as fast as possible"[10] and to take a rest break if needed, but do not stop the timer. The observer then gives encouragement after the first minute with standardised responses: "You're doing well" and "One minute left"[8].

The 2MWT requires two practice walks before it is measured due to a training effect[1][8][11].

Evidence

Reliability

Studies have shown that the 2MWT is consistently reproducible[1][8][11].

Validity

The 2MWT shows good construct validity with similar walking measures. The 2MWT correlates highly with the six and 12 minute walk tests indicating they are similar measures of gait and exercise tolerance in population-based samples[11] and those with respiratory disease[1] or Multiple Sclerosis[4].

A study conducted in Pediatric population with neuromuscular disorders showed that the 2 MWT had strong correlations with Motor Function Measure-32 and Timed Functional test and can be used interchangebly with 6MWT[5].

Responsiveness

Research shows the 2MWT does not discriminate as well as the longer six and 12 minute walk tests in subjects with respiratory disease[1].

One study reported a minimum detectable change for the distance walked (DW) in the 2MWT was 42.5m[11].

In subjects with COPD undergoing pulmonary rehabilitation, a clinically meaningful change of 5.5m in DW has been reported[2].

A study of subjects post cardiac surgery (for coronary artery bypass grafts) demonstrated that the 2MWT was sensitive to change but could not discriminate between those who developed cardiac or respiratory complications and those who did not[6].

Normative Data

Age and gender explain 51% of variance in the distance walked in the 2MWT[8], i.e. older age and female gender are associated with shorter distances walker. Other studies have found some correlation between DW and height, weight, age and gender[11].

One study[8] has shown that subjects reached 70% of their maximum heart rate which was comparable with similar testing of the 6MWT. Authors hypothesised that this could suggest that a steady state of exertion is reached after only a short period of walking, as both the two and six minute walk tests are self-paced. So the 2MWT is a useful measure instead of the 6MWT if it is not practical to perform.

A 2017 meta-analysis[10] pooled data from four studies to produce the following normative values however the authors recommended further research is needed in multiple nations and populations to add more value to the 2MWT.

Data from Bohannon (2017)[10]		
Gender	**Age (years)**	**Mean Distance with Standard Error (metres)**
Male	20-29	217.9 (5.4)
	30-39	202.1 (3.0)
	40-49	192.1 (2.7)
	50-59	189.8 (2.6)
	60-69	183.0 (7.0)
	70-79	163.1 (5.3)
Female	20-29	194.1 (8.4)
	30-39	181.4 (1.7)
	40-49	180.7 (10.4)
	50-59	169.1 (10.0)
	60-69	163.7 (6.9)
	70-79	150.3 (1.3)

- One study[8] has described, with evidence, an equation to predict the DW, regardless of health condition. It takes into account age and gender. The equation is 2MWTpredicted = 252.583 - (1.165 x age) + (19.987 x gender*), where * is male= 1 and female= 0[8].

- Another study[11] used the following equations for men and women, respectively, with normative values available here.

Men: 2MWTpredicted = 279.096 - (0.998 x age) - (1.426 x BMI)

Women: 2MWTpredicted = 257.177 - (0.723 x age) - (1.688 x BMI)

*where BMI is Body Mass Index where weight (in kilogram) divided by height (in metres) squared

- A third study[13] has reported on normative values for healthy Chinese adults aged 18-85 years old (see here) using the following equations:

Male: 2MWD(m)=123.252−[age(yr)×0.699]+[height(cm)×0.711]

Female:2MWD(m)=108.278−[age(yr)×0.691]+[height(cm)×0.698]

- A fourth study[14] reported an average WD of 182.69 + 32.40 metres in healthy Indian adults (20-80 years, n= 300). The authors found that there was no significant difference between different age strata. The authors did not report separate means for men and women but did note that men walked further than women, in general.

-Researchers have also more recently reported on equations for children and adolescents aged 3 - 17 years[15]:

For boys; 39.69 + 16.11(age) - 0.58(age squared) + 53.56(height) - 0.54(body mass)

For girls; 56.56 + 18.04(age) - 0.67(age squared) - 0.64(body mass) + 36.08(height)

Clinical Significance of 2 MWT:

IN PEDIATRIC POPULATION :

1. The 2MWT is of shorter duration, objective, easily administered, and provides a standardized evaluation of functional capacity in populations with reduced ambulatory capability in adults with neuromuscular disease[16]. This format of the test helps in neurologically affected children with behavioral problems, limited ambulatory capacity, lower muscular strength and increased fatigue levels lower cognition levels to test their functional capacity[5]
2. It is an easy-to-implement measure to establish a baseline level of impairment, monitor disease progression and evaluate the effectiveness of current therapeutic interventions in children with significant illness.

IN ADULT POPULATION:

1. It can used in the aged population, individuals with lower extremity amputations, cystic fibrosis, traumatic brain injury, and neurological disorders as a measure of endurance.
2. It is used as a measure of gait speed, aerobic capacity in patients who are unable to complete 6MWT.

References:

1. Butland RJ, Pang J, Gross ER, Woodcock AA, Geddes DM. Two-, six-, and 12-minute walking tests in respiratory disease. Br Med J (Clin Res Ed). 1982. 29; 284(6329): 1607–1608. Accessed 19 February 2019.
2. Johnston KN, Potter AJ, Phillips AC. Minimal important difference and responsiveness of 2-minute walk test performance in people with COPD undergoing pulmonary rehabilitation. Int J Chron Obstruct Pulmon Dis. 2017:12 2849–2857. Accessed 19 February 2019.
3. Brooks D, Parsons J, Hunter JP, Devlin M, Walker J. The 2-minute walk test as a measure of functional improvement in persons with lower limb amputation. Arch Phys Med Rehab. 2001: 82(10):1478-83
4. Scalzitti DA, Harwood KJ, Maring JR, Leach SJ, Ruckert EA, Costello E. Validation of the 2-Minute Walk Test with the 6-Minute Walk Test and other functional measures in persons with Multiple Sclerosis. Int J MS Care. 2018; 20(4): 158–163. Accessed 19 February 2019.
5. J.W. Witherspoon, R. Vasavada, R.H. Logaraj et al. Two-minute versus 6-minute walk distances during 6-minute walk test in neuromuscular disease: Is the 2-minute walk test an effective alternative to a 6-minute walk test? European journal of Paediatric Neurology; 2019; 165-170
6. Brooks D, Parsons J, Tran D, Jeng B, Gorczyca B, Newton J, Lo V, Dear C, Silaj E, Hawn T. The two-minute walk test as a measure of functional capacity in cardiac surgery patients. Arch Phys Med Rehabil. 2004;85: 1525-30. Accessed 23 February 2019.
7. Upton CJ, Tyrrell JC, Hiller EJ. Two minute walking distance in cystic fibrosis. Arch Dis Child 1988;63:1444e8.
8. Selman, JPR, de Camargi AA, Santos J, Lanza FC, Dal Corso S. Reference Equation for the 2-Minute Walk Test in Adults and the Elderly. Respir Care. 2014; 59 (4): 525-530. Accessed 19 February 2019.
9. Connelly DM, Thomas BK, Cliffe SJ, Perry WM, Smith RE. Clinical utility of the 2-Minute Walk Test for older adults living in long-term care. Physiother Can. 2009; 61(2):78-87.
10. Bohannon RW. Normative reference values for the two-minute walk test derived by meta-analysis. J Phys Ther Sci. 2017 Dec; 29(12): 2224–2227. Accessed 25 February 2019.
11. Bohannon RW, Wang Y, Gershon RC. Two-Minute Walk Test performance by adults 18 to 85 years: normative values, reliability, and responsiveness. Arch Phys Med Rehab. 2015; 96:472-7. Accessed 19 February 2019.
12. Mac ICU Rehab. 2 Minute Walk Test Tutorial. Available from: http://www.youtube.com/watch?v = hhgQw7hd_RY
13. Zhang J, Chen X, Huang S, Wang Y, Lin W, Zhou R, Zou H. Two-minute walk test: Reference equations for healthy adults in China. PLoS One. 2018; 13(8): e0201988. Published online 2018 Aug 9. doi: 10.1371/journal.pone.0201988. Accessed 23 February 2019.
14. Priya TK, Verma S. A study to determine the reference values for Two Minute Walk Distance in healthy Indian adults. Int J Physiother Res 2015, Vol 3(5):1208-14. Accessed 25 February 2019.
15. Bohannon RW, Wang Y, Bubela D, Gershon RC. Normative Two-Minute Walk Test distances for boys and girls 3 to 17 years of age. Phys Occup Ther Pediatr. 2018; 38:1, 39-45. Accessed 23 February 2019.
16. Rossier P, Wade DT. Validity and reliability comparison of 4 mobility measures in patients presenting with neurologic impairment. Arch Phys Med Rehabil 2001;82:9e13.

❑❑❑

10

2 Minute Walk Test

Objective

The General Health Questionnaire (GHQ) is a screening device for identifying minor psychiatric disorders in the general population and within community or non-psychiatric clinical settings such as primary care or general medical out-patients. Suitable for all ages from adolescent upwards (but not children), it assesses the respondent's current state and asks if that differs from his or her usual state. It is therefore sensitive to short-term psychiatric disorders but not to long-standing attributes of the respondent.

Intended Population

The self-administered questionnaire focuses on two major areas:

- The inability to carry out normal functions
- The appearance of new and distressing phenomena.

Method of Use

The self-administered questionnaire is an ideal screening device for identifying non-psychotic and minor psychiatric disorders to help inform further intervention.

GHQ-28: a 28 item scaled version – assesses somatic symptoms, anxiety, and insomnia, social dysfunction and severe depression.

GHQ28 4/5* (max score 28)

Reference

1. Michele Sterling, General Health Questionnaire 28; Journal of Physiotherapy Vol 57, 2011-59. Clinimetrics Appraisal

Have You Recently	Better than usual / same as usual		Worse than usual / much worse than usual	
	No	%	No	%
Been feeling perfectly well and in good health?				
Been feeling in need of a good tonic?				
Been feeling run down and out of sorts?				
Felt that you are ill?				
Been getting any pains in your head?				
Been getting a feeling of tightness or pressure in your head?				
Been having hot or cold spells?				
Lost much sleep over worry?				
Had difficulty in staying asleep once you are off?				
Felt constantly under strain?				
Been getting edgy and bad tempered?				
Been getting scared or panicky for no good reason?				

Found everything getting on top of you?				
Been feeling nervous and strung up all the time?				
Felt on the whole you were doing things well?				
Been satisfied with the way you've carried out your task?				
Felt that you are playing a useful part in things?				
Been able to enjoy your normal day – to – day activities?				
Been thinking of yourself as a worthless person?				
Felt that life is entirely hopeless?				
Felt that life isn't worth living?				
Thought of the possibility that you might make away with yourself?				
Found at times you couldn't do anything because your nerves were too bad?				
Found yourself wishing you were dead and away from it all?				
Found that the idea of taking your own life kept coming into your mind?				

❑❑❑

11 International Consultation on Incontinence Modular Questionnaires (ICIQ)

About the ICIQ

The International Consultation of Incontinence (ICIQ) has developed a series of international questionnaires and is striving to validate these questionnaires for the investigation lower urinary tract dysfunction, vaginal symptoms and lower bowel dysfunction in research and clinical settings.[1] Requests to use any of the developed ICIQs in research or clinical practice can be made by visiting ICIQ Contact Us. The following page presents information on the International Consultation on Incontinence Questionnaire for Urinary Incontinence.

Objective

This short questionnaire can be used by clinicians to screen for incontinence, to obtain a brief yet comprehensive summary of the level, impact and perceived cause of symptoms of incontinence and to facilitate patient-clinician discussions.[2]

Intended Population

Adult females and males[2]

Method of Use

A patient-reported questionnaire that can be done by the patient independently or during an assessment with a practitioner.

Time to complete: a few minutes[3]

Question Items[3]

- Frequency of urinary incontinence
- Amount of leakage
- Overall impact of urinary incontinence
- Self-diagnostic item

Scoring System

The ICIQ-UI Short form provides a score ranging from 0-21. With a higher score indicating greater severity of symptoms.[1] The "self-diagnostic" portion of the questionnaire is not given a score.[1]

Evidence

Reliability

Stability: Test-retest reliability range from good to very good (Kappa value = 0.67-0.90) for all items except "overall quality of life which was found to be moderate (Kappa value = 0.58).[2]

Internal consistency has been found to be excellent (Cronbach's alpha coefficient = 0.95).[2]

Validity

Content validity: Items in the ICIQ-UI Short form have been found to be easily interpreted by patients and appear to cover all important domains of incontinence with good response rates from community volunteers.[2]

Construct validity: The ICIQ-UI has been found to differentiated between males and females, with females reporting more incontinence than males (58.9% and 25.2% respectively, $p < 0.001$).[2]

Convergent validity: There currently is no "gold standard" questionnaire for incontinence, but agreement between responses to ICIQ-UI and Bristol Female Lower Urinary Tract Symptoms (BFLUTS)[4] as been investigated.[2] Questions on the 'frequency' and 'usual amount' of leakage ranged from moderate to strong (r=0.53-0.86), questions assessing the perceived causes of incontinence ranged from weak to moderate (r=0.29-0.55).[2]

Sensitivity to change

A statistically significant reduction in symptoms have been found between baseline scores and scores following conservative treatment in both males and females in all items ($p<0.0001$) except for "overall quality of life" (females, $p=0.12$; males, $p=0.24$).[2]

A statistically significant decrease in symptoms has also been found between baseline scores and scores after surgical intervention in both females and males ($p<0.0001$).[2]

References

1. Bristol Urological Institute.The International Consultation of Incontinence Modular Questionnaire. http://www.iciq.net/ (accessed 15 June 2018).
2. · Avery K, Donovan J, Peters TJ, Shaw C, Gotoh M, Abrams P. ICIQ: a brief and robust measure for evaluating the symptoms and impact of urinary incontinence. Neurourology and urodynamics. 2004 Jan 1;23(4):322-30.
3. · Bristol Urological Institute. ICIQ Structure Short Form. http://www.iciq.net/ICIQ-UIshortform.html (accessed 15 June 2018).
4. Jackson S, Donovan J, Brookes S, Eckford S, Swithinbank L, Abrams P. The Bristol female lower urinary tract symptoms questionnaire: development and psychometric testing. BJU International. 1996 Jun 1;77(6):805-12.

❑❑❑

12 Self-Report Urinary Incontinence Questionnaire

Objective

To assess and to evaluate urinary function the for patients at different levels of urinary function using 21-item UIQ in patients seeking outpatient physical therapy services due to PFD.

Intended Population

Patients with urinary urgency, urinary frequency.

Method of Use

The UIQ consists of 21 items: 17 related to urinary leakage problems, 2 related to frequency problems, and 2 related to retention problems. Each item has its own Likert rating scale structure and operational definition.

Urinary Incontinence Questionnaire

Urinary Leakage Items

1. **How often does urine leak for no obvious reason when you are awake?**
   1. Never
   2. Once or less per week
   3. More than once a week
   4. Once a day
   5. Several times a day
   6. Continuously
2. **How much urine usually leaks for no obvious reason when you are awake?**
   1. A few drops
   2. Enough to make underpants/pads wet
   3. Enough to wet outer clothes
   4. Urine runs down legs onto floor
3. **How often does urine leak when you are asleep?**
   1. Never
   2. Once or less per week
   3. More than once a week
   4. Once a day
   5. Several times a day
   6. Continuously
4. **How much urine usually leaks while you are sleeping?**
   1. A few drops
   2. Enough to make pajyamas /pads wet
   3. Enough to wet all clothes and bedding
5. **How often do you leak urine after you thought you had finished urinating?**
   1. Never
   2. Once or less per week
   3. More than once a week
   4. Once a day
   5. Several times a day
   6. Every time
6. **How much urine usually leaks after you thought you had finished urinating?**
   1. A few drops
   2. Enough to make underpants/pads wet
   3. Enough to wet outer clothes
   4. Urine runs down legs onto floor
7. **How often does urine leak before you can get to the toilet?**
   1. Never
   2. Once or less per week
   3. More than once a week
   4. Once a day

5. Several times a day
6. Every time

8. How much urine usually leaks before you can get to the toilet?
1. A few drops
2. Enough to make underpants/pads wet
3. Enough to wet outer clothes
4. Urine runs down legs onto floor

9. How often does urine leak when you are physically active, including coughing or sneezing?
1. Never
2. Once or less per week
3. More than once a week
4. Once a day
5. Several times a day

10. Describe the level of activity that causes urine leakage.
1. Vigorous activity, such as running, exercise, coughing, or sneezing
2. Moderate activity, such as household chores or lifting
3. Light activity, such as walking, bending, or rising
4. Leak even without activity

11. How much urine usually leaks when you are physically active or coughing or sneezing?
1. A few drops
2. Enough to make underpants/pads wet
3. Enough to wet outer clothes
4. Urine runs down legs onto floor

12. What type of protection do you use for your urine leakage?
1. None
2. Underpants liners or mini-pads
3. Maxi-pads
4. Incontinence pads
5. Incontinence briefs
6. Diapers

13. Select the number of protective garments for urine leakage you use per day.

1. 1   2. 2
3. 3   4. 4
5. ≥ 5

14. Overall, how much does leaking urine interfere with your life?
1. Does not interfere with my life
2. Minor inconvenience
3. Slight problem
4. Moderate problem

15. To what extent do you feel your sex life has been affected by urine leakage?
1. Has not affected my sex life
2. A little
3. Somewhat
4. A great deal

16. Describe your level of confidence in your ability to control your urine leakage problem.
1. Complete confidence
2. Moderate confidence
3. Little confidence
4. No confidence

17. How well do you control your urine leakage? (0 being "no control" to 10 being "full control")

0 (no control)   1. 1   2. 2
3. 3   4. 4   5. 5
6. 6   7. 7   8. 8
9. 9   10. 10 (full control)

Urination Frequency Items

18. What is the frequency of your daytime urination?

1–4 times per day   5–8 times per day
9–12 times per day   ≥13 times per day

19. How often do you urinate at night?
1. Do not urinate at night
2. 1 time per night
3. 2 times per night
4. 3 times per night
5. 4 or more times per night

Urinary Retention Items

20. How long can you delay urination from the first time you feel the urge?
1. 1 or more hours
2. 30 minutes
3. 15 minutes
4. less than 10 minutes
5. 1–2 minutes
6. Cannot delay urination

21. After starting to urinate, can you:
1. Stop urine flow completely
2. Maintain a change to the urine stream
3. Partially deflect or change the urine stream
4. Unable to deflect, change, or slow urine stream

13 Fecal Incontinence and Constipation Questionnaire

Background

Fecal incontinence (FI) is defined as the involuntary loss of solid or liquid feces or mucus[1]. Fecal constipation (FC) is a decreased frequency of bowel actions (<1 every 3 days) that also may be associated with excessive straining during the passage of stool.[2] Fecal incontinence and functional constipation are relatively common symptoms in the community, particularly in the elderly[3] affecting approximately 2.2–11.3% and 15% of the population respectively.[4][5]. Moreover, the prevalence of both FI and FC increases with age[6][7][8][9][10][11] and is more frequent in women than men.[11] Several scales measure the severity of fecal incontinence, but the best measure is unknown. Furthermore, there is an increasing demand for patient-reported outcome measures during routine clinical practice to assist with planning patient outcomes.[11][12][13]

Objective

The Fecal Incontinence and constipation questionnaire (FICQ), developed by Focus on Therapeutic Outcomes Inc. in conjunction with a physical therapist, aims to evaluate how bowel dysfunction affects patient-perceived functional status related to pelvic floor dysfunction.[11]

Intended Population

Patients above 18 years with Pelvic-floor dysfunction.

Method of Use

The FICQ is a self-report questionnaire that consists of 20 items: 15 items related to bowel leakage problems and 5 items related to constipation problems.[11] Each item on the questionnaire has its own Likert scale and definition.[11]

Question Items

The bowel leakage items include:*[11]*

- Frequency of bowel leakage while awake and while asleep (FI-OFTENWAKE, FI-OFTENSLEEP)
- The extent bowel leakage affects the individual while awake and while asleep (FI-PROBLEMWAKE, FI-PROBLEMSLEEP)
- Frequency of bowel leakage after defecation and before getting access to a toilet (FI- FINISH,FI-TOILET)
- Frequency of bowel leakage during physical activity and with what intensity of physical activity leakage occurs (El-ACTIVE, Fl-ACTIVITY)
- The protection gamier used and the amount of protection used throughout the day (FI-TYPEPROTC, FI-NUMPROTECT)
- Overall impact of bowel leakage on life, sex, and confidence (Fl-LIFE, Fl-SEX, Fl-CONFIDENCE)
- Voluntary control over bowel leakage and ability to delay defecation (FI-CONTROL,FI-DELAY)

The constipation items include:*[11]*

- Frequency of bowel movements (FC-OFTEN)
- Frequency of use of enemas and laxatives per month (FC-ENEMAS, EC- LAXATIVE)
- The level of strain during a bowel movement and whether manual assistance is required (FC-STRAIN, FC-MANUAL)

As mentioned above, the FICQ asks patients to subjectively rate their symptoms with a Likert scale.[11] A Likert Scale allows individuals to express how much they agree or disagree with a statement. A example of how the scale is used in this questionnaire is written below:

Item #19 of the FICQ: "Do you have strain to have a bowel movement?"[11]

1. Rarely or never
2. Occasionally
3. Sometimes
4. Always

Evidence

Research regarding the psychometric properties of the FICQ is limited. A study by Wang and colleagues (2014) [11] conducted a preliminary analysis of the psychometric properties of the FICQ in patients seeking outpatient rehabilitation services due to pelvic floor dysfunction.[11] The following psychometric properties were assessed:[11]

1. **Unidimensionality:** The scale or questionnaire represents only one construct.[11][14]
2. **Local Independence:** The items in a scale are independent of each other.[14] An individual's response to one item should not be correlated with the response of another item.[14]This quality can be measured via residual correlations, whereby a residual correlation of greater than 0.10 suggests local dependency.[11]
3. **Differential Item Functioning (DIF):** All individuals should have an equal probability of scoring positively on each item regardless of patient groupings (i.e. age).[15]Items are marked as "significant DIF" when this requirement is not met.[11]
4. **Item Hierarchical Structure:** This assesses the difficulty of each item in the questionnaire in a hierarchical order.[11] It helps to measure the construct validity of the questionnaire, which indicates how well a questionnaire measures what it is supposed to.[11]
5. **Precision Testing:** Precision testing provides the reliability or the degree of consistency of a measure.[11] Test information function, which is the amount of information provided by the item responses on a questionnaire about the construct being measured (i.e. bowel function), and standard error can be used to estimate precision testing.[11] [16]

Wang and colleagues (2014)[11] reported unidimensionality in the questionnaire. However, the researchers suggested that refinement of the items is needed to further improve unidimensionality.[11] In regards to local independence, only 5 items on the questionnaire were free of local dependency.[11] No differential item functioning was observed when grouped by sex, age group, acuity, and the number of pelvic floor co-morbid conditions, except for 2 items assessing functional incontinence.[11] When assessing the individual's ability level to complete the questionnaire, the FI and FC items were at the individual's overall ability level.[11] No ceiling effect or floor effects were observed while using the FICQ.[11] As well, the FICQ produced reliable and precise measurements of functional status related to bowel function.[11] Overall, Wang and colleagues (2014)[11] supported the use of the FICQ in an outpatient rehabilitation setting, yet, stated that test developers should aim to improve the quality of existing FICQ items, especially for the fecal constipation dimension.[11] Furthermore, they suggested that more fecal constipation items should be added to increase content coverage.[11] Further research is still required to validate this questionnaire.[11]

References

1. Markland AD, Goode PS, Burgio KL, et al. Incidence and risk factors for fecal incontinence in black and white older adults: a population-based study. J Am Geriatr Soc.2010;58:1341–1346.
2. Brady CM. Constipation and fecal incontinence. In: Munsat TL, ed. Neurologic Bladder, Bowel and Sexual Dysfunction.Vol 1. Oxfordshire, United Kingdom: Elsevier Science Ltd; 2001:27–37.
3. Bharucha A. Fecal Incontinence Gastroenterology 2003; 124: 1672–85.
4. Drossman DA, Li Z, Andruzzi E, et al.US householder survey of functional gastrointestinal disorders. Prevalence, sociodemography, and health impact. Dig Dis Sci 1993; 38: 1569–80.
5. Nelson R, Norton N, Cautley E, Furner S. Community-based prevalence of anal incontinence. JAMA 1995; 274: 559–61.
6. Perry S, Shaw C, McGrother C, Matthews RJ, Assassa RP, Dallosso H, Williams K, Brittain KR, Azam U, Clarke M, Jagger C. Prevalence of faecal incontinence in adults aged 40 years or more living in the community. Gut. 2002 Apr 1;50(4):480-4.
7. Bharucha AE, Zinsmeister AR, Locke GR, Seide BM, McKeon K, Schleck CD, Melton III LJ. Prevalence and burden of fecal incontinence: a population-based study in women. Gastroenterology. 2005 Jul 1;129(1):42-9.
8. Botlero R, Bell RJ, Urquhart DM, Davis SR. Prevalence of fecal incontinence and its relationship

with urinary incontinence in women living in the community. Menopause. 2011 Jun 1;18(6):685-9.

9. Mugie SM, Benninga MA, Di Lorenzo C. Epidemiology of constipation in children and adults: a systematic review. Best Pract Res Clin Gastroenterol. 2011;25:3–18.
10. Harari D, Gurwitz JH, Avorn J, et al. Bowel habit in relation to age and gender: find- ings from the National Health Interview Survey and clinical implications. Arch Intern Med. 1996;156:315–320.
11. Wang YC, Deutscher D, Yen SC, Werneke MW, Mioduski JE. The self-report fecal incontinence and constipation questionnaire in patients with pelvic-floor dysfunction seeking outpatient rehabilitation. Physical therapy. 2014 Feb 1;94(2):273-88.
12. Abrams P, Avery K, Gardener N, Donovan J, ICIQ Advisory Board. The international consultation on incontinence modular questionnaire: www. iciq. net. The Journal of urology. 2006 Mar;175(3):1063-6.
13. Coyne K, Kelleher C. Patient reported outcomes: the ICIQ and the state of the art. Neurourology and Urodynamics: Official Journal of the International Continence Society. 2010 Apr;29(4):645-51.
14. Lord FM. Applications of item response theory to practical testing problems. Routledge; 1980.
15. Holland PW, Wainer H. Differential Item Functioning. Lawrence Erlbaum Associates Ince, New Jersey. 1993.
16. Hambleton RK, Swaminathan H, Rogers HJ. Fundamentals of item response theory. Sage; 1991.

❑❑❑

14 30 Seconds Sit To Stand Test

Objective

The 30 Second Sit to Stand Test is also known as 30 second chair stand test (30CST), is for testing leg strength and endurance in older adults. It is part of the Fullerton Functional Fitness Test Battery. This test was developed to overcome the floor effect of the five or ten repetition sit to stand test in older adults.[1]

Intended Population

- Adults 18-64 years
- Older adults and geriatric care (65 years and above)
- People with osteoarthritis

Method of Use

- The 30-Second Chair Test is administered using a folding chair without arms, with seat height of 17 inches (43.2 cm). The chair, with rubber tips on the legs, is placed against a wall to prevent it from moving.
- The participant is seated in the middle of the chair, back straight; feet approximately a shoulder width apart and placed on the floor at an angle slightly back from the knees, with one foot slightly in front of the other to help maintain balance. Arms are crossed at the wrists and held against the chest.
- Demonstrate the task both slowly and quickly.
- Have the patient practice a repetition or two before completing the test.
- If a patient must use their arms to complete the test they are scored 0.
- The participant is encouraged to complete as many full stands as possible within 30 seconds. The participant is instructed to fully sit between each stand.
- While monitoring the participant's performance to ensure proper form, the tester silently counts the completion of each correct stand. The score is the total number of stands within 30 seconds (more than halfway up at the end of 30 seconds counts as a full stand). Incorrectly executed stands are not counted.
- The 30-second chair stand involves recording the number of stands a person can complete in 30 seconds rather then the amount of time it takes to complete a pre-determined number of repetitions. That way, it is possible to assess a wide variety of ability levels with scores ranging from 0 for those who can not complete 1 stand to greater then 20 for more fit individuals.[1]

Chair stand – Number of stands by age group

A below average number of stands for the patient's age group indicates a high risk of falls.

WOMEN

Age group (years) Figures represent: Below Average; Average; Above Average

- 60 – 64: < 12; 12 – 17; >17
- 65 – 69: < 11; 11 – 16; >16
- 70 – 74: < 10; 10 – 15; >15
- 75 – 79: < 10; 10 – 15; >15
- 80 – 84: < 9; 9 – 14; >14
- 85 – 89: < 8; 8 – 13; >13
- 90 – 94: < 4; 4 – 11; >11

MEN

Age group (years) Below Average Average Above Average

- 60 – 64: < 14; 14 – 19; >19
- 65 – 69: < 12; 12 – 18; >18
- 70 – 74: < 12; 12 – 17; >17
- 75 – 79: < 11; 11 – 17; >17
- 80 – 84: < 10; 10 – 15; >15
- 85 – 89: < 8; 8 – 14; >14
- 90 – 94: < 7; 7 – 12; >12[3]

Evidence

Community-dwelling Elderly Adults

Test/ Retest Reliability in Community-dwelling Elderly

- Excellent test-retest reliability total number of participants: r = 0.89 (95% Confidence interval 0.79-0.93)[4]

Interrater/Intrarater Reliability in Community-dwelling Elderly

A pilot study using a subsample of 15 participants shows excellent interrater reliability: r = 0.95 (95% CI = 0.84-0.97)[4]

Criterion Validity: Predictive /Concurrent

- Excellent criterion validity of the chair stand compared to weight adjusted leg press performance for all participants: r = 0.77, 95% CI = 0.64-0.85
- Excellent criterion validity of the chair stand compared to weight adjusted leg press performance of men: r = 0.78, 95% CI = 0.63-0.88
- Excellent criterion validity of the chair stand compared to weight adjusted leg performance of women: r = 0.71, 95% CI = 0.53-0.84[4]

Osteoarthritis

Standard Error of Measurement (SEM) in Hip Osteoarthritis

- SEM= 1.27 [5]

Test/Retest Reliability in Hip and Knee OA

- Established test-retest reliability between two administrations of the test on the same day by the same rater at three time points over 15 weeks in 40 patients awaiting total hip or knee replacement. ICC (1,1) values ranged from 0.97 (95% CI 0.94-0.98) to 0.98 (95% CI 0.97-0.99). [6]

Interrater/Intrarater Reliability in Hip and Knee OA

- Established inter-rater reliability between two administrations of the same test by two different raters on the same day. Reliability was assessed at three time points over 15 weeks in 42 patients awaiting total hip or knee replacement. ICC (1,1) ranged from 0.93 (95% CI 0.87-0.96) to 0.98 (95% CI 0.96-0.99). [6]

Lower Limb Joint Replacement

Construct Validity in OA Individuals Awaiting Joint Replacement of the Hip or Knee

- Excellent correlation to the 50 ft. walk test: ICC = -0.64(95% CI = -0.75 to -0.49)
- Poor correlation to the Patient Specific Function Scale (PSFS): ICC = 0.26 (95% CI 0.04-0.45)
- Adequate correlation to the SF-36 Physical Function (SF-36 PF): ICC = 0.39 (95% CI 0.19-0.56)
- Adequate correlation to the SF-36 Physical Component Summary (SF-36 PCS): ICC = 0.35 (0.14-0.53)
- Excellent correlation to the Western Ontario and McMaster Universities Arthritis Index (WOMAC): ICC = -0.62 (95% CI -0.74 to -0.47)
- Adequate correlation to the SF-36 Mental Health (SF-36 MH): ICC = 0.33 (95% CI 0.12-0.51) [7]

Responsiveness in OA Individuals Awaiting Joint Replacement of the Hip or Knee

- Significantly higher scores for individuals who did not ambulate with gait aide compared to individuals who did ambulate with gait aid: p = 0.00, Effect size = 0.64 (95% CI 0.32-0.95)
- Standardized Response Mean (SRM) = 0.84 (95% CI 0.61-1.07)
- Guyatt's Responsiveness Index (GRI) = 0.98 (95% CI 0.73-1.22) [7]

References

1. https://www.sralab.org/rehabilitation-measures/30-second-sit-stand-test (last accessed 17th May 2019)
2. Mac ICU Rehab. 30 Second Sit to Stand Test Tutorial. Available from: http://www.youtube.com/watch?v=RFkz33xwRRA
3. Rikli R, Jones C, Functional fitness normative scores for community-residing older adults, ages 60-94. J Aging Phys Activity 1999;7(2):162-81.Available

from: https://www.hqsc.govt.nz/assets/Falls/PR/005-falls-toolkit-chair-stand-test.pdf(accessed 11.3.2021)

4. Rikli, R.E. and Jones, C.J., 1999. Development and validation of a functional fitness test for community-residing older adults. Journal of aging and physical activity, 7(2), pp.129-161.
5. Wright, A. A., Cook, C. E., et al. 2011. "A comparison of 3 methodological approaches to defining major clinically important improvement of 4 performance measures in patients with hip osteoarthritis." J Orthop Sports Phys Ther 41(5): 319-327.
6. Gill, S. and McBurney, H., 2008. Reliability of performance-based measures in people awaiting joint replacement surgery of the hip or knee. Physiotherapy Research International, 13(3), pp.141-152.
7. Gill, S.D., de Morton, N.A. and Mc Burney, H., 2012. An investigation of the validity of six measures of physical function in people awaiting joint replacement surgery of the hip or knee. Clinical rehabilitation, 26(10), pp.945-951.

❑❑❑

15 Sit and Reach Test

Introduction and Purpose

The Sit and reach test is one of the linear flexibility tests which helps to measure the extensibility of the hamstrings and lower back.[1] It was initially described by Wells and Dillon in 1952 and is probably the mostly used flexibility test. It has a simple procedure, is easy to administer, requires minimal skills training for its application, and the equipment necessary to perform the test is affordable. Furthermore, it is also a field test which is easy to administer in a community setting with a large scale of population size.[2]

A good level of flexibility of the hamstrings and lower back is advocated as it plays a key role in health related fitness. Areas where it is important include:[3]

- Injury prevention - acute or chronic musculoskeletal injuries and lower back problems
- Risk of falling
- Gait limitations
- Postural deviations

Technique

- There are various techniques and variation of the Sit and Reach test. The one which is explained below is based upon the Young Men's Christian Association (YCMA) from the American College of Sports Medicine (ACSM) guideline, 2014.[4]
- Pretest: Clients/Patients should perform a short warm-up prior to this test with some gentle stretches. During the test participants are suggested not to do fast, jerky movements, which may increase the possibility of an injury. The participant's shoes should be removed.
- A yardstick is placed on the floor and tape is placed across it at a right angle to the 15 inches mark. The client/patient sits with the yardstick between the legs, with the legs extended at right angles to the taped line on the floor. Heels of the feet should touch the edge of the taped line and be about 10 to 12 inches apart.
- The client/patient should slowly reach forward with extended arms, placing one hand on top of the other facing palms down, as far as possible, holding this position for approximately 2 seconds. Be sure that the participant keeps the hands parallel and does not lead with one hand. Fingertips can be overlapped and should be in contact with the measuring portion or yardstick of the sit-and-reach box.
- The score is the most distant point (cm or in) reached with the fingertips. The best of three trials should be recorded. To assist with the best attempt, the client/patient should exhale and drop the head between the arms when reaching. Testers should ensure that the knees of the participant stay extended; however, the participant's knees should not be pressed down. The client/patient should breathe normally during the test and should not hold her/his breath at any time.
- Note the zero point at the foot/box interface to use the appropriate norms. So for YCMA the "zero" point is set at the 15 inches mark.[4]

Normative values of Sit and Reach Test

		Age (year)											
Percentile		18–25		26–35		36–45		46–55		56–65		>65	
Gender		M	W	M	W	M	W	M	W	M	W	M	W
90	Well above average	22	24	21	23	21	22	19	21	17	20	17	20
80	Above average	20	22	19	21	19	21	17	20	15	19	15	18
70		19	21	17	20	17	19	15	18	13	17	13	17
60	Average	18	20	17	20	16	18	14	17	13	16	12	17
50		17	19	15	19	15	17	13	16	11	15	10	15
40	Below average	15	18	14	17	13	16	11	14	9	14	9	14
30		14	17	13	16	13	15	10	14	9	13	8	13
20	Well below average	13	16	11	15	11	14	9	12	7	11	7	11
10		11	14	9	13	7	12	6	10	5	9	4	9

M, men; W, women.

Fitness Categories for the YMCA Sit-and-Reach Test (in) by Age and Sex[4]

Variations

- Unilateral sit and reach test
- Back-saver sit and reach test
- Bilateral sit and reach test
- V sit and reach test.
- Modified sit and-reach test
- Toe-touch test
- Canadian Trunk Forward Flexion Test
- Chair sit-and-reach test (CSR test)- It was proposed as an alternative for assessing hamstring flexibility in elderly people with correlation coefficient of 0.76 and 0.81 for older men and women respectively.[2][6]

The choice of the test to be employed is more often based on the examiner's preferences, ease of use, professional discipline, or tradition, rather than scientific evidence as there is still no convincing proof or conclusively provided evidence of which test is the most appropriate to use to assess hamstring and low-back flexibility.[2]

Evidence

Lemmink et al. (2003) showed moderate inter class correlation co-efficient(r) of 0.57 and 0.74 in middle aged older men and women respectively.[7]

Ayala F et al. (2011) showed acceptable reproducibility measures for the sit and reach test with 8.74% coefficient of variation (CV) and 0.92 intraclass correlation coefficient (ICC).[8]

According to the meta-analysis done by Vega et al. (2014), Sit-and-reach tests had a moderate mean criterion-related validity for estimating hamstring extensibility (mean correlation coefficient, r= 0.46-0.67), but they had a low mean for estimating lumbar extensibility (r = 0. 16-0.35). [1]

Thus, evidences shows that sit-and-reach tests have a moderate mean criterion-related validity for estimating hamstring extensibility and classic sit and reach test protocol seems to be best to estimate hamstring flexibility.[1]

References

1. Mayorga-Vega D, Merino-Marban R, Viciana J. Criterion-related validity of sit-and-reach tests for estimating hamstring and lumbar extensibility: A meta-analysis. Journal of sports science & medicine. 2014 Jan;13(1):1.
2. Baltaci G, Un N, Tunay V, Besler A, Gerçeker S. Comparison of three different sit and reach tests for measurement of hamstring flexibility in female university students. British journal of sports medicine. 2003 Feb 1;37(1):59-61.
3. Cuberek R, Machová I, Lipenská M. Reliability of V sit-and-reach test used for flexibility self-assessment in females. Acta Gymnica. 2013 Dec 18;43(1):35-9.

4. http://antoinedl.com/fichiers/public/ACSM-guidelines-2014.pdf. Last assessed: December 20, 2019
5. University of Delaware Exercise Science. ACSM Sit and Reach Test. Available from: https://www.youtube.com/watch?v=q23yXIYoagk [last assessed: 2019-12-20]
6. Jones CJ, Rikli RE, Max J, Noffal G. The reliability and validity of a chair sit-and-reach test as a measure of hamstring flexibility in older adults. Research quarterly for exercise and sport. 1998 Dec 1;69(4):338-43.
7. Lemmink KA, Kemper HC, Greef MH, Rispens P, Stevens M. The validity of the sit-and-reach test and the modified sit-and-reach test in middle-aged to older men and women. Research quarterly for exercise and sport. 2003 Sep 1;74(3):331-6.
8. Ayala F, de Baranda PS, Croix MD, Santonja F. Reproducibility and criterion-related validity of the sit and reach test and toe touch test for estimating hamstring flexibility in recreationally active young adults. Physical Therapy in Sport. 2012 Nov 1;13(4):219-26.

❑❑❑

16 Five Times Sit to Stand Test

Introduction

Double leg lowering test (DLLT) general test to assess the core muscles, is like curl up and sit-up test used to assess the abdominal muscles. DLLT is more challenging test than curl-up developed to assess and examine lower abdominal muscle fibers and will be more representative to be used in the lumbar stabilization program but unlike crul-up or sit-up in which they work to flex the trunk against gravity, during DLLT the muscles work eccentrically during lowering the limbs[1][2].

Purpose

The purpose of the test to assess abdominal muscles and the ability of muscles to maintain the posterior pelvic tilting position against the load (lowering both lower limbs from the vertical position).

The test shows great association for rectus abdominis muscle, moderate association with the external oblique, internal oblique, and transversus abdominis[3].

Technique

It is important to be a landmark to ensure if the abdominal muscles can contract enough and keep the pelvis in the posterior tilting position or not. We can use a pressure cuff, or our hand to palpate a bony landmark.

Procedures:

- The subject lies supine on a flat surface, both arms rested across his chest or under the head. Head, and arms be fixed.
- First, the examiner raises the patient's lower leg vertically as high as it is possible to assess the flexibility of the hamstring.
- The examiner explains the procedure to the patient and he/she try it once.
- Blood pressure cuff placed at the pelvis level and inflated for about 40 mmHg.
- The subject is instructed to lower both legs with the extended knee from the vertical position down while keeping the pelvis in the posterior tilting position, and the pressure cuff used as feedback to try to maintain the starting inflated pressure.
- During the test, if the pressure on your hand or the cuff is decreased, stop the test and the angle should be measured as follows (angle measure from the table before pelvis tilt anterior):

  starting position: 900° from the table

  Poor(2/2): Able to reach 75-90° from the table.

  Fair(3/3): Able to reach 46-75° from the table.

  Good(4/4): Able to reach 16-45° from the table.

  normal(5/5): 0-15° from the table[2].

Hip flexors and abdominal muscles work eccentrically together to control the lowering of the limb, as legs lower there is an increase in the resistance to hold the pelvis in position.

Evidence

Reliability

Intraclass correlation coefficient.98[1].

A prospective descriptive study carried on to investigate the kinematic movement of the pelvis during DLLT on a sample consist of 17 young fit adults, divided into two groups, the first group instructed to do the test while trying to control the pelvis, and the second group descends without trying to control the pelvis tilting.

The study concluded, there was a natural tendency for anterior pelvic tilting that increase through the range, anterior pelvic tilt 1° for 3.6° of lower limb lowering from early DLLT[5].

References

1. Krause DA, Youdas JW, Hollman JH, Smith J. Abdominal muscle performance as measured by the double leg-lowering test. Archives of physical medicine and rehabilitation. 2005 Jul 1;86(7):1345-8.
2. O'Sullivan PB, Phyty GD, Twomey LT, Allison GT. Evaluation of specific stabilizing exercise in the treatment of chronic low back pain with radiologic diagnosis of spondylolysis or spondylolisthesis. Spine. 1997 Dec 15;22(24):2959-67.
3. Haladay DE, Denegar CR, Miller SJ, Challis J. Electromyographic and kinetic analysis of two abdominal muscle performance tests. Physiotherapy theory and practice. 2015 Nov 17;31(8):587-93.
4. Lauren Green. Double Leg Lowering Test - A Core Stability Assessment. Available from: http://www.youtube.com/watch?v=tvGf9MwdLCE[last accessed 25/1/2021]
5. Zannotti CM, Bohannon RW, Tiberio D, Dewberry MJ, Murray R. Kinematics of the double-leg-lowering test for abdominal muscle strength. Journal of Orthopaedic & Sports Physical Therapy. 2002 Sep;32(9):432-6.

❑❑❑

17

Thomas Test

Purpose

The Thomas Test (also known as Iliacus Test or Iliopsoas Test) is used to measure the flexibility of the hip flexors, which includes the iliopsoas muscle group, the rectus femoris, pectineus, gracillis as well as the tensor fascia latae and the sartorius.[1]

Impaired range of motion of the hip may be an underlying cause to other conditions such as patellofemoral pain syndrome[2], lower back pain[3], osteoarthritis and rheumatoid arthritis.[4]

Clinically Relevant Anatomy

The hip joint is a diarthroidal ball and-socket style joint, formed from the head of the femur as it articulates with the acetabulum of the pelvis. It serves as the main connection between the lower extremity and the trunk, and typically works in a closed kinematic chain.

There are various muscles making up the hip flexor group being tested in the Thomas Test:

Iliopsoas muscle group	Main Function	Additional movement
Iliopsoas	Hip flexion	External rotation
Rectus femoris	Hip flexion	Knee extension
Tensor fascia lata	Hip flexion	Internal rotation, abduction
Sartorius	Hip flexion	Knee flexion

Technique

The patient should be supine on the examination table, maximally flex both knees, using both arms to ensure that the lumbar spine is flexed and flat on the table and avoids an anterior tilt of the pelvis.[1]

The patient then lowers the tested limb toward the table, whilst the contralateral hip and knee is still held in maximal flexion to stabilize the pelvis and flatten out the lumbar lordosis.[5] The length of the iliopsoas is measured by the angle of the hip flexion.[6]

A modified version of the test is one in which the patient lies down on their back, at the very edge of the table, with both legs hanging freely. The patient must then flex their knee and pull it back to their chest as close as they can, using both arms while doing so. The other leg can hang down.[6] The lumbar spine must remain flat and in contact with the table during the test.[1] The physiotherapist controls the opposite leg to ensure that it maintains full contact with the table.

Interpretation

The Thomas test is negative when the subject's lower back and the sacrum is able to remain on the table. The hip can make a 10° posterior tilt or a 10° hip extension. The knee must be able to make a 90° flexion.[8]

The test is positive when:

- Subject is unable to maintain their lower back and sacrum against the table
- Hip has a large posterior tilt or hip extension greater than 15°
- Knee unable to meet more than 80° flexion

The following structures may be considered during a positive test;

Sign	Structures affected
Extended knee	Quadriceps, rectus femoris
Flexed hip	Psoas muscles
Abducted hip	Tensor fascia lata, iliotibial band
Tibia lateral rotation	Biceps femoris

Reliability

Studies that test the reliability of the Thomas study are very limited.

One study has demonstrated that the modified Thomas test has a very good inter-rater reliability.[9] Another has demonstrated that the modified Thomas test, has an average of only moderate levels of reliability.[10] Further research is required to prove or to refute the reliability of the Thomas test.

Peeler and Anderson conducted a study in 2006 examining the reliability of the Thomas test for assessing hip range. Their study calls into question the reliability of the technique when used to score range of motion and iliopsoas muscle flexibility about the hip joint using both goniometer and pass/fail scoring methods.[11]

References

1. Harvey D. Assessment of the flexibility of elite athletes using the modified Thomas test. British Journal of Sports Medicine 1998;32(1):68-70.
2. Tyler TF, Nicholas SJ, Mullaney MJ, McHugh MP. The role of hip muscle function in the treatment of patellofemoral pain syndrome. The American journal of sports medicine 2006;34(4):630-6.
3. Marrè-Brunenghi G, Camoriano R, Valle M, Boero S. The psoas muscle as cause of low back pain in infantile cerebral palsy. Journal of Orthopaedics and Traumatology 2008;9(1):43-7.
4. Adams JC, Hamblen DL. Outline of Orthopaedics. 13th edition. Churchill Livingstone, 2001. p.459.
5. Konin JG, Brader H. Lumbar Spine Special tests for orthopedic examination. Third edition. USA: Slack Incorporated. 2006. p170.
6. Dr. Jeffrey Tucker. The Psoas and Iliacus: Functional Testing. Available from: https://drjeffreytucker.com/2009/09/the-psoas-and-iliacus-functional-testing/ (accessed 28/11/2020).
7. Liverpool Chiropractic & Sports Injury Clinic. Hip Mobility Assessment | Modified Thomas Test. Available from https://www.youtube.com/watch?v=9fdHMryWbpI (accessed 28/11/2020).
8. McKean M. Postural Screening using the Thomas Test, Part 1. Australian Pistol Shooters' Bulletin. 2005:11-13.
9. Gabbe BJ, Bennell KL, Wajswelner H, Finch CF. Reliability of common lower extremity musculoskeletal screening tests. Physical Therapy in Sport 2004;5(2):90-7.
10. Clapis PA, Davis SM, Davis RO. Reliability of inclinometer and goniometric measurements of hip extension flexibility using the modified Thomas test. Physiotherapy theory and practice 2008;24(2):135-41.
11. Peeler J, Anderson JE. Reliability of the Thomas test for assessing range of motion about the hip. Physical Therapy in Sport. 2007;8(1):14-21.

❑❑❑

18 "FABER Test"

Definition/Description

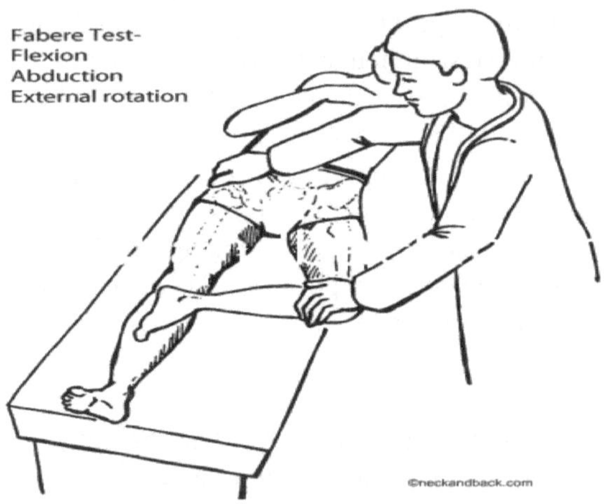

FABERs test. Attribution to "Dr. Donald Corenman, MD - Colroado Spine Doctor".

The FABER (Patrick's) Test stands for: Flexion, Abduction and External Rotation. These three movements combined result in a clinical pain provocation test to assist in diagnosis of pathologies at the hip, lumbar and sacroiliac region. [1]

Clinically Relevant Anatomy

Hip articulation is true diarthroidal ball and-socket style joint.

Formed from the head of the femur as it articulates with the acetabulum of the pelvis. This joint serves as the main connection between the lower extremity and the trunk, and typically works in a closed kinematic chain.[2] Thus is designed for stability and weight-bearing – rather than a large range of movement.

Movements available at the hip joint are flexion, extension, abduction, adduction, internal rotation and external rotation. The ligaments of the hip joint act to increase stability. They can be divided into two groups – intracapsular and extracapsular.

For more detailed information on the anatomy of the hip, lumbar spine and Sacroiliac Joint.

Purpose

The FABER test is used to identify the presence of hip pathology by attempting to reproduce pain in the hip, lumbar spine or sacroiliac region. The test is a passive screening tool for musculoskeletal pathologies, such as hip, lumbar spine, or sacroiliac joint dysfunction, or an iliopsoas spasm.[3][1]

The test also assesses the hip, due to forces being transferred through the joint. The position of flexion, abduction, and external rotation, when combined with overpressure, stresses the femoral-acetabular joint and produces pain, if irritated.[4][5]

In conjunction with other tests such as range of movement and hip quadrant test, FABERs can be a useful tool to guide practitioners when to refer for further imaging in patients with persistent hip or groin pain.[6]

When the FABER test is clustered, it can provide highly useful information in identifying those suffering from sacroiliac joint dysfunction. This tests the sacroiliac joint, as the horizontal abduction force goes through the femur, the soft tissues under tension transfer the forces to the sacroiliac joint. Hence, this test can indicate pathology located in the hip or sacroiliac joint.

Technique

The patient is positioned in supine. The leg is placed in a figure-4 position (hip flexed and abducted with the lateral ankle resting on the contralateral thigh proximal to the knee. [7] While stabilizing the opposite side of the pelvis at the anterior superior iliac spine, an external rotation, abduction and posterior force is then lightly applied to the ipsilateral knee until the end range of motion is achieved. A further few small-amplitude oscillations can be applied to check for pain provocation at the end range of motion. [8] A positive test is one that reproduces the patient's pain or limits their range of movement. [7]

Interpretation

The following findings of a positive FABER test may help to guide your clinical diagnosis;

1. Sarcoiliac Joint Pain on external hip rotation
   - Sacroiliac Joint Dysfunction
   - Sacroiliitis
2. Groin Pain on external hip rotation
   - Iliopsoas Strain or Iliopsoas Bursitis
   - Intraarticular Hip Disorder
     (a) Hip Impingement (femoral acetabular impingement)
     (b) Hip Labral Tear[8]
     (c) Hip loose bodies
     (d) Hip chondral lesion
     (e) Hip Osteoarthritis[10]
3. Posterior Hip Pain on external hip rotation
   - Posterior Hip Impingement

Evidence

- Reliability: FABER measured with a ruler, normalized FABER range of movement, and inclinometry all resulted in excellent intra-rater reliability, with the highest ICC being demonstrated for inclinometry (ICC 0.86, 0.86, and 0.91).[11] The use of an inclinometer may increase reliability when performed by an experienced clinician in comparison with height measutements.
- Sensitivity for identification of hip pathology identified with arthroscopy: 0.89[6]
- Correlation of positive test with OA on radiographs: r = 0.54[10]
- Kappa (95% Confidence interval): 0.63 (0.43-0.83), Kappa Maximum: 0.83, Percent agreement: 84%, Prevalence: 0.37, Bias: 0.07[1]
- Diagnostic value of FABER test compared to MR arthrogra¬phy in labral tear diagnostics: sensitivety: 41%, specificity: 100%, positive predictive value: 100%, negative predictive value: 9%[8]
- The validity and reliability of the FABER test is very contradictory, some say it is an invalid and unreliable test[12] , while others disagree about the outcome and feel physical diagnostic tests do not have enough quality evidence to support the use of them for diagnosis purposes.[13] [14]

Clinical Relevance

The FABER test can be used in assessment of the hip, sacroiliac joint or lumbar spine as a pain provocation test alongside quality subject assessment and basic objective assessment.

The FABER test is quick to perform and can give a measure of range of movement as well as being a pain provocation test, although it may not give a clear diagnosis it may assist the user in clinically reasoning which further tests or exercises to perform.

The evidence supporting this test is varied and more studies are required to fully assess the value of this and other hip pathology tests[15]. Although more evidence is becoming apparent that physical tests are less reliable and subject to user error. [13]

References

1. Martin RL, Sekiya JK. The interrater reliability of 4 clinical tests used to assess individuals with musculoskeletal hip pain. J Orthop Sports Phys Ther. 2008 Feb;38(2):71-7. Epub 2007 Sep 21.
2. Hip Anatomy. (2017, June 6). Physiopedia, . Retrieved 10:17, December 14, 2017 from https://www.physio-pedia.com/index.php?title=Hip_Anatomy&oldid=172875.
3. Dutton M. Orthopaedic: Examination, evaluation, and intervention. 2nd ed. New York: The McGraw-Hill Companies, Inc; 2008.
4. Broadhurst NA, Bond MJ. Pain provocation tests for the assessment of sacroiliac joint dysfunction. Journal of Spinal Disorders. 1998 Aug;11(4):341-5.
5. Philippon MJ, Stubbs AJ, Schenker ML, Maxwell RB, Ganz R, Leunig M. Arthroscopic management of femoroacetabular impingement: osteoplasty technique and literature review. The American journal of sports medicine. 2007 Sep;35(9):1571-80.

6. B, McCroy P, Brukner P, et al. Hip joint pathology: Clinical presentation and correlation between magnetic resonance arthrography, ultrasound, and arthroscopic findings in 25 consecutive cases. Clin J Sports Med. 2003;(13):152-156
7. Flynn T, Cleland J, Whitman J. User's guide to the musculoskeletal examination: Fundamentals for the evidence-based clinician. Buckner, Kentucky: Evidence in Motion; 2008
8. Troelsen A, Mechlenburg I, Gelineck J, Bolvig L, Jacobsen S, Søballe K. What is the role of clinical tests and ultrasound in acetabular labral tear diagnostics? Acta Orthop. 2009 Jun;80(3):314-8.
9. Faber Test | Patrick Faber's Test for Hip Pain Available from:https://www.youtube.com watch?v=nFza4MJv2Uo
10. Theiler R, Stucki G, Schotz R, Hofer H, Seifert B. Parametric and non-parametric measures in the assessment of knee and hip osteoarthritis: interobserver reliability and correlation with radiology. Osteoarthritis Cartilage. 1996:35-42.
11. Bagwell JJ, Bauer L, Gradoz M, Grindstaff TL. The reliability of FABER test hip range of motion measurements. International journal of sports physical therapy. 2016 Dec;11(7):1101.
12. Cattley P, Winyard J, Trevaskis J, Eaton S. Validity and reliability of clinical tests for the sacroiliac joint. A review of literature. Australas Chiropr Osteopathy. 2002 Nov;10(2):73-80.
13. Tijssen M, van Cingel R, Willemsen L, de Visser E. Diagnostics of femoroacetabular impingement and labral pathology of the hip: a systematic review of the accuracy and validity of physical tests. Arthroscopy: The Journal of Arthroscopic & Related Surgery. 2012 Jun 1;28(6):860-71.
14. Vleeming A, Albert HB, Ostgaard HC, Sturesson B, Stuge B.European guidelines for the diagnosis and treatment of pelvic girdle pain. Eur Spine J. 2008 Jun;17(6):794-819. Epub 2008 Feb 8.
15. Reiman MP, Goode AP, Hegedus EJ, Cook CE, Wright AA. Diagnostic accuracy of clinical tests of the hip: a systematic review with meta-analysis. Br J Sports Med. 2013 Sep 1;47(14):893-902.

❑❑❑

19 Flexion, Abduction, External Rotation Test (FABER or Patrick's Test)

Purpose:

To test for the presence of sacroiliac region pain; also, to test for the presence of hip pathology.

Technique:

The patient is supine. The tested LE is placed in a "figure 4" position (hip flexed and abducted, ipsilateral foot resting on the contralateral thigh just above the knee). While stabilizing the opposite side of the pelvis, and external rotation/posteriorly directed force is then applied to the ipsilateral knee.

Positive Test:

The test result is considered to be positive if the patient reports reproduction of buttock or groin pain.

Diagnostic properties/Evidence:

Reference standard anesthetic block of the sacroiliac joint.

Sn= .71, Sp= 1.0, -LR= .23[2], +LR= NA[2]

Reliability:

Inter-examiner Kappa= 0.60-0.62[3,4]

Resources

1. Flynn TW, Cleland JA, Whitman JM. User's Guide to the Musculoskeletal Examination: Fundamentals for an Evidence-based Clinician. EIM. 2008:208.
2. Broadhurst N, Bond M. Pain provocation tests for the assessment of sacroiliac joint dysfunction. J Spinal Disorders 1998;11:341-345.
3. Flynn T, Fritz J, Whitman J, et al. A clinical prediction rule for classifying patients with low back pain who demonstrate short-term improvement with spinal manipulation. Spine 2002:27:2835-2843.
4. Laslett M, Williams M. The reliability of selected pain provocation tests for sacroiliac joint pathology. Spine 1994;19:1243-1249.

❑❑❑

20

"Finkelstein Test"

Introduction

Finkelstein's test is the classic provocative test for diagnosis of De Quervain's disease. Finkelstein hypothesized that the entry of the muscle bellies of the extensor pollicis brevis (EPB) and abductor pollicis longus (APL) tendons into the first extensor compartment was responsible for the findings observed in his now eponymous test.

Clinically Relevant Anatomy

Extensor Pollicis Brevis (EPB)

- Radial abduction of wrist (0-25°)
- Thumb extension (90°)

Abductor Pollicis Longus (APL)

- Wrist radial abduction (0- 25°)
- Thumb abduction (70°- 80°)

Purpose of Testing

The Finkelstein test is used in the diagnosis of De Quervain's syndrome. This fact implies a tenovaginitis and tenosynovitis of the M. extensor pollicis brevis and M. abductor pollicis longus. Finkelstein maneuver is a helpful test to diagnose De Quervain's Tendonitis or first dorsal compartment tendonitis named after the Swiss surgeon Fritz de Quervain. This is a condition brought on by irritation or inflammation of the wrist tendons at the base of the thumb. The inflammation causes the compartment (a tunnel or a sheath) around the tendon to swell and enlarge, making thumb and wrist movement painful.

Testing Position

Sitting or standing.

Technique

To begin, the patient must sit comfortable and relaxed on the examination table. Next, examine the patients hand in the air, while the other hand rests just beside the body. The therapist then asks the patient to make a fist around a thumb and to perform a ulnar deviation.

A modified version of the test is that the patient must sit comfortable and relaxed on the examination table. The patient must hold his afflicted hand in the air, while the other hand should be resting against his/ her body. The therapist grasps the afflicted hand of the patient and rotates it in ulnar deviation. He pulls the patient's thumb across the palm of his/ her hand. This causes additional stress on the extensor tendons of the thumb. [1][2]

The patient actively (or active assistive) flexes thumb maximally and wraps fingers over thumb, making a fist. The patient then ulnarly deviates his/her wrist to stretch the muscles of the 1st extensor compartment. The test is positive if the patient complains of pain over the 1st extensor compartment of the wrist.

Interpretation

- Negative result: The patient doesn't feel any pain radiating up the inside of his/ her arm from the thumb. [1]
- Positive result: Ask the patient if he or she feels pain radiating up the inside of his or her arm from the thumb. If the patient reports noticeable pain then, the Finkelstein's test is positive, what indicates De Quervain's syndrome.[1][3][3][3][4]

Importance of Test

The muscles that cross the wrist are separated into compartments by the extensor retinaculum. In the first compartment, the tendons of the extensor pollicis brevis and abductor pollicis longus pass through to attach distally. According to Neumann, the extensor pollicis brevis attaches distally to the dorsal side of the proximal phalanx and extensor mechanism of the thumb, while the abductor pollicis longus attaches distally to the radial-dorsal side of the 1st metacarpal. The combination of maximum finger flexion and wrist ulnar deviation elongates these tendons and produces pain in symptomatic individuals.[4]

Reliability

- Investigation into the validity of tests are important to know whether our tests are reliable or not.
- Studies that test the reliability of the Finkelstein test are very limited. One research shows that the Finkelstein test has a high reliability [5], but further research is still required.

References

1. Richard Day, John Fox; Neuro- musculoskeletal clinical tests; Churchill Livingstone Elsevier 2009- page 113 (Level of evidence = E)
2. Javier González-Iglesias, Peter Huijbregts, César Fernández-de-las-Peñas, Joshua A. Cleland; Differential Diagnosis and Physical Therapy Management of a Patient With Radial Wrist Pain of 6 Months' Duration: A Case Report; journal of orthopaedic sports physical therapy: volume 40,number 6, June 2010. (level of evidence = C)
3. How to Perform a Finkelstein's Test of the Hand (level of evidence = E)
4. Neumann, Donald. Kinesiology of the Musculoskeletal System: Foundations for Rehabilitation. 2nd edition. St. Louis, MO: Mosby Elsevier, 2010. 303.
5. Javier González-Iglesias, Peter Huijbregts, César Fernández-de-las-Peñas, Joshua A. Cleland; Differential Diagnosis and Physical Therapy Management of a Patient With Radial Wrist Pain of 6 Months' Duration: A Case Report; journal of orthopaedic; sports physical therapy: volume 40, number 6, June 2010.(level of evidence = C)

❑❑❑

21

"Ober's Test"

Purpose

The Ober's test evaluates a tight, contracted or inflamed Tensor Fasciae Latae (TFL) and Iliotibial band (ITB). The Ober's test must not be confounded with Noble's test and the Renne test, two other tests that are commonly used to detect iliotibial band syndrome.

Clinically Relevant Anatomy

Anatomically, the ITB is a continuation of the tendinous portion of the TFL muscle with some contributions from the gluteal muscles. TFL/ITB is a synergist of the gluteus medius muscle in hip abduction[1].

Origin:

- TFL originates[2] from- the anterior part of the external lip of iliac crest, the outer surface of an anterior superior iliac spine, and the deep surface of fascia lata.
- Iliotibial band (ITB) or tract is a lateral thickening of the fascia lata in the thigh[3]. Proximally it splits into superficial and deep layers, enclosing tensor fasciae lata and anchoring this muscle to the iliac crest. It also receives most of the tendon of the gluteus maximus.

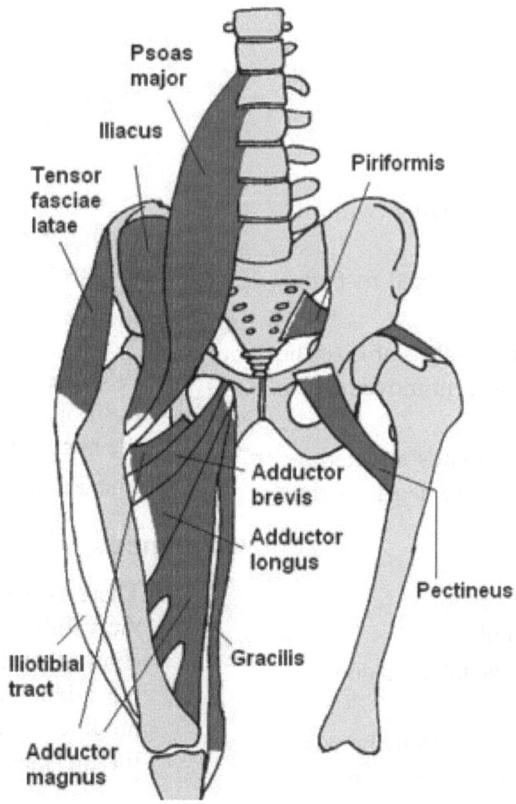

Iliotibial Band and Tensor Fascia Lata

Insertion:

- TFL inserts[2] into the ITB at the anterolateral thigh at the junction of proximal and middle thirds of the thigh.
- ITB is generally viewed as a band of dense fibrous connective tissue that passes over the lateral femoral epicondyle and attaches to Gerdy's tubercle[3] on the anterolateral aspect of the tibia.

Action:

- TFL flexes, medially rotates, and abducts the hip joint; tenses the fascia lata; and may assist in knee extension[2]. Gluteus medius, gluteus minimus, and upper fibers of the gluteus maximus are the primary synergistic muscles of the hip abductors.
- ITB permits the TFL and Gluteus maximus to influence the stability of the extended knee joint, due to the insertion of these muscles into the ITB[4].

Technique

Ober Test

Frank Ober described the test for tightness of TFL and ITB in an article entitled "Back Strain and Sciatica", wherein he discussed the relationship of a contracted TFL and ITB to low backache (May 1935). This was later revised in the year 1937 which cautioned on avoiding hip internal rotation and flexion while carrying out the test[5].

Test position[6][7]:

- The patient should be in side-lying with the affected side up.
- Bottom knee and hip should be flexed to flatten the lumbar curve.
- Stand behind the patient and firmly stabilize the pelvis/greater trochanter to prevent movement in any direction.
- Grasp the distal end of the patient's affected leg with your other hand and flex the leg to a right angle at the knee

Test:

- Extend and abduct the hip joint.
- Slowly lower the leg toward the table -adduct hip- until motion is restricted.
- Ensure that the hip does not internally rotate and flex during the test and the pelvis must be stabilized. As allowing the thigh to drop in flexion and internal rotation would 'give in' to the tight TFL and not accurately test the length[5].

Results:

- If the ITB is normal, the leg will adduct with the thigh dropping down slightly below the horizontal and the patient won't experience any pain; in this case, the test is called negative.
- If the ITB is tight, the leg would remain in the abducted position and the patient would experience lateral knee pain, in this case, the test is called positive.

Modified Ober Test[5]

A modification of the Ober test was first recommended by Kendalls in Posture and Pain. In this test, there is less strain on the medial aspect of the knee joint, less tension on the patella, less interference by a tight Rectus Femoris and it provides a complete stretch on TFL.

Test position:

- The patient is in a side-lying position with underneath leg flexed at hip and knee to flatten the low back.
- The examiner stabilizes the pelvis and keeps the lateral trunk in contact with the table.
- Note: Downward lateral tilt is equivalent to the hip abduction and that would "give in " to a tight TFL.

Test:

The examiner extends the leg. Ensure that leg is not internally rotated.

Results:

- With the knee straight and the pelvis in a neutral position, the thigh drops about 10 degrees below the horizontal. It is suggestive of normal length.
- The leg fails to drop indicates tight ITB and TFL.

Evidence

- There is a limited number of studies to support the validity of this test[10]. A study by Reese et al shows that the use of an inclinometer to measure hip adduction using both the Ober test and the modified Ober test appears to be a reliable method for the measurement of IT band flexibility, and the technique is quite easy to use. It demonstrated a significant difference in ROM between testing with the affected knee flexed vs. extended, with the reliability of .90 and .91 respectively[11]. The modified Ober test allows a significantly greater hip adduction range of motion than the Ober test, the 2 examination procedures should not be used interchangeably for the measurement of the flexibility of the IT band.

- But the study findings in 'An Anatomic Investigation of the Ober Test' [12] by Willet GM et al refutes the hypothesis that the ITB plays a role in limiting hip adduction during either version of the Ober test and question the validity of these tests for determining ITB tightness. The findings underscore the influence of the gluteus medius and minimus muscles as well as the hip joint capsule on Ober test findings. The results of this study suggest that the Ober test assesses the tightness of structures proximal to the hip joint, such as the gluteus medius and minimus muscles and the hip joint capsule, rather than the ITB.

Key Research

- The study in Clinical Biomechanics by Gajdosik RL et al showed the hip adduction movement was restricted more with the knee flexed than with the knee extended for both genders ($P < 0.009$). Thus emphasizing the influence of knee positions and gender on the Ober test for the length of the iliotibial band[13].
- An exercise developed by the Postural Restoration Institute to recruit hamstrings and abdominal muscles showed a significant increase in passive hip-adduction angles ($p<0.01$) and a decrease in pain ($p<0.01$), immediately improve Ober's Test measurements in people with lumbopelvic pain. The study[14] showed hamstring/abdominal activation, rather than iliotibial band stretching, may be an effective intervention for addressing lumbopelvic pain and a positive Ober's Test.
- The study shows the effect of ITB stretching and Hamstring and Abdominal activation on positive Ober test in individuals with lumbopelvic pain[15] The hamstring and abdominal activation showed a greater reduction in pain and increase in hip adduction ROM as compared to only ITB stretching.

References

1. Arab AM, Nourbakhsh MR. The relationship between hip abductor muscle strength and iliotibial band tightness in individuals with low back pain. Chiropractic & osteopathy. 2010 Dec;18(1):1.https://www.ncbi.nlm.nih.gov/pmc/articles/PMC2821316/ (accessed on 25/07/18)
2. Kendall, McCreary, Provance; Muscle Testing and Function with Posture and Pain 4th Edition; Tensor Fascia Latae; Page No.216
3. Fairclough J, Hayashi K, Toumi H, Lyons K, Bydder G, Phillips N, Best TM, Benjamin M. The functional anatomy of the iliotibial band during flexion and extension of the knee: implications for understanding iliotibial band syndrome. Journal of Anatomy. 2006 Mar;208(3):309-16.https://www.ncbi.nlm.nih.gov/pmc/articles/PMC2100245/ (accessed on 25/07/2018)
4. Kendall, McCreary, Provance; Muscle Testing and Function with Posture and Pain 4th Edition; Fascia Latae; Page No.227
5. Kendall, McCreary, Provance; Muscle Testing and Function with Posture and Pain 4th Edition; Modified Ober Test; Page No,56-59.
6. Magee D. Orthopedic Physical Assessment. 2nd ed.Pennsylvania:WB Saunders, 1992. p354-355
7. Hoppenfeld S. Physical Examination of the spine and Extremeities. London: Prentice-Hall International 1976.p167
8. bigesor Ober's Test Available from https://www.youtube.com/watch?time_continue=24&v=A0C0WBw4l4s
9. Modified Ober's Test.Available from https://youtu.be/bFVmNtuH4WU
10. Knee Orthopaedic Test - A Strategic Approach to Assessing the Knee; University of Western States, College of Chiropractic, Clinic Protocol; Ober test; Page No.23; Adopted 12/12. (accessed from Knee_Orthopedic_Tests.pdf on 30/07/18)
11. Reese NB, Bandy WD. Use of an inclinometer to measure flexibility of the iliotibial band using the Ober test and the modified Ober test: differences in magnitude and reliability of measurements. Journal of Orthopaedic & Sports Physical Therapy. 2003 Jun;33(6):326-30.https://www.ncbi.nlm.nih.gov/pubmed/12839207 (accessed on 28/07/2018)

12. Willett GM, Keim SA, Shostrom VK, Lomneth CS. An anatomic investigation of the Ober test. The American journal of sports medicine. 2016 Mar;44(3):696-701.https://www.ncbi.nlm.nih.gov/pubmed/26755689 accessed on 28/07/2018
13. Gajdosik RL, Sandler MM, Marr HL. Influence of knee positions and gender on the Ober test for length of the iliotibial band. Clinical biomechanics. 2003 Jan 1;18(1):77-9.https://www.ncbi.nlm.nih.gov/pubmed/12527250 (accessed on 28/07/2018)
14. Tenney HR, Boyle KL, DeBord A. Influence of hamstring and abdominal muscle activation on a positive Ober's test in people with lumbopelvic pain. Physiotherapy Canada. 2013 Jan;65(1):4-11.https://www.ncbi.nlm.nih.gov/pmc/articles/PMC3563370/ (accessed on 28/07/18)
15. Effect of Iliotibial Band stretching versus Hamstrings and Abdominal muscle activation on a positive Ober's test in subjects with Lumbopelvic Pain: A Randomized Clinical Trial by Vijay Kage, Saitej Kolukula Naidu; July 2015 https://www.ejmanager.com/mnstemps/12/12-1435370486.pdf (accessed on 30/07/18)

❑❑❑

22 "36-Item Short Form Survey (SF-36)"

Objective

The 36-Item Short Form Survey (SF-36) is an oft-used, well-researched, self-reported measure of health. It stems from a study called the Medical Outcomes Study[1].

It comprises 36 questions which cover eight domains of health[2]:

1. Limitations in physical activities because of health problems.
2. Limitations in social activities because of physical or emotional problems
3. Limitations in usual role activities because of physical health problems
4. Bodily pain
5. General mental health (psychological distress and well-being)
6. Limitations in usual role activities because of emotional problems
7. Vitality (energy and fatigue)
8. General health perceptions

The SF-36 is often used as a measure of a person or population's quality of life (QOL).

Intended Population

The original authors designed the SF-36 to measure health at the individual level in clinical practice and research and at the population level for health policy evaluations, and general population surveys[2]. It has been used in thousands of research studies[3]. The SF-36 was originally designed as a generic health measure but has also been applied to specific disease populations.

Method of Use

Patients or individuals are asked to fill out the questionnaire (tick boxes) by themselves and then it is scored by a clinician or researcher. There are variations of the the SF-36; it is both licensed (Optum) and available freely online (Rand). Both sources are from different original authors and contain the same 36 questions and answers only differing slightly in the bodily pain and general health domains[4]. Users should document which version they are using and use the corresponding scoring system.

Scores for the different domains are converted and pooled using a scoring key, for a total score indicating a range of low to high QOL. Two component scores can also be tallied; a physical component summary and a mental component summary[4] but research suggests interpretation can be difficult and should be done in comparison to the overall score or profile[5][6]. Similarly, research also suggests that the SF-36 cannot be used as a single index of over all health-related QOL because it measures two dimensions (physical and mental)[3].

Evidence

Reliability

The SF-36 has been shown to be reliable for people with schizophrenia[7] and long-term survivors of childhood cancer[8].

Validity

The SF-36 has been shown to be valid for people with schizophrenia[7], stroke (the physical and mental health domains, the social functioning less so)[9], mobility disability in the elderly[10], community-dwelling older adults[11] and dyspnea in COPD[12].

Responsiveness

Research has shown the SF-36 to be the most responsive to change in workers with musculoskeletal disorders compared with similar generic health measures[13].

Miscellaneous

The SF-36 is available in multiple languages.

References

1. Ware J. SF-36 Health Survey Update. Spine. 2000. 25; 24: 3130-3139.
2. Ware Jr., J.E. and Sherbourne, C.D. (1992) The MOS 36-Item Short-Form Health Survey (SF-36). I. Conceptual Framework and Item Selection. Medical Care, 30, 473-483.
3. Lins L, Carvalho F. SF-36 total score as a single measure of health-related quality of life: Scoping review. SAGE Open Med. 2016. Published online 2016 Oct 4. doi: 10.1177/2050312116671725. Accessed 16 January 2020.
4. Laucis N, Hays R, Bhattacharyya T. Scoring the SF-36 in Orthopaedics: A Brief Guide. J Bone Joint Surg Am. 2015 Oct 7; 97(19): 1628–1634. Published online 2015 Oct 7. doi: 10.2106/JBJS.O.00030. Accessed 15 January 2020.
5. Taft C, Karlsson J, Sullivan M. Do SF-36 summary component scores accurately summarize subscale scores? Qual Life Res. 2001. 10; 5:395-404.
6. Ware JE, Kosinski M. Interpreting SF-36 summary health measures: a response. Qual Life Res. 2001;10(5):405-13; discussion 415-20.
7. Su, C.-T., Ng, H.-S., Yang, A.-L., & Lin, C.-Y. (2014). Psychometric evaluation of the Short Form 36 Health Survey (SF-36) and the World Health Organization Quality of Life Scale Brief Version (WHOQOL-BREF) for patients with schizophrenia. Psychological Assessment. 2014. 26(3), 980–989
8. Reulen R, Zeegers M, Jenkinson C. The use of the SF-36 questionnaire in adult survivors of childhood cancer: evaluation of data quality, score reliability, and scaling assumptions. Health Qual Life Outcomes. 2006. 4; 77 doi:10.1186/1477-7525-4-77. Accessed 16 January 2020.
9. Anderson C, Laubscher S, Burns R. Validation of the Short Form 36 (SF-36) Health Survey Questionnaire Among Stroke Patients. Stroke. 1996;27:1812–1816. Accessed 16 January 2020.
10. Syddall H, Martin H, Harwood R, Cooper C, Aihie Sayer A. The SF-36: A simple, effective measure of mobility-disability for epidemiological studies. J Nutr Health Aging. 2009; 13: 57-62.
11. Walters S, Munro J, Brazier J. Using the SF-36 with older adults: a cross-sectional community-based survey. Age and Ageing. 2001; 30: 337-343. Accessed 16 January 2020.
12. Mahler D, Mackowiak J. Evaluation of the Short-Form 36-Item Questionnaire to Measure Health-Related Quality of Life in Patients With COPD. Chest. 1995. 107; 6: 1585-1589.
13. Beaton D, Hogg-Johnson S, Bombardier C. Evaluating changes in health status: Reliability and responsiveness of five generic health status measures in workers with musculoskeletal disorders. J Clin Epidemiol. 1997. 50; 1:79-93

SF-36 QUESTIONNAIRE

Name:____________________

Ref. Dr:____________________

Date:_______ ID#:__________

Age: _______ Gender: M / F

Please answer the 36 questions of the Health Survey completely, honestly, and without interruptions.

GENERAL HEALTH:

1. **In general, would you say your health is:**
   a. Excellent
   b. Very Good
   c. Good
   d. Fair
   e. Poor
2. **Compared to one year ago, how would you rate your health in general now?**
   - Much better now than one year ago
   - Somewhat better now than one year ago
   - About the same
   - Somewhat worse now than one year ago
   - Much worse than one year ago

LIMITATIONS OF ACTIVITIES:

The following items are about activities you might do during a typical day. Does your health now limit you in these activities? If so, how much?

3. **Vigorous activities, such as running, lifting heavy objects, participating in strenuous sports.**
   a. Yes, Limited a lot
   b. Yes, Limited a Little
   c. No, Not Limited at all

4. **Moderate activities, such as moving a table, pushing a vacuum cleaner, bowling, or playing gol.**
   a. Yes, Limited a lot
   b. Yes, Limited a Little
   c. No, Not Limited at all
5. **Lifting or carrying groceries**
   a. Yes, Limited a lot
   b. Yes, Limited a Little
   c. No, Not Limited at all
6. **Climbing several flights of stairs**
   a. Yes, Limited a lot
   b. Yes, Limited a Little
   c. No, Not Limited at all
7. **Climbing one flight of stairs**
   a. Yes, Limited a lot
   b. Yes, Limited a Little
   c. No, Not Limited at all
8. **Bending, kneeling, or stooping**
   a. Yes, Limited a lot
   b. Yes, Limited a Little
   c. No, Not Limited at all
9. **Walking more than a mile**
   a. Yes, Limited a lot
   b. Yes, Limited a Little
   c. No, Not Limited at all
10. **Walking several blocks**
   a. Yes, Limited a lot
   b. Yes, Limited a Little
   c. No, Not Limited at all
11. **Walking one block**
   a. Yes, Limited a lot
   b. Yes, Limited a Little
   c. No, Not Limited at all
12. **Bathing or dressing yourself**
   a. Yes, Limited a lot
   b. Yes, Limited a Little
   c. No, Not Limited at all

PHYSICAL HEALTH PROBLEMS:

During the past 4 weeks, have you had any of the following problems with your work or other regular daily activities as a result of your physical health?

13. **Cut down the amount of time you spent on work or other activities** (Yes/No)
14. **Accomplished less than you would like** (Yes/No)
15. **Were limited in the kind of work or other activities** (Yes/No)
16. **Had difficulty performing the work or other activities (for example, it took extra effort)** (Yes/No)

EMOTIONAL HEALTH PROBLEMS:

During the past 4 weeks, have you had any of the following problems with your work or other regular daily activities as a result of any emotional problems (such as feeling depressed or anxious)?

17. **Cut down the amount of time you spent on work or other activities** (Yes/No)
18. **Accomplished less than you would like** (Yes/No)
19. **Didn't do work or other activities as carefully as usual** (Yes/No)

SOCIAL ACTIVITIES:

20. **Emotional problems interfered with your normal social activities with family, friends, neighbors, or groups?**
   a. Not at all
   b. Slightly
   c. Moderately
   d. Severe
   e. Very Severe

PAIN:

21. **How much bodily pain have you had during the past 4 weeks?**
   a. None
   b. Very Mild
   c. Mild
   d. Moderate
   e. Severe
   f. Very Severe
22. **During the past 4 weeks, how much did pain interfere with your normal work (including both work outside the home and housework)?**
   a. Not at all

b. A little bit
c. Moderately
d. Quite a bit
e. Extremely

ENERGY AND EMOTIONS:

These questions are about how you feel and how things have been with you during the last 4 weeks. For each question, please give the answer that comes closest to the way you have been feeling.

23. Did you feel full of pep?
a. All of the time
b. Most of the time
c. A good Bit of the Time
d. Some of the time
e. A little bit of the time
f. None of the Time

24. Have you been a very nervous person?
a. All of the time
b. Most of the time
c. A good Bit of the Time
d. Some of the time
e. A little bit of the time
f. None of the Time

25. Have you felt so down in the dumps that nothing could cheer you up?
a. All of the time
b. Most of the time
c. A good Bit of the Time
d. Some of the time
e. A little bit of the time
f. None of the Time

26. Have you felt calm and peaceful ?
a. All of the time
b. Most of the time
c. A good Bit of the Time
d. Some of the time
e. A little bit of the time
f. None of the Time

27. Did you have a lot of energy?
a. All of the time
b. Most of the time
c. A good Bit of the Time
d. Some of the time
e. A little bit of the time
f. None of the Time

28. Have you felt downhearted and blue?
a. All of the time
b. Most of the time
c. A good Bit of the Time
d. Some of the time
e. A little bit of the time
f. None of the Time

29. Did you feel worn out?
a. All of the time
b. Most of the time
c. A good Bit of the Time
d. Some of the time
e. A little bit of the time
f. None of the Time

30. Have you been a happy person?
a. All of the time
b. Most of the time
c. A good Bit of the Time
d. Some of the time
e. A little bit of the time
f. None of the Time

31. Did you feel tired?
a. All of the time
b. Most of the time
c. A good Bit of the Time
d. Some of the time
e. A little bit of the time
f. None of the Time

SOCIAL ACTIVITIES:

32. During the past 4 weeks, how much of the time has your physical health or emotional problems interfered with your social activities (like visiting with friends, relatives, etc.)?
a. All of the time
b. Most of the time
c. A good Bit of the Time
d. Some of the time
e. A little bit of the time
f. None of the Time

GENERAL HEALTH:

How true or false is each of the following statements for you?

33. I seem to get sick a little easier than other people

Definitely true
Mostly true
Don't know
Mostly false
Definitely false

34. I am as healthy as anybody I know

Definitely true
Mostly true
Don't know
Mostly false
Definitely false

35. I expect my health to get worse

Definitely true
Mostly true
Don't know
Mostly false
Definitely false

36. My health is excellent

Definitely true
Mostly true
Don't know
Mostly false
Definitely false

❑❑❑

23 "4-item Dynamic Gait Index"

Objective

The purpose of this measure is to test the psychometric properties of a short form of the Dynamic Gait Index (DGI) for the clinical measurement of walking function in people with balance and vestibular disorders.

Intended Population

People with balance and vestibular disorders having difficulty walking.

This test was specifically constructed to be administered without using any equipment (cf. DGI requires cones etc.).

Test

4 items were selected for the reduced-item DGI:

1. horizontal head turns
2. vertical head turns
3. gait on level surfaces
4. changes in gait speed

Scoring

With regard to the use of the 4-item DGI as a screening tool for falls, the higher specificity of the 4-item DGI suggests that a closer evaluation of fall risk factors is indicated if an individual has a score of less than 10 of 12.

Original Reference

Marchetti GF, Whitney SL. Construction and validation of the 4-item dynamic gait index. Physical Therapy, 2006 Dec;86(12):1651-60.[1]

Evidence

The clinical psychometric properties of the 4-item DGI were equivalent or superior to those of the 8-item test. The 4-item DGI can be used by clinicians to measure gait in people with balance and vestibular disorders without compromising important clinical measurement characteristics[1].

Reliability

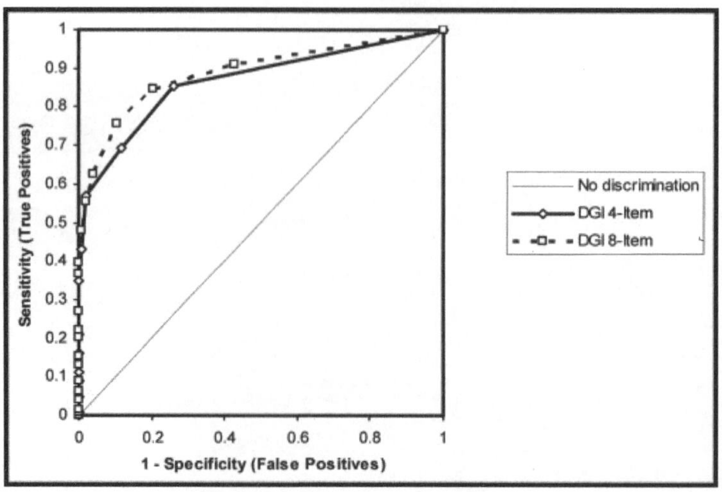

Validity

Table 2 – Rasch Analysis Results for 4-Item Dynamic Gait Index (DGI) for 131 Test and Control Subjects					
Item	**Item Measure**	**SE**	**Infit ZSTD**	**Outfit ZSTD**	**PTBis**
Horizontal Head turns	73.9	1.8	1.6	1.4	0.90
Vertical Head turns	59.2	1.8	0.9	0.9	0.89
Gait on level surface	35.4	2.2	-1.7	-0.2	0.87
Gait with speed changes	31.5	2.3	-1.6	-1.7	0.85

Test subjects had vestibular and balance dysfunction. Data include item and total mean transformed measures scores, standard errors (SE), infit and outfit standardized scores (ZSTD), and point biserial correlation coefficients (PTBis). The DGI items are listed in order of decreasing difficulty. Data for 20 test subjects and 75 control subjects were omitted because of maximum scores. Transformed scale (X) = 17.43, range for subjects = 4.2 – 128.4

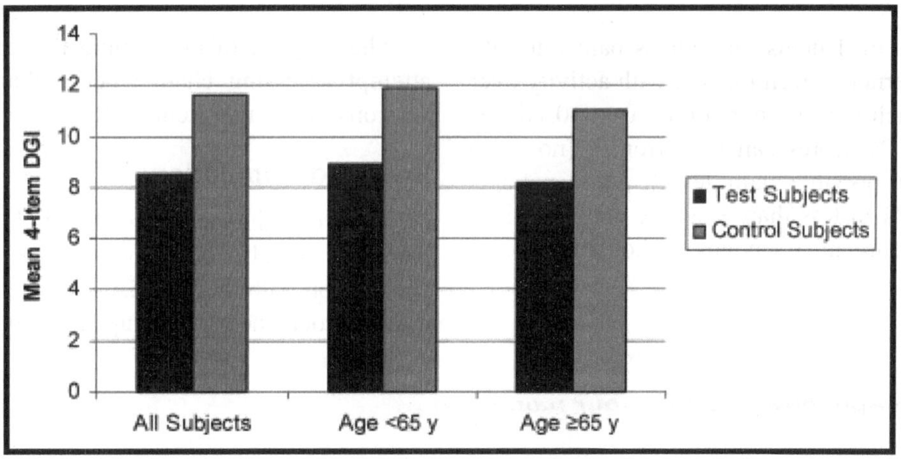

References

1. Marchetti GF, Whitney SL. Construction and validation of the 4-item dynamic gait index. Physical Therapy, 2006 Dec;86(12):1651-60.
2. Lin JH, Hsu MJ, Hsu HW, Wu HC, Hsieh CL. Psychometric Comparisons of 3 Functional Ambulation Measures for Patients With Stroke. Stroke. 2010 Jul 29; online article ahead of print

❑❑❑

24 "4-Item Pain Intensity Measure (P4)"

The P4 consists of 4 items that adress pain intensity in the morning, afternoon, evening, and with activity over the past 2 days. Each item is scored on a 0-to-10 NPRS, therefore the total P4 scores can vary from 0 (no pain) to 40 (the highest possible pain level). Most patients can complete the P4 in less than a minute and clinicians can score the measure in 5 seconds without the use of computational aids.[1]

The purpose of developing this questionnaire was to attempt assessing change better than the two different versions of a single-item NPRS.[1]

Intended Population:

Those over the age of 16 with non-chronic musculoskeletal pain.[1] It has also been shown to be valid when used in conjunction with the WOMAC in people with osteoarthritis awaiting total knee or total hip replacements.[2]

Method of Use

On average, how bad has your pain been ...

	No Pain										Pain as bad as it can be
In the morning over the past 2 days?	0	1	2	3	4	5	6	7	8	9	10
In the afternoon over the past 2 days?	0	1	2	3	4	5	6	7	8	9	10
In the evening over the past 2 days?	0	1	2	3	4	5	6	7	8	9	10
With activity over the past 2 days?	0	1	2	3	4	5	6	7	8	9	10

Patients are asked to circle a single number that corresponds to their pain at each time of day and with activity over the previous 2 days. The numbers are then totaled to yield a score out of 40.

Evidence

Reliability : Test-retest reliability = 0.78[1]

Validity

Longitudinal validity = 0.63 and 0.57 between the retrospective rating of change and the P4 and 24-hour NPRS ($z = 1.73$, $P_1 = .043$), and 0.61 and 0.56 between the retrospective rating of change and the P4 and 2-day NPRS ($z = 2.53$, $P_1 = .006$), respectively.[1]

Responsiveness : MDC_{90} = 9.1 points or 22.2% of the scale range[1]

References

1. Spadoni GF, Stratford PW, Solomon PE, Wishart LR. The Evaluation of Change in Pain Intensity: A Comparison of the P4 and Single-Item Numeric Pain Rating Scales. J Orthop Sports Phys Ther, 2004: 34(4): 187-93.
2. Stratford PW, Dogra M, Woodhouse L, Kennedy DM, Spadoni GF. Validating Self-Report Measures of Pain and Function in Patients Undergoing Hip or Knee Arthroplasty. Physiother Can, 2009: 61; 189-194.

❑❑❑

25

"8-Item Sports Subscale"

The 8-items Sports Measure is part of the Foot and Ankle Ability Measure (FAAM). The FAAM is a self-report outcome instrument developed to assess physical function for individuals with foot and ankle related impairments. This self-report outcome instrument is available in English, German, French and Persian. The Foot and Ankle Ability Measure is a 29-item questionnaire divided into two subscales: the Foot and Ankle Ability Measure, 21-item Activities of Daily Living Subscale and the Foot and Ankle Ability Measure, 8-item Sports Subscale. The Sports subscale assesses more difficult tasks that are essential to sport, it is a population-specific subscale designed for athletes[1][2][3].

For the most valid results it is suggested that scores for the FAAM ADL and Sports subscales be generated only when subjects completed 90% or more of the items (19 of 21 for the ADL and 7 of 8 for the Sports subscales respectively)[1]

Scoring the FAAM

- The response to each item on the Sports subscale is scored from 4 to 0, with 4 being "no difficulty" and 0 being "unable to do".
- If an activity is limited by something other than their foot or ankle is scored as N/A - N/A responses are not counted.
- The scores on each item are added together to get the item score total.
- The number of items with a response is multiplied by 4 to get the highest potential score.
- If the subject answers all 8 items the highest potential score is 32. If one item is not answered the highest potential score is 28, if two are not answered the highest potential score is 24, etc.
- The item score total is divided by the highest potential score. This value is multiplied by 100 to get a percentage.
- A higher score represents a higher level of physical function.

References

1. Martin RL, Hutt DM, Wukich DK. Validity of the Foot and Ankle Ability Measure (FAAM) in Diabetes Mellitus. Foot Ankle Int. 2009 Apr;30(4):297-302
2. Walmsley et al. The rheumatoid foot: a systematic literature review of patient-reported outcome measures. Journal of Foot and Ankle Research 2010, 3:12.
3. RobRoy L. Martin. Evidence of Validity for the Foot and Ankle Ability Measure (FAAM). 2005

Questionnaire:

1. Running

No difficulty at all	Slight difficulty	Moderate difficulty	Extreme difficulty	Unable to do	N/A
(+4)	(+3)	(+2)	(+1)	(0)	(X)

2. Jumping

No difficulty at all	Slight difficulty	Moderate difficulty	Extreme difficulty	Unable to do	N/A
(+4)	(+3)	(+2)	(+1)	(0)	(X)

3. Landing

No difficulty at all	Slight difficulty	Moderate difficulty	Extreme difficulty	Unable to do	N/A
(+4)	(+3)	(+2)	(+1)	(0)	(X)

4. Starting and Stopping Quickly

No difficulty at all	Slight difficulty	Moderate difficulty	Extreme difficulty	Unable to do	N/A
(+4)	(+3)	(+2)	(+1)	(0)	(X)

5. Cutting Lateral Movements

No difficulty at all	Slight difficulty	Moderate difficulty	Extreme difficulty	Unable to do	N/A
(+4)	(+3)	(+2)	(+1)	(0)	(X)

6. Ability to perform activity with your normal techniques

No difficulty at all	Slight difficulty	Moderate difficulty	Extreme difficulty	Unable to do	N/A
(+4)	(+3)	(+2)	(+1)	(0)	(X)

7. Ability to participate in your desired sport as long as you would like

No difficulty at all	Slight difficulty	Moderate difficulty	Extreme difficulty	Unable to do	N/A
(+4)	(+3)	(+2)	(+1)	(0)	(X)

8. How would you rate your current level of function during your sports related activities from 0 to 100 being your level of function prior to your foot and ankle problem and 0 being the inability to perform any of your usual daily activities.

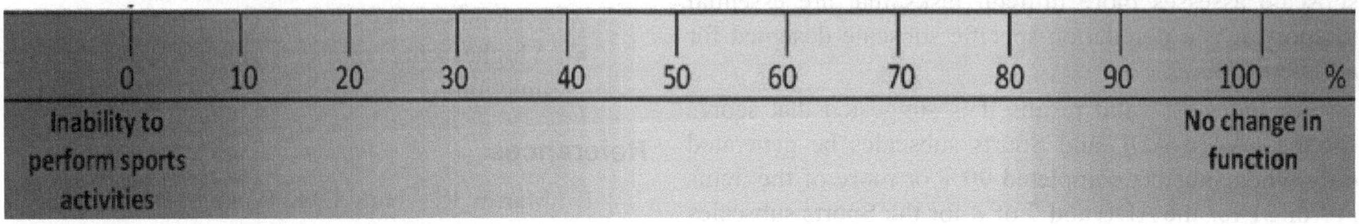

9. How would you rate your current level of function

Normal

Nearly Normal

Abnormal

Severely Abnormal

❑❑❑

26 "Abbey Pain Scale"

Objective

For caregivers to assess the pain experience of people with end-stage dementia who are non-verbal.

Background

Pain assessment can be extremely complex in individuals with dementia, particularly toward the end stages of dementia when an individual may become nonverbal. Pain is a significant experience for those with dementia and it is widely believed to be under reported in the dementia population. In the absence of self-reported pain, caregivers and clinicians must rely on their observation and the knowledge they have of the person in questions usual behaviours.

As a result, the Abbey Pain Scale (APS) was designed to assist in the assessment of pain in the nonverbal individual suffering from end-stage dementia[1].

Like many pain scales for use with people with dementia, there is not a lot of evidence regarding the APS. This is probably because of the nature of the group the scale is designed for. However, the APS has been incorporated into Australian pain guidelines and is recommended by researchers[2][3]

It is easy to use and no training is required[2]. It is easily accessible online and provides some sort of formalised pain assessment for this complex group of dementia sufferers.

Intended Population

Individuals with progressed dementia where they are unable to verbalise pain, and their caregivers.

Methods of Use

The APS requires the caregiver or clinician to observe the individual with dementia for signs of pain.

The Australian Pain Society recommends using this as a movement-based assessment[4], i.e. that observations are made when the individual is moving for daily cares e.g. dressing or pressure area care. Pain may become more obvious on movement, compared to at rest.

The Australian Pain Society also recommends that the scale is completed again one hour post any intervention[4]. If pain appears to persist then a comprehensive assessment of the person's care must be done to identify causes of pain and any corresponding treatments to ease pain. If pain appears to persist beyond 24 hours medical help should be sought.

Each item is rated and rate the following six items on a scale of absent=0, mild=1, moderate=2 or severe=3.

The six items to be observed are:

1. Vocalisation
2. Facial expression
3. Change in body language
4. Behavioural change
5. Physiological change
6. Physical changes

Scores are then added to create a total score which can then be compared to the following to give an overall description of the person's perceived pain experience.

0-2 = No pain

3-7 = Mild pain

8-13 = Moderate pain

>14 = Severe pain

Versions

Swedish[5] / Danish[6] / Japanese[7][8]

Evidence

Reliability

The original authors[1] reported satisfactory reliability of the APS. The Danish version showed good inter-rater reliability[6] and the Japanese version reported good reliability[7].

Validity

Discriminant validity: significant differences observed pre/post treatment[2][6].

The Australian Pain Society notes that the APS does not discriminate between pain and distress so careful observation after pain relief is also needed[4].

References

1. Abbey J, Piller N, De Bellis A, Esterman A, Parker D, Giles L, Lowcay B. The Abbey pain scale: a 1-minute numerical indicator for people with end-stage dementia. Int J Palliate Nurs. 2004; 10: 1: 6-13. Accessed 11 January 2019.
2. Lichtner V, Dowding D, Esterhuizen P, Closs SJ, Long AF, Corbett A, Briggs M. Pain assessment for people with dementia: a systematic review of systematic reviews of pain assessment tools. BMC Geriatr. 2014; 14: 138. Accessed 10 January 2019.
3. Schofield P. The Assessment of Pain in Older People: UK National Guidelines. Age Ageing. 2018; 47(Suppl 1): i1–i22. Accessed 10 January 2019.
4. The Australian Pain Society. Abbey Pain Scale. Available from https://apsoc.org.au/PDF/Publications/Abbey_Pain_Scale.pdf. Accessed 10 January 2019.
5. Karlson C. Reliability and utility of the Abbey Pain Scale-SWE for pain assessment among people with dementia (in progress). Available from https://www.oru.se/english/research/research-projects/rp/?rdb=p1701. Accessed 10 January 2019.
6. Gregersen M, Melin AS, Nygaard IS, Nielsen CH, Beedholm-Ebsen M. Reliability of the Danish Abbey Pain Scale in severely demented and non-communicative older patients. Int J Palliat Nurs. 2016. 22;10:482-488.
7. Takai Y, Yamamoto-Mitani N, Chiba Y, Nishikawa Y, Hayashi K, Sugai Y. Abbey Pain Scale: development and validation of the Japanese version. Geriatr Gerontol Int. 2010.10;2:145-53.
8. Takai Y, Yamamoto-Mitani N, Chiba Y, Kato A. Feasibility and clinical utility of the Japanese version of the Abbey pain scale in Japanese aged care. Pain Manag Nurs. 2014;15: 2:439-48.

❑❑❑

27 "ABILHAND Assessment"

Objective

The ABILHAND is an interview-based assessment of a patient-reported measure of the perceived difficulty in using their hand to perform manual activities in daily activities. The assessment considers the active function of the upper limbs and measures the ability to perform bimanual tasks, regardless of the way in which these tasks are carried out.[1] All of the versions of the assessment are available for from the following website[2] and contain all of the assessment information, downloads of the pack and also the link to the Rasch analysis.

There are currently versions specifically validated for

Chronic stroke, Rheumatoid Arthritis, Systemic sclerosis, Hand Surgery

These test packs are also available in many languages such as English, French, Dutch, Italian, Swedish, Brazilian-Portuguese, Chinese, Canadian English, Canadian French, Czech, Hungarian, Polish, Russian, Serbian, Spanish, UK English, Spanish USA, Bulgarian, Austrian German, Swiss German, Swiss-French, Norwegian, Slovak, Argentinian Spanish, Mexican Spanish.

Instructions

This is an interview-based assessment where the patient is asked to estimate the ease or difficulty of performing a list of activities when carried out without assistance. This can involve any strategy used to carry out the activity, and is self-report and not a physical demonstration of the activity.

The questionnaire is downloaded from the website and one of the 10 random orders of questions. These are read to the patient and scored as either "impossible", "difficult" or "easy". If a task has not been attempted in the last 3 months then it is marked as N/A.

Scoring & Interpretation

Analysis of the answers is via a Rasch model of online analysis, which converts the raw scores into a linear measure.

The output of the online analysis is presented as the patient's manual ability (indicated by a red line) alongside the 95% confidence interval. The better the patient's ability, the more the line will be located on the right. From the output scoresheet, items are ordered from the easiest task at the bottom, to the hardest task at the top.

The most likely score according to the difficulty is given and changes according to the patient's manual ability. This allows the score to be used for treatment planning as easier tasks should have recovered first.

Summary of score versions

ABILHAND in chronic stroke patients

- 23 bimanual activities.
- Each item is answered on a 3-level scale (impossible, difficult, easy).
- The item difficulty increases with bimanual involvement.
- Measurement range: approx. 7 logits.
- Measurement error: 0.36 logits in the centre of the scale.
- Least measurable difference: 0.13 logit in the centre of the scale.
- Separation reliability: 0.90 in our sample of 103 chronic stroke patients.
- Invariant item hierarchy across gender, age, the side affected, delay since CVA, level of depression, overall ability in our sample of 103 chronic stroke patients.

ABILHAND in rheumatoid arthritis patients

- 27 bimanual activities.
- Each item is answered on a 3-level scale (impossible, difficult, easy).
- The item difficulty increases with constraints in the upper limb joints.
- Measurement range: approx. 8 logits.
- Measurement error: 0.42 logits in the centre of the scale.
- Least measurable difference: 0.15 logit in the centre of the scale.
- Separation reliability: 0.95 in our sample of 112 patients with rheumatoid arthritis.
- Invariant item hierarchy across: gender, age, disease duration, number of DMARDs, tender and swollen joint counts, number of hands affected, DAS score, HAQ score, overall ability and time in our sample of 112 patients with rheumatoid arthritis.

ABILHAND in systemic sclerosis patients

- 26 uni- and bimanual activities.
- Each item is answered on a 3-level scale (impossible, difficult, easy).
- Measurement range: approx. 9 logits.
- Measurement error: 0.41 logits in the centre of the scale.
- Least measurable difference: 0.18 logit in the centre of the scale.
- Separation reliability: 0.96 in our sample of 156 patients with systemic sclerosis.
- Invariant item hierarchy across: gender, age, language community, systemic sclerosis subsets, disease duration from the onset of Raynaud phenomenon, Finger-to-palm distance, Total Skin Score, presence of digital pit scars and digital ulcers, score of Health assessment Questionnaire (HAQ), disease activity score and total disease severity score (Total DSS)
- Test-retest reliability: ICC = 0.96 after a delay of 1 month
- Construct validity: ABILHAND vs HAQ (ρ = -0.73), and vs Total DSS(ρ = -0.53).

ABILHAND in hand surgery

- 22 bimanual activities, one uni-manual activity
- Each item is answered on a 3-level scale (impossible, difficult, easy).
- The item difficulty increases with bimanual involvement.
- Measurement range: approx. 9 logits.
- Measurement error: 0.38 logits in the centre of the scale.
- Least measurable difference: 0.15 logit in the centre of the scale.
- Separation reliability: 0.90 in our sample of 305 hand surgery patients.
- Invariant item hierarchy across: gender, age, dominant hand involvement, level of education, diagnosis, follow-up.
- Construct validity: ABILHAND vs QuickDASH (ρ = -0.77), vs Numerical pain scale (ρ = -0.49), vs SF-12 PCS (ρ = 0.56) and vs SF-12 MCS (ρ = 0.31).

References

1. Ashford, Stephen, Mike Slade, Fabienne Malaprade, and Lynne Turner-Stokes. "Evaluation of functional outcome measures for the hemiparetic upper limb: a systematic review." Journal of rehabilitation medicine 40, no. 10 (2008): 787-795.
2. http://rssandbox.iescagilly.be/abilhand.html
3. http://rssandbox.iescagilly.be/abilhand instructions.html
4. Ashford S, Slade M, Malaprade F, Turner-Stokes L. Evaluation of functional outcome measures for the hemiparetic upper limb: a systematic review. Journal of rehabilitation medicine. 2008 Nov 5;40(10):787-95.
5. Basakci Calik B, Gur Kabul E, Tasci M, Erel S, Simsek E, Demir P, Cobankara V. Reliability and Validity of the Turkish Version of the ABILHAND. 2019 Arch Rheumatol 26;34(4)395-405
6. CleanthousS, StrzokS, PompilusF, CanoS, Marquis P, Cohan S, Goldman MD, Kresa-Reahl K, Petrillo J, Castrillo-Viguera C, Cadavid D. Addressing the targeting range of the ABILHAND-56 in relapsing–remitting multiple sclerosis: A mixed methods psychometric study. Multiple Sclerosis Journal–Experimental, Translational and Clinical. 2018 May;4(2):2055217318776990.
7. Penta M, Tesio L, Arnould C, Zancan A, Thonnard JL. The ABILHAND questionnaire as a measure of manual ability in chronic stroke patients: Rasch-based validation and relationship to upper limb impairment. Stroke. 2001 Jul;32(7):1627-34.

28 "The Amyotrophic Lateral Sclerosis Functional Rating Scale (ALSFRS)"

Objective:

Its an instrument for assessing the activities of daily living of patients with Amyotrophic Lateral Sclerosis. Its also used to record disease progression in patients with ALS against other functional scales, quantitative isometric muscle testing, and global assessment scales.

Intended Population:

All the patients with amyotrophic lateral sclerosis.

Method of Use:

It consist of 10 items of functional rating scale which includes activities of daily living, speech, salivation, and swallowing. Each item is scored from 0 to 4. 4 is given if person is normal, and 0 for poor performance Following items are included in the assessment scale-

1. Speech
2. Salivation
3. Swallowing
4. Handwriting
5. Cutting food and handling utensils (with or without gastrostomy)
6. Dressing and hygiene
7. Turning in bed and adjusting bed clothes
8. Walking
9. Climbing stairs
10. Breathing

Interpretation:

minimum score: 0
maximum score: 40

The higher the score the more function is retained.

Reliability: Test-retest Reliability:

It showstest-retest reliability (ICC = 0.95) and is consistent.

Interrater/Intrarater Reliability

Kaufmann et al, 2007

- Excellent interrater reliability when administered by a primary rater; (ICC = 0.93)
- Excellent interrater reliability when administered by a back-up rater, n = 9 (ICC = 0.93)
- Excellent intrarater reliability, n = 41 (ICC = 0.95)
- Excellent reliability when test is administered on telephone, n = 27 (ICC = 0.97)

Validity

Criterion Validity

1. Brooks, B., Sanjak, M., et al. (1996). "The amyotrophic lateral sclerosis functional rating scale-Assessment of activities of daily living in patients with amyotrophic lateral sclerosis." Archives of Neurology 53(2): 141-147.
2. The sensitivity of ALSFRS scores to change in 53 patients' statuses over time was assessed in this two phased trial. The ALSFRS scores declined together in motor and pulmonary function indicating its sensitivity to change.

❑❑❑

29 "Achilles Tendon Total Rupture Score"

Objective:

A patient-reported instrument for measuring outcome after treatment for total Achilles tendon rupture. There is a need for a patient-relevant instrument to evaluate outcome after treatment in patients with a total. Achilles tendon rupture.To develop and validate a new patient-reported instrument for measuring outcome after treatment for total Achilles tendon rupture.

Intended Population:

Patients with a total Achilles tendon rupture after treatment.

Questionnaire:

Items asked:

- Are you limited because of decreased strength in the calf/ Achilles tendon/foot?
- Are you limited because of fatigue in the calf/ Achilles tendon/foot?
- Are you limited due to stiffness in the calf/Achilles tendon/foot?
- Are you limited because of pain in the calf/ Achilles tendon/foot?
- Are you limited during activities of daily living?
- Are you limited when walking on uneven surfaces?
- Are you limited when walking quickly upstairs or uphill?
- Are you limited during activities that include running?
- Are you limited during activities that include jumping?
- Are you limited in performing hard physical labor?

Subjects are asked to grade from 0 to 10 according to their level of limitations and/or difficulties.

Evidence [1]

Reliability

According to the study Validity and Reliability of the Achilles Tendon Total Rupture Score done by Ann Ganestam, et al noted good agreement on reassessment of patients using the ATRS and have concluded that the score is reliable and as such a valid health measurement.

Validity

The Danish version of the ATRS showed good criterion validity because it correlated moderately strongly with the physical component score and physical functioning subscores of the SF-36 and VISA-A.

Responsiveness

A floor or ceiling effect in more than 15% of the respondents was not found for the ATRS or VISA-A scores. The physical functioning subgroup of the SF-36 did, however, show a ceiling for this outcome measure in 24% of the respondents.

Miscellaneous

The Danish version of the ATRS showed moderately strong criterion validity. For study and follow-up purposes, the ATRS seems reliable for the comparison of groups of patients but has limited usability for the repeated assessment of individual patients in the clinic. For future use, the development of analysis guidelines would be desirable.

Contact

Katarina Nilsson-Helander, MD, Department of Orthopaedics, Sahlgrenska University Hospital/Östra, SE-416 85 Göteborg, Sweden (e-mail: ina.nilsson@telia.com).

References

1. Ann Ganestam, Kristoffer Barfod, Jakob Klit, Anders Troelsen. Validity and Reliability of the Achilles Tendon Total Rupture Score; The Journal of Foot and Ankle Surgery, Available online 18 August 2013
2. Nilsson-Helander, K., R. Thomee, et al. (2007). "The Achilles Tendon Total Rupture Score (ATRS): Development and Validation." Am J Sports Med 35(3): 421-426.

❑❑❑

30 "Action Research Arm Test (ARAT)"

Objective

The Action Research Arm Test (ARAT) is a 19 item observational measure used by physical therapists and other health care professionals to assess upper extremity performance (coordination, dexterity and functioning) in stroke recovery, brain injury and multiple sclerosis populations. The ARAT was originally described by Lyle in 1981 as a modified version of the Upper Extremity Function Test and was used to examine upper limb functional recovery post damage to the cortex.[1]

Items comprising the ARAT are categorized into four subscales (grasp, grip, pinch and gross movement) and arranged in order of decreasing difficulty, with the most difficult task examined first, followed by the least difficult task. Lyle proposed that this hierarchical ordering would improve efficiency of testing, as normal movement on the most difficult items would be indicative of successful performance on proceeding items.[1] Task performance is rated on a 4-point scale, ranging from 0 (no movement) to 3 (movement performed normally).[1]

Intended Population

The ARAT has been standardized for individuals with stroke, brain injury, multiple sclerosis, and Parkinson's disease. The test can be administered to individuals 13 years of age and older.[2]

Method of Use

Required Equipment

The following materials (Figure 1) are required for testing:[3]

- Chair without armrests
- Table
- Wooden blocks of various sizes
- Cricket ball
- Sharpening stone
- Alloy tubes
- Washer and bolt
- 2 glasses
- Sharpening stone
- Marbles
- Ball bearings
- Tin lid

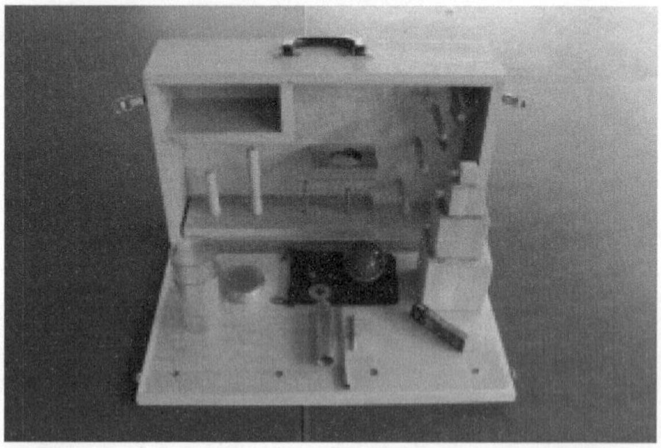

Positioning

Standard positioning for the ARAT has the subject seated upright in a chair with a firm back and no armrests. The head should be in a neutral position, with feet in contact with the floor. This body posture must be maintained throughout the testing period, with the trunk contacting the back of the chair. Feedback is provided as required, to prevent the subject from standing up, shifting laterally or leaning forward.[1]

Instructions

To ensure that test items are performed unilaterally and that the non-test hand remains visible throughout the assessment, the subject is instructed to begin with both forearms pronated and hands resting on the table. Exceptions to this rule are for tasks within the gross movement category which require that the subject begins with bilateral forearm pronation and hands resting on the lap.[1]

The administrator then provides instructions to the subject to perform tasks within the grasp, grip, pinch and gross movement subscales, while scoring the individual based on their performance of each task. The administrator follows instructions provided on the scoring sheet when instructing the subject about the required task.

For grasp tasks (6 items), the subject is instructed to lift testing materials from the surface of the table to a shelf located 37 cm above the starting point. For grip related tasks (4 items), the individual grips testing materials and moves them from one side of the table to the other. Pinching tasks (6 items) require the subject to perform similar movements to those in the grip subscale, but with the use of a fine motor pincer grip instead. Gross movement tasks (3 items) require the individual to move their testing arm to different resting positions including on top of their head, behind their head or to their mouth.[3][5]

Scoring & Interpretation

The 19 items comprising the ARAT are scored using a 4 point ordinal scale, as follows:

0 = no movement

1= movement task is partially performed

2 = movement task is completed but takes abnormally long

3 = movement is performed normally

As outlined by Lyle:[6]

Subjects are first asked to perform the most difficult task within a subscale. If a subject performs the task adequately with normal movement, they are scored a 3 on this item and all remaining items within a subscale. A score between 0-2 on the first item suggests that the second task (least difficult) must be evaluated. Subjects scoring 0 on the second task item are unlikely to be successful on subsequent scale items and are scored 0 for remaining tasks within a category.[3] Remaining moderate level tasks within a subscale are thus not evaluated. Otherwise, all test items within a category must be performed. Consequently, subjects may be asked to perform anywhere from 4 tasks to 19 tasks depending on their performance.[3]

Scores on the ARAT may range from 0-57 points, with a maximum score of 57 points indicating better performance.[3] There are no cut off scores as this assessment is continuous and based on a subject's observed mobility. The ARAT can be used to predict the functional recovery of the upper extremity in stroke rehabilitation. Scores of less that 10 points, between 10-56 points, and 57 points correlate with poor, moderate, and good recovery respectively.[7]

Evidence

Reliability

The ARAT has been shown to have strong psychometric properties. Many domains of reliability have been tested for the ARAT, with studies unanimously showing high reliability, including test-retest reliability ranging from 0.965-0.968 and inter-rater reliability ranging from 0.996-0.998.[2][9] The reliability of ARAT use in the Parkinson's patient population has also been thoroughly tested. The test-retest reliability was found to be 0.99, with a grip reliability of 0.93 and a gross movement reliability of 0.99.[10]

Validity

The ARAT has proven to have strong validity when compared with other upper extremity function scales. Concurrent validity was shown to be high for the ARAT when the assessment was measured against the upper extremity component of the Fugl-Meyer Assessment (FMA) and the Motor Assessment Scale (MAS).[9] In a study comparing scores on the ARAT in stroke populations with scores on the Wolf Motor Function Test, Motor Activity Log and Stroke Impact Scale, results showed good to moderate correlation, indicating a good predictive validity.[11]

Responsiveness

The ARAT has high responsiveness and the ability to detect clinically significant changes in the motor functioning of an individual's upper extremities, particularly in stroke recovery populations.[9]

Limitations

While the ARAT has many strengths, it is also plagued by limitations that can be improved upon in the future to render the tool more trustworthy and applicable to a larger population. One limitation of the ARAT is that scoring is subjective and based on the administrators' interpretation of the client's ability to do the task, with details of test item positioning and maximum time allocated for each item omitted and open to interpretation.[9][12] Scoring may also be impacted by lack of specification of the amount of time defining "abnormally long" used to differentiate a score of 2 or score of 3. Lack of standardization regarding the weight, size and source of testing materials may also result in variability in scoring.[1]

Also, while the ARAT is known for accurately measuring moderate to high degrees of motor impairments, it has shown to have poor sensitivity for measuring mild impairments.[12] Factors that decrease the comprehension of the instructions, such as cognitive impairments or Wernicke's aphasia, may also affect the quality of the results.

References

1. Yozbatiran N, Der-Yeghiaian L, Cramer SC. A standardized approach to performing the action research arm test. Neurorehabilitation and Neural Repair. 2008;22:78-90 doi:10.1177/1545968307305353
2. Shirley Ryan AbilityLab. Action Research Arm Test. 2016 [cited 1 May 2018]. Available from: https://www.sralab.org/rehabilitation-measures/action-research-arm-test
3. Heart and Stroke Foundation. Evaluation Summary-ARAT. Stroke Engine. 2018 [cited 1 May 2018]. Available from: https://www.strokengine.ca/en/quick/arat_quick/
4. Rehab Solutions. ARAT Kits. Rehab Solutions. 2014 [cited 1 May 2018]. Available from: http://www.aratkits.com/about/
5. SaliaRehab Action Research Arm Test. 2012 [Last accessed 30 January 2021]. Available from: https://www.youtube.com/watch?time_continue=3&v=bhkCB0qojZk
6. Lyle RC. A performance test for assessment of upper limb function in physical rehabilitation treatment and research. International Journal of Rehabilitation Research. (1981);4(4), 483-492. doi:10.1097/00004356-198112000-00001
7. Buma FE, Raemeakers M, Kwakkel G, Ramsey NF. Brain Function and Upper Limb Outcome in Stroke: A Cross-Sectional fMRI Study. PLoS ONE. 2015;10:10. doi: 10.1371/journal.pone.0139746
8. Action Research Arm Test. Internet Stroke Center. 2018 [cited 1 May 2018]. Available from: http://www.strokecenter.org/wp-content/uploads/2011/08/action_research_arm_test.pdf
9. McDonnell M. Action Research Arm Test. Australian Journal of Physiotherapy. 2008;54(3):220. PMID: 18833688
10. Song CS. Intrarater Reliability of the Action Research Arm Test for Individuals with Parkinson's Disease. J. Phys. Ther. Sci. 2012;24:1355-1357. https://doi.org/10.1589/jpts.24.1355
11. Chen HF, Lin KC, Wu CY, Chen CL. Rasch validation and predictive validity of the action research arm test in patients receiving stroke rehabilitation. Arch Phys Med Rehabil. 2012;93(6):1039-1045. doi: https://doi.org/10.1016/j.apmr.2011.11.033
12. Carpinella I, Cattaneo D, Ferrarin M. Quantitative assessment of upper motor function in Multiple Sclerosis using an instrumented Action Research Arm Test. Journal of Neuroengineering and Rehabilitation. 2014; 11:67. PMID: 24745972

Action Research Arm Test

Name Age/Gender

Date

Instructions

There are four subtitles: Grasp, Grip, Pinch and Gross Movements. Items in each are ordered so that:

- If the subject passes the first no more need to be administrated and he scores top marks for that sub-test
- If the subject fails to the second, he scores zero and again no more test needed to be performed in that subtest
- Otherwise he needs to compile all tasks within the subtest

Activity	Score

Grasp

1. Block, Wood, 10 cm cube (If score = 3, total = 18 and to Grip)
   Pick up a 10 cm block ________
2. Block, wood, 2.5 cm cube (If score = 0, total = 0 and go to Grip)
   Pick up 2.5 cm block ________
3. Block, Wood, 5cm cube ________
4. Block, Wood, 7.5 cm cube ________

5. Ball (Cricket), 7.5 cm diameter ________
6. Stone 10 × 2.5 × 1 cm ________

Coefficient of Reproducibility = 0.98
Coefficient of Scalability = 0.98

Grip

1. Pour water from glass to glass (If score = 3, total = 12, and go to Pinch) ________
2. Tube 2.25 cm (If score = 0 and go to Pinch) ________
3. Tube 1 × 16 cm ________
4. Washer (3.5 cm diameter) over bolt ________

Coefficient of reproducibility = 0.99
Coefficient of scalability = 0.98

Pinch

1. Ball bearing, 6mm, 3rd finger and thumb (If score = 3, total = 18 and go to Grossmt) ________
2. Marble, 1.5cm, index finger and thumb (If score = 0, total = 0 and go to Grossmt) ________
3. Ball bearing 2nd finger and thumb ________
4. Ball bearing 1st finger and thumb ________
5. Marble 3rd finger and thumb ________
6. Marble 2nd finger and thumb ________

Coefficient of reproducibility = 0.99
Coefficient of scalability = 0.98

Grossmt (Gross Movement)

1. Place hand behind head (If score = 3, total = 9 and finish) ________
2. (If score = 0, total and finish ________
3. Place hand on top of head ________
4. Hand to Mouth ________

Coefficient of reproducibility = 0.98
Coefficient of scalability = 0.97

Subscales on ARAT	Numbers of items per subscale	Score ranges per subscale
Grasp subscale	6 items	Score 0 – 18
Grip subscale	4 items	Score 0 – 12
Pinch subscale	6 items	Score 0 -18
Gross Movement subscale	3 items	Score 0 - 9

❑❑❑

31 "Activities-Specific Balance Confidence Scale"

Objective

Activities-specific balance confidence (ABC) scale is a structured questionnaire that measures an individual's confidence during ambulatory activities without falling or experiencing a sense of unsteadiness. It was developed in 1995 by Powell and Myers, and consists of 16 questions gauging the individual's confidence while doing activities[1].

Intended Population

The ABC scale is reported to be an accurate measure to identify individuals with a fall risk in populations of stroke, multiple sclerosis, Parkinson's, vestibular disorders, in elderly, and in other neurological conditions that can affect balance.

Method of Use

- Its a 16-item questionnaire where patients' rate their confidence while doing activities.
- Scoring from 0-100 (0 is no confidence and 100 is full confidence)
- Paper survey, 5-10 mins for administration.
- No Training required.
- Permission needs to be obtained before use from the authors.

Questionnaire

The ABC Scale has 16 questions that require the patient to rate his/her confidence that he/she will not lose balance or become unsteady while performing the following activities:

1. Walking around the house
2. Walking up or down stairs
3. Bending over to pick up a slipper from the front of a closet floor
4. Reaching for a small can off a shelf at eye level
5. Standing on tiptoes and reaching for something above his/her head
6. Standing on a chair to reach for something
7. Sweeping the floor
8. Walking outside the house to a car parked in the driveway
9. Getting into or out of a car
10. Walking across a parking lot to the mall
11. Walking up or down a ramp
12. Walking in a crowded mall where people rapidly walk past
13. Being bumped into people as they walk through the mall
14. Stepping on to or off an escalator while holding onto a railing
15. Stepping onto or off an escalator while holding onto parcels (so that they are not able to hold the railing)
16. Walking outside on icy sidewalks

Myers et al. (1998) use the following cut-off scores to define level of functioning among active older adults[2]:

1. Lower than 50 %: low level of physical functioning
2. 50-80 %: moderate level of physical functioning
3. Above 80 %: high level of physical functioning

Versions

Apart from the 16-item questionnaire, there are two other versions of the scale:

1. ABC-6 : https://statepi.jhsph.edu/wihs/wordpress/wp-content/uploads/2016/04/ABC6-1015.pdf

The scale has also be translated to multiple languages like chines, german etc.

Psychometric Properties

Reliability

- Internal Consistency: high Internal consistency (a = 0.96) in geriatric population, high Internal consistency (a=0.94) in Stroke[3]
- Test-Retest reliability: excellent overall test-retest reliability ($r=0.92$, $p<0.001$) in elderly, excellent test-retest reliability of the overall score (ICC = 0.85; 95% CI 0.68-0.93), and adequate to excellent item level test-retest reliability (ICC ranged from 0.53 – 0.93) in stroke[3].

Validity

- Criterion validity and construct validity: adequate in stroke patients[4].

References

1. Moiz JA, Bansal V, Noohu MM, Gaur SN, Hussain ME, Anwer S, Alghadir A. Activities-specific balance confidence scale for predicting future falls in Indian older adults. Clin Interv Aging. 2017 Apr 10;12:645-651. doi: 10.2147/CIA.S133523. PMID: 28435236; PMCID: PMC5391867.
2. Myers AM, Fletcher PC, Myers AH, Sherk W. Discriminative and evaluative properties of the activities-specific balance confidence (ABC) scale. J GerontolABiolSciMedSci.1998Jul;53(4):M287-94. doi: 10.1093/gerona/53a.4.m287. PMID: 18314568.
3. Botner, E.M., Miller, W.C., & Eng, J. J. Measurement properties of the Activities-specific Balance Confidence scale among individuals with stroke. Disability and Rehabilitation,2009; 27(4), 156-63.
4. Filiatrault, J., Gauvin, L., Fournier, M., Parisien, M., Robitaille, Y., Laforest, S., Corriveau, H., & Richard, L. Evidence of the psychometric qualities of a simplified version of the Activities-specific Balance Confidence scale for community-dwelling seniors. Archives of Physical Medicine and Rehabilitation, 2007; 88, 664-72.

❑❑❑

32 "The Activities-specific Balance Confidence (ABC) Scale Questionnaire Format"

The ABC can be self-administered or administered via personal or telephone interview. Larger typeset should be used for self-administration, while an enlarged version of the rating scale on an index card will facilitate in-person interviews. Regardless of method of administration, each respondent should be queried concerning their understanding of instructions, and probed regarding difficulty answering specific items.

Instructions to Participants:

For each of the following, please indicate your level of confidence in doing the activity without losing your balance or becoming unsteady from choosing one of the percentage points on the scale form 0% to 100%. If you do not currently do the activity in question, try and imagine how confident you would be if you had to do the activity. If you normally use a walking aid to do the activity or hold onto someone, rate your confidence as it you were using these supports. If you have any questions about answering any of these items, please ask the administrator.

Instructions for Scoring:

The ABC is an 11-point scale and ratings should consist of whole numbers (0-100) for each item. Total the ratings (possible range = 0 – 1600) and divide by 16 to get each subject's ABC score. If a subject qualifies his/her response to items #2, #9, #11, #14 or #15 (different ratings for "up" vs. "down" or "onto" vs. "off"), solicit separate ratings and use the lowest confidence of the two (as this will limit the entire activity, for instance the likelihood of using the stairs.)

- 80% = high level of physical functioning
- 50-80% = moderate level of physical functioning
- < 50% = low level of physical functioning

Myers AM (1998)

- < 67% = older adults at risk for falling; predictive of future fall

LaJoie Y (2004)

1. Powell, LE & Myers AM. The Activities-specific Balance Confidence (ABC) Scale. J Gerontol Med Sci 1995; 50(1): M28-34
2. Myers AM, Fletcher PC, Myers AN, Sherk W. Discriminative and evaluative properties of the ABC Scale. J Gerontol A Biol Sci Med Sci. 1998;53:M287-M294.
3. Lajoie Y, Gallagher SP. Predicting falls within the elderly community: comparison of postural sway, reaction time, the Berg balance scale and ABC scale for comparing fallers and non-fallers. Arch Gerontol Geriatr. 2004;38:11-26.

The Activities-specific Balance Confidence (ABC) Scale

For each of the following activities, please indicate your level of self-confidence by choosing a corresponding number from the following rating scale:

0% 10 20 30 40 50 60 70 80 90 100%

no confidence completely confident

"How confident are you that you will not lose your balance or become unsteady when you…

…walk around the house? ____%

…walk up or down stairs? ____%

…bend over and pick up a slipper from the front of a closet floor ____%

...reach for a small can off a shelf at eye level? ____%

...stand on your tiptoes and reach for something above your head? ____%

...stand on a chair and reach for something? ____%

...sweep the floor? ____%

...walk outside the house to a car parked in the driveway? ____%

...get into or out of a car? ____%

...walk across a parking lot to the mall? ____%

...walk up or down a ramp? ____%

...walk in a crowded mall where people rapidly walk past you? ____%

...are bumped into by people as you walk through the mall?____%

... step onto or off an escalator while you are holding onto a railing? ____%

... step onto or off an escalator while holding onto parcels such that you cannot hold onto the railing? ____%

...walk outside on icy sidewalks? ____%

❑❑❑

33 "The Lawton Instrumental Activities of Daily Living (IADL) Scale"

The assessment of functional status is critical when caring for older adults. Normal aging changes, acute illness, worsening chronic illness, and hospitalization can contribute to a decline in the ability to perform tasks necessary to live independently in the community. The information from a functional assessment can provide objective data to assist with targeting individualized rehabilitation needs or to plan for specific in home services such as meal preparation, nursing care, home-maker services, personal care, or continuous supervision. A functional assessment can also assist the clinician to focus on the person's baseline capabilities, facilitating early recognition of changes that may signify a need either for additional resources or for a medical work-up (Gallo, 2006).

The Lawton Instrumental Activities of Daily Living Scale (IADL) is an appropriate instrument to assess independent living skills (Lawton & Brody, 1969). These skills are considered more complex than the basic activities of daily living as measured by the Katz Index of ADLs (See Try this: Katz Index of ADLs). The instrument is most useful for identifying how a person is functioning at the present time, and to identify improvement or deterioration over time. There are eight domains of function measured with the Lawton IADL scale. Women are scored on all 8 areas of function; historically, for men, the areas of food preparation, housekeeping, laundering are excluded. Clients are scored according to their highest level of functioning in that category. A summary score ranges from 0 (low function, dependent) to 8 (high function, independent) for women, and 0 through 5 for men.

TARGET POPULATION:

This instrument is intended to be used among older adults, and can be used in community or hospital settings. The instrument is not useful for institutionalized older adults. It can be used as a baseline assessment tool and to compare baseline function to periodic assessments.

VALIDITY AND RELIABILITY:

Few studies have been performed to test the Lawton IADL scale psychometric properties. The Lawton IADL Scale was originally tested concurrently with the Physical Self-Maintenance Scale (PSMS). Reliability was established with twelve subjects interviewed by one interviewer with the second rater present but not participating in the interview process. Inter-rater reliability was established at .85. The validity of the Lawton IADL was tested by determining the correlation of the Lawton IADL with four scales that measured domains of functional status, the Physical Classification (6-point rating of physical health), Mental Status Questionnaire (10-point test of orientation and memory), Behavior and Adjustment rating scales (4-6-point measure of intellectual, person, behavioral and social adjustment), and the PSMS (6-item ADLs). A total of 180 research subjects participated in the study, however, few received all five evaluations. All correlations were significant at the .01 or .05 level. To avoid potential gender bias at the time the instrument was developed, specific items were omitted for men. This assessment instrument is widely used both in research and in clinical practice.

STRENGTHS AND LIMITATIONS:

The Lawton IADL is an easy to administer assessment instrument that provides self-reported information about functional skills necessary to live in the community. Administration time is 10-15 minutes. Specific deficits identified can assist nurses and other disciplines in planning for safe discharge. Limitations of the instrument can include the self-report or surrogate report method of administration rather than a demonstration of the functional task. This may lead either to over-estimation or under-estimation of ability. In addition, the instrument may not be sensitive to small, incremental changes in function.

FOLLOW-UP:

The identification of new disabilities in these functional domains warrants intervention and further assessment to prevent ongoing decline and to promote safe living conditions for older adults. If using the Lawton IADL tool with an acute hospitalization, nurses should communicate any deficits to the physicians and social workers/case managers for appropriate discharge planning.

References

1. www.ConsultGeriRN.org.
2. Gallo, J.J., & Paveza, G.J. (2006). Activities of daily living and instrumental activities of daily living assessment. In J.J. Gallo, H.R. Bogner, T. Fulmer,& G.J. Paveza (Eds.), Handbook of Geriatric Assessment (4th ed., pp. 193-240). MA: Jones and Bartlett Publishers.
3. Graf, C. (2006). Functional decline in hospitalized older adults. AJN, 106(1), 58-67.
4. Lawton, M.P., & Brody, E.M. (1969). Assessment of older people: Self-maintaining and instrumental activities of daily living. The Gerontologist, 9(3), 179-186.
5. Pearson, V. (2000). Assessment of function. In R. Kane, & R. Kane (Eds.), Assessing Older Persons. Measures, Meaning and Practical Applications (pp. 17-48). New York: Oxford University Press

The Lawton Instrumental Activities of Daily Living (IADL) Scale

Patient Name:____________________ **Date:**___________ **Patient ID #**____________________

LAWTON - BRODY INSTRUMENTAL ACTIVITIES OF DAILY LIVING SCALE (I.A.D.L.)			
Scoring: For each category, circle the item description that most closely resembles the client's highest functional level (either 0 or 1).			
A. Ability to Use Telephone		**E. Laundry**	
1. Operates telephone on own initiative-looks up and dials numbers, etc.	1	1. Does personal laundry completely	1
2. Dials a few well-known numbers	1	2. Launders small items-rinses stockings, etc.	1
3. Answers telephone but does not dial	1	3. All laundry must be done by others	0
4. Does not use telephone at all	0		
B. Shopping		**F. Mode of Transportation**	
1. Takes care of all shopping needs independently	1	1. Travels independently on public transportation or drives own car	1
2. Shops independently for small purchases			
3. Needs to be accompanied on any shopping trip	0		
4. Completely unable to shop	0	2. Arranges own travel via taxi, but does not otherwise use public transportation	1
	0	3. Travels on public transportation when accompanied by another	1
		4. Travel limited to taxi or automobile with assistance of another	0
		5. Does not travel at all	0

C. Food Preparation		G. Responsibility for Own Medications	
1. Plans, prepares and serves adequate meals independently	1	1. Is responsible for taking medication in correct dosages at correct time	1
2. Prepares adequate meals if supplied with ingredients	0	2. Takes responsibility if medication is prepared in advance in separate dosage	0
3. Heats, serves and prepares meals, or prepares meals, or prepares meals but does not maintain adequate diet	0	3. Is not capable of dispensing own medication	0
4. Needs to have meals prepared and served	0		
D. Housekeeping		**H. Ability to Handle Finances**	
1. Maintains house alone or with occasional assistance (e.g. "heavy work domestic help")	1	1. Manages financial matters independently (budgets, writes checks, pays rent, bills, goes to bank), collects and keeps track of income	1
2. Performs light daily tasks such as dish washing, bed making	1	2. Manages day-to-day purchases, but needs help with banking, major purchases, etc. 3. Incapable of handling money	1
3. Performs light daily tasks but cannot maintain acceptable level of cleanliness	1		
4. Needs help with all home maintenance tasks	1		
5. Does not participate in any housekeeping tasks	0		0
Score		**Score**	
Total score__________________			
A summary score ranges from 0 (low function, dependent) to 8 (high function, independent) for women and 0 through 5 for men to avoid potential gender bias.			
Source: Best Practices in Nursing Care to Older Adults, The Hartford Institute for Geriatric Nursing, New York University, College of Nursing, www.hartfordign.org.			

❑❑❑

34 "Bristol Activities of Daily Living Scale"

Synonyms	BADLS
Purpose	ability of daily living activity(those with dementia)

The Bristol Activities of Daily Living Scale (BADLS) is a 20-item questionnaire designed to measure the ability of someone with dementia to carry out daily activities such as dressing, preparing food and using transport.[1][2][3]

References

1. Bucks, RS; Ashworth, DL; Wilcock, GK; Siegfried, K (1996). *"Assessment of activities of daily living in dementia: development of the Bristol Activities of Daily Living Scale"*. Age and Ageing. 25 (2): 113–120. *doi:10.1093/ageing/25.2.113. PMID 8670538.*
2. Burns, Alistair; Lawlor, Brian; Craig, Sarah (2002). *"Rating scales in old age psychiatry"*. British Journal of Psychiatry. 180 (2): 161–167. *doi:10.1192/bjp.180.2.161. PMID 11823329.*
3. Bucks, RS; Haworth, Judy (2002). *"Bristol Activities of Daily Living Scale: a critical evaluation"*. Expert Review of Neurotherapeutics. 2 (5): 669–676. *doi:10.1586/14737175.2.5.669. PMID 19810983.*

Bristol Activities of Daily Living Scale

Bucks, R. S., Ashworth, D. L., Wilcock, G. K., and Siegfried, K. (1996)

Name of patient:...

Patient number:

Carer's Name:.......................

Assessment date: ....../....../.....

Relationship:................................

This questionnaire is designed to reveal the everyday ability of people who have memory difficulties of one form or another.

For each activity (No. 1 - 20), statements a - e refer to a different level of ability.

Thinking of the last 2 weeks, tick the box that represents your relative's/friend's AVERAGE ability. (If in doubt about which box to tick, choose the level of ability which represents their average performance over the last 2 Weeks. Tick 'Not applicable' if your relative never did that activity when they were well).

1. PREPARING FOOD		
	☐	(a) Selects and prepares food as required
	☐	(b) Able to prepare food if ingredients set out
	☐	(c) Can prepare food if prompted step by step
	☐	(d) Unable to prepare food even with prompting and supervision
	☐	(e) Not applicable

2. EATING	☐	(a) Eats appropriately using correct cutlery
	☐	(b) Eats appropriately if food made manageable and /or uses spoon
	☐	(c) Uses fingers to eat food
	☐	(d) Needs to be fed
	☐	(e) Not applicable
3. PREPARING DRINK	☐	(a) Selects and prepares drinks as required
	☐	(b) Can prepare drinks if ingredients left available
	☐	(c) Can prepare drinks if prompted step by step
	☐	(d) Unable to make a drink even with prompting and supervision
	☐	(e) Not applicable
4. DRINKING	☐	(a) Drinks appropriately
	☐	(b) Drinks appropriately with aids, beaker/straw etc.
	☐	(c) Does not drink appropriately even with aids but attempts to
	☐	(d) Has to have drinks administered (fed)
	☐	(e) Not applicable
5. DRESSING	☐	(a) Selects appropriate clothing and dresses self
	☐	(b) Puts clothes on in wrong order and /or back to front and /or dirty clothing
	☐	(c) Unable to dress self but moves limbs to assist
	☐	(d) Unable to assist and requires total dressing
	☐	(e) Not applicable
6. HYGIENE	☐	(a) Washes regularly and independently
	☐	(b) Can wash self if given soap, flannel, towel, etc.
	☐	(c) Can wash self if prompted and supervised
	☐	(d) Unable to wash self and needs full assistance
	☐	(e) Not applicable

7. TEETH	☐ ☐ ☐ ☐ ☐	(a) Cleans own teeth/dentures regularly and independently (b) Cleans teeth/dentures if given appropriate items (c) Requires some assistance, toothpaste on brush, brush to mouth etc (d) Full assistance given (e) Not applicable
8. BATH/ SHOWER	☐ ☐ ☐ ☐ ☐	(a) Bathes regularly and independently (b) Needs bath to be drawn/shower turned on but washes independently (c) Needs supervision and prompting to wash (d) Totally dependent, needs full assistance (e) Not applicable
9. TOILET/ COMMODE	☐ ☐ ☐ ☐ ☐	(a) Uses toilet appropriately when required (b) Needs to be taken to the toilet and given assistance (c) Incontinent of urine or faeces (d) Incontinent of urine and faeces (e) Not applicable
10. TRANSFERS	☐ ☐ ☐ ☐ ☐	(a) Can get in/out of chair unaided (b) Can get into a chair but needs help to get out (c) Needs help getting in and out of a chair (d) Totally dependent on being put into and lifted from chair e) Not applicable
11. MOBILITY	☐ ☐ ☐ ☐ ☐	(a) Walks independently (b) Walks with assistance i.e. furniture, arm for support (c) Uses aids to mobilise i.e. frame, sticks etc. (d) Unable to walk (e) Not applicable

12. ORIENTATION - TIME	☐ ☐ ☐ ☐ ☐	(a) Fully orientated to time/day/date etc. (b) Unaware of time/day etc but seems unconcerned (c) Repeatedly asks the time/day/date (d) Mixes up night and day (e) Not applicable
13. ORIENTATION - SPACE	☐ ☐ ☐ ☐ ☐	(a) Fully orientated to surroundings (b) Orientated to familiar surroundings only (c) Gets lost in home, needs reminding where bathroom is, etc. (d) Does not recognize home as own and attempts to leave (e) Not applicable
14. COMMUNICATION	☐ ☐ ☐ ☐ ☐	(a) Able to hold appropriate conversation (b) Shows understanding and attempts to respond verbally with gestures (c) Can make self understood but difficulty understanding others (d) Does not respond to, or communicate with others (e) Not applicable
15. TELEPHONE	☐ ☐ ☐ ☐ ☐	(a) Uses telephone appropriately, including obtaining correct number (b) Uses telephone if number given verbally/visually or predrilled (c) Answers telephone but does not make calls (d) Unable/unwilling to use telephone at all (e) Not applicable
16 HOUSEWORK / GARDENING	☐ ☐ ☐ ☐ ☐	(a) Able to do housework/gardening to previous standard (b) Able to do housework/gardening but not to previous standard (c) Limited participation with a lot of supervision (d) Unwilling/unable to participate in previous activities (e) Not applicable

17. SHOPPING	☐	(a) Shops to previous standard
	☐	(b) Only able to shop for 1 or 2 items with or without a list
	☐	(c) Unable to shop alone, but participates when accompanied
	☐	(d) Unable to participate in shopping even when accompanied
	☐	(e) Not applicable
18. FINANCES	☐	(a) Responsible for own finances at previous level
	☐	(b) Unable to write cheque. Can sign name & recognises money values
	☐	(c) Can sign name but unable to recognise money values
	☐	(d) Unable to sign name or recognise money values
	☐	(e) Not applicable
19. GAMES/HOBBIES	☐	(a) Participates in pastimes/activities to previous standard
	☐	(b) Participates but needs instruction/supervision
	☐	(c) Reluctant to join in, very slow needs coaxing
	☐	(d) No longer able or willing to join in
	☐	(e) Not applicable
20. TRANSPORT	☐	(a) Able to drive, cycle or use public transport independently
	☐	(b) Unable to drive but uses public transport or bike etc.
	☐	(c) Unable to use public transport alone
	☐	(d) Unable/unwilling to use transport even when accompanied
	☐	(e) Not applicable

❑❑❑

35 "Activities of Daily Living (ADLs)"

Activities of daily living (ADLs or ADL) is a term used in healthcare to refer to people's daily self-care activities. Sidney Katz et al first came up with the term in the 1950s and the term has been revised since. Physiotherapists and other health professionals often use a person's ability or inability to perform ADLs as a measurement of their functional status, particularly in regard to people post-injury, with disabilities and the elderly.[1]

A 2016 National Health Interview Survey in the USA found that 20.7% of adults 85 or older, 7% of those aged 75 to 84 and 3.4% of those aged 65 to 74 needed help with ADLs. Overall, 6.4% of adults aged more than 65 years needed help with personal care in 2016.[2]

A clear trend is emerging of increased caregiving due to rapid growth in the number of older adults and because of the faster-growing cohort of older adults are those age 80 and older. More than half of 85- to 89-year-olds (59 per cent) need caregiving because of health or functioning reasons. From age 90 on, only a minority of individuals (24 per cent) do not need help from others. Dementia is a reason often for needing a family caregiver. In 2011 in the USA, 3.5 million of the 4.9 million older adults who received help for health or functioning reasons were classified as having probable dementia.[3]

Basic and Instrumental ADLs

Generally, older adults need to be able to manage ADLs and IADLs in order to live independently without the assistance of another person.

Basic ADLs- these are the basic self-care tasks

- Walking (ambulating) ability to get around the home or outside.
- Feeding, ability to get food from a plate into one's mouth.
- Dressing and grooming, ability to select clothes, putting them on, and adequately managing one's personal appearance.
- Toileting, ability to get to and from the toilet, using it appropriately, and cleaning oneself.
- Bathing, ability to wash one's face and body in the bath or shower.
- Transferring, ability to move from one body position to another. This includes being able to move from a bed to a chair, or into a wheelchair. This can also include the ability to stand up from a bed or chair in order to grasp a walker or other assistive device.

Instrumental ADLs- require more complex thinking skills, including organisational skills.

- Managing finances, such as paying bills and managing financial assets.
- Managing transportation, either via driving or by organising other means of transport.
- Shopping and meal preparation. ie everything required to get a meal on the table. It also covers shopping for clothing and other items required for daily life.
- Housecleaning and home maintenance. Cleaning kitchens after eating, maintaining living areas reasonably clean and tidy, and keeping up with home maintenance.
- Managing communication, eg telephone and mail.
- Managing medications, ie obtaining medications and taking them as directed.[5]

Physiotherapy

Physiotherapists assess ADLs and IADLs as part of

assessing an older person's "function." Problems with ADLs and IADLs usually reflect problems with physical health and/or cognitive health. Identifying functional difficulties can help us diagnose and manage problems affecting their everyday life.

Physiotherapists help people perform ADLs through exercise therapy and improving strength and joint mobility. Improving gait speed, grip strength, pain reduction, improved balance etc all improve a persons ability to perform ADLs. A physiotherapists role is also to encourage exercise, prescribe exercises and were appropriate refer to exercise programs eg Otago exercise program. These activities can all help in the performance of ADL. Help is also achieved through advice and teaching the use of assistive devices eg 4 wheel walkers, orthotics

A 2016 study on the effects of inpatient physiotherapy on the ADL status of elderly persons demonstrated the high effectiveness of the hospital physical therapy program in terms of reducing the risk of falls, improving physical ability, increasing handgrip strength, and improving subjective parameters such as pain intensity, self-reported well-being and mobility. [6]

A 2014 systematic review of functional training on muscle strength, physical functioning, and activities of daily living in older adults concluded that functional training may be a better option than muscle strength training alone if the goal is to reduce ADL disability in older adults.[7]Thus to improve ADLs balance programs are a good option.

Outcome Measures

Various outcome measures are available:1. ADL specific outcomes and 2. General outcome measures " ADL specific: eg Katz ADL, Barthel index, Lawton IADL scale, Bristol Activities of Daily Living Scale, FIM. General: eg TUG, 10 metre walk, grip strength, Berg balance scale, Romberg test, BOOMER.

References

1. Wikipedia. Activities of daily living. Available from: https://en.wikipedia.org/wiki/Activities_of_daily_living (last accessed 6.5.2019)
2. McKnights Senior Living. Dec. 20 2017. CDC: More than 20% of 85+ adults need ADL assistance Available from: https://www.mcknightsseniorliving.com/home/news/cdc-more-than-20-of-85-adults-need-adl-assistance/ (last accessed 6.5.2019)
3. Committee on Family Caregiving for Older Adults; Board on Health Care Services; Health and Medicine Division; National Academies of Sciences, Engineering, and Medicine; Schulz R, Eden J, editors. Families Caring for an Aging America. Washington (DC): National Academies Press (US); 2016 Nov 8. 2, Older Adults Who Need Caregiving and the Family Caregivers Who Help Them. Available from: https://www.ncbi.nlm.nih.gov/books/NBK396397/ (last accessed 6.5.2019)
4. Audiopedia ADL. Available from: https://www.youtube.com/watch?v=7C0FFUG0Bk4 (last accessed 6.5.2019)
5. Better health while aging. What are Activities of Daily Living (ADLs) & Instrumental Activities of Daily Living (IADLs)? Available from: https://betterhealthwhileaging.net/what-are-adls-and-iadls/ (last accessed 6.5.2019)
6. Zasadzka E, Kropińska S, Pawlaczyk M, Krzymińska-Siemaszko R, Lisiński P, Wieczorowska-Tobis K. Effects of inpatient physical therapy on the functional status of elderly individuals. Journal of physical therapy science. 2016;28(2):426-31. Available from: https://www.ncbi.nlm.nih.gov/pmc/articles/PMC4792984/ (last accessed 7.5.2019)
7. Liu CJ, Shiroy DM, Jones LY, Clark DO. Systematic review of functional training on muscle strength, physical functioning, and activities of daily living in older adults. European review of aging and physical activity. 2014 Oct;11(2):95. Available from: https://eurapa.biomedcentral.com/articles/10.1007/s11556-014-0144-1#Abs1 (last accessed 7.5.2019)

❑❑❑

36

"American College of Rheumatology Criteria for the Fibromyalgia Classification (1990)"

Based on comparing patients with similar but non-fibromyalgia pain complaints, the American College of Rheumatology (ACR) - committee found that the presence of widespread pain (WSP) combined with at least 11 of 18 tender points best separated patients with fibromyalgia (FM)and controls, even though some combinations of symptoms (e.g., fatigue, cognitive problems) were not evaluated. This occurred because the authors did not recognize the importance of these symptoms at the time of the study. The authors suggested that the presence of 11 of 18 tender points and the simultaneous presence of WSP for at least 3 months should be the classification criteria for FM[1].

Intended Population: Patients suffering from Fibromyalgia

Method of Use: Initially intended for research purposes, the criteria were later widely used in clinical diagnosis, particularly among rheumatologists; they were also used in basic science and clinical studies. The endorsement by the ACR aided in establishing FM as a respectable clinical diagnosis.

Evidence: The reliability and validity of the TP examination outside the context of FMS specialized rheumatology settings was never tested.

ACR Criteria for Fibromyalgia

- **ACR criteria**
  - History of chronic widespread pain ≥ 3 months
  - Patients must exhibit ≥ 11 of 18 tender points
- **Inclusion of other symptoms did not improve the accuracy of the criteria**
- **No exclusions for other diseases or abnormal laboratory/radiographic findings**
- **ACR criteria are both sensitive (88.4%) and specific (81.1%)**

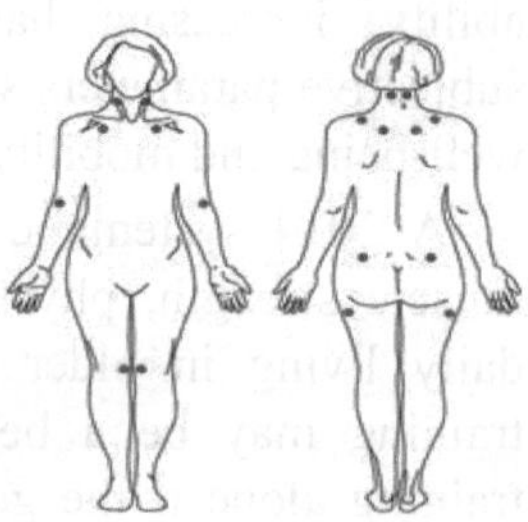

Wolfe F, et al. *Arthritis Rheum.* 1990:33:160-172.

References

1. Häuser W, Wolfe F. Diagnosis and diagnostic tests for fibromyalgia (syndrome)Rheumatismo, 2012; 64 (4): 194-205

❑❑❑

37 Amputee Mobility Predictor

Amputee mobility predictor (AMP) is a quick and easily administered assessment tool designed to measure the functional status of lower-limb amputees with (AMPPRO) and without (AMPnoPRO) the use of a prosthesis. The test was also designed to be clinically feasible in that it takes less than 10 to 15 minutes to administer and requires very little equipment. AMP can be used before prosthetic fitting to predict functional mobility after prosthetic fitting. Although the AMP can be administered both with (AMPPRO) and without (AMPnoPRO) a prosthesis, the AMPnoPRO has the greatest potential to assist in prosthetic prescription.

The AMP was also designed to assess the specific tasks identified in the 5-level Medicare functional classification system (MFCL). MFCL was developed in 1995 by the US Health Care Financing Administration (HCFA) to describe the functional abilities of persons who had undergone lower-limb amputation. (K0, K1, K2, K3, K4)[1]

K-Level 0: Does not have the ability or potential to ambulate or transfer safely with or without assistance, and a prosthesis does not enhance quality of life or mobility.

K-Level 1: Has the ability or potential to use a prosthesis for transfers or ambulation in level surfaces at a fixed cadence. Typical of the limited and unlimited household ambulator

K-Level 2: Has the ability or potential for ambulation with the ability to transverse low-level environmental barriers such as curbs, stairs, or uneven surfaces. Typical of the limited community ambulator.

K-Level 3: Has the ability or potential for ambulation with variable cadence. Typical of the community ambulator who has the ability to transverse most environmental barriers and may have vocational, therapeutic, or exercise activity that demands prosthetic use beyond simple locomotion.

K-Level 4: Has the ability or potential for prosthetic ambulation that exceeds basic ambulation skills, exhibiting high impact, stress, or energy levels. Typical of the prosthetic demands of the child, active adult, or athlete.

Intended Population: Unilateral or Bilateral Lower limb amputees. However, bilateral amputee subjects with amputation levels higher than trans-tarsal foot amputations may be tested only with the AMPPRO because it is not physically possible for them to perform the AMPnoPRO.[1] However, an AMP-Bilat was developed that adapted the scoring for people with bilateral limb loss. These changes included not deducting points for using hands to rise from a chair or immediate balance in standing. In the AMPPRO people with bilateral limb loss will score lower and thus show a lower potential for ambulation, these factors are taken into consideration in the AMP-Bilat.[2] Example of the AMP-Bilat Form.

Methods of Use: The total score range for the AMP is 0 to 42 points. In its AMPnoPRO configuration, the highest possible score is 38 points because item 8, single-limb standing, is eliminated (standing on the prosthetic side is impossible). By using an assistive device, the subjects' potential total score possibilities increase by 5 points (to 43 and 47 points for the AMPnoPRO and AMPRO, respectively), depending on the type of assistive device used during testing.

Most AMP items offer 3 scoring choices: 0 indicates inability to perform the task, 1 implies minimal level of achievement or that some assistance was required in completing the task, and 2 denotes complete independence or mastery of the task

The items are organized with an increasing level of difficulty to allow for the progressive assessment of the amputee.

Items 1 and 2 test the ability to maintain sitting balance. The sitting reach test assesses the ability to displace one's center of mass (COM) and to return to balanced sitting without falling. If the amputee subject does not have the ability to sit and reach in sitting independently, then the possibility for even limited prosthetic use is remote and the amputee subject therefore would be classed as a level K0.

Items 3 through 7 are designed to examine the amputee subject's ability to maintain balance while performing the relatively simple task of transferring from chair to chair and standing unchallenged. These skills are necessary for a level 1 amputee subject who would receive a prosthesis for transfers and simple standing activities. The ability to perform these test items safely would probably suggest that the patient could manage a prosthesis in limited situations, especially in a supervised environment.

Items 8 through 13 are more challenging activities related to standing balance. Subject performs several tests including; single-limb balance, modified standing reach test, nudge test, and check reactive balance. In order to maintain balance during these tests subject requires adequate somatosensory and vestibular systems. Succeeding these tests means that the amputee subject has the potential to be a safe household ambulator; that is, he/she can function at level K2

AMP items 14 through 20 evaluate the quality of gait and the ability to negotiate specific obstacles. These qualities are defined as k3 ambulator or level 4 suggesting, the amputee subject can perform all skills with greater ease.

Item 21 accounts for the use of particular assistive devices.[1]

Validity

The concurrent validity of the AMP was tested against 2 known tests, the 6-minute walk, which is a rehabilitation standard, and the Amputee Activity Survey (AAS), which has been shown to be a valid subjective instrument for amputee subjects. The 6-minute walk distance showed a moderate to high positive relationship with both the AMPnoPRO and AMPPRO ($r = .69$, $P < .0001$; $r = .82$, $P < .0001$, respectively). The AAS had a high to moderate positive correlation to the AMPnoPRO and AMPPRO ($r = .67$, $P < .0001$; $r = .77$, $P < .0001$, respectively).

Predictive validity of the AMP was also examined by first determining the relationship between the 6-minute walk distance and the AMPnoPRO test, age, time after amputation, and comorbidity. The overall model was statistically significant ($P < .0001$) indicating that together these variables do a fairly good job of explaining the variance in the 6-minute walk distance.[1]

Another study with 82 patients with lower limb loss compared the predictive ability of the AMPnoPRO to a single limb balance test, and the Lower-Extremity Motor Coordination Test. They measured outcome with the TUG, the 2-min Walking Test, and K levels. The AMPnoPRO was found to be the best statistical predictor for mobility outcome with a prosthesis. Further research is needed as this was a small sample size. [4]

Reliability

Gailey et al tested the intra and inter-rater reliability of the AMP with and without a prosthesis using Intra-class correlation coefficients (ICCs). The inter-rater score demonstrated excellent reliability (.99) for the AMPPRO and the AMPnoPRO. Test-retest intra-rater reliability also had excellent reliability, with rater 1 and rater 2 ICC scores of .96 and .98, respectively, for the AMPPRO. ICC scores for the AMPnoPRO were .97 and .86, respectively, for rater 1 and rater 2.[1]

Resources

Predictor, A. M., Index, L. C., Group, S. I., Medicine, A., Index, R. M., Index, T. B., … Classification, I. (2005). Lower Limb Prosthetic Outcome Measures: A Review of the Literature 1995 to 2005 Elizabeth Condie, Grad Dip Phys, FCSP, Helen Scott, Grad Dip Phys, MCSP, and Shaun Treweek, BSc, PhD American Academy of Orthotists and Prosthetists Lower Limb Prosthetic Outcome Measures: A Review of the Literature 1995 to 2005.

Kaluf, B. (2014). Evaluation of Mobility in Persons with Limb Loss Using the Amputee Mobility Predictor and the Prosthesis Evaluation Questionnaire Y Mobility Subscale: A Six-Month Retrospective Chart Review, 26(2).

References

1. Gailey, R. S., Roach, K. E., Applegate, E. B., Cho, B., Cunniffe, B., Licht, S., … Cho, B. (2002). The Amputee Mobility Predictor: An Instrument to Assess Determinants of the Lower-Limb Amputee's Ability to Ambulate, 83 (May). https://doi.org/10.1053/apmr.2002.32309
2. Raya MA, Gailey RS, Gaunaurd IA, Ganyard H, Knapp-Wood J, McDonough K, Palmisano T. Amputee mobility predictor-bilateral: a performance-based measure of mobility for people with bilateral lower-limb loss. Journal of Rehabilitation Research & Development. 2013 Nov 1;50(7).
3. Mission Gait. Amputee Mobility Predictor - Setup and Instruction. Sep 2019. Available from: https://youtu.be/goN4j6WRRWE.
4. Spaan MH, Vrieling AH, van de Berg P, Dijkstra PU, van Keeken HG. Predicting mobility outcome in lower limb amputees with motor ability tests used in early rehabilitation. Prosthetics and orthotics international. 2017 Apr;41(2):171-7.

□□□

38 Arthritis Hand Function Test (AHFT)

The Arthritis Hand Function Test (AHFT) is an 11-item performance-based test designed to measure hand strength and dexterity in persons with arthritis and rheumatoid arthritis. It deals with the areas of self-care, work and leisure in such patients[1].

This test is divided into 4 subscales and tests are performed bilaterally:

1. Strength,
2. Applied Strength,
3. Dexterity, and
4. Applied Dexterity

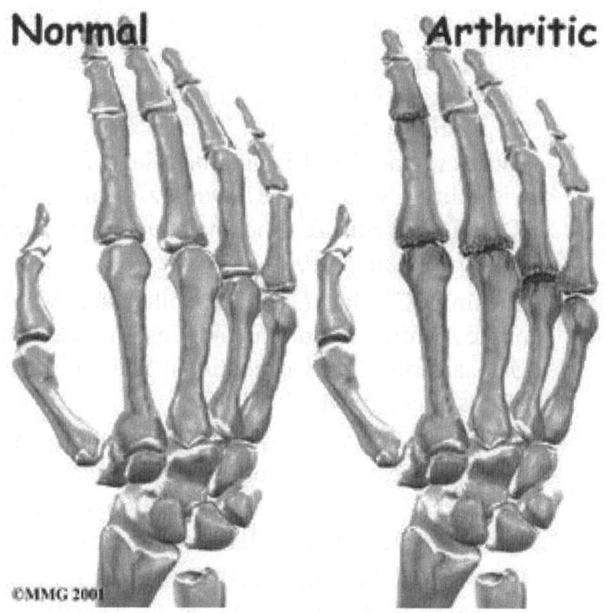

It was developed by Catherine Backman and Hazel Mackie in 1997 and requires purchasing the scoring forms from The University of British Columbia, Canada[2].

Intended Population

Useful in both research and clinical applications, the AHFT can be used for pre- and post-operative evaluations, and to measure treatment outcomes pertaining to hand function. It is particularly targeted towards:

1. Osteo-arthritis
2. Rheumatoid arthritis
3. Systemic Sclerosis

Procedure

Equipment Required

The equipment required is:

1. Sphygmomanometer,
2. pinch meter,
3. 9-hole pegboard,
4. shoe,
5. button board,
6. 2 safety pins,
7. theraplast,
8. plate,
9. knife and fork,
10. coins and a box,
11. wooden tray,
12. 12 cans of soup,
13. pitcher and a glass,
14. 1 litre container,
15. measuring cup,
16. stopwatch.

Training Required

AFHT comes with a scoring and instruction Manual that describes the purpose of the test, the procedure for each item, and instructions for assembly of the test kit. It is not difficult to administer and does not require additional training.

Time Required

The test can be administered in approx. 20 minutes.

Method

The 4 sub-scales are to be administered bilaterally and the scoring noted down on the manual sheet.

Dexterity: performed one hand at a time, 1 time, 1 item

1. 9-hole peg test timed for place and removal in a 9-hole pegboard.

Strength: performed one hand at a time, 3 trials, 3 items

1. gross grip strength (mm Hg)
2. tip pinch with the thumb and index (kg)
3. three-point pinch strength with the thumb, index and middle finger (kg)

Applied Dexterity: bilateral actions, 5 items

1. Fasten and unfasten 4 buttons
2. Lace a shoe and tie a bow;
3. Pin and unpin two safety pins in a cloth;
4. Pick up and manipulate four coins into a slot;
5. Cut a piece of putty with a knife and fork into four pieces.

Applied Strength: bilateral actions, 2 items

1. Individual lifts a tray with six filled tin cans, which added or subtracted depending on the patients' lifting ability. Scored on the no. of cans filled (0-12)
2. Individual lifts one liter of water. Water is added or subtracted depending on the patients' lifting ability. Scored on the total amount of water obtained.

Scoring

Scoring is according to the manual provided. the acquired scores are compared to established normative values.

Evidence

Reliability

1. Interrater Reliability: In RA, intra-class correlation coefficient (ICC) ranged from 0.89 to 1.0. In OA, ICC ranged from 0.99 to 1.0. shows strong interrater reliability[3][4].
2. Test Re-test Reliability: ICC of 0.53 to 0.95 in RA; ICC 0.74 – 0.96 in OA[3][4].

Validity

1. with Jebson's Hand function Test: The AHFT correlated well (r=.63)for the right hand, but poorly (r=.08) for the left hand[5].
2. with Arthritis Impact Measurement Scales: The AHFT correlated well (r=.71) with the dexterity component on the AIMS[5]

References

1. Poole JL. Measures of hand function: Arthritis Hand Function Test (AHFT), Australian Canadian Osteoarthritis Hand Index (AUSCAN), Cochin Hand Function Scale, Functional Index for Hand Osteoarthritis (FIHOA), Grip Ability Test (GAT), Jebsen Hand Function Test (JHFT), and Michigan Hand Outcomes Questionnaire (MHQ). Arthritis Care Res (Hoboken). 2011 Nov;63 Suppl 11:S189-99. doi: 10.1002/acr.20631. PMID: 22588744.
2. Poole, J.L. (2003), Measures of adult hand function: Arthritis Hand Function Test (AHFT), Grip Ability Test (GAT), Jebsen Test of Hand Function, and The Rheumatoid Hand Functional Disability Scale (The Duruöz Hand Index [DHI]). Arthritis & Rheumatism, 49: S59-S66. doi:10.1002/art.11406
3. Backman C, Mackie H. Reliability and Validity of the Arthritis Hand Function Test in Adults with Osteoarthritis. The Occupational Therapy Journal of Research, 1997. 17:1,55-66.
4. Backman C, Mackie M, Harris J. Arthritis Hand Function Test: Development of a Standardized Assessment Tool. The Occupational Therapy Journal of Research, 1991.11:4, 245-256
5. Duruöz MT, Poiraudeau S, Fermanian J, Menkes C, Amor B, Dougados M, et al. Development and validation of a rheumatoid hand functional disability scale that assesses functional handicap. J Rheumatol 1996; 23: 1167– 72.

❑❑❑

39 Back Pain Functional Scale

Back pain is a vast topic to discuss as it shows its impacts on a patient's physical, emotional, and social quality of life[1]. Furthermore, treating back pain involves considering the biopsychosocial model into aspect [1]. Besides treating back pain, there is a need for using appropriate and suitable outcome measures in clinical practice. However, none of the single outcome measures can include and assess all perspectives of pain considering the patient's quality of life into aspects. In addition, there are different outcome measures used based on the needs of patients, their severity of symptoms, and their clinical presentations[2]. Therefore, it is necessary for Health Care Professionals to use valid and reliable outcome measures to evaluate and treat back pain effectively. Consecutively, an outcome measure that has psychometric properties in terms of good validity, reliability, sensitivity, and utility should be considered in clinical practices[2]. Hence, it is necessary to know the psychometric property of an outcome measure prior to its implication. Moreover, there are lists of outcome measures used to quantify back pain scores. These are the Numerical rating scale (NRS), Roland-Morris disability questionnaire (RMDQ), Back pain functional score, Oswestry disability index (ODI), Pain self-efficacy Questionnaire (PSEQ) and the patient-specific functional scale (PSFS) in order to assess and treat back pain efficiently.

However, it is not possible to use all these diagnostic tools to examine back pain functional scores. Besides, to assess the patient's quality of pain and physical function, the 'Back pain functional scale' is widely used in practice[3].

Back Pain Functional Scale

The Back Pain Functional Scale (BPFS) is a subjective scale used to measure the patient's physical function after low back pain. This scale was developed by Stratford et al. (2000). It is simple and easy to understand and administer by the patients. This scale is based upon the International Classification of Function (ICF) model proposed by the World Health Organisation. It is used to evaluate the patient's level of physical independence during the initial two weeks of low back pain. However, it is not used for backpain after two weeks. This scale consists of a total score of 60. Moreover, the patient's score can be measured from the responses obtained on the Likert scale (0 to 5), and accordingly, a total score is summed up out of 60. Furthermore, the maximum score obtained indicates the maximum physical abilities of the patients. In addition, this scale also has an 'Adjusted score' ranging from 0 (0%)-unable to perform any activity to 60 (100%)-no difficulty in any activity[4].

Method of Use

The BPFS consists of 12 items:

1. Usual work, housework, or school activities
2. Usual hobbies, recreational, or sporting activities
3. Performance of heavy activities around your home
4. Bending or stooping
5. Putting on your shoes or socks
6. Lifting a box of groceries from the floor
7. Sleeping
8. Standing for 1 hour
9. Walking 1 mile
10. Going up or down 2 flights of stairs (about 20 steps)
11. Sitting for 1 hour
12. Driving for 1 hour

Responses	Points
Unable to perform activity	0
Extreme difficulty	1
Quite a bit of difficulty	2
Moderate difficulty	3
A little bit of difficulty	4
No difficulty	5

Total Score = Sum of points from all 12 measures

Adjusted Total Score = Total Score / 60

Interpretation

- Minimum Score: 0
- Maximum Score: 60
- Maximum Adjusted Score: 1 (100%)
- The higher the score the greater the patient's functional ability

Total Score (Adjusted)	Interpretation
0 (0%)	unable to perform any activity
60 (100%)	no difficulty in any activity

Psychometric properties of Back Pain Functional Scale (BPFS)

According to Stratford et al. (2000), this scale has a minimal detectable change of 22.2% with a standard error of measure of 6.5% at a 95% confidence interval. In addition, this scale has excellent test-retest reliability with an intra-class correlation coefficient of 0.88 at a confidence interval of 77%. Thus, this representation indicates that this scale can be used in the clinical setting to measure the functional outcome of patients after low back pain[4].

However, there are other functional scales used to measure physical function in patients with low back pain besides back pain functional scale. These are 'Roland-Morris disability scale', 'Oswestry disability scale', and 'Short form 36 surveys'. Therefore, it is necessary to consider the relative efficacy and effectiveness of 'Back Pain Functional Scale' as compared to other scales.

Evidence

There is one study aim to evaluate the correlation of back pain functional scale with other functional scales. This study has examined correlation of 'Back pain functional scale with 'Roland and Morris', 'Oswestry disability scale', and 'Short form 36 surveys'.

Advantages and Disadvantages of Back Pain Functional scale

Advantages

- Easy to demonstrate and administer
- Good psychometric properties
- Used for assessing physical functions during stages weeks of back pain
- The patient can easily understand and use this scale

Disadvantages

- Cannot be used in patients having back pain after two weeks

Recommendations

Further research is required to know the sensitivity of this scale over time. In addition, the aforementioned study was performed considering only 120 back pain patients[3]. However, there are approximately one-quarter of patients affected by back pain annually[2], Thus, the results obtained from this study cannot be generalizable to overall population. Hence, further research on larger population is required to prove the generalisability of the results obtained from this study[3].

References

1. Allegri M, Montella S, Salici F, Valente A, Marchesini M, Compagnone C, Baciarello M, Manferdini ME, Fanelli G. Mechanisms of low back pain: a guide for diagnosis and therapy. F1000Research. 2016:5
2. Maughan EF, Lewis JS. Outcome measures in chronic low back pain. European Spine Journal. 2010 Sep 1:19(9): 1484-94.
3. Koc M, Bayar B, Bayar K. A comparison of Back pain functional scale with Roland Morris disbility questionnaire, Oswestry disability index, and short form 36-health survey. Spine. 2018 Jun 15:43(12):877-82
4. Stratford, P. W. and Binkley, J. M. "A comparison study of the back pain functional scale and Roland Morris Questionnaire. North American Orthopaedic Rehabilitation Research Network." J Rheumatol 2000 27(8): 1928-1936.

❑❑❑

40 Bangla Clubfoot Tool

The Bangla clubfoot tool [1] was developed to suit the context of the large Walk For Life clubfoot program in Bangladesh. It was largely developed from components of existing validated clubfoot assessment measures (such as the Roye Score), and adapted for local use. It is accurate, expedient, and inexpensive and has been shown to be a very reliable evaluation instrument[1].

Intended Population

This tool is used to assess outcomes for children with clubfoot in Bangladesh and may be a suitable measure to use across other lower and middle income settings. It is designed for use in busy clinics to assess results of clubfoot management in children of walking age, ie mid-term to longer-term results[1].

Method of Use

Three areas of examination are included: parent satisfaction, gait, clinical examination of the clubfoot[1]. The subjective elements of parents' assessment addressed satisfaction with their child's treatment (five questions). The gait and clinical aspects of assessment included the children's physical ability to squat, walk, run, and use stairs, (four items) and objective assessment of heel position and ankle range (two items)[2].

A. Partial Rating	Yes	Don't Know	No	Mean Score (%)	Rating
	+1	0	-1		#
1. Happy with child's feet?					
2. Recommend to others?					
3. Does child play with others?					
4. Does child wear shoes of choice?					
5. Does child have pain?					
Parental rating scale (– / 5)					
B. Gait Assessment	**Yes**	**Not fully / with assistance**	**No**	**Mean Score (%)**	**Rating**
	+1	0	-1		#
6. Squatting					
7. Walking					
8. Running					
9. Up / Down steps					
Gait assessment score (- / 4)					
C. Clinical examination	**Valgus**	**Straight**	**Varus**	**Means Score(%)**	
	+1	0	-1		#
10. Heel position Left					
Heel Position Right					

	>0 dorsiflexion	0/90 degrees	<0 dorsiflexion	Means Score(%)	
	+1	0	-1		#
11. Ankle range Left					
Ankle range Right					
Clinical examination sub score (- / 2)				Left / Right	
Total Score (- / 11)					

The scoring system provides easily understood categories.

Total score guide (after Porecha, ([7])				
Clubfoot	11	9	7	0
'Grading'	Very good	Good	Fair	Poor
%	85 - 100	70 - 85	60 - 70	<50

Reference: Evans AM, Perveen R, Ford-Powell VA, Barker S. The Bangla clubfoot tool: a repeatability study. Journal of foot and ankle research. 2014 May 6;7(1):27.

Evidence

Evans *et al*[1] demonstrated this simple tool to feature good reliability both within and between examiners. A more recent study by Smythe et al, in 2018, comparing outcome measures after the Ponsetti method had good inter-observer agreement between the two expert physiotherapists. The study found that Bangla score had a sensitivity of 79.2% (95%CI: 57.8-92.9%) and a specificity of 79.5% (95%CI: 64.7-90.2%) in predicting the need for referral with positive and negative predictive values of 67.9% and 87.5% respectively[3]

References

1. Evans AM, Perveen R, Ford-Powell VA, Barker S. The Bangla clubfoot tool: a repeatability study. Journal of foot and ankle research. 2014 May 6;7(1):27.
2. Evans AM, Chowdhury MM, Kabir MH, Rahman MF. Walk for life-the National Clubfoot Project of Bangladesh: the four-year outcomes of 150 congenital clubfoot cases following Ponseti method. Journal of foot and ankle research. 2016 Nov 9;9(1):42.
3. Smythe T, Gova M, Muzanuwi R, Foster A, Lavy C. A Comparison of outcome measures used to report clubfoot treatment with the Ponseti method: results from a cohort in Harare, Zimbabwe. BMC Musculoskeletal Disorders (2018) 19:450

❑❑❑

41 Assessing Children with Clubfoot

Not all Clubfeet are the same and it is important that all people treating Clubfoot use the same terms to describe the different types. The causes of clubfoot are not clearly understood. Most commonly, it is classified as "Idiopathic Clubfoot" which means there is no known cause. "Secondary Clubfoot" which occurs when there is another disease or condition that is causing or is linked to the clubfoot, such conditions are usually neurological or syndromic disorders such as Arthrogyposis or Spina Bifida. There is also a condition known as "Positional Clubfoot", which is not really a true clubfoot as the foot is fully correctable. [1] Each type of clubfoot has unique characteristics and may need specific treatment. Early recognition of the type of clubfoot one is dealing with can help guide appropriate treatment. Individuals with clubfoot experience bone and soft tissues deformation and this abnormality can be presented through a range of abnormal alignments.

Assessment

When a child with clubfoot presents for the first time it is important to do a full assessment to check for any other neuromuscular abnormalities. This should include:

- Upper limbs and hands for range of movement, tone and deformity
- Cervical spine, head and face for signs of torticollis or facial features that may indicate a syndrome
- Full check from top to base of spine (child in prone) for any abnormality, particularly spina bifida
- The hips for any sign of Development dysplasia of the hip
- Both lower limbs including limb length, range of movement, tone and deformity

Classification

Although there is no classification system universally used for clubfoot, clubfoot can be classified according to the nature of the deformity: [2]

Idiopathic Clubfoot

Most commonly, Clubfoot is classified as "Idiopathic Clubfoot" meaning there is no known cause for the deformity. In Idiopathic Clubfoot, there can also be a definite hereditary influence, in that if a person has a relative, parent, or sibling that has Clubfoot, then they are more likely to have Clubfoot or have a child with it (3-10% chance). Within the group of Idiopathic Clubfeet there is a wide spectrum of impairment depending on severity, as well as whether the Clubfoot has been untreated, partially treated, poorly treated, or successfully treated.[3]

Untreated Clubfoot

All clubfeet from birth up to 2 years of age that have had very little or no treatment can be considered as untreated clubfeet.[3]

If clubfoot is not treated successfully, it can progress to a severe deformity causing lifelong disability. As the child grows and puts weight on their feet they will bear weight through the sides, or even the tops of their feet. A large callus of thickened skin forms on the weight-bearing surface and the deformed position causes pain and leaves the feet open to injury and infection. The person will not be able to wear normal footwear and in most cases will experience severe difficulty in walking by the time they are in their 20s or 30s. Having such a visible deformity can cause people with clubfoot to be discriminated against, and they may not be able to access education and employment. As well as being very difficult for the individual and their family, this has an effect on society as a whole, as it means that people born with clubfoot may not be able to work and contribute economically. [3]

Treated Clubfoot

Untreated clubfeet that have been corrected with Ponsetti treatment are termed "treated clubfeet". Treated clubfeet are usually braced full-time for 3 months and at night up to age 4 or 5 years.[3]

Recurrent Clubfoot

This is a Clubfoot which has achieved a good result with Ponsetti treatment, but the deformity has recurred. Recurrence means the reappearance of any or all of the components of the original clubfoot deformity after successful treatment. It is common in the first and second years after treatment especially if bracing has not been continued, but can happen at any time until skeletal maturity is reached. The most common reason is due to abandoning the braces early. [3]

Neglected Clubfoot

The Neglected Clubfoot is in a child older than 2 years, where little or no treatment has been performed. The Neglected Clubfoot may respond to Ponsetti Treatment, but also may have bony deformity that requires surgical correction.[3]

Atypical Clubfoot

This is a Clubfoot which involves a foot that is often swollen, has a plantar flexed first metatarsal and an extended big toe. Some children are born with atypical clubfoot, but we believe others become atypical because of poor treatment, most often occurring as a result of slippage of a cast.[3]

Complex Clubfoot

Any foot with deformity that has received any type of treatment other than the Ponseti method may have added complexity because of additional pathology or scarring from surgery.[3]

Resistant Clubfoot

This is a Clubfoot where Ponseti Treatment has been correctly performed but there has been no significant improvement. It is often found that this type of Clubfoot is not in fact idiopathic after all and is secondary or syndromic.[3]

Secondary Clubfoot

Secondary Clubfoot, on the other hand, occurs when there is another disease or condition that is causing or linked to the development of Clubfoot. Such conditions are usually Neurological such as Spina Bifida associated with concurrent sensory and or motor impairments or Syndromic Disorders such as Arthrogryposis associated with more global findings and involvement of other musculoskeletal issues:

Spina Bifida

A congenital, neurological condition where there is failure of the formation of the bone or skin or both to cover the lower end of the spinal cord and nerves. It is often associated with neurological problems in the legs, and clubfoot. If cases present to the clubfoot clinic it is important to find out what the long-term prognosis is, and whether the child is likely to walk. If the child is likely to survive and walk then it is worth trying Ponseti Clubfoot Treatment. The success rate with simple manipulation is not high and surgery may be considered. Even if the child has a low likelihood of walking the parents might still like to try to get the feet corrected so that shoes can be worn.[4]

Arthrogryposis

A congenital condition where the child is born with a number of deformities of the joints. A severe case can have stiffness of the elbows, wrists, hips, knees, and feet. People with severe cases are often unable to walk. Clubfoot is a relatively common association. Ponseti treatment can be tried and is often partially successful.[4]

Amniotic Band Syndrome

The cause of amniotic band syndrome is not fully clear, but children with this condition are born with tight skin and soft tissue bands around their limbs, constricting blood and lymph flow and causing swelling. Some cases are associated with clubfoot although in the one illustrated here it is only mild. Treatment of the tight band often involves surgery. If there is a clubfoot associated, then Ponseti treatment should only be done with extreme care as blood supply to the foot can be affected and there is a risk of gangrene. These cases are best referred to a centre with surgical experience.[4]

Tibial Agenesis

Failure in the formation of the tibia. There is a spectrum of presentations from complete absence to a slightly short tibia. In this case there is only a very short tibia and the foot therefore adopts a varus deformity pointing to the midline. This is not a clubfoot deformity even though there is a similarity in the appearance. If there is doubt about the diagnosis, an X-ray should be taken. Treatment is very complicated and many surgeons recommend an amputation with below-knee prosthesis. There is little benefit in starting clubfoot treatment.[4]

Assessment

The underlying deformity of clubfoot can be most easily understood if it is divided into four components, whose first letters make up the Acronym CAVE. These components are: Cavus, Adductus, Varus, and Equinus. We will look at them in turn. Treatment will then address Cavus first, then Adductus, then Varus, and lastly Equinus. So the Acronym CAVE is useful both to describe the deformity and to outline the treatment.

Cavus

The picture below shows a medial view of the plastic model of a clubfoot. You can see that the arch of the foot is higher than normal. This is because the first metatarsal (blue line) is plantarflexed in relation to the calcaneum and hindfoot (red line).

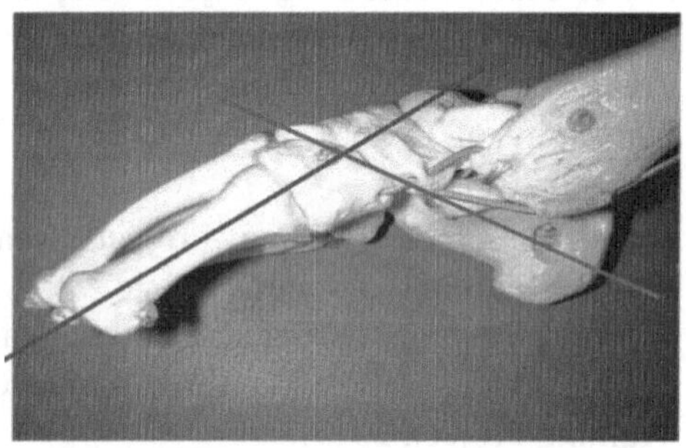

Remember: Correct Cavus First

Adductus

Adductus is movement towards the midline. In both the pictures above it can be seen that the forefoot is adducted towards the midline. This is the second part of the deformity of clubfoot.

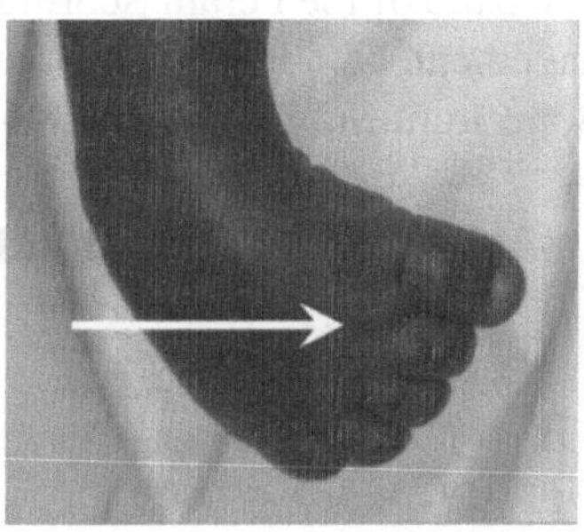

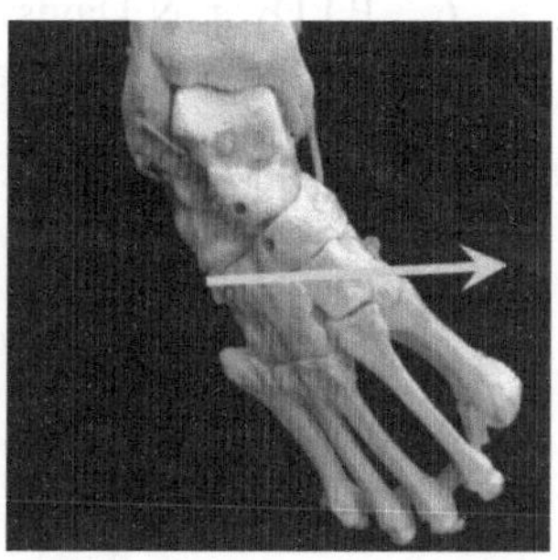

Components of the Adductus

The pictures below show on the left a normal foot, in the middle a model of the clubfoot, and on the right a dissection of an infant's clubfoot. In the two clubfoot pictures it can be seen that the navicular moves medially and starts to dislocate off the talus. The calcaneum also rotates medially under the talus as part of the adductus deformity.

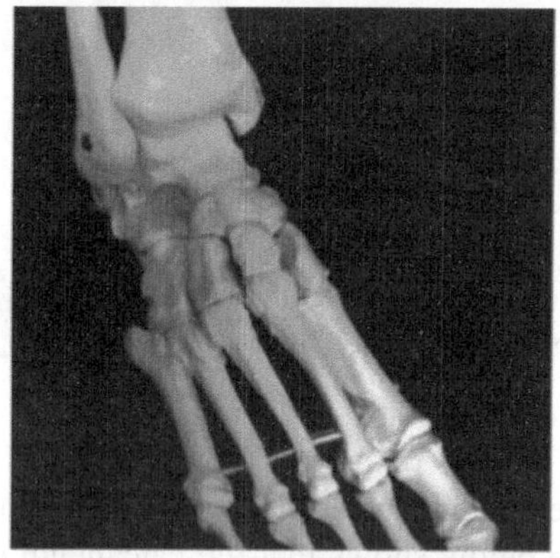

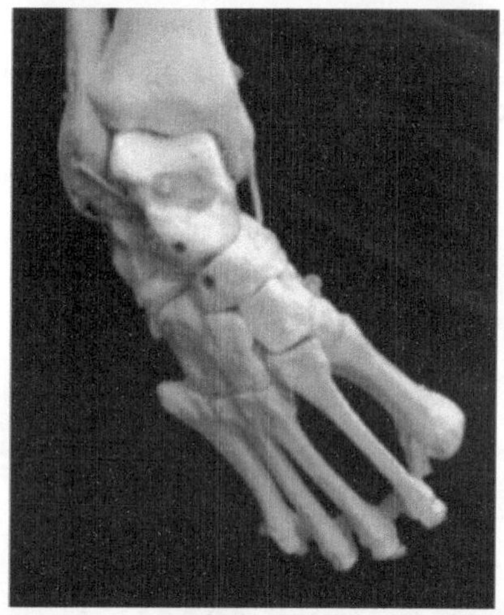

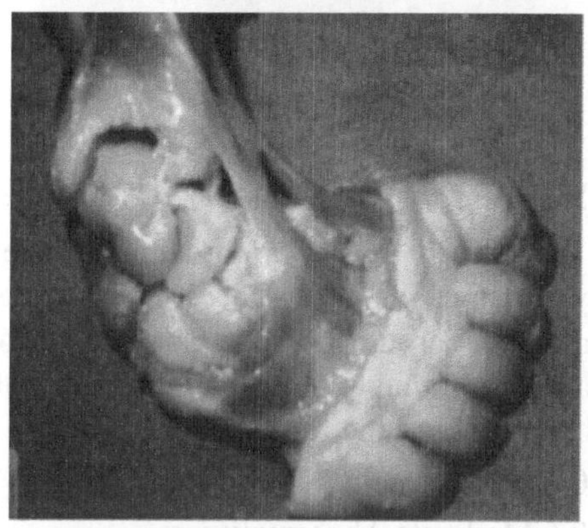

Varus

Varus means movement towards the midline. The pictures above show that the heel in the clubfoot is in varus and angled towards the midline.

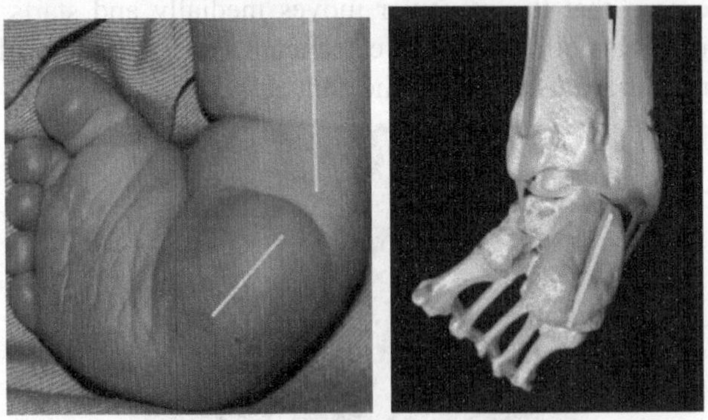

Equinus

Equinus means an increase in the plantarflexion of the foot. The picture below shows that the calcaneum (red line) is plantarflexed in relation to the tibia (blue line). This is the final part of the CAVE deformity and will be the last part to be corrected.

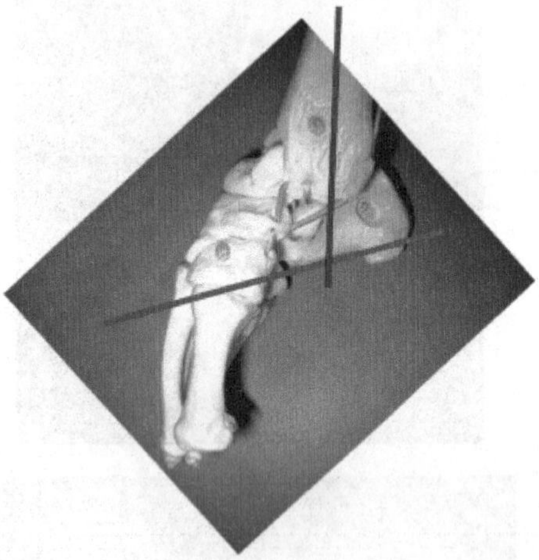

Severity

There is no agreed method of grading the severity of deformity, Pirani et al[5][6] devised a simple scoring system, the Pirani Score, based on six clinical signs of contracture that research has found to be both valid and reliable. Each is scored according to the following principle:

- 0 No Abnormality
- 0.5 Moderate Abnormality
- 1.0 Severe Abnormality

The six signs are separated into three related to the hindfoot (severity of the posterior crease, emptiness of the heel and rigidity of then equinus) and three related to the mid foot (curvature of the lateral border of the foot, severity of the medial crease and position of the lateral part of the head of the talus). Thus each foot can receive a Hindfoot Score between 0 to 3, a Midfoot Score between 0 to 3 and Total Score between 0 to 6.

Tools and Measures

- Pirani Score
- Roye Score
- Bangla Clubfoot Tool

References

1. Africa Clubfoot Training Project. Chapter 1 Africa Clubfoot Training Basic & Advanced Clubfoot Treatment Provider Courses - Participant Manual. University of Oxford: Africa Clubfoot Training Project, 2017.
2. Clubfoot,http://emedicine.medscape.com/article/1237077-overview#a4 (accessed 28 June 2017)
3. Africa Clubfoot Training Project. Chapter 2 Africa Clubfoot Training Basic & Advanced Clubfoot Treatment Provider Courses - Participant Manual. University of Oxford: Africa Clubfoot Training Project, 2017.
4. Africa Clubfoot Training Project. Chapter 15 Africa Clubfoot Training Basic & Advanced Clubfoot Treatment Provider Courses - Participant Manual. University of Oxford: Africa Clubfoot Training Project, 2017.
5. Pirani S, Hodges D & Sekeramayi F (2003) A reliable and valid method of assessing the amount of deformity in the congenital clubfoot deformity (The Canadian Orthopaedic Research Society and the Canadian Orthopaedic Association conference proceeding) in The Journal of Bone and Joint Surgery 90 (B) SUPP_1, 53
6. P.J.Dyer, N.Davis, The Role of the Perani Scoring System in the Management of Clubfoot by the Ponseti Method, J Bone Joint Surg [Br] 2006;88-B:1082-4.

❑❑❑

42 Assessing Clubfoot Treatment (ACT) Tool

The Assessing Clubfoot Treatment (ACT) score was developed for clubfoot therapists to assess the results of Ponseti treatment in children of walking age, in low resource settings, where access to qualified therapists may be limited. In many of these settings treatment is being offered by non-specialised health workers[1]. It is helpful in predicting the need for referral for further intervention, whether that is a specialist opinion or referral for further manipulation and casting[2]. The use of the ACT score is to accurately inform and predict future management. It answers such questions as:

1. Does the child need more treatment?
2. Has the child been successfully treated?
3. Will the child's quality of life be improved?

Intended Population

An evaluation tool, for clubfoot therapists (non-specialised health workers) in low resource settings, to assess the results of Ponseti treatment of congenital talipes equinovarus (CTEV) in children of walking age.[2]

Method

The ACT tool consists of 4 questions; each scored from 0 to 3, giving a total from 0 to 12 where 12 is the ideal result. The 4 questions consist of one physical assessment and three parent reported outcome measures. It takes 5 minutes to administer and has been observed to have excellent inter-observer agreement.[3]

- The question about the plantigrade position of the foot should be answered first with physical examination of the child in supine, with the knee extended and measurement of passive range of dorsiflexion of the hindfoot.
- The remaining three questions of the ACT score should be answered by the carers about the child's pain, ability to wear shoes and satisfaction. The child is then given verbal instructions to complete the functional performance review.

Table 1: ACT questions and score[4]

Score	1.The foot is plantigrade	2.Does your child complain of pain in their affected foot?	3.Can your child wear shoes of your/ their choice?	4.How satisfied are you with your child's foot?
0	Does not reach plantigrade, with additional adduction, cavus or varus	Yes and it often limits their activity	Never	Very dissatisfied
1	Does not reach plantigrade, no additional deformity	Yes and it sometimes limits their activity	Sometimes	Somewhat dissatisfied
2	Plantigrade achieved	Yes but it does not limit their activity	Usually	Somewhat satisfied
3	More than plantigrade i.e. some dorsiflexion	No	Always	Very Satisfied

A score of 8 or less indicates that the child needs a referral,

- A score between 9-10 indicates that the child would benefit from a referral of surgical/medical review
- A score of 11 or 12 indicated the child had a good outcome.

Evidence

T Smythe developed a tool that has good reliability both within and between examiners and is helpful in predicting the need for referral for further intervention (specialist opinion or for further manipulation and casting)[1]. A study by Smythe et al, in 2018, comparing outcome measures after the Ponsetti method had good inter-observer agreement between the two expert physiotherapists. The study found that the ACT score had 79.2% (95%CI: 57.8–92.9%) sensitivity and 100% (95%CI: 92–100%) specificity in predicting the need for referral, with positive and negative predictive values of 100 and 89.8% respectively.[2]

References

1. Smythe T, Wainwright A, Foster A, Lavy C. What is a good result after clubfoot treatment? A Delphi-based consensus on success by regional clubfoot trainers from across Africa. PLoS ONE,2017 12(12): e0190056. https://doi.org/10.1371/journal.pone.0190056
2. Smythe T, Gova M, Muzarurwi R, Foster A, Lavy C. A comparison of outcome measures used to report clubfoot treatment with the Ponseti method: results from a cohort in Harare, Zimbabwe. BMC Musculoskeletal Disorders. 2018, 19:450
3. Smythe, TH; (2018) Evidence to improve clubfoot services in Africa with Zimbabwe as a case study. PhD (research paper style) thesis, London School of Hygiene & Tropical Medicine. DOI: https://doi.org/10.17037/PUBS.04649940
4. Smythe T, PhD Thesis - Evidence to improve clubfoot services in Africa with Zimbabwe as a case study London School of Hygiene & Tropical Medicine. DOI: https://doi.org/10.17037/PUBS.04649940

❑❑❑

43 Barthel Index

Objective

The Barthel Scale/Index (BI) is an ordinal scale used to measure performance in activities of daily living (ADL). Ten variables describing ADL and mobility are scored, a higher number being a reflection of greater ability to function independently following hospital discharge.Time taken and physical assistance required to perform each item are used in determining the assigned value of each item. The Barthel Index measures the degree of assistance required by an individual on 10 items of mobility and self care ADL. [1]

Intended Population

Patients with stroke, patients with other neuromuscular or musculoskeletal disorders, oncology patients.

Method of Use

Time to administer- Self report: 2-5 minutes; Direct observation: 20 minutes, Times may vary depending on clients tolerance and abilities. The MBI/BI is simple to administer. Requires training if administered by direct observation. It has been developed in many forms that can be administered in many situations and can be used for longitudinal assessment. The Barthel includes 10 personal activities: feeding, personal toileting, bathing, dressing and undressing, getting on and off a toilet, controlling bladder, controlling bowel, moving from wheelchair to bed and returning, walking on level surface (or propelling a wheelchair if unable to walk) and ascending and descending stairs. The original Index is a three-item ordinal rating scale completed by a therapist or other observer in 2-5 minutes. Each item is rated in terms of whether the patient can perform the task independently, with some assistance, or is dependent on help based on observation (0=unable, 1=needs help, 2=independent). The final score is x 5 to get a number on a 100 point score. Proposed guidelines for interpreting Barthel scores are that scores of 0-20 indicate "total" dependency, 21-60 indicate "severe" dependency, 61-90 indicate "moderate" dependency, and 91-99 indicates "slight" dependency.2 Most studies apply the 60/61 cutting point. Note- the Barthel Index should not be used alone for predicting outcomes.[2]

Versions

Modified 10-item version (MBI); 5-item short form; The expanded 15-item version; The extended BI (EBI); The 3-item BI; Self-rating BI (SB); Early Rehabilitation Barthel Index (ERI)Level of measurements are limited to either complete independence or needing assistance. Each performance item is scored on an ordinal scale with a specified number of points assigned to each level or ranking.

Reliability

The MBI amd BI are reliable tests to administer. Five studies of the MBI reported excellent internal consistency: one study of the MBI reported excellent test-retest reliability; one study of the MBI and 4 studies of BI reported excellent inter-rater reliability; and 1 study of the BI reported adequate inter-rater reliability[6]. As a predictive tool the the MBI predicted instrumental ADL performance at 6-months post-stroke: likelihood a patient will regain continence following stroke; risk for falls in patients with stroke; functional recovery following stroke; and acute care hospital length following stroke.[6]

Responsiveness

Ability to detect change in patients is poor in highly functional individuals, a ceiling effect being noted.

Resources

Heart and Stroke Foundation; Canadian Partnership for Stroke Recovery. Stroke Engine. **Barthel Index.** This website has an excellent summary of the Barthel Index, its use and its psychometric properties.

References

1. Wikipedia. Barthel Scale. Available from: https://en.wikipedia.org/wiki/Barthel_scale (last accessed 27.4.2019)
2. Elite learning. The original Barthel index of ADLs. Available from: https://www.elitecme.com/resource-center/rehabilitation-therapy/the-original-barthel-index-of-adls/ (last accessed 30.4.2019)
3. Scribd. Barthel index. Available from: https://www.scribd.com/document/101609741/Barthel-Index-0-20 (last accessed 27.4.2019)
4. RACGP. Barthel Index. Available from: https://www.racgp.org.au/clinical-resources/clinical-guidelines/key-racgp-guidelines/view-all-racgp-guidelines/silver-book/tools/barthel-index (last accessed 27.4.2019)
5. John Adamson. How to Interpret - The Barthel Index. Available from: https://www.youtube.com/watch?v=0TyPiuvgfho&feature=youtu.be (last accessed 27.4.2019)
6 Heart and Stroke Foundation; Canadian Partnership for Stroke Recovery. Stroke Engine. Barthel Index. Accessed 24 June 2019.

The Barthel Index Items and Scoring:

Bowels

0 = Incontinent (or needs to be given enema)

1 = occasional accident (once/week)

2 = continent

Bladder

0 = incontinent, or catheterized and unable to manage

1 = occasional accident (max. once per 24 hours)

2 = continent (for over 7 days)

Grooming

0 = needs help with personal care

1 = independent face/hair/teeth/shaving (implements provided)

Toilet use

0 = dependent

1 = needs some help, but can do something alone

2 = independent (on and off, dressing, wiping)

Feeding

0 = unable

1 = needs help cutting, spreading butter, etc.

2 = independent (food provided within reach)

Transfer

0 = unable – no sitting balance

1 = major help (one or two people, physical), can sit

2 = minor help (verbal or physical)

3 = independent

Mobility

0 = immobile

1 = wheelchair independent, including corners, etc.

2 = walks with help of one person (verbal or physical)

3 = independent (but may use any aid)

Dressing

0 = dependent

1 = needs help, but can do about half unaided

2 = independent (including buttons, zips, laces etc)

Stairs

0 = unable

1 = needs help (verbal, physical, carrying aid)

2 = independent up and down

Bathing

0 = dependent,

1 = independent (or in shower)

❑❑❑

44 Facial Disability Index

Introduction

It was developed by Dr. Jessie Van Swearingen with Dr. Jennifer Brach in order to evaluate the disability resulting from disorders of the facial nerve.[1]

Method of Use

It is a patient-rated outcome measure. There are 10 items from which items 1-5 constitute the Physical Function subscale, while items 6-10 constitute the Social/Well-being Function subscale. Each item in the Physical Function subscale is rated from 5 to 0 while items in the Social/Well-being Function subscale are rated from 6 to 1. The individual subscales are scored out of a total of 100 where the highest score is the best result.[1]

Evidence

It has been validated and is reliable for use in clinical studies with the theta reliability coefficients for Physical Function = .88 and Social/Well-being function = .83. Additionally, compared to SF-36, the FDI was able to satisfactorily correlate impairments, disability, and psychosocial status.[1] A prospective follow-up study comparing patient-reported facial and psychosocial function (FaCE scale and FDI outcome measures) with physician-graded facial function (Sunnybrook and House-Brackmann grading) in early and follow-up stages in Bell's palsy patients showed low to fair correlation between FaCE/FDI and Sunnybrook score in early stages, suggesting a quality of life (QOL) designs are less suited for the acute stage, and higher correlations at follow-ups suggest using of questionnaires for QoL evaluation with time[9].

References

1. VanSwearingen JM, Brach JS. The Facial Disability Index: reliability and validity of a disability assessment instrument for disorders of the facial neuromuscular system. Phys Ther. 1996 Dec;76(12):1288-98; discussion 1298-300. doi: 10.1093/ptj/76.12.1288.
2. Pavese C, Cecini M, Camerino N, De Silvestri A, Tinelli C, Bejor M, Dalla Toffola E. Functional and social limitations after facial palsy: expanded and independent validation of the Italian version of the facial disability index. Phys Ther. 2014 Sep;94(9):1327-36. doi: 10.2522/ptj.20130254.
3. Gonzalez-Cardero E, Infante-Cossio P, Cayuela A, Acosta-Feria M, Gutierrez-Perez JL. Facial disability index (FDI): adaptation to Spanish, reliability and validity. Med Oral Patol Oral Cir Bucal. 2012 Nov 1;17(6):e1006-12. doi: 10.4317/medoral.18054.
4. Graciano AJ, Bonin MM, Mory MR, Tessitore A, Paschoal JR, Chone CT. Translation, cultural adaptation and validation of the facial disability index into Brazilian Portuguese. Braz J Otorhinolaryngol. 2020 Sep-Oct;86(5):602-608. doi: 10.1016/j.bjorl.2019.04.003.
5. Özden F, Karaman ÖN, Tuğay N, Savaş Ö, Sözen T, Üçüncü H. The reliability and validity of the Turkish version of the Facial Disability Index. Disabil Rehabil. 2020 May 15:1-10. doi: 10.1080/09638288.2020.1762768.
6. Barry P, Mancini J, Alshukry A, Salburgo F, Lavieille JP, Montava M. Validation of French versions of the Facial Disability Index and the Facial Clinimetric Evaluation Scale, specific

quality of life scales for peripheral facial palsy patients. Clin Otolaryngol. 2019 May;44(3):313-322. doi: 10.1111/coa.13294.

7. van Veen MM, Bruins TE, Artan M, Mooibroek-Leeuwerke T, Beurskens CHG, Werker PMN, Dijkstra PU. Health-related quality of life in facial palsy: translation and validation of the Dutch version Facial Disability Index. Health Qual Life Outcomes. 2020 Jul 31;18(1):256. doi: 10.1186/s12955-020-01502-0.
8. Volk GF, Steigerwald F, Vitek P, Finkensieper M, Kreysa H, Guntinas-Lichius O. Facial Disability Index und Facial Clinimetric Evaluation Skala: Validierung der Deutschen Versionen [Facial Disability Index and Facial Clinimetric Evaluation Scale: validation of the German versions]. Laryngorhinootologie. 2015 Mar;94(3):163-8. German. doi: 10.1055/s-0034-1381999.
9. Bylund N, Hultcrantz M, Jonsson L, Marsk E. Quality of Life in Bell's Palsy: Correlation with Sunnybrook and House-Brackmann Over Time. The Laryngoscope. 2021 Feb;131(2):E612-8.

Facial Disability Index

Please circle the most appropriate response to the following questions related to problems associated with the function of your facial muscles. For each question, consider your function during the past month:

Physical Function

1. How much difficulty did you have did you have keeping food in your mouth, moving food around in your mouth, or getting food stuck in your cheek while eating?

Usually did with	Usually did not eat because:
5 -- no difficulty	1 -- of health
4 -- a little difficulty	0 -- of other reasons
3 -- some difficulty	2 - much difficulty

2. How much difficulty did you have drinking from a cup?

Usually did with:	Usually did not drink because
5 -- no difficulty	1 -- of health
4 -- a little difficulty	0 -- of other reasons
3 -- some difficulty	
2 – much difficulty	

3. How much difficulty did you have saying specific sounds while speaking?

Usually did with:	Usually did not speak because:
5 -- no difficulty	1 -- of health
4 -- a little difficulty	0 -- of other reasons
3 -- some difficulty	
2 – much difficulty, slurring of speech	

4. How much difficulty did you have with your eye tearing excessively or becoming dry?

Usually did with:	Usually did not tearing because:
5 -- no difficulty	1 -- of health
4 -- a little difficulty	0 -- of other reasons
3 -- some difficulty	
2 – much difficulty	

5. How much difficulty did you have with brushing your teeth or rinsing your mouth?

Usually did with:	Usually did not brusing or rinsing because:
5 -- no difficulty	1 -- of health
4 -- a little difficulty	0 -- of other reasons
3 -- some difficulty	
2 – much difficulty	

Social Function

6. How much of the time have you felt calm and peaceful?

6 – all of the time	5 – most of the time
4 – a good bit of the time	3 – some of the time
2 – a little bit of the time	1 – none of the time

7. How much of the time did you isolate yourself from people around you?

6 – all of the time	5 – most of the time
4 – a good bit of the time	3 – some of the time
2 – a little bit of the time	1 – none of the time

8. How much of the time did you get irritable toward those around you?

6 – all of the time	5 – most of the time
4 – a good bit of the time	3 – some of the time
2 – a little bit of the time	1 – none of the time

9. How often did you wake up early or wake up several times during your nighttime sleep?

6 – all of the time	5 – most of the time
4 – a good bit of the time	3 – some of the time
2 – a little bit of the time	1 – none of the time

10. How often has your facial function kept you from going out to eat, shop, or participate in family or social activities?

6 – all of the time	5 – most of the time
4 – a good bit of the time	3 – some of the time
2 – a little bit of the time	1 – none of the time

DO NOT COMPLETE THIS SECTION – TO BE COMPLETED BY YOUR THERAPIST

Scoring:

Physical Function Social Function

Total Score (questions 1-5) – N × 110

Total Score (questions 6-10) × 100

N 4 N 5

N = Number of questions answered

45 Bath Assessment of Walking Inventory

Objective

Chronic pain has widespread detrimental effects on normal functioning. Patients commonly complain of unwelcome changes in their capacity, ability and quality of movement. Although the measurement of function is a frequent component of clinical assessment, instruments often rely on patient self-report of remembered global function on specific tasks of physical capacity or are global measures of bodily awareness. To date walking assessment has relied on a laboratory setting. No unobtrusive, clinically easy to use instruments exist to measure the quality of walking when in pain. An abnormal gait is not of itself a clinically significant problem. Indeed many patients report a lack of awareness of how they walk. Walking is often only a means to achieve a goal. However, the social context of pain behaviour and the effect of pain behaviour on observers are often clinically important. Judgements about pain are known to be based on verbal and facial behaviour. we do not know what the critical factors are which, when therapeutically manipulated, can lead to sustained improvements in walking quality. Establishing instruments to measure the quality of walking is a critical first step in enabling future research into the 'biopsychosocial' influences on walking quality. Understanding the complexity of walking is essential in clinical formulation and treatment planning; achieving a reliable measure of walking quality will also allow for the further investigation of pain-related function. The primary objective is to develop an assessment tool designed specifically to assess the quality of walking in adults with chronic pain for use in clinical and research settings.

Intended Population

Adults over 17 years of age, reporting pain of at least six months in duration, with intact limbs and without any structural impairment that restricted range or pattern of movement.

Document

Measures used were:

1. Two minute timed walk test (TMTWT)
2. One minute sit to stand (STS)
3. Sickness impact profile (SIP)

Evidence

Reliability

Clarke and Eccleston (2009)[1]

Demonstrates good internal consistency (Cronbach 0.71) and adequate intra- (Kappa 0.61–0.98) and inter-rater reliability (Kappa 0.61–0.98).

Validity

Clarke and Eccleston (2009)[1]

Validity was established in comparison with well-used measures of functioning.

Responsiveness

Further independent study is required to develop this instrument.

Resources

Jane E. Clarke and Christopher Eccleston (2009). Assessing the quality of walking in adults with chronic pain: The development and preliminary psychometric evaluation of the Bath Assessment of Walking Inventory, European Journal of Pain, 13(3), 305-311

References

1. Jane E. Clarke and Christopher Eccleston (2009). Assessing the quality of walking in adults with chronic pain: The development and preliminary psychometric evaluation of the Bath Assessment of Walking Inventory, European Journal of Pain, 13(3), 305-311

❑❑❑

46 Male Urogenital Distress Inventory (MUDI)

Objective

The Male Urogenital Distress Inventory (MUDI) can be used in clinical practice and research to measure the effect of interventions for urinary incontinence on health-related quality of life in men.[1]

Intended Population

Community-dwelling, racially diverse men with continence problems.[1]

Method of Use

The MUDI contains 27 items that are each coded on the following 5-point scale: 1 = symptom not present, 2 = symptom present but not bothersome, 3 = symptom present and slightly bothersome, 4 = symptom present and moderately bothersome, and 5 = symptom present and greatly bothersome. Total scores range from 27 (no symptoms) to 135 (maximum degree of associated bother).[1] It takes about 20 minutes to complete by either self-administration or interview.[1]

Evidence

Reliability: Internal consistency score with Cronbach's coefficient was .89.[1]

Validity

Content validity agreement scores were 97% for item clarity and 95% for item fit.[1]

Responsiveness

Miscellaneous

The MUDI captures the dimension of physical health, focusing on bother from multiple symptoms associated with urinary incontinence. Further testing should be done on test-retest reliability and sensitivity to change. Concurrent validity should also be evaluated further by comparing to a generic health-related quality of life instrument.[1]

References

1. Robinson J, Shea S. Development and testing of a measure of health-related quality of life for men with urinary incontinence. J Am Geriat Soc 2002;50:935-945.

❑❑❑

47 Pelvic Floor Distress Inventory (PFDI - 20)

Objective

The Pelvic Floor Distress Inventory Questionnaire-20 (PFDI-20) is the short-form version of the Pelvic Floor Distress Inventory (PFDI).[1] Similar to the PFIQ-7, it is a health-related quality of life questionnaire for women with pelvic floor conditions to fill out.[1] The PFDI-20 is comprised of 3 scales, which include the Urinary Distress Inventory-6 (UDI-6), Pelvic Organ Prolapse Distress Inventory-6 (POPDI-6), and the Colorectal-Anal Distress Inventory-8 (CRADI-8).[1]

Intended Population

Women over the age of 18 with disorders of the pelvic floor including urinary incontinence, pelvic organ prolapse, and fecal incontinence.[1]

Method of Use

Since it is comprised of the UDI-6, POPDI-6, and the CRADI-8, the PFDI-20 includes 20 questions.[1] Each question begins with a "yes" or "no" response. If "yes," the patient must indicate how much bowel, bladder, or pelvic symptoms have been bothering them in the past 3 months on a 4-point scale that ranges from "not at all" (0) to "quite a bit" (4).[1] The scale scores are found individually by calculating the mean value of their corresponding questions and then multiplying by 25 to obtain a value that ranges from 0 to 100.[1] The sum of the 3 scales are added together to get the PFDI-20 summary score, which ranges from 0 to 300.[1]

Evidence

Correlation: Correlation, represented by r, ranges from -1.0 to +1.0. If the r value is 0 that means there is no correlation. If the r value is close to -1.0 that means that both values will decrease linearly. If the r value is close to +1.0 that means that both values will increase linearly. Correlation of the short-form versions with the long-form versions:[1]

- UDI-6 r=0.86[1]
- POPDI-6 r=0.92[1]
- CRADI-8 r=0.93[1]

Reliability: The test-retest reliability, represented by intraclass correlation coefficients (ICC):[1]

- PFDI-20 ICC=0.93[1]
- UDI-6 ICC=0.82[1]
- POPDI-6 ICC=0.91[1]
- CRADI-8 ICC=0.84[1]

Validity: The PFDI-20 demonstrates construct validity as it demonstrates a significant association with appropriate measures of symptom severity and pelvic floor diagnoses.[1]

Responsiveness: Each of the 3 scales of the PFDI-20 demonstrated moderate to excellent responsiveness with effect size and standardized response mean values ranging from 0.70 to 1.28.[1] The sensitivity of the PFDI-20 as a whole was excellent with an effect size of 1.48 $P < .0001$ and standardized response mean of 1.09 $P < .0001$.[1] The ability of the PFDI-20 to discriminate between subjects who indicated that they were "worse" after surgery from those who indicated they were "better" was excellent with c-statistic of .95.[1]

Clinically Meaningful Change: At the time of creation, the clinically meaningful change in quality of life (MCID) [2] needed to be studied in larger populations.[1] Studies have found minimal importance changes (MIC) ranging from 23 to 45.[1][3][4] For example, in their small sample size, Barber and colleagues (2004)[1] found a change in the summary score of 45 points or more to be meaningful after surgery.[1]

However, it is important to consider that patients undergoing surgery also generally have higher scores at baseline.[5] More recently, Wiegersma and colleagues (2017)[5] aimed to determine the MIC in women undergoing conservative pelvic organ prolapse treatments for mild symptoms.[5] They found that an improvement of 13.5 points to be helpful when evaluating the effects of conservative treatment strategies.[5]

Miscellaneous: The strength of the PFDI-20 is that it is a short form that gives a comprehensive assessment of the effect of pelvic floor disorders on the quality of life of women, rather than assessing just one aspect of pelvic floor function such as urinary incontinence. A more generic quality-of-life form as the SF-36 has demonstrated poor responsiveness in patients undergoing treatment for urinary incontinence. In these patient populations, it may be important to use both a generic quality-of-life instrument and a condition-specific instrument that has demonstrated responsiveness. The PFDI-20 is easy to use in both clinical and research settings.[1]

References

1. Barber MD, Walters MD, Bump RC. Short forms of two condition-specific quality-of-life questionnaires for women with pelvic floor disorders (PFDI-20 adn PFIQ-7). Am J Obstet Gynecol 2005;193:103-113.
2. Crosby RD, Kolotkin RL, Williams GR. Defining clinically meaningful change in health-related quality of life. Journal of clinical epidemiology. 2003 May 1;56(5):395-407.
3. Gelhorn HL, Coyne KS, Sikirica V, Gauld J, Murphy M. Psychometric evaluation of health-related quality-of-life measures after pelvic organ prolapse surgery. Female pelvic medicine & reconstructive surgery. 2012 Jul 1;18(4):221-6.
4. Utomo E, Blok BF, Steensma AB, Korfage IJ. Validation of the pelvic floor distress inventory (PFDI-20) and pelvic floor impact questionnaire (PFIQ-7) in a Dutch population. International urogynecology journal. 2014 Apr 1;25(4):531-44.
5. Wiegersma M, Panman CM, Berger MY, De Vet HC, Kollen BJ, Dekker JH. Minimal important change in the pelvic floor distress inventory-20 among women opting for conservative prolapse treatment. American journal of obstetrics and gynecology. 2017 Apr 1;216(4):397-e1.

Pelvic Floor Distress Inventory Questionnaire

		If yes, how much does it bother you?			
	Yes / No	**Not at all**	**Somewhat**	**Moderately**	**Quite a bit**
1.Do you usually experience pressure in the lower abdomen?					
2.Do you usually experience heaviness or dullness in the lower abdomen?					
3.Do you usually have a bulge or something falling out that you can see or fell in the vaginal area?					
4.Do you usually have to push on the vagina or around the rectum to have a complete bowel movement?					
5.Do you usually experience a feeling of incomplete bladder emptying?					
6.Do you ever have to push up in the vaginal area with your fingers to start or complete urination?					
7.Do you feel you need to strain too hard to have a bowel movement?					
8.Do you feel you have not completely emptied your bowels at the end of a bowel movement?					
9.Do you usually lose stool beyond your control if your stool is well formed?					
10.Do you usually lose stool beyond your control if you stool is loose or liquid?					

11.Do you usually lose gas from the rectum beyond your control					
12.Do you usually have pain when you pass your stool?					
13.Do you experience a strong sense of urgency and have to rush to the bathroom to have a bowel movement?					
14.Does part of your stool ever pass through the rectum and bulge outside during or after a bowel movement?					
15.Do you usually experience frequent urination					
16.Do you usually experience urine leakage associated with a feeling of urgency; that is, a strong sensation of needing to go to the bathroom?					
17.Do you usually experience urine leakage related to laughing, coughing, or sneezing>					
18.Do you usually experience small amounts of urine leakage (that is, drops)?					
19.Do you usually experience difficulty emptying your bladder?					
20.Do you usually experience pain of discomfort in the lower abdomen or genital, region?					

48 Pelvic Floor Impact Questionnaire (PFIQ - 7)

Objective

The Pelvic Floor Impact Questionnaire-7 (PFIQ-7) is a shortened, less comprehensive version of the Pelvic Floor Impact Questionnaire (PFIQ).[1] It was created by Barber and colleagues (2004)[1] to save time, yet remain effective, in clinical and research encounters. It is a health-related quality of life questionnaire for women with pelvic floor conditions to fill out.[1] It includes scales from the Urinary Impact Questionnaire (UIQ-7), Pelvic Organ Prolapse Impact Questionnaire (POPIQ-7), and the Colorectal-Anal Impact Questionnaire-7 (CRAIQ-7),[1] which are short-forms of their the longer versions. It is useful to determine changes in symptom-severity over time and before and after treatments.[1]

Intended Population

Women over the age of 18 with pelvic floor conditions including urinary incontinence, pelvic organ prolapse, and fecal incontinence.[1]

Method of Use

The PFIQ-7 consists of 7 questions that need to be answered 3 times each (corresponds to the scales previously mentioned) considering symptoms related to the bladder or urine, vagina or pelvis, and bowel or rectum and their effect on function, social health, and mental health in the past 3 months.[1] The responses for each question range from "not at all" (0) to "quite a bit" (3).[1] To get scale scores, the mean of each of the 3 scales is individually calculated, which ranges from 0-3, this number is then multiplied by 100 and then divided by 3.[1] The scale scores are then added together to get the total PFIQ-7 score, which ranges from 0-300. A lower score means there is a lesser effect on quality of life.[1]

Evidence

Correlation: Correlation, represented by r, ranges from -1.0 to +1.0. If the r value is 0 that means there is no correlation. If the r value is close to -1.0 that means that both values will decrease linearly. If the r value is close to +1.0 that means that both values will increase linearly.

Correlation of the short-form versions with the long-form versions:[1]

- UIQ-7 r=0.96[1]
- POPIQ-7 r=0.94[1]
- CRAIQ-7 r=0.96[1]

Reliability: The test-retest reliability, represented by intraclass correlation coefficients (ICC):[1]

- PFIQ-7 ICC=0.77[1]
- UIQ-7 ICC=0.81[1]
- POPIQ-7 ICC=0.70[1]
- CRAIQ-7 ICC=0.81[1]

Validity: The PFIQ-7 demonstrates construct validity as it demonstrates a significant association with appropriate measures of symptom severity and pelvic floor diagnoses.[1]

Responsiveness: The PFIQ-7 has shown moderate responsiveness between the pre- and post-operative periods for pelvic and continence surgeries.[1] The standardized response mean (SRM) for all the sub scales fell within the range of 0.5 to 0.7.[1] It showed an effect size of 0.67 and a SRM of 0.63.[1] However, the responsiveness has been shown to be vary amongst different patients.[2] The highest SRMs have been found in the UIQ-7 and the CRAIQ-7 and the lowest SRMs have been found in the POPIQ-7.[2] However, the SRM for the POPIQ-7 increased at 3 and 12 months in patients who underwent surgery for pelvic organ prolapse.[2]

Clinically Meaningful Change: At the time of creation, the clinically meaningful change in quality of life (MCID) [3] needed to be studied in larger populations.[1] However, in their small sample size, Barber and colleagues (2004)[1] found a change in the summary score of 36 points (12%) or more to be meaningful after surgery.

Miscellaneous: The PFIQ-7 demonstrated a statistically significant improvement at 3 to 6 months after surgery, but the responsiveness was somewhat less than the PFDI-20.[1]

References

1. Barber MD, Walters MD, Bump RC. Short forms of two condition-specific quality-of-life questionnaires for women with pelvic floor disorders (PFDI-20 and PFIQ-7). American journal of obstetrics and gynecology. 2005 Jul 1;193(1):103-13.
2. Barber MD, Chen Z, Lukacz E, Markland A, Wai C, Brubaker L, Nygaard I, Weidner A, Janz NK, Spino C. Further validation of the short form versions of the Pelvic Floor Distress Inventory (PFDI) and Pelvic Floor Impact Questionnaire (PFIQ). Neurourology and urodynamics. 2011 Apr;30(4):541-6.
3. Crosby RD, Kolotkin RL, Williams GR. Defining clinically meaningful change in health-related quality of life. Journal of clinical epidemiology. 2003 May 1;56(5):395-407.

Pelvic Floor Impact Questionnaire—short form 7 (PFIQ-7)

How do symptoms or conditions in the following usually affect your	Bladder or urine	Bowel or rectum	Vagina or pelvis
1. Ability to do household chores (cooking, laundry housecleaning)?	• Not at all • Somewhat • Moderately • Quite a bit	• Not at all • Somewhat • Moderately • Quite a bit	• Not at all • Somewhat • Moderately • Quite a bit
2. Ability to do physical activities such as walking, swimming, or other exercise?	• Not at all • Somewhat • Moderately • Quite a bit	• Not at all • Somewhat • Moderately • Quite a bit	• Not at all • Somewhat • Moderately • Quite a bit
3. Entertainment activities such as going to a movie or concert?	• Not at all • Somewhat • Moderately • Quite a bit	• Not at all • Somewhat • Moderately • Quite a bit	• Not at all • Somewhat • Moderately • Quite a bit
4. Ability to travel by car or bus for a distance greater than 30 minutes away from home?	• Not at all • Somewhat • Moderately • Quite a bit	• Not at all • Somewhat • Moderately • Quite a bit	• Not at all • Somewhat • Moderately • Quite a bit
5. Participating in social activities outside your home?	• Not at all • Somewhat • Moderately • Quite a bit	• Not at all • Somewhat • Moderately • Quite a bit	• Not at all • Somewhat • Moderately • Quite a bit
6. Emotional health (nervousness, depression, etc)?	• Not at all • Somewhat • Moderately • Quite a bit	• Not at all • Somewhat • Moderately • Quite a bit	• Not at all • Somewhat • Moderately • Quite a bit
7. Feeling frustrated?	• Not at all • Somewhat • Moderately • Quite a bit	• Not at all • Somewhat • Moderately • Quite a bit	• Not at all • Somewhat • Moderately • Quite a bit

Total × 100 × 100 × 100

Scoring the PFIQ-7: =

All of the items use the following response scale:

0, Not at all; 1, somewhat; 2, moderately; 3, quite a bit PFIQ-7 Score Scales:

Urinary Impact Questionnaire (UIQ-7): 7 items under column heading "Bladder or urine"

Colorectal-Anal Impact questionnaire (CRAIQ-7): 7 items under column heading "Bowel / rectum"

Pelvic Organ Prolapse Impact Questionnaire (POPIQ-7): Items under column "Pelvis / Vagina" Scale Scores: Obtain the mean value for all of the answered items within the corresponding scale (possible value 0 – 3) and then multiply by (100/3) to obtain the scale score (range 0-100). Missing items are dealt with by using the mean from answered items only. PFIQ-7 Summary Score: Add the scores from the 3 scales together to obtain the summary score (range 0-300).

❑❑❑

49 Fingertips to Floor Distance - Special Test

Objective

To assess the total mobility of the lumbo-pelvic region in clients presenting with lumbo-pelvic pain. It is a test that is simple to administer with excellent inter and intra-rater reliability, validity, and responsiveness.

Intended Population

Musculoskeletal conditions of the lumbar-pelvic region eg

1. Chronic Low Back Pain
2. Ankylosing Spondylitis (Axial Spondyloarthritis)
3. Radiculopathic Low Back Pain
4. Osteoarthritis of the Lumbo-pelvic region

Method of Use

The patient is asked to bend forward and attempt to reach for the floor with their fingertips. The physical therapist then measures the distance between the patient's right long finger and the floor using a standard measuring tape. Ask the client whether pain, stiffness or both limited the Fingertips to floor (FTF) test. If the FTF test is limited by pain, the location and pain score out of 10 should be documented. If the FTF test is 0 cm or the patient is able to place their palms to the floor with no pain, a different outcome measure should be considered. As forward bending flexibility is highly variable even in the asymptomatic population no normative values exist. Note- Patients with LBP with or without neural symptoms often present with FTF test measures of greater than 20cm.

Reliability: The intra- and interobserver reliability were excellent ICC (intraclass correlation coefficient) = .99)[2].

Validity: Spearman's correlation coefficient for trunk flexion assessed by the test and the radiologic measure are excellent (rs =.96).[2]

Responsiveness

97 for SRM (standardized response mean) and .87 for effect size.

Miscellaneous

FTF test has been criticized for not measuring isolated lumbar flexion ROM, as forward bending range involves pelvic, hip, thoracic spine, dural and shoulder mobility. However pure lumbar flexion active ROM measures should not be used as an outcome measure to monitor patient progress, as they have been shown to be weakly correlated to the patients' level of disability.[3]

Rainville J et al also found total lumbosacral flexion may be as equally relevant as true lumbar flexion in the measurement of trunk mobility in the clinical examination of patients with chronic low back pain. In regards to their relationship t oa self-reported disability, total flexion seemed to be more relevant to outcome following intensive rehabilitation[4].

References

1. G Gellerman Finger to Floor Test- Lumbo-Pelvic Mobility Available from: https://www.youtube.com/watch?v=8_f9FpyRSsU (last accessed 22 October 2019)
2. Perret C, Poiraudeau S, Fermanian J, Colau MM, Benhamou MA, Revel M. Validity, reliability, and responsiveness of the fingertip-to-floor test. Archives of physical medicine and rehabilitation. 2001;82(11):1566-70.
3. Sullivan MS, Shoaf LD, Riddle DL. The relationship of lumbar flexion to disability in patients with low back pain. Physical therapy. 2000;80(3):240-50.
4. Rainville J, Sobel JB, Hartigan C. Comparison of total lumbosacral flexion and true lumbar flexion measured by a dual inclinometer technique. Spine. 1994 Dec;19(23):2698-701. Available from: https://www.ncbi.nlm.nih.gov/pubmed/7899966 (accessed 22 October 2019)

50 Beighton Score

Objective

The Beighton score is a popular screening technique for hypermobility. This is a nine – point scale and requires the performance of 5 maneuvers, four passive bilateral and one active unilateral performance. It was originally introduced for epidemiological studies involving the recognition of hypermobility in populations. Therefore the scale was well suited, being easy and quick to perform in large numbers of people [1]. The criteria of the Beighton score were the first used to recognize hypermobility, and this method has been in use for 30 years. It involves evaluation of only a few joints and does not include other involved systems [2][3][4].

The Beighton score is a modification of the Carter and Wilkinson scoring system (1964) [5]. Because passive extension of the fingers was too severe, it was replaced by passive extension of just the little finger beyond 90° with the forearm flat on a table [6].

Disadvantages:

1. It samples only a small number of joints for examination, so that hypermobile joints outside this selected group will inevitably and invariably be overlooked.
2. It is an "all-or-none" test. It gives no indication of the degree of hypermobility, merely an expression of the widespread nature of its distribution. An alternative scale that offers a wider view of joint laxity (including the shoulder, hip, patella, ankle, foot and toes) is the 10 – point hospital Del Mar criteria (Barcelona) (Bulbena et al, 1992) [1][3]

Etiology

The Beighton score has subsequently been used internationally to define generalized joint laxity in all populations and all age groups. Most of the available prevalence studies used different cutoffs, ranging from >3 hypermobile joints to > 6 hypermobile joints of 9 assessed (both thumbs, both little fingers, both elbows, both knees and the trunk), and in some, only the dominant side was assessed. The most frequent choice of cutoff was > 4 hypermobile joints [7]

Beighton and Horan (1969) revised the test to measure joint laxity in people with Ehlers – Danlos syndrome [6].

Clinical Use

Components of the Beighton scale [6]:

	LEFT	RIGHT
1. Passive dorsiflexion and hyperextension of the fifth MCP joint beyond 90°	1	1
2. Passive apposition of the thumb to the flexor aspect of the forearm	1	1
3. Passive hyperextension of the elbow beyond 10°	1	1
4. Passive hyperextension of the knee beyond 10°	1	1
5. Active forward flexion of the trunk with the knees fully extended so that the palms of the hands rest flat on the floor	1	1
TOTAL	/9	

The first four elements can be given a maximum score of 2, because these are performed bilateral. The last element is scored with 0 or 1. The maximum score for ligament laxity is 9. A score of 9 means hyperlax. A score of zero is tight. Several researchers appoint a score of 0-3 as normal and a score of 4-9 as representing ligamentous laxity (Al - Rawi et al 1985, Diaz et al 1993, Klemp et al 1984). According to child (1986), a score of 4 or more out of 9 indicates generalized hypermobility of the joints [6].The spinal forward flexion criterion differs from the other criteria, in that it measures hamstring flexibility and anatomic proportions to ligamentous laxity [5]. According to the Beighton and Horan criteria, generalized joint laxity is present when four or more of five tests are positive, including contralateral knee hyperextension [7]. In fact there is no universal agreement on a threshold for BJHMS, some researchers use a Beighton scale score of 5/9, other researchers use a score of 6/9 and still others use a modified score of 3/9 [1][8][9][10][11].

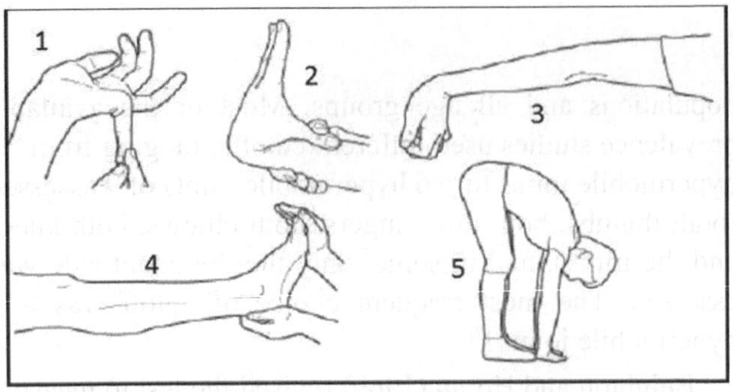

Instructions during the performance of the Beighton scale:

1. I am going to bend your little finger up at 90° to the back of your hand
2. I am going to bend your thumb back on the front of your forearm
3. I am going to bend your elbow backwards
4. I am going to bend your knee backwards
5. Can you put your hands flat on the floor with your knees straight [7]

Evidence of Use

Reliability

Clinch J et al (2011) showed that the prevalence of hypermobility in UK children is high, possibly suggesting that the Beighton score cutoff of >4 is too low or that this scoring is not appropriate for use in subjects whose musculoskeletal system is still developing. These results provide a platform to evaluate the relationships between the Beighton criteria and key clinical features (including pain), thereby testing the clinical validity of this scoring system in the pediatric population [7]

According to Remvig et al., the Beighton and Horan method for diagnosis of generalized joint laxity showed high kappa values (intraobserver: 0.75; interobserver: 0.78) [13].

Kyndall L. Boyle investigated the intrarater and interrater reliability of the Beighton and Horan Joint Mobility Index for women aged 15 to 45 years. His purpose was to determine the intrarater and interrater reliability of composite BHJMI scores (overall 0-9) and categorized scores (0-2, 3-4, 5-9). The percentage agreement and the Spearman rho for the intrarater and interrater reliability of the composite scores were 69% and 0.86 and 51% and 0.87, respectively. The percentage agreement and the Spearman rho for the intrarater and interrater reliability of the category scores were 81% and 0.81 and 89% and 0.75, respectively. This concluded that the reliability of BHJMI was good to excellent [14][9][10].

Validity

Smits – Engelsman B. et al.Objective was to evaluate the validity of the Beigthon score as a generalized measure of hypermobility and to measure the prevalence of hypermobility and pain in a random population of school age children between 6 and 12 years. Method. Children's joints and movements were assessed according to the Beighton score by qualified physiotherapists and by use of goniometry measuring 16 passive ranges of motion of joints on both sides of the body. Conclusion. There were no significant differences in Beighton score for sex in this population. They also concluded that the Beigton score, when goniometry is used, is a valid instrument to measure generalized joint mobility in children 6 to 12 years. In white children between 6 and 12 years of age, it is recommended that 7/9 be the cutoff for the Beighton score. [15]

Responsiveness

There may be a need to devise a new, more specific assessment tool to evaluate joint laxity in the developing musculoskeletal system—one that can be used to identify children at risk of symptoms such as pain and pathology such as connective tissue disease and, as importantly, to reassure those who do not need further medical intervention [7]. Bravo J. et al (2006) concluded that the Beighton score is an insufficient method for JHS diagnosis. They recommend that a validated hypermobility criteria set (i.e., the Brighton criteria or the Hospital del Mar criteria) be routinely used in the evaluation of rheumatology patients [2].

According to Schubert-Hjalmarsson E et al (2012) pain appears to affect activity and participation in children with HMS. Balance is also increased compared with healthy controls [16].

Fatoye F et al. concluded that pain and Quality of Life might form important components of clinical examination for children diagnosed with HMS. These children may benefit from appropriate treatment programmes to alleviate pain intensity and improve quality of life [17].

Engelbert RH et al concluded that in children with generalized joint hypermobility and hypomobility, the maximal exercise capacity is significantly decreased compared with age- and gender-matched control subjects. The most probable explanation for the reduced exercise tolerance in our patients is deconditioning [18]

References

1. Keer R., Grahame R. Hypermobility Syndrome: Recognition and Management for Physiotherapists. Elsevier 2003; page 2 – 4
2. Bravo JF. Wolff C. Clinical study of hereditary disorders of connective tissues in a chilean population. Arthritis & Rheumatism, 2006
3. HMSA: the beighton score (internet: http://www.hypermobility.org/beighton.php)
4. Pasinato F., Souza J.A., Rodrigues Corrêa E.C., Toniolo da Silva A.M. Temporomandibular disorder and generalized joint hypermobility application of diagnostic criteria. Braz J Otorhinolaryngol. 2011;77(4):418-25.
5. Frontera W., Slovik D., Dawson D. Exercise in Rehabilitation Medicine. Sheridan books 2006; page 41
6. Alter M. Science of Flexibility. Sheridan books 2004 (third edition); page 89
7. Clinch J. et al. Epidemiology of Generalized Joint Laxity (Hypermobility) in Fourteen-Year-Old Children From the UK. Arthritis & Rheumatism, 2011
8. Russek L.N. Hypermobility Syndrome. Physical Therapy, Journal of the American Physical Therapy Association; 1999; 79:591-599.
9. Quatman C.E., Ford K.R., Myer G.D., Paterno M.V., Hewett T.E. The Effects of Gender and Maturational Status on Generalized Joint Laxity in Young Athletes. J Sci Med Sport. 2008 June; 11(3):257-263.
10. Evans A.M., Rome K., Peet L. The foot posture index, ankle lunge test, Beighton scale and the lower limb assessment score in healthy children - a reliability study. Journal of Foot and Ankle Research 2012, 5:1.
11. Yazici M., Ataoglu S., Makarc S., Sari I., Erbilen E., Albayrak S., Yazici S., Uyan C. The relationship between echocardiographic features of mitral valve and elastic properties of aortic wall and beighton hypermobility score in patients with mitral valve prolapse. JPN Heart J, may 2004.
12. Physiotutors. The Beighton Score | Generalized Joint Hypermobility . Available from:https://www.youtube.com/watch?v=ZwWts_P-Xws
13. Remvig L, Jensen DV, Ward RC. Are diagnostic criteria for general joint hypermobility and benign joint hypermobility syndrome based on reproducible and valid tests? A review of the literature. J Rheumatol. 2007; 34: 798–803.
14. Boyle K.L., Witt P., Riegger-Krugh C. Intrarater and Interrater Reliability of the Beighton and Horan Joint Mobility Index.
15. Smits – Engelsman B et al. Beighton score: a valid measure for generalized hypermobility in children. J Pediatr. 2011 Jan; 158(1): 119, 123.
16. Schubert-Hjalmarsson E. et al. Pain, balance, activity, and participation in children with hypermobility syndrome. Pediatr Phys Ther. 2012: 24(4):339-44.
17. Fatoye F. et al. Pain intensity and quality of life perception in children with hypermobility syndrome. Rheumatol Int. 2012 May; 32(5): 1277-84.
18. Engelbert RH. et al. Exercise tolerance in children and adolescents with musculoskeletal pain in joint hypermobility and joint hypomobility syndrome. Pediatrics. 2006 Sep; 118(3)

❑❑❑

51 Oxford Knee Score

Objective

The Oxford Knee Score (OKS) was developed in 1998 and validated to measure pain and function after total knee replacement[1].

Intended Population

The OKS was originally developed and validated for use with individuals undergoing knee arthroplasty but has also been used to measure outcomes in pharmacological treatments, after osteotomies, following rehabilitation or with fractures[2]. It is a primary outcome measure of choice for national audits of knee replacements[3]. It has also been used to predict revisions six months after replacement[4].

Method of Use

The OKS is a patient reported outcome measure that consists of 12 questions obout an individual's activities of daily living and how they have been affected by pain over the preceding four weeks.

Questions

The patient is first asked to date their questionnaire and confirm which side/leg they are receiving treatment for. If both knees are involved, a questionnaire is done for each leg[5].

From Dawson et al 1998[1] and Oxford University Innovation[5]	
Questions	**Scoring**
1. How would you describe the pain you usually have from your knee?	None Very mild Mild Moderate Severe
2. Have you had any trouble with washing and drying yourself (all over) because of your knee?	No trouble Very little trouble Moderate trouble Extreme difficulty Impossible to do
3. Have you had any trouble getting in and out of a car or using public transport because of your knee? (whichever you tend to use)	No trouble Very little trouble Moderate trouble Extreme difficulty Impossible to do

4. For how long have you been able to walk before the pain from your knee becomes severe (with or without a stick)	No pain/more than 30 minutes 16 to 30 minutes 5 to 15 minutes Around the house only Not at all/pain severe when walking
5. After a meal (sat at a table), how painful has it been for you to stand up from a chair because of your knee?	Not at all painful Slightly painful Moderately painful Very painful Unbearable
6. Have you been limping when walking, because of your knee?	Rarely/ never Sometimes, or just at first Often,not just at first Most of the time All of the time
7. Could you kneel down and get up again afterwards?	Yes, easily With little difficulty With moderate difficulty With extreme difficulty No, impossible
8. Have you been troubled by pain from your knee in bed at night?	No nights Only 1 or 2 nights Some nights Most nights Every night
9. How much has pain from your knee interfered with your usual work (including housework)?	Not at all A little bit Moderately Greatly Totally
10. Have you felt that your knee might suddenly "give way" or let you down?	Rarely/ never Sometimes, or just at first Often, not just at first Most of the time All of the time
11. Could you do the household shopping on your own?	Yes, easily With little difficulty With moderate difficulty With extreme difficulty No, impossible
12. Could you walk down a flight of stairs?	Yes, easily With little difficulty With moderate difficulty With extreme difficulty No, impossible

Scoring

When the OKS was originally developed, it was designed to be as simple as possible in order to promote use. The original scoring system was a 1-5 where one represented the best outcome[5]. However, clinicians found this confusing in practice and adaptations began to appear so the original authors developed a new scoring system from 0-4 where four is the best outcome and total scores range from 0 (worst outcome) to 48 (best outcome)[5].

If there are more than two missing answers, it is recommended that the overall score should not be calculated. In the event one or two questions are unanswered, it is recommended that clinicians put in a mean answer from the patient's other answer, If a question has more than one answer, the worst response i.e. smallest number is used for calculations[5].

Equipment

Pen and paper, or online calculator.

Reference

Original article by Dawson et al 1998.

Useful information on background and use of The Oxford Knee Score by Oxford University Innovation.

Evidence

Reliability: The OKS has demonstrated strong test-retest reliability in its original testing[1]. A 2016 systematic review of 23 studies found good evidence of its reproducibility[6].

Validity: OKS shows significant correlation with similar measures (American Knee Society Score, SF-36, Health Assessment Questionnaire), particularly the pain and physical function domains[1]. A 2016 systematic review (23 studies) found good evidence for its internal consistency and construct validity[6].

Responsiveness: Research suggests the OKS is responsive to change post operatively [1][6] and a change of four or more points represents "real" change for an individual while a change of seven or more points represents "clinically relevant"[7].

Miscellaneous

Research[8] suggests that the OKS should not be used to decide whether or not an individual should have surgery because it can be biased in regards to gender, older age and to individuals reporting worse symptoms in order to meet criteria for surgery. Instead, the individual's pain symptoms should be used to determine surgery.

References

1. Dawson J, Fitzpatrick R, Murray D, Carr A. Questionnaire on the perceptions of patients about total knee replacement surgery. J. Bone Joint Surg 1998; 80-B:63-69. Accessed 15 January 2020.
2. Murray D, Rogers K, Pandit H, Beard D, Carr A, Dawson, J. The use of the Oxford Hip and Knee Scores. The Journal of Bone and Joint Surgery. 2007. 89; 8: 1010-4. Accessed 2 December 2019.
3. Browne J, Lewsey L, Van Der Muelen J, Black N. Report to the Department of Health. London, UK: London School of Hygiene & Tropical Medicine; 2007. Patient Reported Outcome Measures (PROMS) in Elective Surgery.
4. Rothwell A, Hooper G, Hobbs A, Frampton C. An analysis of the Oxford hip and knee scores and their relationship to early joint revision in the New Zealand Joint Registry. J Bone Joint Surg Br. 2010 Mar;92(3):413-8. Accessed 15 January 2020.
5. Oxford University Innovation. The Oxford Knee Score (OKS). 2016. Accessed online from https://innovation.ox.ac.uk/outcome-measures/oxford-knee-score-oks/ on 15 January 2020.
6. Harris K, Dawson J, Gibbons E, Lim C, Beard D, Fitzpatrick R, Price A. Systematic review of measurement properties of patient-reported outcome measures used in patients undergoing hip and knee arthroplasty. Patient Relat Outcome Meas. 2016; 7: 101–108. Published online 2016 Jul 25. doi: 10.2147/PROM.S97774. Accessed 15 January 2020.
7. Beard D, Harris K, Dawson J, Doll H, Murray DW, Carr AJ, Price AJ. Meaningful changes for the Oxford hip and knee scores after joint replacement surgery. J Clin Epidemiol. 2015 Jan;68(1):73-9. doi: 10.1016/j.jclinepi.2014.08.009. Epub 2014 Oct 31. Accessed 15 January 2020.
8. Robb C, McBryde C, Caddy S, Thomas A, Pynser P. Oxford scores as a triage tool for lower limb arthroplasty lead to discrimination and health inequalities. Ann R Coll Surg Engl (Suppl) 2013; 95. Accessed 15 January 2020.

❑❑❑

52 Berg Balance Scale

Objective

The Berg balance scale is used to objectively determine a patient's ability (or inability) to safely balance during a series of predetermined tasks. It is a 14 item list with each item consisting of a five-point ordinal scale ranging from 0 to 4, with 0 indicating the lowest level of function and 4 the highest level of function and takes approximately 20 minutes to complete. It does not include the assessment of gait.

Intended Population

Elderly population with impairment of balance, patients with acute stroke (Berg et al 1995, Usuda et al 1998).

Method of Use

Equipment required

1. A ruler
2. 2 standard chairs (one with arm rests, one without)
3. A footstool or step
4. 15 ft walkway
5. Stopwatch or wristwatch
6. The scale

Name: ______________ **Date:** ___________________
Location: _______________ **Rater:** _________________

ITEM DESCRIPTION SCORE (0-4)

Sitting to standing ________
Standing unsupported ________
Sitting unsupported ________
Standing to sitting ________
Transfers ________
Standing with eyes closed ________
Standing with feet together ________
Reaching forward with outstretched arm ________
Retrieving object from floor ________
Turning to look behind ________
Turning 360 degrees ________
Placing alternate foot on stool ________
Standing with one foot in front ________
Standing on one foot ________
Total ________

General instructions for completing the scale

Please document each task and/or give instructions as written. When scoring, please record the lowest response category that applies for each item.

In most items, the subject is asked to maintain a given position for a specific time. Progressively more points are deducted if:

- the time or distance requirements are not met
- the subject's performance warrants supervision
- the subject touches an external support or receives assistance from the examiner

The subject should understand that they must maintain their balance while attempting the tasks. The choices of which leg to stand on or how far to reach are left to the subject. Poor judgment will adversely influence the performance and the scoring.

Equipment required for testing is a stopwatch or watch with a second hand, and a ruler or other indicator of 2, 5, and 10 inches. Chairs used during testing should be a reasonable height. Either a step or a stool of average step height may be used for item # 12.

Interpretation

Cut-off scores for the elderly were reported by Berg et al 1992 [2] as follows :

1. A score of 56 indicates functional balance.
2. A score of < 45 indicates individuals may be at greater risk of falling.

It has been reported more recently that in the elderly population a change of 4 points is needed to be 95% confident that true change has occurred if a patient scores within 45–56 initially, 5 points if they score within 35–44, 7 points if they score within 25–34 and, finally, 5 points if their initial score is within 0–24 on the Berg Balance Scale [3].

Evidence

Reliability: Studies of various elderly populations (N = 31–101, 60–90 + years of age) have shown high intrarater and interrater reliability (ICC =.98,14,15 ratio of variability among subjects to total = .96–1.0,16 rs =.8817). Test-retest reliability in 22 people with hemiparesis is also high (ICC [2,1]=.98).

Berg K et al (1995) The Balance Scale: reliability assessment for elderly residents and patients with an acute stroke Scandinavian Journal of Rehabilitation Medicine 27, 27-36

Validity: Content validity of the BBS was established in a 3-phase development process involving 32 health care professionals who were experts working in geriatric settings. Criterion-related validity has been supported by moderate to high correlations between BBS scores and other functional measurements in a variety of older adults with disability.

Berg K, Wood-Dauphine SL, Williams JL, Gayton D (1992) Measuring balance in the elderly: validation of an instrument Canadian Journal of Public Health S2: s7-s11.

Usuda S, Araya K, Umehara K, Endo M, Shimizu T, Endo F (1998) Construct validity of functional balance scale in stroke inpatients Journal of Physical Therapy Science 10, 53-56.

Whitney, S., D. Wrisley, et al. (2003). Concurrent validity of the Berg Balance Scale and the Dynamic Gait Index in people with vestibular dysfunction. Physiother Res Int 8(4): 178-86.

Responsiveness: Increasing age has not been shown to correlate with decreasing BBS scores.

Steffen, T. M., T. A. Hacker, et al. (2002). Age- and gender-related test performance in community-dwelling elderly people: Six-Minute Walk Test, Berg Balance Scale, Timed Up and Go Test, and gait speeds. Phys Ther 82(2): 128-37.

Mao, H. F., I. P. Hsueh, et al. (2002). Analysis and comparison of the psychometric properties of three balance measures for stroke patients. Stroke 33(4): 1022-7.

Stevenson, T. J. (2001). Detecting change in patients with stroke using the Berg Balance Scale. Aust J Physiother 47(1): 29-38.

Salbach, N. M., N. E. Mayo, et al. (2001).

Responsiveness and predictability of gait speed and other disability measures in acute stroke. Arch Phys Med Rehabil 82(9): 1204-12.

Limitations: In ataxic clients it cannot, however, reflect problems in the performance of daily living activities, which are caused by the effects of ataxia on the upper extremities, because none of the items are designed to do this.

References

1. Kembe Frederick. 5253 Assessment Process Berg Balance Scale F.H.F. Available from: http://www.youtube.com/watch?v=i_Jlc5kL6KU[last accessed 08/02/13]
2. Berg K, Wood-Dauphinee S, Williams JI, Maki, B: Measuring balance in the elderly: Validation of an instrument. Can. J. Pub. Health, July/August supplement 2:S7-11, 1992.
3. Donoghue, D. and Stokes, E.K., (2009). How much change is true change? The minimum detectablefckLRchange of the Berg Balance Scale in elderly people. Journal of Rehabilitation Medicine, 41(5), pp.fckLR343-346.

❑❑❑

53 Community Balance and Mobility Scale

Objective

The Community Balance and Mobility Scale (CB&M) was developed to evaluate the balance and mobility of patients who may be ambulatory, yet still have balance deficits that affect their engagement in the community[1]. This test can be beneficial for patients that have reached a ceiling effect on other objective measures, such as the Berg Balance Test and Timed Up and Go, due to the challenging nature of the tasks[2]. The purpose of the CB&M is not to indicate a need for a gait aid, falls risk, or discharge placement, but to reflect the balance and mobility skills necessary for full participation in the community[2].

Intended Population

The CB&M is intended for assessing the balance and mobility of higher functioning ambulatory individuals with ABI, including children and adolescents. Other populations that have been validated for its use include patients with stroke or cerebral palsy, and older adults[3]. This test may be especially useful for individuals who are in the process of returning to living in the community.

Method of Use

Test Setting & Equipment Required

The CB&M is completed using a set 8-meter measured track and a full flight of stairs is required. This test requires approximately 20-30 minutes to administer. It is recommended that the assessor instructs the patient verbally as well as demonstrates all of the items to ensure proper understanding[2].

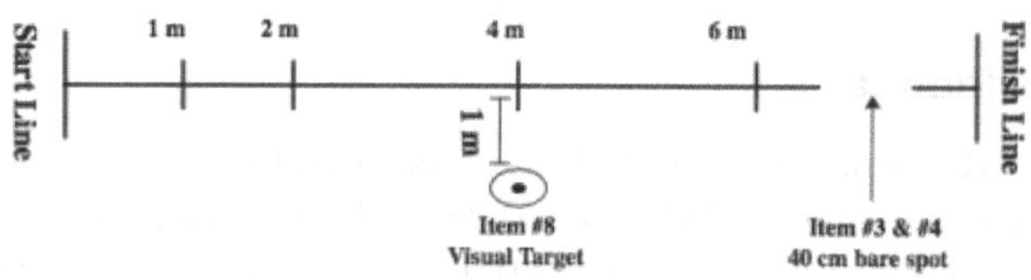

CB&M scale 8-meter track setup[2]

Other materials include:[2]

- Stopwatch
- Laundry basket or large rigid box of the same dimensions
- 2 lb. and 7.5 lb. weights
- A visual target (a paper circle 20 cm in diameter with a 5 cm black circle in the middle)
- A bean bag

Scoring

The CB&M is comprised of 13 items, and 6 of the tasks are to be performed bilaterally. Scoring is based on a scale of 0 to 5, with a score of 0 reflecting complete inability to perform the task and a score of 5 reflecting the most successful completion of the task possible[2]. CB&M scores range from 0 to 96, and items are scored upon completion of the first trial of an item. The only exceptions are if it is clear that the individual did not understand the task, in which case re-instruction and a second trial are allowed[2]. Items are to be completed without use of a gait aid, with exception for #12, although orthoses are allowed to be worn[2]. If the patient is unable to complete the task or the therapist deems the task would not be safe for the patient to complete, a score of zero should be recorded[2].

List of Items

- Unilateral Stance
- Tandem Walking
- 180 Tandem Pivot
- Lateral Foot Scooting
- Hopping Forward
- Crouch and Walk
- Lateral Dodging
- Walking & Looking
- Running with Controlled Stop
- Forward to Backward Walking
- Walk, Look and Carry
- Descending StairsStep-Ups x 1 Step

Evidence

Reliability: In adults, intraclass correlation coefficients (ICCs) of 0.977 (95% CI = 0.957 – 0.986) for intra-rater reliability, 0.977 (95% CI = 0.972 – 0.988) for inter-rater reliability, 0.898 (95% CI = 0.624 – 0.953) for 5 day apart reliability, and 0.975 (95%CI = 0.810 – 0.991) for immediate test-retest reliability were established[1].

In children and youth, ICCs of 0.93 (95% CI = 0.87 - 0.97) for inter-rater and 0.90 (95% CI = 0.81 - 0.95) for test-retest reliability (3 - 14 days apart, with a mean interval of 8.4 days) were established within a live-rating setting[4]. In the video-rating setting, ICCs of 0.95 (95% CI = 0.89 - 0.97) for inter-rater reliability and 0.90 (95% CI = 0.79 - 0.95) for test-retest reliability were demonstrated[4].

Validity: Construct validity was established by Howe et al. (2006) with a significant correlation with self-paced gait velocity at $r = 0.53$ ($p = 0.001$) and maximal gait velocity $r = 0.64$ ($p = 0.001$)[1]. In addition, mean CB&M scores were statistically significant ($p < 0.03$) between different care settings, demonstrating the measure's ability to differentiate amongst various settings and the continuum of rehabilitation[1].

CB & M can be used to determine if a patient will be able to return to community living and is considered a valid outcome measure in order to determine dynamic instability[2].

Considerations

1. Administration of the CB&M scale does not require specific training, but therapists should be familiar with the tool and have a good understanding of it prior to use. While therapists reported difficulty with observing all required criteria simultaneously when first using the scale, over time and with practice it became easier[1].
2. The CB&M items represent skills that are required for community living. As a result, the environmental context in which the items are performed should be considered to provide a complete assessment of the patient's mobility[1].
3. The test can be administered within 20-30 minutes depending on familiarity for therapist and patient. The test may require more time if the therapist is unfamiliar with the administration or when a patient is first introduced to the scale. In addition, the scale may take longer to administer in children[2].

References

1. owe JA, Inness EL, Venturini A, Williams JI, Verrier MC. The Community Balance and Mobility Scale-a balance measure for individuals with traumatic brain injury. Clinical Rehabilitation. 2006 Oct;20(10):885-95.
2. Howe J, Inness E, Wright V. The Community Balance and Mobility Scale [Internet]. Tbims.org. 2011 [cited 5 May 2018]. Available from: http://www.tbims.org/cbm/index.html
3. Community Balance and Mobility Scale [Internet]. Shirley Ryan AbilityLab - Formerly RIC. 2013 [cited 5 May 2018]. Available from: https://www.sralab.org/rehabilitation-measures/community-balance-and-mobility-scale#stroke
4. Wright F, Ryan J, Brewer K. Reliability of the Community Balance and Mobility Scale (CB&M) in high-functioning school-aged children and adolescents who have an acquired brain injury. Brain Injury. 2010;24(13-14):1585-1594.

❑❑❑

54

Borg Rating of Perceived Exertion

Objective

Borg rating of perceived exertion (RPE) is an outcome measure scale used in knowing exercise intensity prescription. It is use in monitoring progress and mode of exercise in cardiac patients as well as in other patient population undergoing rehabilitation and endurance training.

Borg RPE scale was developed by Gunnar Borg[1] for rating exertion and breathlessness during physical activity; that is, how hard the activity is as shown by high heart and respiration rate, profuse perspiration and muscle exertion.

Versions And Scoring

Borg original version is a scale of 6-20; it has a high correlation to heart rate and multiplying each number by 10 gives the training heart rate as at the time of scoring. It was later reconstructed to category (C) ratio (R) scale, termed Borg CR10 Scale or modified Borg Dyspnoea Scale which is mostly used in diagnosis of breathlessness and dyspnea, chest pain and musculo-skeletal pain. The CR-10 scale is best used in a specific area of the body sensation such as muscle pain or from pulmonary responses.[2]

Borg RPE Scale		Borg CR10 Scale	
Scoring	**Level of Exertion**	**Scoring**	**Level of Exertion**
6	No Exertion	0	No Exertion
7	Extremely Light	0.5	Very very Slight
8		1	Very Slight
9	Very Light	2	Slight
10		3	Moderate
11	Light	4	Somewhat Severe
12		5	Severe
13	Somewhat Hard	6	
14		7	Very Severe
15	Hard (Heavy)	8	
16		9	Very very Severe
17	Very Hard	10	Maximal
18			
19	Extremely Hard		
20	Maximal Exertion		

In Borg RPE;

- 9 = 'very light' exercise which equals walking slowly for few minutes at own pace of a healthy individual..
- 13 = 'somewhat hard' but the individual is still able to continue the activity.
- 17 = 'very hard'. A healthy person can continue but must push themselves beyond their comfort of being very fatigued.
- 19 = extremely strenuous exercise.for most people, the hardest they have ever experienced.

Intended Population

It is intended for all patient under rehabilitation. and for monitoring exercise prescription in athletes.It may not be suitable for children's use as the scoring is difficult to interpret in this age group.[3]

Method of Use

The scale is a very simple numerical list. Participants are asked to rate their exertion on the scale during the activity, taking into consideration feelings of physical stress and fatigue, disregarding any factor such as leg pain or breathlessness but focusing on the whole feeling of exertion. This number chosen connotes the intensity of activity allowing the participant to speed up or slow down movements/activity. The scale takes few seconds to complete, can be self or researcher administered in single occasion or multiple times.

Evidence

Reliability: Testing of the subject twice was used in ascertaining reliability in a study and Borg RPE was found to be reliable in rating exertion[4][5] The verbal anchor using VAS of the scale when tested in different clinical group and setting was found to have no significant difference in meaning in the groups except for the group that has a brain injury.[6]

Validity: Originally RPE was validated against heart rate.[7] With time, RPE has since been researched extensively in a variety of different conditions and population groups.

Borg RPE scores were positively associated with heart rate in adults during exercise sessions using the Wii Fit Plus.[8]

Skinner et al, found no significant differences in any of the physiological and perceptual variables in work intensity when the work load was presented in a random order and compared with those obtained during the progressive exercise test.[4]

A recent study reported that the Borg RPE scale may be used in individuals with Parkinson's disease in which formal exercise testing may not be available.[9]

Responsiveness: A work[11] done in a laboratory setting comparing physiological measurements and actual lifting tasks in the workplace found a relationship between perceived physical exertion and individual physical capacity; in both cardiovascular[12]and muscular work[13].

However, a research by by Village et al.[14] shows a weak relationship between perceived physical exertion and workload

References

1. Rating of perceived exertion. Available from: https://en.wikipedia.org/wiki/Rating_of_perceived_exertion(accessed 24 May 2019)
2. Williams N. The Borg Rating of Perceived Exertion (RPE) scale. Occupational Medicine.2017; 67(5):404–405, https://doi.org/10.1093/occmed/kqx063
3. Pfeiffer K, Pivarnik JM, Womack CJ, Reeves MJ, Robert MM. Reliability and validity of the Borg and OMNI RPE Scales in adolescent girls. Medicine and science in sports and exercise. 2003; 34(12):2057-61.
4. Skinner JS, Hutsler R, Bergsteinová V, Buskirk ER. The validity and reliability of a rating scale of perceived exertion. Medicine and science in sports. 1973;5(2): 94-6.
5. Lamb KL, Eston RG, Corns D. Reliability of ratings of perceived exertion during progressive treadmill exercise.Br J Sports Med 1999;33:336–339
6. Dawes, Helen N. et al. Borg's Rating of Perceived Exertion Scales: Do the Verbal Anchors Mean the Same for Different Clinical Groups? Archives of Physical Medicine and Rehabilitation. 2005;86(5): 912 - 916
7. American College of Sports Medicine. ACSM's guidelines for exercise testing and prescription. Lippincott Williams & Wilkins; 2013 Mar 4.
8. Pollock BS, Barkley JE, PotenzinI N, Desalvo RM, Buser SL, Otterstetter et al. Validity of Borg Ratings of Perceived Exertion During Active Video Game Play. Int J Exerc Sci. 2013; 6(2): 164–170.
9. PENKO AL, BARKLEY JE, KOOP MM, ALBERTS JL. Borg scale is valid for ratings of perceived exertion for individuals with Parkinson's disease. International journal of exercise science. 2017;10(1):76.
10. Vivo Phys-Evan Mathews. RPE - Rating of Perceived Exertion. Available from: http://www.youtube.com/watch?v=HgEHl0-IB14[last accessed 30/4/2019]
11. akobsen MD, Sundstrup E, Persson R, Andersen CH, Andersen LL. Is Borg's perceived exertion scale a useful indicator of muscular and cardiovascular load in blue-collar workers with lifting tasks? A cross-sectional workplace study. Eur J Appl Physiol 2014;114(2):425–434.
12. Scherr J, Wolfarth B, Christle JW, Pressler A, Wagenpfeil S, Halle M. Associations between Borg's Rating of Perceived Exertion and physiological measures of exercise intensity. Eur J Appl Physiol 2013;113(1):147–155
13. Fontes EB, Smirmaul BP, Nakamura FY, Pereira G, Okano AH, Altimari LR et al. The relationship between rating of perceived exertion and muscle activity during exhaustive constant-load cycling. Int J Sports Med 2010;31(10):683–688.
14. Village J, Frazer M, Cohen M, Leyland A, Park I, Yassi A. Electromyography as a measure of peak and cumulative workload in intermediate care and its relationship to musculoskeletal injury: an exploratory ergonomic study. Appl Ergon 2005;36(5):609–618

❑❑❑

55 Box and Block Test

Objective

The Box and Block Test (BBT) measures unilateral gross manual dexterity. It is a quick, simple and inexpensive test. It can be used with a wide range of populations, including clients with stroke.

Intended Population

Those with a range of neurological diagnoses including:

- Stroke
- Multiple Sclerosis
- Traumatic Brain Injury (TBI)
- Neuromuscular Disorders
- Geriatric Spinal Cord Injury (SCI)
- Fibromyalgia

The BBT cannot be used with clients who have severe upper extremity impairment or those with sever cognitive impairment.

Features of the Measure

The BBT is composed of a wooden box divided in two compartments by a partition and 150 blocks. The BBT administration consists of asking the client to move, one by one, the maximum number of blocks from one compartment of a box to another of equal size, within 60 seconds. The box should be oriented lengthwise and placed at the client's midline, with the compartment holding the blocks oriented towards the hand being tested. In order to practice and register baseline scores, the test should begin with the unaffected upper limb.

Additionally, a 15-second trial period is permitted at the beginning of each side. Before the trial, after the standardized instructions are given to clients, they should be advised that their fingertips must cross the partition when transferring the blocks, and that they do not need to pick up the blocks that might fall outside of the box[2]

Method of Use

Equipment Required:

- Stopwatch
- Wooden box dimensioned in 53.7 cm × 25.4 cm × 8.5 cm
- Partition (should be placed at the middle of the box, dividing it in two containers of 25.4 cm each) 150 wooden cubes (2.5 cm in size)

Set-Up:

- A test box with 150 blocks and a partition in the middle is placed lengthwise along the edge of a standard-height table
- The patient should be seated on a standard height chair facing the box
- 150 blocks should be in the compartment of the test box on the side of the patient's dominant hand
- The examiner should face the patient so she or he could view the blocks being transported

Description: The patient is allowed a 15-second trial period prior to testing

- Individuals are seated at a table, facing a rectangular box that is divided into two square compartments of equal dimension by means of a partition.
- One hundred and fifty, 2.5 cm, colored, wooden cubes or blocks are placed in one compartment or the other.
- The individual is instructed to move as many blocks as possible, one at a time, from one compartment to the other for a period of 60 seconds.

- Standardized dimensions for the test materials and procedures for test administration and scoring have been provided by Mathiowetz et al, 1985.
- To administer the test, the examiner is seated opposite the individual in order to observe test performance.
- The BBT is scored by counting the number of blocks carried over the partition from one compartment to the other during the one-minute trial period.
- Patient's hand must cross over the partition in order for a point to be given, and blocks that drop or bounce out of the second compartment onto the floor are still rewarded with a point.
- Multiple blocks carried over at the same time count as a single point.
- Higher scores on the test indicate better gross manual dexterity

Scoring: Clients are scored based on the number of blocks transferred from one compartment to the other compartment in 60 seconds[2]. Score each hand separately. Higher scores are indicative of better manual dexterity. During the performance of the BBT, the evaluator should be aware of whether the client's fingertips are crossing the partition. Blocks should be counted only when this condition is respected. Furthermore, if two blocks are transferred at once, only one block will be counted. Blocks that fall outside the box, after trespassing the partition, even if they don't make it to the other compartment, should be counted.

Patient Instructions:[2]

Detailed patient instructions as outlined by Mathiowetz et al.

"I want to see how quickly you can pick up one block at a time with your right (or left) hand [point to the hand]. Carry it to the other side of the box and drop it. Make sure your fingertips cross the partition. Watch me while I show you how."

Transport three cubes over the partition in the same direction you want the patient to move them. After a demonstration say the following:

"If you pick up two blocks at a time, they will count as one. If you drop one on the floor or table after you have carried it across, it will still be counted, so do not waste time picking it up. If you toss the blocks without your fingertips crossing the partition, they will not be counted. Before you start, you will have a chance to practice for 15 seconds. Do you have any questions?"

"Place your hands on the sides of the box. When it is time to start, I will say ready and then go."

Trial period: Start the stop watch at the word go. When 15 seconds has passed, say "stop." If mistakes are made during the practice period, correct them before the actual testing begins.

On completion of the practice period, transport the cubes to the original compartment.

Continued with the following directions:

"This will be the actual test. The instructions are the same. Work as quickly as you can. Ready." [Wait 3 seconds]

"Go."

"Stop." [After 1 minute, count the blocks and record as described above]

"Now you are to do the same thing with your left (or right) hand. First you can practice. Put your hands on the sides of the box as before. Pick up one block at a time with your hand, and drop it on the other side of the box."

"Ready." [Wait 3 seconds] "Go."

"Stop." [After 15 seconds]

Return the transported blocks to the compartment as described above.

"This will be the actual test. The instructions are the same. Work as quickly as you can."

"Ready." [Wait 3 seconds]

"Go."

"Stop." [After 1 minute, count the blocks and record as described above]

Evidence

Reliability

Test-retest Reliability:

- Acute and Chronic Stroke: (Chen et al, 2009) [3]
  - Excellent test-retest reliability when tested on more affected (r = 0.98) and less affected hand (r = 0.93)
- Upper Limb Impairment: (Desrosiers et al, 1994; n = 35 able bodied subjects; mean age = 71.7(60-89) years; n = 34 subjects with impairment; mean age = 74.5(65-87) years) [4]
  - Excellent test-retest reliability of the right hand for able bodied subjects (ICC= 0.97)
  - Excellent test-retest reliability of the left hand for able bodied subjects (ICC= 0.96)

  - Excellent test-retest reliability of the right hand for subjects with impairment (ICC= 0.90)
  - Excellent test-retest reliability of the left hand for subjects with impairment (ICC= 0.89)
- Upper Extremity Paresis: (Platz et al, 2005; n = 56 people with upper limb paresis as a result of stroke, Multiple Sclerosis (MS), and traumatic brain injury (TBI); median age = 54(13-92) years; n = 37 for stroke; median age = 62(22-92) years; n = 14 for MS; median age = 43(28-60) years; n = 5 for TBI; median age = 34(13-50) years) [5]
  - Excellent test-retest reliability (ICC = 0.96)
- Spastic Hemiplegia: (Siebers et al, 2010) [6]
  - Excellent test-retest reliability (ICC = 0.95)

Interrater/Intrarater Reliability

- Normal Adults: (Mathiowetz et al, 1985) [7]
  - Excellent interrater reliability for the right hand (r = 1.00)
  - Excellent interrater reliability for the left hand (r = 0.99)
- Upper Extremity Paresis: (Platz et al, 2005) [5]
  - Excellent interrater reliability (ICC = 0.99)
- Spastic Hemiplegia: (Siebers et al, 2010) [6]
  - Excellent interrater reliability (r = 0.95)
- Fibromyalgia: (Canny et al, 2009; n = 30 participants with fibromyalgia; mean age = 46.9(range 20-68) years; n = 30 healthy participants; mean age= 41.2(29-52) years) [8]
  - Excellent intrarater reliability for participants with fibromyalgia (ICC = 0.90)
  - Excellent intrarater reliability for healthy participants (ICC = 0.98)
  - Excellent interrater reliability for participants with fibromyalgia (ICC = 0.85)
  - Excellent interrater reliability for healthy participants (ICC = 0.80)

Validity: Criterion Validity (Predictive/Concurrent):

Stroke: (Lin et al, 2010; n = 59 patients with stroke; sex = 47 males, 12 females; mean age = 55.5(11.66) years)

Concurrent Validity Pre- and Post- Treatment

Measure	Pretreatment (r)	Posttreatment (r)
NHPT	-0.80 (Excellent)	-0.71 (Excellent)
ARAT	0.63 (Excellent)	0.64 (Excellent)
FMA	0.44 (Adequate)	0.35 (Adequate)
MAL-AOU	-0.37 (Adequate)	0.49 (Adequate)
MAL-QOM	0.52 (Adequate)	0.52 (Adequate)
SIS	0.59 (Adequate)	0.52 (Adequate)

(ARAT = Action Research Arm Test, BBT = Box and Block Test, CI = confidence interval, FMA = Fugl-Meyer Assessment, MAL-AOU = Motor Activity Log-Amount of Use, MAL-QOM = Motor Activity Log-Quality of Movement, NHPT = Nine-Hole Peg Test, SIS = Stroke Impact Scale)

Construct Validity (Convergent/Discriminant)

- Upper Limb Impairment: (Desrosiers *et al*, 1994)[4]
  - Excellent convergent validity with the Action Research Arm Test (r = 0.80)
  - Adequate convergent validity with Functional Autonomy Measurement System (r (right hand) = 0.47; r (left hand) = 0.51)
- Upper Extremity Paresis: (Platz et al, 2005)[5]
  - Excellent convergent validity with the Action Research Arm Test (r = 0.95)
  - Excellent convergent validity with the Fugl-Meyer Test (r = 0.92)
  - Excellent convergent validity with the Hemispheric Stroke Scale (r = -0.67)
  - Adequate convergent validity with the Passive Joint motion/Joint pain sub-scale of Fugl-Meyer Test (r = 0.43)
  - Poor convergent validity with the Modified Barthel Index (r = 0.04)
- Central Paresis: (Platz et al, 2008; n = 33 neurological patients with central paresis due to stroke, ischemic/anoxic brain damage, traumatic brain injury, or spinal cord injury; n=3 patients with SCI(C3,C4,T8), 6 patients with TBI, and 23 patients with stroke; sex = 20 males, 13 females; mean duration of disease = 19.4 months; mean age = 49.7(17.3) years) [5]
  - Excellent convergent validity with Resistance to Passive Movement (r = -0.680)

References

1. Mathiowetz, V., G. Volland, et al. (1985). "Adult norms for the Box and Block Test of manual dexterity." Am J Occup Ther 39(3160243): 386-391.
2. Mathiowetz, V., G. Volland, et al. (1985). "Adult norms for the Box and Block Test of manual

dexterity." Am J Occup Ther 39(3160243): 386-391.
3. Chen, H. M., Chen, C. C., et al. "Test-retest reproducibility and smallest real difference of 5 hand function tests in patients with stroke." Neurorehabil Neural Repair 2009 23(5): 435-440
4. Desrosiers, J., Bravo, G., et al. "Validation of the Box and Block Test as a measure of dexterity of elderly people: reliability, validity, and norms studies." Arch Phys Med Rehabil 1994 75: 751-755
5. Platz, T., Pinkowski, C., et al. "Reliability and validity of arm function assessment with standardized guidelines for the Fugl-Meyer Test, Action Research Arm Test and Box and Block Test: a multicentre study." Clin Rehabil 2005 19(4): 404-411
6. Siebers, A., Oberg, U., et al. "The effect of modified constraint-induced movement therapy on spasticity and motor function of the affected arm in patients with chronic stroke." Physiother Can 2010 62(4): 388-396
7. Mathiowetz, V., Volland, G., et al. "Adult norms for the Box and Block Test of manual dexterity." Am J Occup Ther 1985 39(3160243): 386-391
8. Canny, M. L., Thompson, J. M., et al. "Reliability of the box and block test of manual dexterity for use with patients with fibromyalgia." Am J Occup Ther 2009 63(4): 506-510

❑❑❑

56 Brief Pain Inventory-Short Form

The Brief Pain Inventory - Short Form (BPI-sf) is a 9 item self-administered questionnaire used to evaluate the severity of a patient's pain and the impact of this pain on the patient's daily functioning. The patient is asked to rate their worst, least, average, and current pain intensity, list current treatments and their perceived effectiveness, and rate the degree that pain interferes with general activity, mood, walking ability, normal work, relations with other persons, sleep, and enjoyment of life on a 10 point scale. The BPI-sf is a modification of the Brief Pain Inventory - Long Form, which includes additional questions on demographics (date of birth, marital status, education, employment), pain history, aggravating and easing factors, treatment and medication, pain quality, and response to treatment.

The brevity of the BPI-sf makes it suitable for settings in which pain is assessed on a daily basis (e.g. in a randomized control trial), whereas the long-form may be more appropriate as a baseline measure. The questionnaire exists within the biopsychosocial model of pain, as it addresses sensory, emotional, and functional aspects of the pain experience[1]. Thus, the tool is responsive to changes in pain associated with both pharmacological, physical, and psychological interventions[2].

Intended Population

Originally intended for use in epidemiological studies and clinical trials involving patients with cancer-related pain, the BPI-sf is now widely used in a range of chronic cancer-related and non-malignant pain conditions, including HIV/AIDS, phantom limb pain, critical limb ischemia, neuropathy, low back pain, and osteoarthritis. The tool has also been used to assess individuals experiencing acute pain, for example post-operatively. The questionnaire has been translated into numerous languages including Vietnamese, Chinese, Italian, German, Taiwanese, Greek, Norwegian, French, Hindi, Japanese, and Spanish[3].

Method of Use

The questionnaire can be completed via self-report or interview. The short form version takes 5 minutes for the patient to complete.

Evidence

Reliability: The psychometric properties of the tool have been analyzed in a range of populations with cancer and non-cancer related pain. Acceptable reliability has been reported in studies of patients with advanced cancer pain[4], osteoarthritis pain[5][6], and chronic pain in neuropathic and nociceptive pain patients (Turkish translation)[7].

Validity: Kumar reports that the BPI has been validated in patient populations with bone metastases, breast cancer and postoperative cancer patients and in a variety of languages including Brazilian, Chinese, Greek, Hindi, Italian, Japanese, Korean, Malay, Norwegian, Polish, Russian, Spanish, Taiwanese and Thai[8].

A number of studies have utilized a confirmatory factor approach (CFA) to determine the construct validity of the BPI. A three factor representation (pain intensity, activity interference, and affective interference) was compared with a two factor (pain intensity, activity interference) and one-factor (pain intensity) approach. Research by Atkinson and colleagues supports both two- and three-factor representations in the HIV/AIDS and cancer populations[9]. Lapane and colleagues and Tan and colleagues report that a two-factor model has greater validity for patients with non-cancer pain (including arthritis, back/neck pain, injury-/trauma-related pain, neuropathic pain, and fibromyalgia-related pain)[10][3].

Responsiveness: Studies have reported on the responsiveness of the BPI with respect to change in patient's self-reported pain over time and change with treatment[3]. The tool was able to detect change in pain and impact of pain in patients with hip osteoarthritis up to one year following total hip replacement[5]. No minimum clinically important change (MCIC) has been reported in the literature regarding patients with cancer-related pain[8]. Kumar suggests future studies employ a patient-rated global impression of change as a criterion measure to determine an MCIC in this population.

References

1. Mendoza T, et al. Reliability and validity of a modified Brief Pain Inventory short form in patients with osteoarthritis. Eur J Pain 2006;353-361.
2. Hwang SS, Chang VT, Kasimis B. Dynamic cancer pain management outcomes: the relationship between pain severity, pain relief, functional interference, satisfaction and global quality of life over time. J Pain Symptom Manage 2002;23:190–200.
3. Tan G, et al. Validation of the Brief Pain Inventory for chronic nonmalignant pain. J Pain 2004;5(2):133-137.
4. Pelayo-Alvarez M, Perez-Hoyos S, Agra-Varela Y. Reliability and concurrent validity of the Palliative Outcome Scale, the Rotterdam Symptom Checklist, and the Brief Pain Inventory. J Palliat Med 2013;16(8):867-874.
5. Kapstad H, Rokne B, Stavem K. Psychometric properties of the Brief Pain Inventory among patients with osteoarthritis undergoing total hip replacement surgery. Health Qual Life Outcomes 2010;8(1):1-8.
6. Williams VS, Smith MY, Fehnel SE. The validity and utility of the BPI interference measures for evaluating the impact of osteoarthritic pain. J Pain Symptom Manage 2006;31(1):48-57.
7. Erdemoglu AK, Koc R. Brief Pain Inventory score identifying and discriminating neuropathic and nociceptive pain. Acta Neurologica Scandinavica 2013;128(5):351-358.
8. Kumar SP. Utilization of brief pain inventory as an assessment tool for pain in patients with cancer: a focused review. Indian J Palliat Care 2001;17(2).
9. Atkinson TM, et al. Using confirmatory factor analysis to evaluate construct validity of the Brief Pain Inventory (BPI). J Pain Symptom Manage 2011;41(3):558-565.
10. Lapane KL, et al. One, two, or three? Constructs of the Brief Pain Inventory among patients with non-cancer pain in the outpatient setting. J Pain Symptom Manage 2013.
11. Tyler EJ, Jensen MP, Engel JM, Schwartz L. The reliability and validity of pain interference measures in persons with cerebral palsy. Arch Phys Med Rehabil 2002:83(2),236-239.

Brief Pain Inventory (Short Form)

Study Id **Hospital Name**

Date **Time**

Name:

1. Throughout our lives, most of us have had pain from time to time (such as minor headaches, sprains, and toothaches). Have you had pain other than these everyday kinds of pain today?

   Yes No

2. On the diagram, shade in the areas where you feel pain. Put an X on the area that hurts the most.

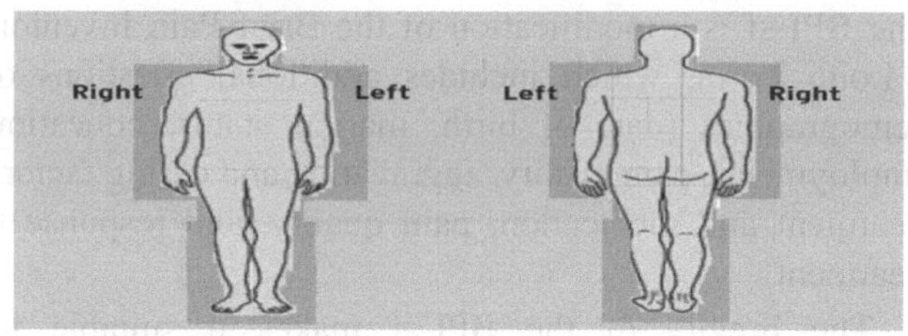

3. Please rate your pain by circling the one number that best describes your pain at its WORST in the past 24 hours.

   0 No Pain 1 2 3 4 5 6 7 8 9 10 Pain as bad as you can imagine

4 Please rate your pain by circling the one number that best describes your pain at its LEAST in the past 24 hours.

   0 No Pain 1 2 3 4 5 6 7 8 9 10 Pain as bad as you can imagine

5. Please rate your pain by circling the one number that best describes your pain on the AVERAGE.

   0 No Pain 1 2 3 4 5 6 7 8 9 10 Pain as bad as you can imagine

6. Please rate your pain by circling the one number that tell how much pain you have RIGHT NOW

0 No Pain	1	2	3	4	5	6	7	8	9	10 Pain as bad as you can imagine

7. What treatments or medications are you receiving for your pain?

____

____

____

8. In the past 24 hours, how much RELIEF have pain treatments or medications provided? Please circle the one percentage that most shows how much relief you have received.

0% No Relief	10%	20%	30%	40%	50%	60%	70%	80%	90%	100% Complete Relief

9. Circle the one number that describes how, during the past 24 hours. PAIN HAS INTERFERED with your:

A. General Activity:

0	1 Does not Interfere	2	3	4	5	6	7	8	9	10 Completely interferes

B. Mood

0	1 Does not Interfere	2	3	4	5	6	7	8	9	10 Completely interferes

C. Walking Ability

0	1 Does not Interfere	2	3	4	5	6	7	8	9	10 Completely interferes

D. Normal work (Includes both work outside the home and housework)

0	1 Does not Interfere	2	3	4	5	6	7	8	9	10 Completely interferes

E. Relation with other people

0	1 Does not Interfere	2	3	4	5	6	7	8	9	10 Completely interferes

F. Sleep

0	1 Does not Interfere	2	3	4	5	6	7	8	9	10 Completely interferes

G. Enjoyment of life

0	1 Does not Interfere	2	3	4	5	6	7	8	9	10 Completely interferes

❑❑❑

57 Brigham and Women's Carpal Tunnel Questionnaire

Objective

The purpose of the test: In 1993, Levine et al developed The Brigham and Women's Hospital Symptom Severity Scale (SSS) and Functional Status Scale (FSS) to measure symptom severity and functional status in patients with carpal tunnel syndrome (CTS)[1].

Intended Population

Levine et al[1]

- Purpose of this study: development of the SSS and FSS and to assess reliability, validity, and responsiveness to clinical change
- 77 pts with CTS were included in this study, 39 evaluated pre-op and 1 yr post op carpal tunnel release (CTR), 28 were managed non-op
- 17 men, 50 women, 9 pt's receiving workman's compensation
- median age 57

  median duration of symptoms: 18 mo

Amadio et al[2]

- Purpose of this study: to compare SSS and FSS responsiveness to clinical change to the following generic questionnaires: the DASH, AIMS2, and the SF-36 and to clinical examination findings and electrophysiological testing
- 22 pt with CTS, evaluated 1 day prior and 3 mo post op CTR
- all patients had failed non-op therapy
- mean age 60

Katz et al [3]

- Purpose of this study: to compare reliability, validity, and responsiveness of SSS and FSS in recipients and non-recipients of worker's compensation
- 268 pts, 155 work comp, SSS and FSS were measured pre op CTR and 6 months post op CTR
- 197 women, 71 men
- mean age: 40
- mean symptom duration: work comp 2.2 mo, non work comp 5.6 mo

Ozyurekoglu et al[4]

- Purpose of this study: to calculate the MCID of the SSS in patients with CTS
- 28 pts included, results from SSS were analyzed prior to a carpal tunnel injection and 3 mo after a carpal tunnel injection
- 19 women, 9 men, no workmen's compensation claims
- mean age: 38
- inclusion criteria: c/o intermittent hand numbness and waking at night due to numbness, no previous treatment of CTS

Method of Use

Constructs or items the test was designed to measure: The SSS and FSS are self-administered questionnaires that were designed to measure symptom severity and functional status in patients with CTS.[1] The SSS consist of 11 questions based on six domains thought to be critical by experts for evaluating CTS: pain, paresthesia, numbness, weakness, nocturnal symptoms, and over all functional status. The FSS contains 8 functional activities that are commonly affected by CTS and that are performed by a wide variety of patients.[1]

Evidence

Reliability

Levine et al[1]: Test- retest reliability: researchers measured scores on the SSS and FSS 2 days apart and calculated pearson correlation coefficients: SSS was 0.91 FSS was 0.93 (excellent).

Internal consistency: SSS Chronbach alpha 0.89, FSS Chronbach alpha 0.91

Katz et al[3]: Internal consistency: SSS Chronbach alpha for the non work comp group was 0.89, work comp group 0.89 . FSS Chronbach alpha for the non work comp group was 0.88, work comp group 0.89

Validity: Levine et al stated "there is no universally accepted measurement of the severity of symptoms or functional status of the hand.[1]" Therefore, they examined validity by assessing traditional objective measures of disability and impairment found in patients with CTS: grip, pinch strength, median nerve sensory conduction, 2 pt discrimination, and Semmes Weinstein monofilament testing. However, as expected they found mod-weak correlations because the SSS and FSS measure disability not usually captured by objective findings. Since objective findings in patients with CTS often do not correlate with symptom and functional improvements, these researchers also analyzed validity by looking at patient satisfaction. Greater satisfaction with results correlated with greater improvement in the SSS and FSS scores.[1]

Spearman Coefficients from Levine et al [1]:

	Grip strength	Pinch Strength	2 pt discrimination	Semmes Weinstein	Pt. Satisfaction (patients in the retrospective cohort)	Pt. Satisfaction (patients in the prospective cohort)
SSS	0.38 ($p<0.05$)	0.47 ($p<0.01$)	0.15	0.17	0.52 ($p=0.0007$)	0.50 ($p<0.01$)
FSS	0.50 ($p<0.001$)	0.60 ($p<0.001$)	0.42 ($p<0.01$)	0.24	0.29 ($p=0.09$)	0.54 ($p<0.01$)

Amadio et al evaluated patients pre op and post op CTR and measured the following objective findings: sensation, grip strength, pinch strength, dexterity, and motion.[2] Their results found the only objective finding improved after a CTR was dexterity. No other physical measurement improved despite significant improvements on the SSS and FSS.[2] These findings support claims made by Levine et al that establishing validity of the SSS and FSS cannot be solely based on objective findings since improvements in symptoms and function do not always correlate with a change in objective findings. Katz et al assessed validity by looking at patient satisfaction, perceived improvement in quality of life and perceived improvement in symptoms.[3] The following Spearman Coefficients were reported by Katz et al[3]:

	Patient satisfaction		Perceived improvement in quality of life		perceived improvement in symptoms	
	WC	NWC	WC	NWC	WC	NWC
SSS	0.69	0.37	0.68	0.37	0.59	0.31
FSS	0.55	0.21	0.54	0.41	0.48	0.19

WC-patients receiving workman's compensation, NWC patients not receiving workman's compensation

Responsiveness

Levine et al[1]

- Patient satisfaction post op CTR was highly correlated with improvements in the SSS and mod correlated with an improvement in the FSS
- 38 pts evaluated retrospectively mean SSS pre-op was 3.4 and 1.9 post op, effect size 1.4; mean FSS 3.0 pre op and 2.0 post op, effect size 0.82 - 28 pts evaluated prospectively mean SSS pre-op was 3.1 and 2.0 post op, effect size 1.13; Mean FSS 32.7 pre op and 2.1 post op, effect size 0.71

Amadio et al[2]

- The SSS and FSS both showed a significant change $p<0.01$ in the direction of improved health status from pre-op to post-op
- The SSS and FSS were found to be more responsive to clinical change than all clinical examination findings including electrophysiological testing and the DASH, AIMS2 and the SF-36

Minimal Clinical Important Difference (MCID)

The MCID is the smallest amount of change between two outcome measure scores that has clinical meaning to a patient. Ozyurekoglu et al determined the MCID of the SSS by using a ROC curve and analyzing the relationship between change scores on the SSS and the clinical result of a carpal tunnel injection. The clinical result of each injection was judged as satisfactory if the patient was satisfied with their results and did not require any additional care.[4] The MCID of the SSS was determined to be 1.04 in this study. For practical purposes, the researchers suggest using 1.0 as the MCID.[4] . The MCID of the FSS has not been determined.

References

1. Levine DM, Simmons BP, Koris MJ, Daltroy LH, Hohl GG, Fossel AH, Katz JN. A self-administered questionnaire for the assessment of severity of symptoms and functional status in carpal tunnel syndrome. J Bone Joint Surg Am. 1993; 75: 1585-1592
2. Amadio PC, Silverstein MD, Ilstrup DM, Schleck BS, Jensen LM. Outcome Assessment for Carpal Tunnel Surgery: The Relative Responsiveness of Generic, Arthritis-Specific, Disease-Specific, and Physical Examination Measures. JHand Surg (Am). 1996; 21A: 338-346.
3. Katz JN, Punnett L, Simmons BP, Fossel AH, Mooney N, Keller RB. Worker's Compensation Recipients with Carpal Tunnel Syndrome: The Validity of Self-Reported Health Measures. Am J Public Health. 1996; 86(1): 52-56
4. Ozyurekoglu T, McCabe S, Goldsmith LJ, LaJoie AS. The Minimally Clinically Important Difference of the Carpal Tunnel Syndrome Symptom Severity Scale. J Hand Surg (Am). 2006; 31(5): 733-738.
5. Wainner RS, Fritz JM, Irrgang JJ, Delitto A, Allison S, Bonninger M. Development of a Clinical Prediction Rule for the Diagnosis of Carpal Tunnel Syndrome. Arch Phys Med Rehab. 2005; 86(4): 609-618

□□□

58 Brodie–Trendelenburg Test

Introduction

This technique was originally described in the in 1846 by Brodi an popularized by Trendelenburg in 1891. The primary aim of this test was to identify an incompetency in the sapenofemoral junction.

Technique

The affected leg is raised so that the veins are emptied by gravity. Around the upper thigh region a tourniquet is applied, sufficiently tightly to constrict the saphenous vien. The femoral vein blood flow is'nt obstructed. The subject is then asked to stand and the degree of filling of he saphenous vein is noted.

Interpretation

If the test is negative, with the tourniquet in place the veins fill within a period of 30 seconds, ad upon removal of the tourniquet n increased rate of filling is observed. There is no retrograde flow taking place through the saphenofemoral junction, and the filling occurs due to incompetency of the communicating veins. If the test is positive, While the patient stands with a tourniquet is placed, the varicosities will remain collapsed throughout the 30second period. Once the tourniquet is removed the internal saphenous vein rapidly fills with blood from above. This indicates that the valves of the saphenous vein at the saphenofemoral junction are incompetent, but the valves of the communicating veins are still intact. Doubly positive, If the veins rapidly fill on standing and again as the tourniquet is removed is there is further distension of the veins. This indicates incompetency of the valves of both the saphenous and communicating systems of veins.

Nil, the tourniquet is applied and even after removal there is only slow filling of the veins from below. This indicates that both the saphenous veins and the communicating veins are competent.

Thus this test serves 2 purposes, firstly demonstrates any backward flow at the saphenofemoral junction and secondly it establishes if there are incompetent communicating veins between the deep ad superficial venous systems.[1][2][3][4]

References

1. Steiner CA, Palmer LH. A simplification of the diagnosis of varicose veins. Ann Surg. 1948 Feb;127(2):362.
2. Bhasin N, Scott DJ. How should a candidate assess varicose veins in the MRCS clinical examination? A vascular viewpoint. The Annals of The Royal College of Surgeons of England. 2006 May;88(3):309-12.
3. BERGAN J. Risk Factors, Manifestations, and Clinical Examination of the Patient with Primary Venous Insufficiency. InThe Vein Book 2007 Jan 1 (pp. 119-124). Academic Press.
4. Shilpa K, Lakshmi DV, Divya Gorur K. Evaluation of Varicose Veins. Sclerotherapy in Dermatology. 2018 May 31:29.

❑❑❑

59 Burn Specific Health Scale -Brief (BSHS-B)

The Burns Specific Health Scale-Brief (BSHS-B) questionnaire is an appropriate measurement tool for the assessment of general, physical, mental, and social health aspects of the burn survivor. [1] It is commonly used to quantify the recovery of quality of life (QoL) after a burn.[2] In response to the lack of a specific instrument to assess the health of patients with burns, Blades et al. in 1979 recorded the first 114-item version of BSHS-Abbreviated (BSHS-A) instrument[3]; and after its construction, modified versions of BSHS-Reviewed (BSHS-R)[4] and a short version of BSHS-B were created.[5]

Intended Population

To measure burn specific health outcomes in survivors of burn injury[5].

Scoring

The instrument measures psychosocial difficulties and physical difficulties using nine domains (Table 1). The participant is asked to choose from a 5-point scale of severity, where "0" is extreme and "4" is none at all. It has a total obtainable score of 40.[6]

Table 1: Domains of the Burn Specific Health Scale -Brief (BSHS-B)[6]

Physical(8)	Burn specific (10)	Social and emotional (22)
Hand function(5)	Heat specificity (5)	Affect (7)
Simple abilities (3)	Treatment regimens (5)	Work (4)
		Sexuality (3)
		Interpersonal relationship (4)
		Body image (4)

The 40-item questionnaire, aims to assess QOL specific to postburn topics, requires about 15 minutes to complete. Higher BSHS-B score indicates fewer problems and, accordingly, a higher QoL.[6]

Evidence

Reliability and validity: Internal consistency of the BSHS-B has been shown to be excellent with a Cronbach's factor alphas ranging between 0.75-0.93.[5] There is evidence of concurrent validity for the BSHS-B when compared with the abbreviated and revised versions.[7] It is claimed that the BSHS-B exhibits construct validity in its association with a variety of aspects of burn-related health.[8][9]

The BSHS-B has been used to establish criterion validity for the QuickDASH in an Australian sample with upper limb burns and it was found that while mean scores improved over the period of the study for both measures, the effect sizes were greater for the QuickDASH.[10] When used in conjunction with the SF-36, the BSHS-B was found to provide more useful information regarding fear-avoidance and post-traumatic stress disorder in relation to return to work.[11]

References

1. Kvannli L, Finlay V, Edgar DW, Wu A, Wood FM. Using the Burn Specific Health Scale-Brief as a measure of quality of life after a burn—What

score should clinicians expect?. Burns. 2011 Feb 1;37(1):54-60.

2. Edgar DW, Katsu A, Group AAH. Burn survivor rehabilitation: principles and guidelines for the allied health professional. In: Edgar DW, editor. ANZBA concensus document. Brisbane, Queensland, Australia: Australian and New Zealand Burns Association; 2007.
3. Blades B, Mellis N, Munster AM. A burn specific health scale. The Journal of trauma 1982; 22(10) : 872-5.
4. Blalock SJ, Bunker BJ, DeVellis RF. Measuring health status among survivors of burn injury: revisions of the Burn Specific Health Scale. The Journal of trauma 1994;36(4):508-15.
5. Kildal M, Andersson G, Fugl-Meyer AR, Lannerstam K, Gerdin B. Development of a brief version of the Burn Specific Health Scale (BSHS -B). The Journal of trauma 2001;51(4):740-6. Blades B, Jones C, Munster A. Quality of life after major burns. J Trauma 1979;19:556–8.
6. Murphy ME, Holzer CE, Richardson LM, Epperson K, Ojeda S, Martinez EM, Suman OE, Herndon DN, Meyer WJ. Quality of Life of Young Adult Survivors of Pediatric Burns Using World Health Organization Disability Assessment Scale II and Burn Specific Health Scale-Brief: A Comparison. J Burn Care Res. 2015 Sep-Oct;36(5) 521-533. doi:10.1097/bcr.0000000000000156. PMID: 25167373; PMCID: PMC4362787.
7. Kildal M, Andersson G, Gerdin B. Health status in Swedish burn patients: Assessment utilising three variants of the Burn Specific Health Scale. Burns. 2002 Nov 1;28(7):639-45.
8. Willebrand M, Kildal M. A simplified domain structure of the burn-specific health scale-brief (BSHS-B): a tool to improve its value in routine clinical work. Journal of Trauma and Acute Care Surgery. 2008 Jun 1;64(6):1581-6.
9. Wikehult B. Use of healthcare, perceived health and patient satisfaction in patients with burns (Doctoral dissertation, Universitetsbiblioteket).
10. Wu A, Edgar DW, Wood FM. The QuickDASH is an appropriate tool for measuring the quality of recovery after upper limb burn injury. Burns. 2007 Nov 1;33(7):843-9. Dyster-Aas J, Kildal M, Willebrand M. Return to work and health-related quality of life after burn injury. Journal of rehabilitation medicine. 2007 Jan 5;39(1):49-55.

❑❑❑

60 Central Sensitization Inventory

Introduction

The Central Sensitization Inventory (CSI) is a self-report outcome measure designed to identify patients who have symptoms that may be related to central sensitization (CS) or central sensitivity syndromes (CSS) such as fibromyalgia, neck injury, temporomandibular joint disorder or migraine/ tension headaches.[1]

The CSI consists of two parts.

- Part A includes 25 questions related to common CSS symptoms.
- Part B determines if the patient has been diagnosed with certain CSS disorders or related disorders, such as anxiety and depression.[2] The CSI has been validated in various languages.[3]

Intended Population

Chronic pain populations[2]

Method of Use

In Part A of the CSI patients are asked various questions designed to assess central sensitization symptoms. The patient scores each answer on a scale of 0 (never) to 4 (always). A score of more than 40 indicates the presence of central sensitization. Only Part A is scored. Part B asks for the patient to circle any specific diagnosis they have received. The full questionnaire can be found here.

Evidence

Reliability: Mayer et al (2012) found the CSI has strong psychometric properties (test-retest reliability = 0.817; Cronbach's alpha = 0.879).[2]

In 2018 these results were replicated in a large multi-country sample (Cronbach's αlpha= 0.92).[3]

Validity: The CSI has been shown to be a useful and valid measure for screening patients with CSS.[4] A 2014 study by Neblett et al found the CSI accurately identified 82.8% of participants as having CSS whereas 54.8% participants were correctly identified as not having CSS. However, this study also found that the likelihood of false-positives increases when the CSI is used on patients who have both complex pain and psychophysiological disorders.[4]

References

1. Neblett, R. The central sensitization inventory: A user's manual. Journal of Applied Biobehavioral Research. 2018; 23(2).
2. Mayer, TG, Neblett, R, Cohen, H, Howard, KJ, Choi, YH, Williams, MJ, Perez, Y, Gatchel, RJ. The Development and Psychometric Validation of the Central Sensitization Inventory (CSI). Pain Pract 2012; 12(4): 276-85.
3. Cuesta-Vargas, A, Neblett, R, Chiarotto, A, Kregel, J, Nijs, J, Van Wilgen, CP. Dimensionality and Reliability of the Central Sensitization Inventory (CSI) in a Pooled Multi-Country Sample. Journal of Pain 2018; 19(3): 317-29.
4. Neblett, R, Hartzell, MM, Cohen, H, Mayer, TG, Williams, M, Choi, YH. Ability of the Central Sensitization Inventory to Identify Central Sensitivity Syndromes in an Outpatient Chronic Pain Sample. The Clinical Journal of Pain 2014; 31(4).

❑❑❑

61 Cerebral Palsy Outcome Measures

Introduction

An Outcome Measure is the result of a test that is used to objectively determine the baseline function of a patient at the beginning of treatment. Once treatment has commenced, the same instrument can be used to determine progress and treatment efficacy. With the move towards Evidence Based Practice (EBP) in the health sciences, objective measures of outcome are important to provide credible and reliable justification for treatment. The instrument should also be convenient to apply for the therapist and comfortable for the patient. An integral part of evaluating clinical practice is to objectively assess the intervention and measure it against a set of outcomes to determine its efficacy. Prior to determining any orthotic intervention, the careful choice of treatment goals and aims is essential in children with complex neuromuscular disability in order to identify and determine appropriate outcome measures.[1]

This means the therapist can ensure they are providing the most appropriate intervention that meets the treatment goals and expectations of the child, parent/caregiver and the clinical team. Change is inevitable in growing and developing children with Cerebral Palsy and the change that occurs is nonlinear and variable by subset of Cerebral Palsy.[2] The outcomes of interventions should be based on the expectations for children with Cerebral Palsy of the same age and gross motor function, rather than the established norms for children without developmental delays.[3]

Reliability, Validity, Specificity and Responsiveness

Selecting the appropriate outcome measures can be used to establish more efficient and effective methods of intervention for children with varying presentations of Cerebral Palsy.[4] The elements that constitute effective outcome measures include:

1. Reliability: measures are constant over time and when used by different raters. [1] [5]
2. Validity: appropriate to assess what the clinician or researcher wants to assess in a manner that makes intrinsic sense. [1] [5]
3. Specificity: the ability to distinguish between the presence or absence of a certain condition in people. [1] [5]
4. Responsiveness: the ability to detect minimal, but clinically relevant changes. [1] [5]

The International Classification of Function, Disability and Health (ICF) is the World Health Organization›s framework for measuring health and disability at both individual and population levels. The ICF has shifted the focus of the impairments in children with Cerebral Palsy from restriction in joint ROM or abnormal muscle tone to the evaluation of functions by assessing the quantitative and qualitative aspects of a child's Activities of Daily Living (ADL). [6] It states that the focus of rehabilitation should be shifted from identifying a person's disability to focusing on enhancing a person's function, ability and performance quality for each individual in a contextual manner. The ICF identified domains that should be evaluated in children with Cerebral Palsy to include body function and structure, activity and participation. A consensus-based survey of clinicians, parents and youth with Cerebral Palsy supported these domains as relevant to the evaluation of all health care interventions in children with Cerebral Palsy. [7]

The primary goal of orthotic treatment of ambulant children with Cerebral Palsy (GMFCS I-III) is to optimise their gait. This is with the expectation that it will preserve or improve their physical function and provide them with the ability to increase their participation in physical activities, recreation and sport. [8] Evaluating orthotic intervention requires the use of outcome measures that will not only assess the function and quality of walking, but also the health related quality of life. Quality of life is frequently used as a 'catch all' expression for any self-reported measure, even when the instrument is capturing information objectively verifiable as functional ability, activities or participation. [9]

Clinician Reported Outcome Measures (CROMs) used in the literature to evaluate the efficacy of orthoses and specifically AFOs for children with Cerebral Palsy include the Timed Up and Go test (TUG), the 88 and 66 item Gross Motor Function Measure (GMFM-88 and GMFM-66 respectively), Gross Motor Performance Measure (GMPM), Clinical Gait Assessment Score (CGAS), Pediatric Balance Scale (PBS) and the Standardised Walking Obstacle Course (SWOC). All of these outcome measures have been proven to be valid and reliable to evaluate motor function and performance in children with Cerebral Palsy. [10] [1] [2] [3] [4] [5]

The TUG is a basic test of functional mobility that evaluates an individual›s ability to manoeuvre his or her body capably and independently to accomplish everyday tasks.[6] The standard TUG test requires a child to rise from a seat with assistance of their arms and where the knees are flexed at 90°, stand momentarily, walk 3m, turn, return to the same seat, and sit down.[7] Statistically significant differences in TUG scores have been observed in children across the GMFCS levels I-III, meaning it can act as a predictor of gross motor function. [6] [8] The TUG has displayed excellent reliability, validity and repeatability in children aged 3-18 years who can understand instructions and do not have cognitive deficits.[6] [8] It is an outcome measure that can quickly and easily evaluate the common orthotic treatment goal of improving the efficiency of gait and also has the potential to monitor change over time. It is also possible to employ the TUG in the child's own environment, closely aligning with values of the ICF domains.

The Gross Motor Functional Measure (GMFM) is a criterion-referenced measure expressly constructed for the purpose of assessing capacity to perform specific functions and evaluate change in the gross motor function of children with CP. [3] The GMFM-88 and 66 item tools were especially developed to assess the gross motor function in children with CP and are among the few outcome measures that have displayed sensitivity to change when evaluating orthotic intervention. There have also been strong correlations established between a child's GMFCS level and the scores attained in the GMFM sections D and E. [9] A large study with 257 participants conducted by Russell et al. [10], described the 'D' dimension of standing and 'E' dimension of walking, running and jumping of the GMFM to be sensitive to functional change in children with CP when using AFOs.

The 88 and 66 item GMFM cover the five dimensions of lying and rolling, sitting, crawling and kneeling, standing, and walking running and jumping. Administering the full five dimensions of the GMFM 88 or 66 item scales is a time consuming process, often taking in excess of 45 minutes, which means clinical utility is often low. The particular dimensions 'D' and 'E' of the GMFM may be assessed separately when evaluating a specific area of function in order to save time, while still retaining reliability, validity and sensitivity of the full measure. However, after 5 years of age, changes in a child's motor abilities are more related to developing and refining motor functions in specific environments, rather than the development of basic gross motor skills. [1] Ceiling effects have been identified in older or more able children assessed with the GMFM. [1] This may explain why some studies described larger improvements in gross motor function in children younger than 5 years of age when compared with older children.

While CROMs are very good at assessing the ICF domain of body function and structure, they do not necessarily correlate with the components of function in the ICF domains of activity and participation. An important feature of outcome measures is the extent to which they reflect a person's activity in everyday life. Environmental factors influence health conditions such as Cerebral Palsy and these factors can have an impact on the performance of activities. [2] A Patient Reported Outcome Measure (PROM) such as the Pediatric Outcomes Data Collection Instrument (PODCI), the Pediatric Evaluation of Disability Inventory (PEDI) or Gillette Functional Assessment Questionnaire (FAQ), permits the child and family to provide information from their own everyday environment that relates not only to the function of the child's gait but also to quality of life issues. It is not always possible for healthcare professionals to observe children in their own environment, which makes the PROM a powerful and valuable evaluation tool.

The PODCI is a parent-reported outcome measure that assesses the mobility, physical function, comfort, happiness and expectations of the healthcare interventions in children with musculoskeletal health issues. [8] In accordance with the ICF values, it not only focuses on assessing function and performance following healthcare interventions, but also evaluates quality of life issues. The PODCI has good reliability and validity when evaluating quality of life issues and walking function in children with Cerebral PalsyP, but does have floor and ceiling effects in the transfer and mobility scales. [3] [3] It demonstrates only a modest sensitivity to detect changes of walking function in children with CP following orthopaedic surgery as the scoring system is considered too expansive to detect subtle changes. [8] [3] Lee et al. [3] found statistically significant improvements in PODCI scores following orthopaedic surgery, but only minimal clinically relevant results. This may mean the PODCI may not be sensitive enough to evaluate the effects of orthotic intervention on mobility and provide results that are clinically relevant.

The PEDI is a parent reported outcome measure administered by a clinician that has shown to be reliable, repeatable and valid in children and adolescents with CP from ages 2-18 to evaluate motor function, self-care and participation. [1] [3] Its clinical relevance is further supported by evidence that motor skills are not necessarily representative of overall functional improvements following healthcare interventions as it assesses not only capability but also quality of performance. [1] The mobility scales in the PEDI have less detail than the GMFM scales. As a result, the PEDI demonstrates only moderate responsiveness to change in motor skills and should not be used in isolation to evaluate the ICF domain of body function and structure. [4] However, unlike the GMFM, it does have the advantage of being able to assess a child's gross motor function in their everyday environment and is therefore more reflective of community function. Despite the PEDI being a patient-reported outcome measure, it still requires a trained healthcare professional to administer the evaluation. The PEDI covers the broad range of motor function, self-care and participation and is very thorough. It can take more than 30 minutes to complete, which may take up already valuable clinical time.

The Gillette Functional Ability Questionnaire (FAQ) is a reliable, repeatable and valid condition-specific functional scale that was developed especially for children with Cerebral Palsy. [8] (TABLE 4) Similar to the PEDI, it assesses a child's walking ability across different domains. However it only focuses on the ability to achieve a particular level and not the capability. No training or equipment is necessary to administer the 10-level, parent-reported questionnaire and it is quick and easy to apply. It has shown sensitivity to change in children with Cerebral Palsy who have undergone orthopaedic surgery, but it is unclear as to whether it would be sensitive and responsive to change following orthotic intervention. [5] [6]

Given the heterogeneous nature of the Cerebral Palsy population, the goals of rehabilitation are often widely distributed across the ICF domains. This may result in problems interpreting the outcome when using standardised outcome measures alone. [7] [8] Items in a standardised outcome measure may not match the individual treatment goals and even if they do, the outcome may not necessarily represent goal attainment. To breach this gap and complement standardised outcome measures, Goal Attainment Scales (GAS) have been successfully used to measure the extent to which individual goals are attained for ambulant children with Cerebral Palsy. [7] [9] The use of GAS measures allows the orthotist to not only perform the clinical evaluation of the orthotic intervention, but also ensure that patient and family satisfaction is measured. The clinician, parents and child are able to identify specific areas for evaluation, quickly perform the assessment and provide a score from a predetermined ordinal scale. In heterogeneous populations, GAS measures have exhibited increased responsiveness to the ICF domain of activity and participation than those of traditional standardised outcome measures. [9] [10] [1]

References

1. Debuse D, Brace H. Outcome measures of activity for children with cerebral palsy: a systematic review. Pediatr Phys Ther. 2011 Fall;23(3):221-31
2. Rosenbaum PL, Walter SD, Hanna SE, Palisano RJ, Russell DJ, Raina P, et al. Prognosis for gross motor function in cerebral palsy: creation of motor development curves. Jama. [Multicenter Study Research Support, Non-U.S. Gov't Research Support, U.S. Gov't, P.H.S.]. 2002 Sep 18;288(11):1357-63
3. Palisano RJ, Hanna SE, Rosenbaum PL, Russell DJ, Walter SD, Wood EP, et al. Validation of a model of gross motor function for children with cerebral palsy. Phys Ther. [Research Support, Non-U.S. Gov't Research Support, U.S. Gov't, P.H.S. Validation Studies]. 2000 Oct;80(10):974-85
4. Stanger M, Oresic S. Rehabilitation approaches for children with cerebral palsy: overview. J Child Neurol. [Review]. 2003 Sep;18 Suppl 1:S79-88
5. Jerosch-Herold C. An evidence-based approach to choosing outcome measures: a checklist for the critical appraisal of validity, reliability and responsiveness studies. British Journal of Occupational Therapy. 2005;68(8):347-53

6. World Health Organisation. International Classifiaction of Functioning, Disability and Health (ICF). Geneva, Switzerland: World Health Organization 2001
7. Vargus-Adams JN, Martin LK. Measuring what matters in cerebral palsy: a breadth of important domains and outcome measures. Arch Phys Med Rehabil. [Research Support, N.I.H., Extramural]. 2009 Dec;90(12):2089-95
8. Narayanan UG. Management of children with ambulatory cerebral palsy: an evidence-based review. J Pediatr Orthop. [Review]. 2012 Sep;32 Suppl 2:S172-81
9. Morris C, Kurinczuk JJ, Fitzpatrick R. Child or family assessed measures of activity performance and participation for children with cerebral palsy: a structured review. Child Care Health Dev. [Evaluation Studies]. 2005 Jul;31(4):397-407
10. Yi SH, Hwang JH, Kim SJ, Kwon JY. Validity of pediatric balance scales in children with spastic cerebral palsy. Neuropediatrics. 2012 Dec;43(6):307-13

❑❑❑

62 Chronic Pain Grade Scale (CPGS)

Chronic pain grade questionnaire (CPG),a questionnaire for grading pain, was established several years ago before the publication of the World Health Organization's International Classification of Functioning Disability and Health (ICF). The purpose of the ICF was to give doctors a standard with which to work when comparing pain and health. The researchers in this study wanted to see if the two could be used together in assessing pain and disability.[1]

Purpose

The CPGS is a multidimensional measure that assesses 2 dimensions of overall chronic pain severity: pain intensity and pain-related disability. It is suitable for use in all chronic pain conditions, including chronic musculoskeletal (MSK) and low back pain[2]

Content

Subscale scores for pain intensity and disability are combined to calculate a chronic pain grade that enables classification of chronic pain patients into 5 hierarchical categories: grades 0 (no pain) to IV (high disability-severely limiting) [2].

Items: The CPGS is comprised of 7 items[1]:

1. How would you rate your pain on a 0-10 scale at the present time, this is right now, where 0 is 'no pain' and 10 is 'pain as bad as it could be'?
2. In the past 6 months, how intense was your worse pain rated on a 0-10 scale (rated as above)?
3. In the past 6 months, on average, how intense was your pain rated on a 0-10 scale (rated as above)? (That is your usual pain at times you were experiencing pain.)
4. About how many days in the last 6 months have you been kept from your usual activities (work, school, housework) because of this pain?
5. In the past 6 months, how much has this pain interfered with your daily activities on a 0-10 scale where 0 is 'no interference' and 10 is 'extreme change'?
6. In the past 6 months, how much has this pain changed your ability to take part in recreational, social, and family activities where 0 is 'no change' and 10 is 'extreme change'?
7. In the past 6 months, how has this pain changed your ability to work (including housework) where 0 is 'no change' and 10 is 'extreme change'?

Recall Period: Pain in the past 3–6 months

Obtaining the Scale: The scale is available in the original reference [1], as well as directly from the author.

Administration: The CPGS is an interview-administered questionnaire that can also be self-completed by respondents [3]

Scoring

All items are scored on an 11-point Likert scale, with responses ranging from 0–10. Scores are calculated for 3 subscales: the characteristic pain intensity score, which ranges from 0–100, is calculated as the mean intensity ratings for reported current, worst, and average pain; the disability score, which ranges from 0–100, is calculated as the mean rating for difficulty performing daily, social, and work activities; and the disability points score, which ranges from 0–3, is derived from a combination of ranked categories of number of disability days and disability score. [3]

Interpretation

The 3 subscale scores (characteristic pain intensity, disability score, and the disability points score) are used to classify subjects into 1 of the 5 pain severity grades: grade 0 for no pain, grade I for low disability-low intensity, grade II for low disability-high intensity, grade III for high disability-moderately limiting, and grade IV for high disability-severely limiting.

Merits and Demerits

- The CPGS is a valid and reliable tool that is useful for the evaluation of chronic MSK pain
- It allows for grading of the global severity of chronic pain and therefore analysis of the qualitative changes in chronic pain over time
- Further, the CPGS assesses not only aspects of the pain itself, but also the impact of the pain on daily, social, and work activities, which is a significant advantage over many other pain questionnaires
- Time to complete the CPGS does not exceed 10 minutes
- Easy to administer
- The CPGS has been adapted into UK English [4]. An Italian version has been developed to evaluate severity in chronic pain patients [5].
- A limitation of the CPGS relative to the other scales is the complexity of scoring
- Additionally, further research is needed to be able to compare scoring methods and cut points

Psychometric Information

Development: Interviews were conducted with primary care patients with back pain, headache, and temporomandibular disorder [6]. The development of the graded classification drew on concepts by Turk and Rudy of chronic pain severity [7] [8]. Two of the items used in the disability score were adapted from their Multidimensional Pain Inventory [9]. The Guttman scaling method was used to develop the graded classification of chronic pain [2].

Acceptability: The CPGS is easy to understand and complete based on a high response rate (76.3%) to a postal survey sent to general practice patients in the UK [4]. Among MSK chronic pain patients, missing values were only noted in<3% of each of the questions in an Italian version of the CPGS [2].

Reliability: For internal consistency, Cronbach's alpha was shown to be = 0.74 among patients with chronic back pain [2]. In an Italian version of CPGS, Cronbach's alpha ranged from 0.81–0.89 for subscales and global scores in patients with chronic MSK pain [5]. In UK general practice patients with low back pain, test–retest reliability was high after a 2-week interval.

Validity: For construct validity, cross-sectional and longitudinal studies of general practice patients have shown that higher scores on the CPGS, indicating greater chronic pain, are significantly associated with higher rates of unemployment, greater pain impact scale scores, greater use of opioid analgesics and physician visits, depressed mood, and lower self-rated health status [2] [4] [10]. Comparisons of CPGS scores with the Short Form 36 Health Survey (SF-36) indicate that a higher chronic pain grade using the CPGS is associated with poorer physical, psychological, social, and general health as measured by the SF-36 (P= 0.001) [10] and worse scores on the SF-36 bodily pain scale (p = 0.545,P<0.0001) (95). Spearman's correlation coefficients for the CPGS scores and the various dimensions of SF-36 were highest for the pain dimension (r = -0.71 to -0.84) and lowest for the mental health dimension (r=-0.28 to-0.38) [4].

Ability to detect change: Among patients with moderate to severe chronic MSK pain, the CPGS has been shown to be modestly responsive to changes after 12 months of treatment with an efficacious pain intervention, with standardized effect sizes for the intensity and disability sub-scales of 0.41 and 0.43, respectively. Among participants with chronic knee or hip pain, the standardized effect size for the CPGS intensity was 0.32 [11].

References

1. Diane Dixon, Beth Pollard, and Marie Johnston. What does the chronic pain questionnaire measure? In Pain. July 2007. Vol. 130. Pp. 249-253.
2. Von Korff M, Ormel J, Keefe FJ, Dworkin SF. Grading the severity of chronic pain. Pain 1992;50:133–49.
3. HAWKER GA. Measures of Adult Pain. Arthritis Care Research 2011; 63,S240–S252
4. Smith BH, Penny KI, Purves AM, Munro C, Wilson B, Grimshaw J,et al. The Chronic Pain Grade questionnaire: validation and reliability in postal research. Pain 1997;71:141–7.
5. Salaffi FF, Stancati AF, Grassi W. Reliability and validity of the Italian version of the Chronic Pain Grade questionnaire in patients with musculoskeletal disorders. Clin Rheumatol 2006; 25:619–31
6. Von Korff M, Dworkin SF, Le RL. Graded chronic pain status: an epidemiologic evaluation. Pain 1990;40:279–91

7. Turk DC, Rudy TE. Towards a comprehensive assessment of chronic pain patients. Behav Res Ther 1987;25:237–49
8. Turk DC, Rudy TE. Toward an empirically derived taxonomy of chronic pain patients: integration of psychological assessment data. J Consult Clin Psychol 1988;56:233–8.
9. Kerns RD, Turk DC, Rudy TE. The West Haven-Yale Multidimensional Pain Inventory (WHYMPI). Pain 1985;23:345–56.
10. Penny KI, Purves AM, Smith BH, Chambers WA, Smith WC. Relationship between the chronic pain grade and measures of physical, social and psychological well-being. Pain 1999;79:275–9
11. Elliott AM, Smith BH, Smith WC, Chambers WA. Changes in chronic pain severity over time: the Chronic Pain Grade as a valid measure. Pain 2000;88:303–8

❑❑❑

63 Clinical Outcome Assessment

Introduction

A clinical outcome assessment (COA) is a measure that describes or reflects how a patient feels, functions, or survives. Types of COAs include[1]:

1. Patient-reported outcome (PRO) measures
2. Observer-reported outcome (ObsRO) measures
3. Clinician-reported outcome (ClinRO) measures
4. Performance outcome (PerfO) measures.[2]

Types of Clinical Outcome Assessments

Patient-Reported Outcomes (PRO)

- Outcome where the patient is the rater
- Rely on a patient's direct responses to questions
- Responses may be recorded by the patient in a variety of ways such as on paper, via computerized questionnaire forms, or via interviews where the patient's observations or reports are recorded exactly as spoken, without any interpretation (judgment) on the part of the interviewer.
- Patient's direct report can capture a wide range of feelings and functions, as well as provide a direct measurement of how a patient feels, e.g., pain or low mood

Increasing interest in developing PRO COAs. FDA guidance on the topic [3] has highlighted the regulatory agency's interest in these instruments[2]

Clinician-Reported Outcomes (ClinRo)

- Reflects the evaluation of a patient's condition by a healthcare professional
- Based on the report that comes from a trained health care professional after observation of a patient's condition. a good example of this is the pain rating scale

Observer-Reported Outcomes (ObsRo)

- Measurement based on an observation by someone other than the patient or a health professional.
- Usually done by patient's non-clinical care giver, family or anyone living around patient and observes the patient in daily life. A good example is the assessment of a patient's cognition.

Performance Outcome (PerfO)

- The patient is assessed, but no rater judgment impacts the measurement, categorized as COAs because a patient's motivation or volition is involved in the task performance.
- Based on the patient's performance of a defined task that is quantified in a specified way that does not rely on judgment to determine the rating.
- Include instruments such eg distance walked in 6 minutes and Timed up and go (TUG)
- Clinician or observer is administering and monitoring performance of the PerfO assessment task, this individual does not apply judgment to quantifying the performance..[2]

The Context of Use of the COA

The context of use typically includes the following elements;

- Disease, injury, impairment or condition being treated
- Patient population demographics (age, disease severity, language, culture, education)
- Clinical treatment objectives and plan of treatment

Conclusion

- An outcome assessment, the patient assessment used in an endpoint, is the measuring instrument that provides a rating or score (categorical or continuous) that is intended to represent some aspect of the patient's health status.

- Outcome assessments are used to define efficacy endpoints when developing a therapy for a disease or condition.
- Most efficacy endpoints are based on specified clinical assessments of patients.
- When clinical assessments are used as clinical trial outcomes, they are called clinical outcome assessments (COAs).[2].

References

1. FDA COA Available from:https://www.fda.gov/about-fda/clinical-outcome-assessment-coa-frequently-asked-questions#COADefinition (last accessed 14.5.2020)
2. Walton MK, Powers III JH, Hobart J, Patrick D, Marquis P, Vamvakas S, Isaac M, Molsen E, Cano S, Burke LB. Clinical outcome assessments: conceptual Foundation—Report of the ISPOR clinical outcomes assessment–emerging good practices for outcomes research Task force. Value in Health. 2015 Sep 1;18(6):741-52. Available from:https://www.ncbi.nlm.nih.gov/pmc/articles/PMC4610138/ (last accessed 14.5.2020)
3. US Food and Drug Administration. Patient-Reported Outcome Measures: Use in Medical Product Development to Support Labeling Claims. [Accessed July 20, 2014];2009 Available from:

   http://www.fda.gov/Drugs/Guidance Compliance RegulatoryInformation/Guidances/ucm064981.htm.

❑❑❑

64 Coma Recovery Scale (Revised)

Objective

The Coma Recovery Scale (CRS-R) , also known as the JFK Coma Recovery Scale - revised, is used to assess patients with a disorder of consciousness, commonly coma.[1] It may be used to differentiate between vegetative state (VS) and minimally conscious state (MCS).[2] It can also be used to monitor emergence from minimally conscious state (EMCS or MCS+).[2]

Intended Population

- Traumatic Brain Injury (TBI)
- Stroke (CVA)
- Brain Tumour

Method of Use

The CRS-R consists of 23 items, grouped into 6 sub-scales:

1. Auditory
2. Visual
3. Motor
4. Oromotor
5. Communication
6. Arousal

The lowest score on each sub-scale represents reflexive activity; the highest represents behaviors mediated by cognitive input. The total score ranges between 0 (worst) and 23 (best). This measure takes a minimum of 25 minutes to complete.

Equipment Required

- Instruction Sheet
- Tongue Depressor
- Scoring Sheet
- An object which produces a loud noise
- Brightly Coloured Object
- ADL Items, e.g. toothbrush, phone
- Hand-held Mirror
- Baseball Sized Ball
- Pencil
- 2 Common Functional Objects (often a cup and a hairbrush or comb)

Evidence

Giacino, Kalmar and Whyte [1] studied 80 patients with severe acquired brain injury. These individuals were admitted to an inpatient Coma Intervention Programme with a diagnosis of either vegetative state (VS) or minimally conscious state (MCS). They compared the CRS-R to the Disability Rating Scale (DRS), and found that the total scores showed "significant correlation" between the 2 scales, which indicates acceptable concurrent validity. In addition, the CRS-R was able to distinguish 10 patients in an MCS who were scored as in VS by the DRS.

Reliability

Test-retest Reliability

Disorder of Consciousness Presentation - TBI (Traumatic Brain Injury), CVA (Stroke), hypoxi-ischaemic Brain injury and Tumour[1]:

n=20; mean age=36.7 years (ranging from 17 to 57 years); mean time post injury = 57.15 days (range 22 to 169 days). Excellent test-retest reliability (Spearman rho = .94)

Inter/Intra-rater Reliability

Disorders of Consciousness Presentation (variety of neurological conditions, including TBI (Traumatic Brain Injury)[2]:

n = 77; age range 19-86 years; 43 patients 1-27 days post injury, 34 27 days to 24 years post injury.

- Excellent reliability for total score (k=.80)
- Excellent reliability for subscales:
  Auditory k = .82; Visual k = .85; Motor k = .93; Oromotor k = .92; Communication k = .98; Arousal k = .74.

Validity: This scale shows excellent concurrent validity as it correlates significantly with total scores on the orginal CRS and the DRS[1]:

Concurrent validity with CRS: Spearman rho = .97

In addition, in the original study by Giacino, Kalmar & Whyte[1], which had 80 inpatients with severe ABI, the CRS-R was able to distinguish 10 patients in an MCS who were misclassified as being in a VS by the DRS.

Sensitivity and Specificity: Sensitivity and Specificity of the Coma Recovery Scale-Revised Total Score in Detection of Conscious Awareness.

Bodien et al, 2016[3]:

- CRS-R total score of 10 or higher yielded a sensitivity of .78 for correct identification of patients in MCS or EMCS
- CRS-R total score of 10 or higher gave a specificity of 1.00 for correct identification of patients who did not meet criteria for either of these diagnoses (i.e, were diagnosed with vegetative state or coma)

References

1. Giacino, J. T., K. Kalmar and J. Whyte (2004). "The JFK Coma Recovery Scale-Revised: measurement characteristics and diagnostic utility." Arch Phys Med Rehabil Dec 2004: 2020-9
2. Diagnostic accuracy of the vegetative and minimally conscious state: Clinical consensus versus standardized neurobehavioral assessment fckLRSchnakers C, Vanhaudenhuyse A, Giacino J, et al. "Diagnostic accuracy of the vegetative and minimally conscious state: Clinical consensus versus standardized neurobehavioral assessment". BMC Neurol. 2009; 9:35.
3. Sensitivity and Specificity of the Coma Recovery Scale-Revised Total Score in Detection of Conscious Awareness.fckLRBodien YG, Carlowicz CA, Chatelle C, Giacino JT. Arch Phys Med Rehabil. 2016 Mar;97(3):490-492
4. Giacino, J & Kalmar, K. Coma Recovery Scale-Revised. The Center for Outcome Measurement in Brain Injury 2006 (accessed March 13, 2016).
5. Assessment scales for disorders of consciousness: evidence-based recommendations for clinical practice and research.fckLRAmerican Congress of Rehabilitation Medicine, Brain Injury-Interdisciplinary Special Interest Group, Disorders of Consciousness Task Force1, Seel RT, Sherer M, Whyte J, Katz DI, Giacino JT, Rosenbaum AM, Hammond FM, Kalmar K, Pape TL, Zafonte R, Biester RC, Kaelin D, Kean J, Zasler N. Arch Phys Med Rehabil. 2010 Dec;91(12):1795-813

❑❑❑

65 Copenhagen Neck Functional Disability Scale

Objective

The Copenhagen Neck Functional Disability Scale (CNFDS) is a self-administered questionnaire developed to measure the level of functional disabilities in patients with neck pain. Jordan et al. designed this questionnaire in 1998. [1] It is partially derived from both the Neck Disability Index (NDI) and the Low Back Pain Rating Scale.[2]

The Copenhagen Neck Functional Disability Scale has been developed for those who have neck pain and disabilities due to the pain. The scale includes questions relating to headache, ability to sleep and to concentrate and activities of daily living. There are also questions of a psychosocial nature such as: social contact, emotional relationships and attitudes toward the future.[3]

This scale, together with the NDI, the Northwick Park Pain Questionnaire (NPPQ) and the Neck Pain and Disability Scale (NPDS) are widely used for assessing neck pain or disability. [4]

The scale's original version was developed in Danish. [5][3]

In the meanwhile there are several translations, such as in English, French, Turkish and Polish. All of them are validated and shown to be reliable. [4] [6] [3]

Intended Population

The CNFDS was especially devised to overcome the Neck Disability Index's lack of generalizability to European populations. [7] It was developed on people who had undergone neck surgery for cervical disc herniation, chronic neck pain and chronic mechanical neck pain. (Level of evidence: 2C) [3] The CNFDS is a useful instrument for patients with neck complaints treated by physiotherapy. The questionnaire is available for patient from 20 to 75 years. (Level of evidence: 2A) [7][3]

Method of Use

It's a very easy questionnaire to take off and it can be completed in only 10 minutes. Patients can complete the scale by using pen and paper, mail or telephone. The instrument is useful in the clinical setting, and therefore often used in the practice. [7]

The CNFDS consists of 15 items. These items are individually answered by either 'yes', 'occasionally' or 'no'. For questions one till five, a 'yes' indicates a good function. For questions six till fifteen, a 'no' indicates a good function. A good function receives a score of zero, a poor function receives a score of two and the answer 'occasionally' always receives a score of one. [1]

Afterwards, we add up all the scores of the questions to form the total score. This total score ranges from 0 to 30. [1]

The total score determines the level of functional disability, in which higher numbers represent a higher level of disability. A score of 0 indicates that there are no neck complaints present whereas 30 indicates that the patient is extremely disabled as a result of the neck complaints. [3]

Comparison between repeated scores could be made between raw scores, or as percentage change from baseline (original) score. [3]

Evidence

Reliability: The reliability of the Copenhagen neck functional disability scale was evaluated with short-term (same day) and between-day (2 days later). Respectively the result was Pearson correlation coefficient of 0.99 and 0.98. Which means that the test-retest reliability is very good. (Grades of Recommendation: B) [7]. There is an extremely high internal consistency of the total scores, with a Cronbach alpha coefficient of 0.9. The individual items scored high alpha values uniformly. (Grades of Recommendation: B)[3]

Validity: Construct validity: Construct validity investigates whether the correct variables were measured in relation to the predefined variables. The Copenhagen neck functional disability scale measures the level of disabilities due to the pain. [3]

The construct validity of the English version was assessed by comparing disability scores to self-reported pain scores and to doctors and patients global assessment. The Pearson correlation for pain and disability is high (r = 0.83). The disability score compared with patients global assessment gave a Spearman rank correlation of r = 0.89, high score. The disability score compared with doctors global assessments gave a Spearman rank correlation of r = 0.56, a moderate score. (Grades of Recommendation: B) [3] [7]

External construct/convergent validity: There is a significantly correlation between the CNFDS and other numerical variables. (Grades of Recommendation: B) [8]

- CNFDS and Vas-score for current pain: Spearman's correlation = 0.45
- CNFDS and Vas-score for worst pain: Spearman's correlation= 0.37
- CNFDS and Vas-score for mean pain: Spearman's correlation = 0.19
- CNFDS and SF36 physical: Spearman's correlation = -0.44
- CNFDS and SF36 mental: Spearman's correlation = -0.44 [8]

Responsiveness: The responsiveness of the CNFDS is similar to the responsiveness of the Neck Disability Index, the Northwick Park Pain Questionnaire and the Neck Pain and Disability Scale. All these scales showed good sensitivity to change with nearly identical SRM values. (SRMCNFDS=0,89; p<0,01). (Grades of Recommendation: B) [4] [3]

The short-term and long-term responsiveness correlate very well to self-reported changes in pain. [3] Studies showed that there is a small correlation demonstrated with pain scores at 6 weeks (r=0.49; p<0,0001), 4 months (r=0.48; p<0,0001), and a moderate correlation at 12 months (r=0.54; p<0,0001). (Grades of Recommendation: B) [7][9][3] For the French version of the CNFDS the sensitivity to change is 0.33 in patients with marked worsening, in patients with worsening it is 0.02. In patients with no change and with an improvement and with a marked improvement the sensitivity to change is respectively 0.10, 0.51 and 0.68. (Grades of Recommendation: B) [8] The designer of the questionnaire believes that the CNFDS's possible decreased sensitivity regarding individual questions is compensated for by the greater number of questions included. (Grades of Recommendation: D) [3] No quantification estimated minimal clinically important difference was reported. [7]

References

1. FEJER, R., JORDAN, A. & HARTVIGSEN, J. 2005. Categorising the severity of neck pain: establishment of cut-points for use in clinical and epidemiological research. Pain, 119, 176-82. (level of evidence:2C)
2. PICKERING, P. M., OSMOTHERLY, P. G., ATTIA, J. R. & MCELDUFF, P. 2011. An examination of outcome measures for pain and dysfunction in the cervical spine: a factor analysis. Spine (Phila Pa 1976), 36, 581-8. (level of evidence 2C)
3. JORDAN, A., MANNICHE, C., MOSDAL, C. & HINDSBERGER, C. 1998. The Copenhagen Neck Functional Disability Scale: a study of reliability and validity. J Manipulative Physiol Ther, 21, 520-7. (level of evidence 2C)
4. KOSE, G., HEPGULER, S., ATAMAZ, F. & ODER, G. 2007. A comparison of four disability scales for Turkish patients with neck pain. J Rehabil Med, 39, 358-62. (level of evidence 2C)
5. SCHELLINGERHOUT, J. M., VERHAGEN, A. P., HEYMANS, M. W., KOES, B. W., DE VET, H. C. & TERWEE, C. B. 2012. Measurement properties of disease-specific questionnaires in patients with neck pain: a systematic review. Qual Life Res, 21, 659-70. (level of evidence 2A)
6. MISTERSKA, E., JANKOWSKI, R. & GLOWACKI, M. 2011. Cross-cultural adaptation of the Neck Disability Index and Copenhagen Neck Functional Disability Scale for patients with neck pain due to degenerative and discopathic disorders. Psychometric properties of the Polish versions. BMC Musculoskelet Disord, 12, 84. . (level of evidence 2C)
7. PIETROBON, R., COEYTAUX, R. R., CAREY, T. S., RICHARDSON, W. J. & DEVELLIS, R. F. 2002. Standard scales for measurement of functional outcome for cervical pain or dysfunction: a systematic review. Spine (Phila Pa 1976), 27, 515-22. (level of evidence 2A)

8. FORESTIER, R., FRANCON, A., ARROMAN, F. S. & BERTOLINO, C. 2007. French version of the Copenhagen neck functional disability scale. Joint Bone Spine, 74, 155-9. (level of evidence: 2C
9. FERREIRA, M. L., BORGES, B. M., REZENDE, I. L., CARVALHO, L. P., SOARES, L. P., DABES, R. A., CARVALHO, G., DRUMMOND, A. S., MACHADO, G. C. & FERREIRA, P. H. 2010. Are neck pain scales and questionnaires compatible with the international classification of functioning, disability and health? A systematic review. Disabil Rehabil, 32, 1539-46. (level of evidence 2A)

The Copenhagen Neck Functional Disability Scale

Overview: The Copenhagen Neck Functional Disability Scale can be used to evaluate the disability experienced by patients with neck pain. The scores can be monitored over time to evaluate the disease course and response to any interventions.

Questions:

(1) Can you sleep at night without neck pain interfering?
(2) Can you manage daily activities without neck pain reducing activity levels?
(3) Can you manage daily activities without help from others?
(4) Can you manage putting on your clothes in the morning without taking more time than usual?
(5) Can you bend over the washing basin in order to brush your teeth without getting neck pain?
(6) Do you spend more time than usual at home because of neck pain?
(7) Are you prevented from lifting objects weighing from 2-4 kilograms due to neck pain?
(8) Have you reduced your reading activity due to neck pain?
(9) Have you been bothered by headaches during the time that you have had neck pain?
(10) Do you feel your ability to concentrate is reduced due to neck pain?
(11) Are you prevented from participating in your usual leisure time activities due to neck pain?
(12) Do you remain in bed longer than usual due to neck pain?
(13) Do you feel that neck pain has influenced your emotional relationship with your nearest family?
(14) Have you had to give up social contact with other people during the past two weeks due to neck pain?
(15) Do you feel that neck pain will influence your future?

Direction of questions:

- "positive" (a yes indicates good function): 1-5
- "negative" (a yes indicates poor function): 6 – 12

Response	Points for "Positive" Directed	Points for "Negative" Directed
yes	0	2
occasionally	1	1
no	2	0

disability index = SUM(points for all 15 questions)

Interpretation: •

minimum score: 0 •

maximum score: 30 •

The higher the score the greater the disability.

References: Jordan A Manniche C et al. The Copenhagen Functional Disability Scale: A study of reliability and validity. J Manipulative Physiological Therapeutics. 1998; 21: 520-527.

❑❑❑

66

DASH Outcome Measure

Introduction

The Disabilities of the Arm, Shoulder and Hand (DASH) questionnaire is a 30-item questionnaire that looks at the ability of a patient to perform certain upper extremity activities.[1][2][3] This questionnaire is a self-report questionnaire that patients can rate difficulty and interference with daily life on a 5 point Likert scale.[1][2].

The QuickDASH is an abbreviated version of the original DASH outcome measure. In comparison to the original 30 item DASH outcome measure, the QuickDASH only contains 11 items[4] It is a questionnaire that measures an individual's ability to complete tasks, absorb forces, and severity of symptoms[4] The QuickDASH tool uses a 5-point Likert scale from which the patient can select an appropriate number corresponding to his/her severity/ function level.[5]

Intended Population

- The intended population for the DASH is any person with one or more upper extremity musculoskeletal disorders.[1][2][3]
- The QuickDASH outcome measure is designed to be used on patients presenting with one or more disabilities of the arm, shoulder, and hand.[4][5]

Scoring

DASH and QuickDASH Scoring Formula = ([(sum of n responses)/n] -1)(25) where n represents the number of completed items.[1]

- DASH cannot be computed if greater than three items are missing.[1]

  QuickDASH cannot be computed if greater than one item is missing.[1]

Level of Disability

In both the DASH and QuickDASH a higher scores indicate a greater level of disability and severity, whereas, lower scores indicate a lower level of disability.[1][3] The score on both test ranges from 0 (no disability) to 100 (most severe disability)[4]

Additional Optional Modules

The DASH and QuickDASH have two optional 4-item additional modules that can be used. The two optional additional modules are:

- Work - Used for workman compensation patients or those whose disability is affecting their ability to work
- Sports/Performing Arts - Used for Athletes and Musicians

The optional modules cannot be scored if an answer is missing.[1]

Evidence

Psychometric Property	DASH	QuickDASH
Reliability	ICC(2,1) = 0.96[2]	ICC(2,1) = 0.90[6]
Validity	Pearson r > 0.70[2]	Pearson r > 0.70[7]
Minimal Detectable Change (MDC)	12.75% - 17.23%[3]	11.2%[6]
Minimal Clinical Important Difference (MCID)	10.83-15[8]	15.91-20[8]
Responsiveness	• Good responsiveness to self-rated changes before and after most arm, shoulder, and hand diagnoses and surgeries[3] • Comparable responsiveness compared to other joint and disease-specific measures[2]	Slightly more responsive to the original DASH outcome measure and, clinically, may be preferable due to shorter length[4][7]
Miscellaneous	Available in 27 different languages. Many of these versions have had or are in the process of being tested for their psychometric properties.[1]	QuickDASH measure has more relative efficiency compared with the DASH[7] Recent studies have also analyzed the reliability of a modified QuickDASH outcome measure, from a questionnaire into a visual analog version[5]

(MDC)– the smallest amount of change that has to occur before the change can be considered a true change and not error[3]

(MCID) – the amount of change in the score that has to occur before it signifies an important or beneficial difference in the patient's condition.[6]

References

1. The DASH outcome measure. Available at http://www.dash.iwh.on.ca, Accessed March 12, 2011.
2. Beaton DE, Katz JN, Fossel AH, Wright JG, Tarasuk V, Bombardier C. Measuring the whole or the parts?: validity, reliability, and responsiveness of the Disabilities of the Arm, Shoulder and Hand outcome measure in different regions of the upper extremity. Journal of Hand Therapy. 2001 Apr 1;14(2):128-42.
3. Beaton DE, Davis AM, Hudak P, McConnell S. The DASH (Disabilities of the Arm, Shoulder and Hand) outcome measure: what do we know about it now?. The British Journal of Hand Therapy. 2001 Dec;6(4):109-18..
4. Gummesson C, Ward MM, Atroshi I. The shortened disabilities of the arm, shoulder and hand questionnaire (Quick DASH): validity and reliability based on responses within the full-length DASH. BMC musculoskeletal disorders. 2006 Dec 1;7(1):44.
5. Matheson LN, Melhorn JM, Mayer TG, Theodore BR, Gatchel RJ. Reliability of a visual analog version of the QuickDASH. JBJS. 2006 Aug 1;88(8):1782-7.
6. Mintken PE, Glynn P, Cleland JA. Psychometric properties of the shortened disabilities of the Arm, Shoulder, and Hand Questionnaire (QuickDASH) and Numeric Pain Rating Scale in patients with shoulder pain. Journal of Shoulder and Elbow Surgery. 2009 Nov 1;18(6):920-6.
7. Beaton DE, Wright JG, Katz JN, Upper Extremity Collaborative Group. Development of the QuickDASH: comparison of three item-reduction approaches. JBJS. 2005 May 1;87(5):1038-46.
8. Franchignoni F, Vercelli S, Giordano A, Sartorio F, Bravini E, Ferriero G. Minimal clinically important difference of the disabilities of the arm, shoulder and hand outcome measure (DASH) and its shortened version (QuickDASH). journal of orthopaedic & sports physical therapy. 2014 Jan;44(1):30-9.

The Disabilities of the Arm, Shoulder and Hand (DASH) Score

Clinician's name (or ref)

Patient's name (or ref

Please rate your ability to do the following activities in the last week.

1. Open a tight or new jar	No difficulty	Mild difficulty	Moderate difficulty	Severe difficulty	Unable
2. Write	No difficulty	Mild difficulty	Moderate difficulty	Severe difficulty	Unable
3. Turn a key	No difficulty	Mild difficulty	Moderate difficulty	Severe difficulty	Unable
4. Prepare a meal	No difficulty	Mild difficulty	Moderate difficulty	Severe difficulty	Unable
5. Push open a heavy door	No difficulty	Mild difficulty	Moderate difficulty	Severe difficulty	Unable
6. Place an object on a shelf above your head	No difficulty	Mild difficulty	Moderate difficulty	Severe difficulty	Unable
7. Do heavy household chores (eg wash walls, wash floors)	No difficulty	Mild difficulty	Moderate difficulty	Severe difficulty	Unable
8. Garden or do yard work	No difficulty	Mild difficulty	Moderate difficulty	Severe difficulty	Unable
9. Make a bed	No difficulty	Mild difficulty	Moderate difficulty	Severe difficulty	Unable
10. Carry a shopping bag or briefcase	No difficulty	Mild difficulty	Moderate difficulty	Severe difficulty	Unable
11. Carry a heavy object (over 10 lbs)	No difficulty	Mild difficulty	Moderate difficulty	Severe difficulty	Unable
12. Change a lightbulb overhead	No difficulty	Mild difficulty	Moderate difficulty	Severe difficulty	Unable
13. Wash or blow dry your hair	No difficulty	Mild difficulty	Moderate difficulty	Severe difficulty	Unable
14. Wash your back	No difficulty	Mild difficulty	Moderate difficulty	Severe difficulty	Unable
15. Put on a pullover sweater	No difficulty	Mild difficulty	Moderate difficulty	Severe difficulty	Unable
16. Use a knife to cut food	No difficulty	Mild difficulty	Moderate difficulty	Severe difficulty	Unable
17. Recreational activities which require little effort (eg cardplaying, knitting, etc)	No difficulty	Mild difficulty	Moderate difficulty	Severe difficulty	Unable
18. Recreational activities in which you take some force or impact through your arm, shoulder or hand (eg golf, hammering, tennis, etc)	No difficulty	Mild difficulty	Moderate difficulty	Severe difficulty	Unable
19. Recreational activities in which you move your arm freely (eg playing frisbee, badminton, etc)	No difficulty	Mild difficulty	Moderate difficulty	Severe difficulty	Unable
20. Manage transportation needs (getting from one place to another)	No difficulty	Mild difficulty	Moderate difficulty	Severe difficulty	Unable
21. Sexual activities	No difficulty	Mild difficulty	Moderate difficulty	Severe difficulty	Unable
22. During the past week, to what extent has your arm, shoulder or hand problem interfered with your normal social activities with family, friends, neighbours or groups?	Not at all	Slightly	Moderately	Quite a bit	Extremely
23. During the past week, were you limited in your work or other regular daily activities as a result of your arm, shoulder or hand problem?	Not limited at all	Slightly limited	Moderately limited	Very limited	Unable

Please rate the severity of the following symptoms in the last week					
24. Arm, shoulder or hand pain	None	Mild	Moderate	Severe	Extreme
25. Arm, shoulder or hand pain when you performed any specific activity	None	Mild	Moderate	Severe	Extreme
26. Tingling (pins and needles) in your arm, shoulder or hand	None	Mild	Moderate	Severe	Extreme
27. Weakness in your arm, shoulder or hand	None	Mild	Moderate	Severe	Extreme
28. Stiffness in your arm, shoulder or hand	None	Mild	Moderate	Severe	Extreme
29. During the past week, how much difficulty have you had sleeping because of the pain in your arm, shoulder or hand?	None	Mild	Moderate	Severe	Extreme
30. I feel less capable, less confident or less useful because of my arm, shoulder or hand problem	None	Mild	Moderate	Severe	Extreme

❑❑❑

67 DN4 Questionnaire

It is a clinician-administered questionnaire consisting of 10 items. Seven items related to pain quality (i.e. sensory and pain descriptors) are based on an interview with the patient and 3 items based on the clinical examination. [1] The DN4 (which stands for Douleur Neuropathique 4) is one of the questionnaires that can be useful in diagnosing neuropathic pain. It has components of how the pain feels to the patient but also requires the examining health professional to assess whether there is reduced sensation (hypoaesthesia) to touch or pinprick and whether light brushing increases or causes pain (allodynia).[2] Questionnaire initially written in French but immediately translated into English by the same team. The scale has been widely used since 2005 because of its simplicity. It evaluates neuropathic pain following central and peripheral neurological lesions. It is also used for diagnostic purposes, allowing the clinician to determine if the pain is of neuropathic origin.[3] This questionnaire has been well validated in a number of studies. The DN4 questionnaire was originally developed and validated in French.[4]

Evidence

Reliability: It is a reliable component of the diagnostic work up for painful diabetic polyneuropathy[5] Inter-rater agreement coefficient:0.80 (0.71–0.89), and test-retest intra-class correlation coefficient: 0.95 (0.92–0.97)].[5] The Persian version of DN4 questionnaire is a reliable, valid, feasible, and easily administered tool for precise discrimination neuropathic pain from NNP in Farsi. The characteristics of this test can assist practitioner to diagnose neuropathic pain accurately for both clinical and research purposes.[6] The DN4 is an easy-to-use screening tool that is reliable for discriminating between neuropathic and nociceptive pain conditions in daily practice. [7]

Validity: Valid for a cut-off value ≥ 4 points [5] DN4 is valid for painful diabetic polyneuropathy which supports its usefulness as a screening tool for neuropathic pain in diabetes.[5]

Sensitivity: The DN4 questionnaire has very good sensitivity (83%) [5]

Specificity: It has specificity of (90%) [5]

References

1. http://hqlo.biomedcentral.com/articles/10.1186/1477 - 7525-5-66
2. http://www.gloshospitals.nhs.uk/en/Wards-and-Departments/Departments/Pain-Management/Different-Pains/Nerve-Pain/Assessment-of-Nerve-Pain/DN4-Draft/
3. http://scalelibrary.com/assessment_scale_result.php?echelle=DN4%20Questionnaire&retour=liste&scalage=adulte
4. http://hqlo.biomedcentral.com/articles/10.1186/1477-7525-5-66
5. Validation of DN4 as a screening tool for neuropathic pain in painful diabetic polyneuropathy.fckLRSpallone V1, Morganti R, D'Amato C, Greco C, Cacciotti L, Marfia GA.
6. Validity and reliability of the persian (Farsi) version of the DN4 (Douleur Neuropathique 4 Questions) questionnaire for differential diagnosis of neuropathic from non-neuropathic pains.fckLRMadani SP1, Fateh HR, Forogh B, Fereshtehnejad SM, Ahadi T, Ghaboussi P, Bouhassira D, Raissi GR.
7. Validation of the Dutch version of the DN4 diagnostic questionnaire for neuropathic pain. fckLRvan Seventer R1, Vos C, Giezeman M, Meerding WJ, Arnould B, Regnault A, van Eerd M, Martin C, Huygen F.

DN4 Questionnaire

Please complete this questionnaire by ticking one answer for each item in the 4 questions below:

INTERVIEW OF THE PATIENT

Question 1: Does the pain have one or more of the following characteristics?

	YES	NO
1 – Burning		
2 – Painful cold		
3 – Electric shocks		

Question 2: Is the pain associated with one of more of the following symptoms in the same area?

	YES	NO
4 – Tingling		
5 – Pins and needles		
6 – Numbness		
7 – Itching		

EXAMINATION OF THE PATIENT

Question 3: Is the pain located in an area where the physical examination may reveal one or more of the following characteristics?

	YES	NO
8 – Hypoesthesia to touch		
9 – Hypoesthesia to prick		

Question 4: In the painful area, can the pain be caused or increased by:

	YES	NO
10 – Brushing		

The total score is calculated as the sum of the 10 items and the cut-off value for the diagnosis of neuropathic pain is a total score of 4/10

Total	

Bouhassira D, Attal N, Alchaar H, et al. "Comparison of pain syndromes associated with nervous or somatic lesions and development of a new neuropathic pain diagnostic questionnaire (DN4)." Pain 114.1-2 (2005): 29-36.

68

Edinburgh Handedness Inventory (EHI)

Purpose

The Edinburgh Handedness Inventory (EHI), sometimes referred to as the Edinburgh Handedness Questionnaire (EHQ), was developed by Richard Charles Oldfield to objectively ascertain the handedness of a subject in activities of daily living (ADL).[1] It is the most commonly used screening tool for handedness.[2][3]

Intended population

It has been used in a wide variety of subjects ranging from children with autism to adults with stroke.[2][3]

Method of Use

There is controversy surrounding its use due to the existence of multiple variations of the tool and improper understanding of the original test instructions.[2][4] The older 20-item questionnaire contains instructions to be strictly followed during administration. Items are rated either by direct observation or by self-report.[1] A more commonly used, shorter 10-item version was developed to overcome sociocultural differences that affected the relevance of certain items which limited its universal use.[1][3]

The original 20 items are:

Writing	Drawing	Throwing
Scissors	Comb	Toothbrush
Knife (without fork)	Spoon	Hammer
Screwdriver	Tennis racket	Knife with fork
Cricket bat	Golf club Broom	
Rake Striking a match	Opening a box (lid)	
Dealing cards	Threading a needle	

From the above, items 1, 2, 3, 4, 6, 7, 8, 15, 17, and 18 made it into the ubiquitous 10-item version of the EHI.[1]

Scoring

For each of the items, the subject is asked to specify the side they prefer to perform the given activity (self-rated method), alternatively, the subjects can be made to perform the said activity and the observer can rate the findings (direct observation method). [Refer to the following document: https://rhd.talkbank.org/protocol/handedness.pdf] If the preference is for either the left or the right side, then a "+" is marked on the column for that side.

If the preference for a particular side is so strong that one wouldn't use the other side unless forced, then a "++" is marked on that side.

If there is no preference for any side, then a "+" is marked on both sides.

For items that involve a bimanual task such as striking a match, the hand involved in the usage of the key item (i.e. the match) is considered as the preferred side.

If the subject has no experience of any given task, then that item remains unmarked.

The final score is called the "Laterality Quotient". It is calculated using the formula:

Laterality Quotient = (R-L)/(R+L) X 100

Here, R & L refer to the total number of "+" marked on the right and left side respectively.

The Laterality Quotient value is used to interpret handedness as given below:

- Left-handedness = Less than -40
- Ambidexterity = Between -40 and +40
- Right-handedness = More than +40

Psychometrics

According to Oldfield, results from a self-reported EHI yield less reliable results since subjects usually overestimate the number of tasks carried out by the dominant hand.[1]

References

1. Oldfield RC. The assessment and analysis of handedness: The Edinburgh inventory. Neuropsychologia. 1971; 9: 97-113.
2. Edlin JM, Leppanen ML, Fain RJ, Hackländer RP, Hanaver-Torrez SD, Lyle KB. On the use (and misuse?) of the Edinburgh Handedness Inventory. Brain Cogn. 2015 Mar;94:44-51. doi: 10.1016/j.bandc.2015.01.003.
3. Caplan B., Mendoza JE. Edinburgh Handedness Inventory. In: Kreutzer JS, DeLuca J, Caplan B (eds) Encyclopedia of Clinical Neuropsychology. 2011; Springer: New York, NY. https://doi.org/10.1007/978-0-387-79948-3_684
4. Fazio R, Coenen C, Denney RL. The original instructions for the Edinburgh Handedness Inventory are misunderstood by a majority of participants. Laterality. 2012;17(1):70-7. doi: 10.1080/1357650X.2010.532801.

Edinburgh Handedness Inventory

Surname____________Given Name_________________

Date of Birth______________Sex____________________

Please indicate your preferences in the use of hands in the following activities by putting + in the appropriate column. Where the preference is so strong that you would never try to use the other hand unless absolutely forces to, put ++. If any case you are really indifferent put + in both columns.

Some of the activities require both hands. In these cases the part of the task, or object, for which hand preference is wanted is indicated in brackets.

Please try to answer all the questions, and only leave a blank if you have no experience at all of the object or task.

	YES	NO
1. Writing		
2. Drawing		
3. Throwing		
4. Scissors		
5. Toothbrush		
6. Knife (without fork)		
7. Spoon		
8. Broom (upper hand)		
9. Striking Match (match)		
10. Opening box (lid)		
i. Which foot do you prefer to kick with?		
ii. Which eye do you use when using only one?		

❑❑❑

69

Elderly Mobility Scale

Objective

To measure the function of frail elderly adults[1]. The Elderly Mobility Scale (EMS) was developed in 1994 as part of an assessment package[1]. It is a relatively simple outcome measure and is quick to administer[2].

Intended Population: Frail elderly adults in hospital.

Method of Use: The following is from the Chartered Society of Physiotherapists and can be accessed here (includes instructions, form for recording scores and some simple interpretation of scores).

Equipment: Metre rule, stopwatch, access to a bed and chair, usual walking aid, form to record scores

Physical space needed: Space for bed, chair, wall, space for 6m walk

Evidence

Reliability: Inter-rater reliability: High[3]: two studies[1][4](n=19 and n=15) have shown no significant difference between scores

Intra-rater reliability: No statistically significant differences in scoring by 15 physiotherapists[5].

Validity: Content validity: The items of the test show a hierarchy of difficulty with "lie to sit" being the easiest task to perform and the functional reach being the most difficult task to perform[6]. It has been proposed that the EMS measures two dimensions of mobility: bed mobility and functional mobility [6].

Concurrent validity: EMS scores had highly significant correlations with both the Barthel and Functional Independence Measure (FIM) scores for 36 patients, age 70–93 years. (Spearman's rho for Barthel: 0.962, FIM: 0.948)[1]. A significant correlation between EMS and Barthel scores has been demonstrated in a second study (n=66, aged 66-69 years)[4]. A third study[5] (n=32, aged >55 years) has demonstrated concurrent validity with the Modified Rivermead Mobility Index.

Predictive validity: Is not conclusive. One study has shown that those discharged to home from hospital have higher EMS scores than those discharged to inpatient rehabilitation[2]. Another study has demonstrated the use of EMS scores to classify residential care placements[6]. Although results were limited by the study design (cross-sectional rather than prospective), there appears there may be some useful cut off scores which could correlate the level of mobility with a type of residential care required. As the authors suggest, further research is required to confirm this. A third study[4] found EMS scores showed no predictive validity for placement on discharge from hospital.

Responsiveness: In one study of 83 patients with a mean age of 79 in a clinical day hospital, researchers found the EMS was significantly more likely ($p<0.001$) to detect an improvement in mobility following a course of physiotherapy, compare to two other functional measures[7].

Limitations: The EMS has been shown to have a ceiling effect[2][3]. A correction was published by Smith because of an error in the functional reach measurement in the original publication[8]. See above for correct scale. Evidence for two different modifications to the EMS was published in 2006: the Modified Elderly Mobility Scale (MEMS)[9] and the Swedish version of the Modified Elderly Mobility Scale (Swe M-EMS)[3]. The MEMS has added a stair climbing task to the EMS and increased the walk distance from six metres to 10 metres to minimise the ceiling effect[9]. The Swe M-EMS was translated into Swedish from its original English and research shows high inter-rater reliability and correlations with two other functional measures. Researchers found the EMS was limited in its sensitivity as a single measure to record improvement following an acute stroke[3].

References

1. Smith R. Validation and reliability of the Elderly Mobility Scale. Physiotherapy. 1994; 80 (11): 744-747.
2. de Morton NA, Nolan J, O'Brien M, Thomas S, Govier A, Sherwell K, Harris B, Markham N. A head-to-head comparison of the de Morton Mobility Index (DEMMI) and Elderly Mobility Scale (EMS) in an older acute medical population. 2015. Disabil Rehabil, 37:20, 1881-1887.
3. Linder A, Winkvist L, Nilsson L, Sernert N. Evaluation of the Swedish version of the Modified Elderly Mobility Scale (Swe M-EMS) in patients with acute stroke. Clin Rehabil. 2006; 20 (7): 584-597.
4. Prosser L, Canby A. Further validation of the Elderly Mobility Scale for measurement of mobility of hospitalized elderly people. 1997. Clin Rehabil. 11; 338-343.
5. Nolan JS, Remilton LE, Green MM. The Reliability and Validity of the Elderly Mobility Scale in the Acute Hospital Setting. The Internet Journal of Allied Health Sciences and Practice. 2008; 6 (4):1-7.
6. Yu MSW, Chan CCH, Tsim RKM. Usefulness of the Elderly Mobility Scale for classifying residential placements. Clin Rehabil. 2007; 21(12): 1114–1120.
7. Spilg EG, Martin BJ, Mitchell SL. A comparison of mobility assessments in a geriatric day hospital. Clin Rehabil. 2001; 15: 296-300.
8. Chartered Society of Physiotherapists. EMS section of Outcome Measures manual Version 2. 2012.
9. Kuys SS, Brauer SG. Validation and reliability of the Modified Elderly Mobility Scale. Australas J Ageing. 2006; 25(3): 140-144.

	Elderly Mobility Scale	Score:	Score:	Score:
Lying To Sitting	2 - Independent 1 - Needs help of 1 person 0 - Needs help of 2+ people	____	____	____
Sitting To Lying	2 - Independent 1 - Needs help of 1 person 0 - Needs help of 2+ people	____	____	____
Sitting To Standing	3 - Independent in under 3 seconds 2 - Independent in over 3 seconds 1 - Needs help of 1 person 0 - Needs help of 2+ people	____	____	____
Standing	3 - Stands without support and able to reach 2 - Stands without support but needs support to reach 1 - Stands but needs support 0 - Stands only with physical support of another person	____	____	____
Gait	3 - Independent 2 - Independent with frame 1 - Mobile with walking aid but erratic / unsafe 0 - Needs physical help to walk or constant supervision	____	____	____
Timed Walk (6 meters)	3 - Under 15 seconds 2 - 16-30 seconds 1 - Over 30 seconds 0 - Unable to cover 6 meters	____	____	____
Functional Reach	4 - Over 20 cm 2 - 10 - 20 cm 0 - Under 10 cm	____	____	____
	Total Scores:	/20	/20	/20

EQ-5D

EQ-5D is a standardised measure of health-related quality of life developed by the EuroQol Group to provide a simple, generic questionnaire for use in clinical and economic appraisal and population health surveys. EQ-5D assesses health status in terms of five dimensions of health and is considered a 'generic' questionnaire because these dimensions are not specific to any one patient group or health condition. EQ-5D can also be referred to as a patient-reported outcome (PRO) measure, because patients can complete the questionnaire themselves to provide information about their current health status and how this changes over time. 'EQ-5D' is not an abbreviation and is the correct term to use when referring to the instrument in general.[1]

EQ-5D is widely used around the world in clinical trials and real-world clinical settings, population studies, and health economic evaluations. By mid-2020, the number of EQ-5D studies registered with the EuroQol Group totalled over 39,000. These comprised over 80 clinical areas and related to surgical procedures, hospital waiting lists, physiotherapy, general practice and primary care, and rehabilitation. The number of annual requests to use EQ-5D is approximately 5000, and EQ-5D data have been reported in over 8000 peer-reviewed papers over the past 30 years.[2]

EQ-5D can be used for a variety of purposes. In clinical trials and routine clinical settings, EQ-5D can be used (i) to provide a profile of patient health on the day of questionnaire completion; (ii) to monitor the health status of patient groups at particular times, e.g. at referral, admission, discharge, and follow-up; and (iii) to measure changes in health status over time in individual patients and in cohorts of patients, such as before and after health interventions and treatments. In population studies, EQ-5D can be used to assess population health status at local and national levels and to follow population health status over time. In medical decision-making, EQ-5D can be used (i) to measure the impacts and outcomes of healthcare services; (ii) to provide relevant information for the economic evaluation of health programmes and policies; and (iii) to assist in providing evidence about effectiveness in processes where drugs or procedures require approval. EQ-5D is recommended by many health technology assessment (HTA) bodies internationally as a key component of cost-utility analyses.[3]

EQ-5D was developed by the EuroQol Group, and its distribution and licensing are managed by the EuroQol Research Foundation. The EuroQol website [4] provides detailed information and the latest developments about EQ-5D including guidance for users, a list of available language versions and value sets by country/region, population norms, and key EQ-5D references. It also explains how to obtain the questionnaire. Those wishing to use EQ-5D must first register their study or trial via the website, using the page 'How to obtain EQ-5D',[5] which has more detailed information about registering, including an animated video. EQ-5D is provided without charging a license fee to non-commercial organisations after they have registered (approximately 95% of users), while commercial users are charged a fee. Registering a study does not obligate the purchase of an EQ-5D licence, but it enables the EuroQol Research Foundation to provide further information relevant to the type of study proposed, including terms and conditions

Development

The EuroQol Group first met in 1987 with the goal of identifying a set of standardised questions that could be used to collect data on how people's lives were affected by illness and by health interventions. What was originally termed 'the EuroQol instrument' was developed by 1990 and contained questions on five aspects (or 'dimensions') of health, with three levels of severity in each dimension.[6]

It was constructed simultaneously in five languages:

Dutch, Finnish, Norwegian, Swedish, and English (which was to function as the source, or reference, language).[7] The questionnaire was re-named 'EQ-5D' in 1995 and now comprises a family of questionnaires: the three-level EQ-5D-3L, the five-level EQ-5D-5L, and the youth version EQ-5D-Y.

EQ-5D was designed as a self-completed questionnaire to fulfil two functions: (i) to provide a descriptive profile of current health status; and (ii) to provide a way of assigning a single numerical value to each of the possible health states described by the descriptive system, for use in economic evaluations of health care.[8] The requirements for its design were that (i) the dimensions should be relevant to both patients and members of the general population; (ii) the descriptive system should be simple – with as few dimensions as possible, and as few levels as possible within each dimension; (iii) it should be short and easily self-completed in a range of settings, and simple enough not to require detailed instructions; and (iv) it should be reliable, valid, and able to identify changes in health status related to illness and health interventions.

Components

The EQ-5D essentially consists of two pages: the EQ-5D descriptive system (page 2 of the questionnaire) and the EQ-5D visual analogue scale (EQ VAS) (page 3 of the questionnaire) (Video: Explaining the EQ-5D in about Two and Half Minutes). As noted above, 'EQ-5D' is not an abbreviation and is the correct term to use when referring to the instrument.

Descriptive systems

The EQ-5D descriptive system comprises five dimensions: mobility, self-care, usual activities, pain and discomfort, and anxiety and depression. The number of levels in these dimensions differ in the EQ-5D-3L (three levels) and the EQ-5D-5L (five levels). The EQ-5D-Y has the same five dimensions, but they are worded more appropriately for young people

EQ-5D-3L

In EQ-5D-3L, the five dimensions each have three response levels of severity. The mobility dimension ranges from 'I have no problems walking about' to 'I am confined to bed'. The self-care dimension ranges from 'I have no problems with self-care' to 'I am unable to wash or dress myself'. The usual activities dimension concerns work, study, housework, family, or leisure activities and ranges from 'I have no problems doing my usual activities' to 'I am unable to do my usual activities'. The pain/discomfort dimension ranges from 'I have no pain or discomfort' to 'I have extreme pain or discomfort'. The anxiety/depression dimension ranges from 'I am not anxious or depressed' to 'I am extremely anxious or depressed'.

Respondents are asked to choose the statement in each dimension that best describes their health status on the day they are surveyed. Their responses are coded as a number (1, 2, or 3) that corresponds to the respective level of severity: 1 indicates no problems, 2 some problems, and 3 extreme problems. In this way, a person's health state profile can be defined by a 5-digit number, ranging from 11111 (having no problems in any of the dimensions) to 33333 (having extreme problems in all the dimensions). The health state 12321 would indicate a person having no problems with mobility, having some problems with self-care, being unable to perform their usual activities, having some pain or discomfort, and not being anxious or depressed. In total, the EQ-5D-3L describes 243 ($=3^5$) potential health states.[9]

EQ-5D-5L

EQ-5D-5L was introduced in 2009 with the aim of enhancing instrument sensitivity and providing respondents with the opportunity to provide a more detailed and accurate picture of their health. The EQ-5D-5L descriptive system uses the same five dimensions as the EQ-5D-3L but has two extra levels of severity in each dimension. The five levels in each dimension are worded as (1) 'not /no problems', (2) 'slight problems', (3) 'moderate problems', (4) 'severe problems', and (5) 'unable to' (mobility, self-care, usual activities), 'extreme' (pain/depression), or 'extremely' (anxiety/depression). A few changes in the wording of some levels were also made. For example, in the mobility dimension, the 3L term 'confined to bed' has been replaced with 'unable to walk about' in the 5L; and the first level of self-care in the 5L now refers to washing and dressing, to be consistent with the other levels. Because of the additional levels in EQ-5D-5L, the descriptive system describes 3125 ($=5^5$) potential health states.[10]

EQ-5D-Y

The EQ-5D version (EQ-5D-Y) was introduced by the EuroQol Group in 2009 as a more suitable questionnaire for children and adolescents.[11] It is based on the EQ-5D-3L, but the wording has been modified to be more easily understood and relevant for younger people. The dimensions are: mobility (walking about); looking after myself; doing usual activities (e.g., going to school, hobbies, sports, playing, doing things with family and friends); having pain or discomfort; and feeling worried, sad, or unhappy. The levels for the first four dimensions are: 'none/no problems', 'some (problems)', and 'a lot (of problems)'. The levels in the feeling worried, sad, or unhappy dimension are: 'not', 'a bit', and 'very'. EQ-5D-Y is recommended for use with 8–11-year-olds and for 12–15-year-olds (although the adult version may be appropriate in the older age group, depending on study design; see Table 1.[12] For children aged 4–7 years, a proxy version should be used – i.e. a version of the questionnaire that is suitable for completion by a third party (e.g. a parent, caregiver, or health professional) on the child's behalf.

TABLE 1: Recommended age range of users of the EQ-5D-Y version [12]

Age range	Recommendation
0-3 years	No EQ-5D-Y version is available for this age range
4-7 years	For children aged 4–7, a proxy version should be used No self-reported EQ-5D-Y is available for this age range at present.
8-11 years	Use EQ-5D-Y The EQ-5D-Y is more understandable for children in this age range than an adult version of the EQ-5D
12-15 years	Both the EQ-5D-Y and adult EQ-5D versions can be used An overlapping area. Generally, EQ-5D-Y is recommended. Depending on the study design, however, it might be appropriate to use one of the EQ-5D adult versions. For example, if a study includes both adult respondents and respondents between the ages of 12 and 15, the study team might prefer to use just one version of EQ-5D across the whole study population.
16 years and over	Use an adult version (EQ-5D-3L or EQ-5D-5L) A possible exception would be a study that only includes children up to age 18. In this case, EQ-5D-Y would be recommended across the full age range, to avoid using two different versions of EQ-5D.

EQ VAS

The second part of the questionnaire in all three versions of EQ-5D comprises a standard vertical 20-cm VAS that is calibrated from 'the worst health you can imagine' (scored 0) at its base to 'the best health you can imagine' (scored 100) at its apex. Respondents are asked to 'mark an X on the scale to indicate how your health is TODAY' and to write the number in an adjoining box.

This procedure makes it possible for respondents to provide a rating of their overall health on the day they complete the questionnaire. The VAS can also be used to assess changes in a patient's perception of their own health over time. For example, a patient may rate their current health as 50 on the scale, but after a medical intervention the respondent's rating may be 85, reflecting a substantial improvement in health status. When a group of patients completes the EQ-5D questionnaire before and after treatment, the change in self-rated health can be recorded from the VAS data.

EQ-5D versions

Modes of administration: EQ-5D is available in different formats depending on the mode of administration. The 3L, 5L, and Y versions can be self-completed on paper or by telephone or digitally, e.g., laptop/desktop, tablet, REDCap, interactive voice response (IVR), and smartphone/personal digital assistant (PDA). The EQ-5D can be hosted on local servers or on alternatives such as REDCap, LimeSurvey, Castor EDC, or Qualtrics platforms.

If people are unable to complete the EQ-5D themselves for any reason, e.g. due to ill-health or literacy problems, interviewer-administered versions are available for use in telephone, online, or face-to-face interviews.

It is sometimes appropriate to ask a caregiver (or proxy) to answer on behalf of people who cannot complete the questionnaire themselves (e.g. because they are too young, too ill, or have severe mental health problems or intellectual disability). The EQ-5D has two proxy versions: proxy version 1 asks the proxy to provide their own rating of the other person's health, while proxy version 2 asks the proxy how they think the person being evaluated would describe his/her own health if they were able to complete the questionnaire.

Psychometric properties

The validity, reliability, and responsiveness of EQ-5D-3L have been assessed for EQ-5D versions in many different health conditions, including cardiovascular disease,[41][42] mental health populations,[43] aged care,[44] skin conditions,[45] cancer,[46] and total knee arthroplasty.[47]

The brevity of EQ-5D-3L is likely to be a major factor in its widespread use, but the three-level format can be a limitation in some clinical areas. The EQ-5D-3L descriptive system can be less sensitive to small and medium changes in health status,[48] so it may be less able to detect change in some conditions.[49][50]

The 5L descriptive system has shown improved responsiveness compared to the 3L system, e.g. in a comparison of eight patient groups [25], osteoarthritis,[51] and joint replacement,[52] as well as acceptable psychometric properties in conditions such as stroke,[53] chronic obstructive lung disease,[54] and scoliosis.[55] Some studies have assessed the EQ-5D-3L and EQ-5D-5L together.[56]

References

1. Brooks R, Boye KS, Slaap B. EQ-5D: a plea for accurate nomenclature. J Patient Rep Outcomes. 2020;4(1):52. doi: 10.1186/s41687-020-00222-9. PMID: 32620995; PMCID: PMC7334333.
2. https://pubmed.ncbi.nlm.nih.gov/?term=eq-5d&filter=dates.1990-2020%2F12%2F21 (accessed 21st December 2020).
3. Kennedy-Martin M, Slaap B, Herdman M, van Reenen M, Kennedy-Martin T, Greiner W, Busschbach J, Boye KS. Which multi-attribute utility instruments are recommended for use in cost-utility analysis? A review of national health technology assessment (HTA) guidelines. Eur J Health Econ. 2020;21(8):1245-1257. doi: 10.1007/s10198-020-01195-8. PMID: 32514643; PMCID: PMC7561556.
4. https://euroqol.org
5. https:/euroqol.org/support/how-to-obtain-eq-5d/
6. EuroQol Group. EuroQol--a new facility for the measurement of health-related quality of life. Health Policy. 1990;16(3):199-208. doi: 10.1016/0168-8510(90)90421-9. PMID: 10109801.
7. Brooks R. The EuroQol Group after 25 years. Springer, 2013. Available from: www.springeronline.com. doi: 10.1007/978-94-007-5158-3. ISBN 978-94-007-5158-3
8. Rabin R, de Charro F. EQ-5D: a measure of health status from the EuroQol Group. Ann Med. 2001;33(5):337-43. doi: 10.3109/07853890109002087. PMID: 11491192.
9. EuroQol Research Foundation. EQ-5D-3L User Guide, 2018. Available from https://euroqol.org/publications/user-guides.
10. EuroQol Research Foundation. EQ-5D-5L User Guide, 2019. Available from: https://euroqol.org/publications/user-guides.
11. Wille N, Badia X, Bonsel G, Burström K, Cavrini G, Devlin N, Egmar AC, Greiner W, Gusi N, Herdman M, Jelsma J, Kind P, Scalone L, Ravens-Sieberer U. Development of the EQ-5D-Y: a child-friendly version of the EQ-5D. Qual Life Res. 2010;19(6):875-86. doi: 10.1007/s11136-010-9648-y. PMID: 20405245; PMCID: PMC2892611.
12. EuroQol Research Foundation. EQ-5D-Y User Guide, Version 2.0, 2020. Available from: https://euroqol.org/publications/user-guides/.
13. Rabin R, Gudex C, Selai C, Herdman M. From translation to version management: a history and review of methods for the cultural adaptation of the EuroQol five-dimensional questionnaire. Value Health. 2014;17(1):70-6. doi: 10.1016/j.jval.2013.10.006. PMID: 24438719.
14. Wild D, Grove A, Martin M, Eremenco S, McElroy S, Verjee-Lorenz A, Erikson P; ISPOR Task Force for Translation and Cultural Adaptation. Principles of Good Practice for the Translation and Cultural Adaptation Process for Patient-Reported Outcomes (PRO) Measures: report of the ISPOR Task Force for Translation and Cultural Adaptation. Value Health. 2005;8(2):94-104. doi: 10.1111/j.1524-4733.2005.04054.x. PMID: 15804318.
15. Quality-adjusted life year
16. https://euroqol.org/eq-5d-3l-about/valuation
17. https://euroqol.org/eq-5d-instruments/eq-5d-5l-about/valuation-standard-value-sets/
18. Devlin NJ, Brooks R. EQ-5D and the EuroQol Group: Past, Present and Future. Appl Health Econ Health Policy. 2017;15(2):127-137. doi: 10.1007/s40258-017-0310-5. PMID: 28194657; PMCID: PMC5343080.
19. Brooks R. EuroQol: the current state of play. Health Policy. 1996;37(1):53-72. doi: 10.1016/0168-8510(96)00822-6. PMID: 10158943.
20. Dolan P, Gudex C, Kind P, Williams A. The time trade-off method: results from a general population study. Health Econ. 1996;5(2):141-54. doi: 10.1002/(SICI)1099-1050(199603)5:2<141::AID-HEC189>3.0.CO;2-N. PMID: 8733106.
21. Dolan P. Modeling valuations for EuroQol health states. Med Care. 1997;35(11):1095-108. doi: 10.1097/00005650-199711000-00002. PMID: 9366889.
22. Szende A, Oppe M, Devlin N. (eds.) EQ-5D value sets: Inventory, comparative review and user guide. EuroQol Group Monographs Volume 2. Springer, 2006. doi: 10.1007/1-4020-5511-0. ISBN 978-1-4020-5511-9.
23. Brooks R, Rabin R, de Charro F. (eds). The measurement and valuation of health status using

EQ-5D: a European perspective. Springer, 2003. doi: 10.1007/978-94-017-0233-1. ISBN 978-94-017-0233-1.

24. Oppe M, Rand-Hendriksen K, Shah K, Ramos-Goñi JM, Luo N. EuroQol Protocols for Time Trade-Off Valuation of Health Outcomes. Pharmacoeconomics. 2016;34(10):993-1004. doi: 10.1007/s40273-016-0404-1. PMID: 27084198; PMCID: PMC5023738.
25. Janssen MF, Pickard AS, Golicki D, Gudex C, Niewada M, Scalone L, Swinburn P, Busschbach J. Measurement properties of the EQ-5D-5L compared to the EQ-5D-3L across eight patient groups: a multi-country study. Qual Life Res. 2013;22(7):1717-27. doi: 10.1007/s11136-012-0322-4. PMID: 23184421; PMCID: PMC3764313.
26. van Hout B, Janssen MF, Feng YS, Kohlmann T, Busschbach J, Golicki D, Lloyd A, Scalone L, Kind P, Pickard AS. Interim scoring for the EQ-5D-5L: mapping the EQ-5D-5L to EQ-5D-3L value sets. Value Health. 2012;15(5):708-15. doi: 10.1016/j.jval.2012.02.008. PMID: 22867780.
27. Robinson A, Spencer A. Exploring challenges to TTO utilities: valuing states worse than dead. Health Econ. 2006;15(4):393-402. doi: 10.1002/hec.1069. PMID: 16389652.
28. Devlin N, Buckingham K, Shah K, Tsuchiya A, Tilling C, Wilkinson G, van Hout B. A comparison of alternative variants of the lead and lag time TTO. Health Econ. 2013;22(5):517-32. doi: 10.1002/hec.2819. PMID: 22715069.
29. Attema AE, Versteegh MM, Oppe M, Brouwer WB, Stolk EA. Lead time TTO: leading to better health state valuations? Health Econ. 2013; 22(4): 376-92. doi: 10.1002/hec.2804. PMID: 22396243.
30. Oppe M, Devlin NJ, van Hout B, Krabbe PF, de Charro F. A program of methodological research to arrive at the new international EQ-5D-5L valuation protocol. Value Health. 2014;17(4):445-53. doi: 10.1016/j.jval.2014.04.002. PMID: 24969006.
31. Janssen BM, Oppe M, Versteegh MM, Stolk EA. Introducing the composite time trade-off: a test of feasibility and face validity. Eur J Health Econ. 2013;14 Suppl 1:S5-13. doi: 10.1007/s10198-013-0503-2. PMID: 23900660.
32. Stolk EA, Oppe M, Scalone L, Krabbe PF. Discrete choice modeling for the quantification of health states: the case of the EQ-5D. Value Health. 2010;13(8):1005-13. doi: 10.1111/j.1524-4733.2010.00783.x. PMID: 20825618.
33. Discrete choice
34. Stolk E, Ludwig K, Rand K, van Hout B, Ramos-Goñi JM. Overview, Update, and Lessons Learned From the International EQ-5D-5L Valuation Work: Version 2 of the EQ-5D-5L Valuation Protocol. Value Health. 2019;22(1):23-30. doi: 10.1016/j.jval.2018.05.010. PMID: 30661630.
35. Kreimeier S, Greiner W. EQ-5D-Y as a Health-Related Quality of Life Instrument for Children and Adolescents: The Instrument's Characteristics, Development, Current Use, and Challenges of Developing Its Value Set. Value Health. 2019;22(1):31-37. doi: 10.1016/j.jval.2018.11.001. PMID: 30661631.
36. Ramos-Goñi JM, Oppe M, Stolk E, Shah K, Kreimeier S, Rivero-Arias O, Devlin N. International Valuation Protocol for the EQ-5D-Y-3L. Pharmacoeconomics. 2020;38(7):653-663. doi: 10.1007/s40273-020-00909-3. PMID: 32297224.
37. Prevolnik Rupel V, Ogorevc M; IMPACT HTA HRQoL Group. EQ-5D-Y Value Set for Slovenia. Pharmacoeconomics. 2021 Feb 10. doi: 10.1007/s40273-020-00994-4. Epub ahead of print. PMID: 33565048.
38. Kreimeier S, Oppe M, Ramos-Goñi JM, Cole A, Devlin N, Herdman M, Mulhern B, Shah KK, Stolk E, Rivero-Arias O, Greiner W. Valuation of EuroQol Five-Dimensional Questionnaire, Youth Version (EQ-5D-Y) and EuroQol Five-Dimensional Questionnaire, Three-Level Version (EQ-5D-3L) Health States: The Impact of Wording and Perspective. Value Health. 2018;21(11):1291-1298. doi: 10.1016/j.jval.2018.05.002. PMID: 30442276.
39. Kind P, Klose K, Gusi N, Olivares PR, Greiner W. Can adult weights be used to value child health states? Testing the influence of perspective in valuing EQ-5D-Y. Qual Life Res. 2015;24(10):2519-39. doi: 10.1007/s11136-015-0971-1. PMID: 25894060; PMCID: PMC4564451.
40. Devlin N, Parkin D, Janssen B. Methods for Analysing and Reporting EQ-5D Data. Springer, 2020. Open Access. Available from: www.springeronline.com. doi: 10.1007/978-3-030-47622-9. ISBN 978-3-030-47622-9.
41. Dyer MT, Goldsmith KA, Sharples LS, Buxton MJ. A review of health utilities using the EQ-5D in studies of cardiovascular disease. Health Qual Life Outcomes. 2010;8:13. doi:10.1186/1477-7525-8-13. PMID: 20109189; PMCID: PMC2824714.

42. Batóg P, Rencz F, Péntek M, Gulácsi L, Filipiak KJ, Prevolnik Rupel V, Simon J, Brodszky V, Baji P, Závada J, Petrova G, Rotar A, Golicki D. EQ-5D studies in cardiovascular diseases in eight Central and Eastern European countries: a systematic review of the literature. Kardiol Pol. 2018;76(5):860-870. doi: 10.5603/KP.a 2018. 0033. PMID: 29350378.
43. Brazier J, Connell J, Papaioannou D, Mukuria C, Mulhern B, Peasgood T, Jones ML, Paisley S, O'Cathain A, Barkham M, Knapp M, Byford S, Gilbody S, Parry G. A systematic review, psychometric analysis and qualitative assessment of generic preference-based measures of health in mental health populations and the estimation of mapping functions from widely used specific measures. Health Technol Assess. 2014;18(34):vii-viii, xiii-xxv, 1-188. doi: 10.3310/hta18340. PMID: 24857402; PMCID: PMC4781324.
44. Bulamu NB, Kaambwa B, Ratcliffe J. A systematic review of instruments for measuring outcomes in economic evaluation within aged care. Health Qual Life Outcomes. 2015 Nov;13:179. DOI: 10.1186/s12955-015-0372-8. PMID: 26553129; PMCID: PMC4640110.
45. Yang Y, Brazier J, Longworth L. EQ-5D in skin conditions: an assessment of validity and responsiveness. Eur J Health Econ. 2015; 16(9): 927-939. doi:10.1007/s10198-014-0638-9. PMID :25358263; PMCID: PMC4646948.
46. Schwenkglenks M, Matter-Walstra K. Is the EQ-5D suitable for use in oncology? An overview of the literature and recent developments. Expert Rev Pharmacoecon Outcomes Res. 2016;16(2):207-219.

    doi:10.1586/14737167.2016.1146594.PMID: 26808097.
47. Shim J, Hamilton DF. Comparative responsiveness of the PROMIS-10 Global Health and EQ-5D questionnaires in patients undergoing total knee arthroplasty. Bone Joint J. 2019;101-B (7):832-837. doi:10.1302/0301-620X.101B7. BJJ-2018-1543.R1. PMID: 31256677; PMCID: PMC6616061.
48. Herdman M, Gudex C, Lloyd A, Janssen M, Kind P, Parkin D, Bonsel G, Badia X. Development and preliminary testing of the new five-level version of EQ-5D (EQ-5D-5L). Qual Life Res. 2011;20(10):1727-36. doi: 10.1007/s11136-011-9903-x. PMID: 21479777; PMCID: PMC 3220807.
49. Payakachat N, Ali MM, Tilford JM. Can The EQ-5D Detect Meaningful Change? A Systematic Review. Pharmacoeconomics. 2015;33(11):1137-54. doi: 10.1007/s40273-015-0295-6. PMID: 26040242; PMCID: PMC4609224.
50. Hounsome N, Orrell M, Edwards RT. EQ-5D as a quality of life measure in people with dementia and their carers: evidence and key issues. Value Health. 2011;14(2):390-399. doi:10.1016/j.jval.2010.08.002. PMID: 21402307.
51. Bilbao A, García-Pérez L, Arenaza JC, García I, Ariza-Cardiel G, Trujillo-Martín E, Forjaz MJ, Martín-Fernández J. Psychometric properties of the EQ-5D-5L in patients with hip or knee osteoarthritis: reliability, validity and responsiveness. Qual Life Res. 2018;27(11):2897-2908. doi: 10.1007/s11136-018-1929-x. PMID: 29978346.
52. Jin X, Al Sayah F, Ohinmaa A, Marshall DA, Johnson JA. Responsiveness of the EQ-5D-3L and EQ-5D-5L in patients following total hip or knee replacement. Qual Life Res. 2019;28(9):2409-2417. doi:10.1007/s11136-019-02200-1. PMID: 31089988.
53. Chen P, Lin KC, Liing RJ, Wu CY, Chen CL, Chang KC. Validity, responsiveness, and minimal clinically important difference of EQ-5D-5L in stroke patients undergoing rehabilitation. Qual Life Res. 2016;25(6):1585-1596. doi:10.1007/s11136-015-1196-z. PMID: 26714699.
54. Nolan CM, Longworth L, Lord J, Canavan JL, Jones SE, Kon SS, Man WD. The EQ-5D-5L health status questionnaire in COPD: validity, responsiveness and minimum important difference. Thorax. 2016;71(6):493-500. doi: 10.1136/thoraxjnl-2015-207782.
    PMID: 27030578; PMCID: PMC4893131.
55. Cheung PWH, Wong CKH, Lau ST, Cheung JPY. Responsiveness of the EuroQoL 5-dimension (EQ-5D) in adolescent idiopathic scoliosis. Eur Spine J. 2018;27(2):278-285. doi:10.1007/s00586-017-5330-1. PMID: 28993884.
56. Qian X, Tan RL, Chuang LH, Luo N. Measurement Properties of Commonly Used Generic Preference-Based Measures in East and South-East Asia: A Systematic Review. Pharmacoeconomics. 2020;38(2):159-170. doi: 10.1007/s40273-019-00854-w. PMID: 31761995; PMCID: PMC7081654.

❑❑❑

70

Falls Efficacy Scale-International (FES-I)

Objective

The Falls Efficacy Scale International (FES-I) is a measure of "fear of falling" or "concerns about falling", developed as a part of the Prevention of Falls Network Europe (ProFaNE) project from 2003 to 2006 by Todd et al[1]. It is a 16 item questionnaire, useful to the researchers and clinicians interested in fear of falling, with a score ranging from minimum 16 (no concern about falling) to maximum 64 (severe concern about falling)[2].

Intended Population

The FES-I is intended to be used in adult population to measure the level of concern about falling during social and physical activities inside and outside the home whether or not the person actually does the activity.

Method of Use

Equipment: Pen Paper

Training: no special training required

Mode and Cost of Instrument

It can be administered as self-completion questionnaires, or interview-based questionnaire.

Instrument

It is a 16-item questionnaire where individuals are instructed to score their concern of falling during an activity on a 4 point Likert scale with 1 as not concerned at all and 4 as very concerned. The item scores are summed up to obtain a total, with higher the score, higher being the concern for falling.

The items included are:

1. Cleaning the house (e.g. sweep, vacuum, dust)
2. Getting dressed or undressed
3. Preparing simple meals
4. Taking a bath or shower
5. Going to the shop
6. Getting in or out of a chair
7. Going up or down stairs
8. Walking around in the neighborhood
9. Reaching for something above your head or on the ground
10. Going to answer the telephone before it stops ringing
11. Walking on a slippery surface (e.g. wet or icy)
12. Visiting a friend or relative
13. Walking in a place with crowds
14. Walking on an uneven surface (e.g. rocky ground, poorly maintained pavement)
15. Walking up or down a slope
16. Going out to a social event (e.g. religious service, family gathering, or club meeting)

Psychometric Properties

Reliability and validity

1. In Parkinson's Disease: Internal consistency (α = 0.96, On phase; 0.98, Off phase) and test-retest reliability (0.94; 0.91) were satisfactory in on phase of drug an off phase. There was a a moderate/high correlation (rS = |0.50–0.70|) between FES-I and Visual Analog Scale-Fear of Falling, Berg Balance Scale, and Functional Reach Test[3].
2. In Vestibular disorders: excellent test-retest reliability (ICC=0.94). Excellent validity[4].
3. In Older Adults: Excellent test retest reliability, and validity in both community dwelling and geriatric nursing home dwelling individuals[2].

4. In Multiple sclerosis: Excellent internal consistency ($\alpha = 0.96$) with adequate criterion validity[5].
5. In Joint Pains and fractures: Excellent internal consistency ($\alpha = 0.94$)[6].

References

1. L. Yardley, N. Beyer, K. Hauer, G. Kempen, C. Piot-Ziegler, and C. Todd, "Development and initial validation of the falls efficacy scale-international (FES-I)," Age and Ageing, 2005. vol. 34, no. 6, pp. 614–619.
2. Dewan N, MacDermid J. "Fall Efficacy Scale-International (FES-I)." Journal of Physiotherapy, 2014. vol. 60, no. 1, p. 60.
3. Mehdizadeh M, Martinez-Martin P, Habibi S, Fereshtehnejad S, Abasi A, Khatoon J, et al. "Reliability and Validity of Fall Efficacy Scale-International in People with Parkinson's Disease during On- and Off-Drug Phases", Parkinson's Disease, 2019, Article ID 6505232, 7 pages.
4. Morgan MT, Friscia LA, Whitney SL, Furman JM, Sparto PJ. Reliability and validity of the Falls Efficacy Scale-International (FES-I) in individuals with dizziness and imbalance. Otol Neurotol. 2013 Aug;34(6):1104-8
5. van Vliet R, Hoang P, Lord S, Gandevia S, Delbaere K. Falls efficacy scale-international: a cross-sectional validation in people with multiple sclerosis. Arch Phys Med Rehabil. 2013 May;94(5):883-9.
6. Visschedijk JH, Terwee CB, Caljouw MA, Spruit-van Eijk M, van Balen R, Achterberg WP. Reliability and validity of the Falls Efficacy Scale-International after hip fracture in patients aged ≥ 65 years. Disabil Rehabil. 2015;37(23):2225-32.

Falls Efficacy Scale-International (English)

I would like to ask some questions about how concerned you are about the possibility of falling. For each of the following activities, please circle the opinion closest to your own to show how concerned you are that you might fall if you did this activity. Please reply thinking about how you usually do the activity. If you currently don't do the activity (example: if someone does your shopping for you), please answer to show whether you think you would be concerned about falling IF you did the activity.

1. Cleaning the house (e.g. sweep, vacuum, dust)
2. Getting dressed or undressed
3. Preparing simple meals
4. Taking a bath or shower
5. Going to the shop
6. Getting in or out of a chair
7. Going up or down stairs
8. Walking around in the neighborhood
9. Reaching for something above your head or on the ground
10. Going to answer the telephone before it stops ringing
11. Walking on a slippery surface (e.g. wet or icy)
12. Visiting a friend or relative
13. Walking in a place with crowds
14. Walking on an uneven surface (e.g. rocky ground, poorly maintained pavement)
15. Walking up or down a slope
16 Going out to a social event (e.g. religious service, family gathering, or club meeting)

Not at all concerned (1)

Somewhat concerned (2)

Fairly concerned (3)

Very concerned (4)

Reference: Yardley, L., Beyer, N., Hauer, K., Kempen, G., Piot-Ziegler, C., & Todd, C. (2005). Development and initial validation of the Falls Efficacy Scale-International (FES-I). Age and Ageing, 34(6), 614-619. doi:10.1093/ageing/afi196.

Falls Risk Assessment Tool (FRAT): An Overview to Assist Understanding and Conduction

Introduction

Falls are problematic within the elderly population. Approximately 28.7% of older adults reported falling at least once in the preceding 12 months, resulting in an estimated 29 million falls and 7 million fall injuries in the United States.[1] A study specifies that 44% of falls cause minor injuries such as bruises, abrasions and sprains and 4-5% of falls cause major injuries such as wrist and hip fractures.[2] Within the NHS in 2003 the cost per 10,000 population was £300,000 in the 60–64 age group, increasing to £1,500,000 in the >75 age group. These falls cost the UK government £981 million, of which the NHS incurred 59.2%.[3] According to the NHS long term plan (2019), they aim to increase funding for primary and community care by at least £4.5 billion and reducing falls-related costs could go some way to achieving this[4].

The strongest single predictor of future falls is a history of previous falls. This is probably because an individual's reason for falling the first time is likely to recur. Assessment of physical functioning is the next strongest predictor and so its inclusion is likely to increase a tool's predictive ability[5]. According to NICE (2013) assessment and prevention of falls guidelines, older people in contact with healthcare professionals should be asked routinely whether they have fallen in the past year[6].

Understandably therefore in elderly physiotherapy assessment, there is a lot of focus around patients falls history and often use tools like the Falls Risk Assessment Tool (FRAT). Student and newly qualified physiotherapists, however, don't often understand why the factors included in falls risk assessments contribute to falls. This document aims to increase understanding of the impact of risk factors for falls in the elderly population.

FRAT

It is a 4-item falls-risk screening tool for sub-acute and residential care. The FRAT has three sections:

- Part 1 - falls risk status.
- Part 2 – risk factor checklist.
- Part 3 – action plan[7].

Within the UK there does not appear to be a standardised falls risk assessment[8]. Policies regarding this tend to be trust specific. The NHS website (2018) does provide a self-assessment based on the FRAT, however from personal experience, the conduction of the FRAT and similar falls-related tools requires clarity and understanding.

FALLS RISK ASSESSMENT TOOL (FRAT)		
UR Number	Surname	Given Number
Date of Birth		
Part 1 Fall Risk Status		
Risk Factor	**Level**	**Risk Score**
Recent Falls (To score this, complete history of fall overleaf)	None in last 12 months............. One or more between 3 and 12 months ago .... One or more in last 3 months..... One or more in last 3 months (inpatient / Resident)	2 4 6 8
Medications (Sedatives, Anti-Depressants, Anti-Parkinson's, Diuretics, Anti-Hypertensives, Hypnotics)	Not taking any of these............. Taking one........................... Taking two.......................... Taking more than two..............	1 2 3 4
Psychological (Anxiety, Depression, Cooperation, Insight or Judgement esp. re. mobility	Does not appear to have any of these........... appears mildly affected by one or more......... appears moderately affected by one or more... appears severely affected by one or more......	1 2 3 4
Cognitive Status (AMTS: Hodkinson Abbreviated Mental Test Score)	Intact Mildly impaired Mod Impaired Severely Impared	1 2 3 4
Low Risk = 5 – 11; Medium Risk = 12 – 15 High Risk 16 – 20 Risk Score / 20		
Automatic High-Risk Status (if ticked then circle HIGH risk below)		

Recent change in functional status and / or medications affecting safe mobility (or anticipated) Dizziness / Postural hypotension		
Fall Risk Status: (Circle): Low / Medium / High => List fall status on care plan / Flow chart Important: if High, Commence Fall Alert		
PART 2: Risk Factor Checklist		Yes / No
Vision	Reports / observed difficulty seeing – objects / signs / finding way around	
Mobility	Mobility status unknown or appears unsafe / impulsive / forgets gait aid	
Transfers	Transfer status unknown or appears unsafe / impulsive / forgets gait aid	
Behaviours	Observed or reported agitation, confusion, disorientation Difficulty following instructions or non-complaint (observed or known)	
Activities of Daily Living (ADL's)	Observed risk taking behaviours, or reported from referrer / previous facility Observed unsafe use of equipment Unsafe footwear / inappropriate clothing	
Environment	Difficulties with orientation to environment i.e., areas between bed / bathroom / dining room	
Nutrition	Underweight / low appetite	
Continence	Reported or knows urgency / nocturia / accidents	
Other		

How Does Medication Affect Falls?

Medication has long been known to have side effects that can increase the risk of falling. There are many different medications all with different methods of action and side-effects. It's also important to consider the combinations of different medications that can affect falls. Different classes of drugs can influence falls risks by different mechanisms and thus when combined can majorly increase falls risk. Polypharmacy can typically be defined as a patient using more than 3 or 4 medications at one time and this is important as a study by Dhalwani et al., (2017) found that nearly one-third of the total population taking 5 or more drugs had significantly increased falls rate of 21% in a 2-year period[9].

The CDC produced a resource called "Stopping Elderly Accidents, Deaths & Injuries" (STEADI) to provide material to help offer effective interventions to reduce falls risk. They characterise medicines using a 3 point system which can be seen below[10].

Agency for healthcare research and quality fall risk table		
Point Value	**Medicine Class**	**Potential Side Effects**
3 (High)	Analgesic/opiates, antipsychotics, anticonvulsants, benzodiazepines, nonbenzodiazepines, sedatives, hypoglycaemics	Sedation, dizziness, postural disturbances, altered gait and balance, impaired cognation
2 (Medium)	Antihypertensives, cardiac drugs / antiarrhythmics, antidepressants	Induced orthostasis, confusion, poor health status
1 (Low)	Diuretics	Increased ambulation, Induced orthostasis
Score > 6	Higher risk for fall, medication fall risk evaluation	
Resource: STEADI materials for healthcare providers. Centres for Disease Control and Prevention website. https://www.cdc.gov/stead/materials.html. Updated March 24, 2017.		

Understanding Medication Fall Mechanisms

Any medication acting on the brain (psychotropics) or affecting the function of the cardiovascular system can increase fall risk. Psychotropics including anxiolytics/sedative-hypnotics, antipsychotics, antidepressants, anticonvulsants, and narcotic pain medications typically increase risk due to their effects on cognitive function, resulting in sedation, slower reaction times, and impaired balance[11][12][13]

Cardiovascular medications often either lower blood pressure with subsequent hypotension or affect heart rate, resulting in bradycardia, tachycardia, or periods of asystole[14]. Maintaining consciousness and an upright posture requires adequate blood flow to the brain and so drugs affecting this do carry a risk of potential fall, if blood pressure is not kept in the optimal parameters.

Recent systematic reviews with meta-analyses have confirmed the effects of medications on increased falls, however, there are still some uncertainties regarding whether all drugs in certain sub-groups have the same effect as others and so further work is needed to address this. A systematic review by De Vries et al., (2018) found that loop diuretics were significantly associated with increased falls risk, beta-blockers significant decrease in falls risk[15]. Specific drug properties and method of interaction have an effect. Another recent systematic review by Seppala et al., (2018) found antipsychotics, anti-depressants, benzodiazepines have a significant increase in falls risk[16].

Psychological Status

How Does Psychological State Increase Falls Risk Status?

Anxiety	Anxiety has been defined as feeling of unease, such as worry or fear (NHS UK, 2018) Feelings of anxiety are commonly experienced by most people at some point in their life, but can be symptoms can be experience long term (MHS UK, 2018) Anxiety can affect falls risk through a variety of mechanisms, including gait; individuals taking shorter strides and having a slower gait speed, increasing falls risk (Young and Williams, 2015) Those with anxiety may focus more internally (e.g. their own feet) rather than externally and this further increases falls risk (Young and William, 2015)
Depression	Depression is recognized as a chronic condition in which the sufferer persistently experiences bouts of low mood. It can affect people in a wide variety of ways and can produce a range of symptoms (NHS UK, 2016) Depression and falls are frequently associated, with depression acknowledge as an independent risk factor for falls (Deandrea et al., 2010) Stalehoef et al. (2002) reported four determinants of recurrent falls: postural sway, history of falls, handgrip strength, and depressive symptoms. Isolated symptoms of depression may have a direct role in promoting falls in the elderly such as; insomnia (Stone et al., 2008) and poor appetite and weight loss (Shahar et al. 2009) Depression is also associated with a characteristic pattern of cognitive deficits, affecting mainly attention, executive function, and processing speed (McDermoot & Ebmeier, 2009)

Cognitive Status

Impact of Cognitive Status on Falls

- The motor and sensory systems are linked by higher-order neurological processes and cognition.[17]
- Previous research has demonstrated cognition has a key role in the regulation of gait and balance in older adults:[18]
- Increased levels of cognition are required for movement planning and adapting to environmental changes.[19]
- Therefore, impairments in the cognition increase risk of falling.[20]
- A study ("Gait, Cognition & Decline") on 2700 older adults with and without dementia showed that adults with dementia fall more than when compared to healthy counterparts.[21]
- Mini-Mntal State Examination (MMSE) score ≤ 24 equates to increased falls risk.[22]
- Specifically, subjects scoring < 28 on the MMSE demonstrated a nearly three-fold increased risk for

falls compared to control subjects whose MMSE was 30/30.[23]

- The cognitive test included in the FRAT is the Hodkinson Abbreviated Mental Test Score (ABTS). This test is used to assess for the possibility of dementia and is now sometimes used for other cognitive impairments[24]. Scores indicate the level of impairment, however more rigorous cognitive testing is required to confirm this.

Critique of FRAT

- Risk Factor Checklist (Part 2) fails to appreciate balance specifically. If this was a self-reported concern of the patient, areas of proprioception and the vestibular system could be objectively looked at in more depth within specialist physiotherapy assessment.
- Lacks context – eludes to being objective however fails to provide any guidance on questioning to obtain further information. Area for development – extended box to record subjective and objective measures.
- NICE guidelines state the FRAT does not assess all the risk variables highlighted in their guidelines for falls prevention. Furthermore, NICE state it should not be relied solely on to assess risk of falls and requires further investigation[6]. If high falls risk is identified, more extensive assessment is required – e.g. Elderly Mobility Scale to provide objective measures that guide physiotherapy treatment.
- Nowhere to record a collateral history. Having an area to collect information would allow for exploration into issues and areas highlighted in Part 2.
- 'History of Falls' section lacks ability to record detailed mechanics of fall. Tick boxes can be supported by a descriptive component. (See 'Potential Modifications to the FRAT').
- Cognitive test included is rather outdated and cannot be relied on to confirm cognitive impairment.
- Recommendation: carry out with several members of MDT present to incorporate areas of expertise.

Potential Modifications to the FRAT

During the process of evaluating the FRAT, there is a perceived lack of depth pertaining to the falls section. It is proposed that some amendments could be made to this in order to improve clarity and increase information and reliability.

Current 'History of Falls' Section:

History of Falls (Note: For an accurate history, consult patient/ resident / family / medical records	
Falls prior to this administration (Home or referring facility) and/or during current stay If ticked, detail most recent below	
Circumstances of Recent falls: **(Circle Below)**	**Information Obtained from..................** **(Where ? / Comments)**
Last Fall Time Ago----Trip Slip Lost Balance Collapse Leg/s gave way Dizziness	___________
Previous Time Ago----Trip Slip Lost Balance Collapse Leg/s gave way Dizziness	___________
Previous Time Ago----Trip Slip Lost Balance Collapse Leg/s gave way Dizziness	___________

Potential Developments:

History of falls		
Falls with in last 12 months:	Yes / No	If Yes, How Many? -----------------
Context of most recent fall: Trip / Slip Dizziness	Legs give away LOC	Balance
Other..........		Please Explain-------------------
Baseline Mobility:		**Was aid used at time of fall? Yes / No**
Description of fall:		
Injuries sustained? Yes / No		If Yes, Please Explain

References

1. Cuevas-Trisan R. Balance problems and fall risks in the elderly. Physical Medicine and Rehabilitation Clinics. 2017 Nov 1;28(4):727-37.
2. Hart A. *Falls in the Older Adult Population: Risk Factors, Risk Identification Instruments and Fall Prevention Programs* (Doctoral dissertation, Stern College for Women). 2015
3. Scuffham P, Chaplin S, Legood R. Incidence and costs of unintentional falls in older people in the United Kingdom. Journal of Epidemiology & Community Health. 2003 Sep 1;57(9):740-4.
4. England NH. The NHS long term plan. London: NHS England. 2019.
5. Sherrington C, Tiedemann A. Physiotherapy in the prevention of falls in older people. Journal of physiotherapy. 2015 Apr 1;61(2):54-60.
6. Centre for Clinical Practice at NICE (UK. Falls: Assessment and prevention of falls in older people. 2013
7. Stapleton C, Hough P, Oldmeadow L, Bull K, Hill K, Greenwood K. Four-item fall risk screening tool for subacute and residential aged care: The first step in fall prevention. Australasian Journal on Ageing. 2009 Sep;28(3):139-43.
8. Matarese M, Ivziku D. Falls risk assessment in older patients in hospital. Nursing Standard. 2016 Jul 27;30(48).
9. Dhalwani NN, Fahami R, Sathanapally H, Seidu S, Davies MJ, Khunti K. Association between polypharmacy and falls in older adults: a longitudinal study from England. BMJ open. 2017 Oct 1;7(10):e016358.
10. Centers for Disease Control and Prevention. STEADI (Stopping Elderly Accidents, Deaths & Injuries) tool kit for health care providers. National Institute of Health and Human Services, Atlanta. 2013.
11. De Jong MR, Van der Elst M, Hartholt KA. Drug-related falls in older patients: implicated drugs, consequences, and possible prevention strategies. Therapeutic advances in drug safety. 2013 Aug;4(4):147-54.
12. Johnell K, Jonasdottir Bergman G, Fastbom J, Danielsson B, Borg N, Salmi P. Psychotropic drugs and the risk of fall injuries, hospitalisations and mortality among older adults. International journal of geriatric psychiatry. 2017 Apr;32(4):414-20.
13. Seitz D, Iaboni A, Kirkham J. Psychotropic Drugs and Falls in Older Adults: an Update for the Geriatric Psychiatrist. The American Journal of Geriatric Psychiatry. 2017 Mar 1;25(3):S21.
14. Darowski A, Whiting R. Cardiovascular medication and falls. Reviews in Clinical Gerontology. 2011 May;21(2):170-9.
15. de Vries M, Seppala LJ, Daams JG, van de Glind EM, Masud T, van der Velde N, Blain H, Bousquet J, Bucht G, Caballero-Mora MA, van der Cammen T. Fall-risk-Increasing drugs: a systematic review and meta-analysis: I. cardiovascular drugs. Journal of the American Medical Directors Association. 2018 Apr 1;19(4):371-e1.
16. Seppala LJ, Wermelink AM, de Vries M, Ploegmakers KJ, van de Glind EM, Daams JG, van der Velde N, Blain H, Bousquet J, Bucht G, Caballero-Mora MA. Fall-risk-increasing drugs: a systematic review and meta-analysis: II. Psychotropics. Journal of the American Medical Directors Association. 2018 Apr 1;19(4):371-e11.
17. Purves D, Cabeza R, Huettel SA, LaBar KS, Platt ML, Woldorff MG, Brannon EM. Cognitive neuroscience. Sunderland: Sinauer Associates, Inc; 2008.
18. Herman T, Mirelman A, Giladi N, Schweiger A, Hausdorff JM. Executive control deficits as a prodrome to falls in healthy older adults: a prospective study linking thinking, walking, and falling. Journals of Gerontology Series A: Biomedical Sciences and Medical Sciences. 2010 May 19;65(10):1086-92.
19. Muir SW, Gopaul K, Montero Odasso MM. The role of cognitive impairment in fall risk among older adults: a systematic review and meta-analysis. Age and ageing. 2012 Feb 27;41(3):299-308.
20. Gleason CE, Gangnon RE, Fischer BL, Mahoney JE. Increased risk for falling associated with subtle cognitive impairment: secondary analysis of a randomized clinical trial. Dementia and geriatric cognitive disorders. 2009;27(6):557-63.
21. Allali G, Launay CP, Blumen HM, Callisaya ML, De Cock AM, Kressig RW, Srikanth V, Steinmetz JP, Verghese J, Beauchet O, Biomathics

Consortium. Falls, cognitive impairment, and gait performance: results from the GOOD initiative. Journal of the American Medical Directors Association. 2017 Apr 1;18(4):335-40.

22. Anstey KJ, Von Sanden C, Luszcz MA. An 8-year prospective study of the relationship between cognitive performance and falling in very old adults. Journal of the American Geriatrics Society. 2006 Aug; 54(8): 1169-76.

23. Mahoney JE, Shea TA, Przybelski R, Jaros L, Gangnon R, Cech S, Schwalbe A. Kenosha County Falls Prevention Study: A Randomized, Controlled Trial of an Intermediate-Intensity, Community-Based Multifactorial Falls Intervention. Journal of the American Geriatrics Society. 2007 Apr;55(4):489-98.

24. Hodkinson HM. Evaluation of a mental test score for assessment of mental impairment in the elderly. Age and ageing. 1972 Nov 1;1(4):233-8.

❑❑❑

71

Fatigue Severity Scale

Objective

The Fatigue Severity Scale is a 9-item scale which measures the severity of fatigue and its effect on a person's activities and lifestyle in patients with a variety of disorders. It was originally devised for people with Multiple Sclerosis or systemic lupus erythematosus[1].

Intended Population

Those with a variety of diagnoses including arthritis, fibromyalgia, Multiple sclerosis, Parkinson's disease and stroke.

Method of Use

A self-report scale of nine items about fatigue, its severity and how it affects certain activities. Answers are scored on a seven point scale where 1 = strongly disagree and 7 = strongly agree. This means the minimum score possible is nine and the highest is 63. The higher the score, the more severe the fatigue is and the more it affects the person's activities. It is simple to understand and takes an average of eight minutes to answer[3].

Evidence

Reliability

Test-retest Reliability: One study reported excellent test-retest reliability (ICC = 0.91) in a Brazilian-Portuguese version for people with Parkinson's (n = 30, mean age = 62 (11) years, mean time post- Parkinson's = 7.6 (6.5) years)[4]. Similar results were found in a study of cirrhotic patients[3].

Validity: Able to discriminate between groups (with and without fatigue) in a study of people with cirrhosis[3]. Correlates with depressive symptomology (Beck Depression Inventory) and quality of life (SF-36)[3].

Parkinson's Disease

- Excellent (r = -0.77) negative correlation with Functional Assessment of Chronic Illness Therapy-Fatigue (FACIT-F) scale[5]
- Excellent (r = 0.62) correlation with Nottingham Health Profile (NHP-EN) scale[5]
- Excellent (r = 0.84) correlation with Parkinson's Fatigue (PFS) scale [6]
- Poor-adequate (r = 0.22-0.47) correlation with Parkinson's Disease Questionnaire-39 (PDQ-39) scale; n = 66, mean age = 70.8 (9.9) years, time since Parkinson's = 70.2 (56.1) months) [7]

Responsiveness: No significant changes observed with the scale pre and post liver transplant[3]. The FSS has been reported to have low floor and moderate ceiling effects[8].

References

1. Krupp LB, LaRocca NG, Muir-Nash J, Steinberg AD. Arch Neurol. 1989 Oct;46(10):1121-3. The Fatigue Severity Scale. Application to patients with multiple sclerosis and systemic lupus erythematosus. Arch Neurol. 1989;46(10):1121-3. Accessed 27 June 2019.
2. Mometrix Academy. Fatigue severity scale. Available from: https://www.youtube.com/watch?v=XAwDgczNCO0)last accessed 3.3.2019)
3. Rossi D, Galant LH, Marroni CA. Psychometric property of fatigue severity scale and correlation with depression and quality of life in cirrhotics. Arq Gastroenterol. 2017. 54; 4: 344-348. Accessed 27 June 2019.
4. Valderramas, S., Feres, A. C., et al. "Reliability and validity study of a Brazilian-Portuguese version of the fatigue severity scale in Parkinson's

patients." Arq Neuropsiquiatr 2012 70(7): 497-500

5. Hagell, P., Hoglund, A., et al. "Measuring fatigue in Parkinson's: a psychometric study of two brief generic fatigue questionnaires." J Pain Symptom Manage 2006 32(5): 420-432
6. Grace, J., Mendelsohn, A., et al. "A comparison of fatigue measures in Parkinson's." Parkinsonism Relat Disord 2007 13(7): 443-445
7. Herlofson, K. and Larsen, J. P. "The influence of fatigue on health-related quality of life in patients with Parkinson's." Acta Neurol Scand 2003 107(1): 1-6
8. Amtmann D, Bamer AM, Noonan V, Lang N, Kim J, Cook KF. Comparison of the psychometric properties of two fatigue scales in multiple sclerosis. Rehabil Psychol. 2012. 57; 2: 159–166. Accessed 27 June 2019.
9. Rosti-Otajärvi E, Hämäläinen P, Wiksten A, Hakkarainen T, Ruutiainen J. Validity and reliability of the Fatigue Severity Scale in Finnish multiple sclerosis patients. Brain and Behaviour. 2017. Volume7; Issue7 : e00743. Accessed 27 June 2019.

Fatigue Severity Scale

Date ________________ Name ______________

Please circle the number between 1 and 7 which you feel best fits the following statements. This refers to your usual way of life within the last week. 1 indicates "strongly disagree" and 7 indicates "strongly agree."

Read and circle a number.	**Strongly Disagree → Strongly Agree**
1. My motivation is lower when I am fatigued.	1 2 3 4 5 6 7
2. Exercise brings on my fatigue.	1 2 3 4 5 6 7
3. I am easily fatigued.	1 2 3 4 5 6 7
4. Fatigue interferes with my physical functioning.	1 2 3 4 5 6 7
5. Fatigue causes frequent problems for me.	1 2 3 4 5 6 7
6. My fatigue prevents sustained physical functioning.	1 2 3 4 5 6 7
7. Fatigue interferes with carrying out certain duties and responsibilities.	1 2 3 4 5 6 7
8. Fatigue is among my most disabling symptoms.	1 2 3 4 5 6 7
9. Fatigue interferes with my work, family, or social life.	1 2 3 4 5 6 7

VISUAL ANALOGUE FATIGUE SCALE (VAFS)

Please mark an "X" on the number line which describes your global fatigue with 0 being worst and 10 being normal

1………2………3……….4……….5……….6……….7……….8……….9……….10 --

❑❑❑

72

Fear-Avoidance Belief Questionnaire

Objective

The Fear-Avoidance Beliefs Questionnaire (FABQ) is a patient reported questionnaire which specifically focuses on how a patient's fear avoidance beliefs about physical activity and work may affect and contribute to their low back pain and resulting disability

Description

With the emergence of the biopsychosocial mode of low back pain (LBP) led to the development of the the Fear-Avoidance Beliefs Questionnaire (FABQ) by Waddel et al in 1993[1]. The FABQ is a questionnaire based on the Fear-Avoidance Model of Exaggerated Pain Perception, a model created in attempts to explain why some patients with acute painful conditions can recover while other patients develop chronic pain from such conditions[2][3][4]. The FABQ measures patients' fear of pain and consequent avoidance of physical activity because of their fear[2][3].

Areas of assessment include; ADLs, behaviour, functional mobility, general health, life participation, mental health, motivation, occupational performance, pain, personality, quality of life, self-efficacy, stress and coping.

Intended Population

The FABQ has been proven to be a reliable and valid assessment tool based on patients with chronic low back pain. In recent research, the FABQ is being used in populations with acute low back pain to identify the risk of long-term disability[3]. It is also used in patients with spinal injuries, musculoskeletal conditions and chronic pain.

Methods of Use

The questionnaire consists of 16 items in which a patient rates their agreement with each statement on a 7-point Likert scale. Where 0= completely disagree, 6=completely agree. There is a maximum score of 96. A higher score indicates more strongly held fear avoidance beliefs. [2] There are two subscales within the FABQ; the work subscale (FABQw) with 7 questions (maximum score of 42) and the physical activity subscale (FABQpa) with 4 questions (maximum score of 24).[2][3]. The numbers in parentheses below designate which items from the FABQ are included in each subscale[2].

Subscale	Questions Included	Total Possible Points	High Score
FABQw	6,7,9-12, 15	42	>34[3]
FABQpa	2-5	24	>15[5]

The questionnaire takes approximately 10 minutes to complete.

A strong relationship exists between elevated fear avoidance beliefs and chronic disability secondary to LBP[2][3]. "Avoidance may lead to reduced activity levels, an exacerbation of the fear and avoidance behaviors, prolonged disability, and adverse physical and psychological effects" [3][4][6]. Thus, the FABQ is an outcome measure that serves as a clinically useful screening tool in identifying patients with high fear avoidance beliefs who are at risk for prolonged disability. Management of patients with elevated FABQ scores requires clinicians to tailor interventions to meet those needs. Research suggests multi-disciplinary approach including cognitive behavioral therapy and graded exposure to physical activity[3].

Evidence

Reliability

- Total FABQ test-retest reliability (ICC=0.97)[5]
- FABQ Physical Activity subscale test-retest reliability (ICC=0.72-0.90)[5]
- FABQ Work subscale test-retest reliability (ICC=0.80-0.91)[5]
- The use of the FAbQ as a screening tool for patients with non-work related LBP was not supported[7]
- The FABQ (When 'back' is replaced by 'shoulder') is an adequate predictor of how fear avoidance behaviours contribute to shoulder pain and disability. [8]
- The FABQ may be recommended for test-retest evaluations as 'good' reliability was found, and it has the ability to discriminate between patients with cervical radiculopathy and healthy subjects. [9]

Validity

- Evidence shows that the FABQ is correlated with Roland and Morris Disability Questionnaire. The correlation coefficients for the FABQ, the FABQ Work subscale and the FABQ Physical Activity subscale are 0.52, 0.63, and 0.51, respectively.[5]
- The FABQ was also shown to be correlated with the Tampa Scale of Kinesiophobia, another measure of fear avoidance. The correlation coefficients for the FABQ Work subscale and the FABQ Physical Activity subscale are 0.53 and 0.76, respectively. [5]
- The FABQ is not a good indicator of mental health for patients with pelvic girdle pain and has questionable validity when assessing these patients. [10]

References

1. Waddell et al (1993) Pain 52: 157–168.
2. Waddell C, Newton M, Henderson I, et al. A Fear-Avoidance Beliefs Questionnaire (FABQ) and the role of fear-avoidance beliefs in chronic low back pain and disability. Pain. 1993; 52:157-168
3. Fritz JM, George S. Identifying Psychosocial Variables in Patients With Acute Work-Related Low Back Pain: The Importance of Fear-Avoidance Beliefs. Phys Ther. 2002; 82(10): 973-983.
4. Lethem J, Slade PD, Troup JDG, Bendey G. Outline of a fear avoidance model of exaggerated pain perceptions, Behav Res Ther. 1983;21:401-408.
5. Williamson E. Fear Avoidance Behavior Questionnaire. Austrailian Journal of Physiotherapy. 2006; 52: 149.
6. Vlaeyen JWS, Kole-Snijders AMJ, Boeren RGB, van Eck H. Fear of movement/(re)injury in chronic low back pain and its relation to behavioral performance. Pain. 1995;62: 36, 272.
7. Cleland, Joshua A, Fritz, Julie M, & Brennan, Gerard P. (2008). Predictive validity of initial fear avoidance beliefs in patients with low back pain receiving physical therapy: is the FABQ a useful screening tool for identifying patients at risk for a poor recovery? European Spine Journal, 17(1), 70-79.
8. Mintken, Paul E, Cleland, Joshua A, Whitman, Julie M, & George, Steven Z. (2010). Psychometric properties of the Fear-Avoidance Beliefs Questionnaire and Tampa Scale of Kinesiophobia in patients with shoulder pain. Archives of physical medicine and rehabilitation, 91(7), 1128-1136.
9. Dedering, Åsa, & Börjesson, Tina. (2013). Assessing Fear-avoidance Beliefs in Patients with Cervical Radiculopathy. Physiotherapy Research International, 18(4), 193-202.
10. Grotle, Margreth, Garratt, Andrew M, Jenssen, Hanne Krogstad, & Stuge, Britt. (2012). Reliability and construct validity of self-report questionnaires for patients with pelvic girdle pain. Physical therapy, 92(1), 111-123.

Fear-Avoidance Beliefs Questionnaire (FABQ)
Waddell et al (1993) Pain , 52 (1993) 157 - 168

Here are some of the things which other patients have told us about their pain. For each statement please circle any number from 0 to 6 to say how much physical activities such as bending, lifting, walking or driving affect or would affect your back pain.

	Completely Disagree		Unsure			Completely Agree	
1. My pain was caused by physical act	0	1	2	3	4	5	6
2. Physical activity makes my pain w							
3. Physical activity might harm my							
4. I should not do physical activities which (might) make my pain worse							
5. I cannot do physical activities which (might) make my pain worse							
The following statements are about how your normal work affects or would affect your back pain							
6. My pain was caused by my work or by an accident at wo							
7. My work aggravated my							
8. I have a claim for compensation for my							
9. My work is too heavy for mr							
10. My work makes or would make my pain worse							
11. My work might harm my b							
12. I should not do my normal work with my present pa							
13. I cannot do my normal work with my present pain							
14. I cannot do my normal work till my pain is treated							
15. I do not think that I will be back to my normal work within 3 months							
16. I do not think that I will ever be able to go back to that wo							

Scoring

Scale 1: fear-avoidance beliefs about work – items 6, 7, 9, 10, 11, 12, 15.

Scale 2: fear-avoidance beliefs about physical activity – items 2, 3, 4, 5.

Source: Gordon Waddell, Mary Newton, Iain Henderson, Douglas Somerville and Chris J. Main, A Fear-Avoidance Beliefs Questionnaire (FABQ) and the role of fear-avoidance beliefs in chronic low back pain and disability, Pain, 52 (1993) 157 – 168, 166.

❑❑❑

73 The Bournemouth Questionnaire

Objective

The Bournemouth questionnaire (BQ) is a comprehensive multi-dimensional core outcome tool assessing patients' outcome of care in a routine clinical setting[1][2]. it is a short, self-report questionnaire, developed by J. Bolton. The questionnaire exists in two different versions. The first version measures different dimensions in patients with low back pain, whereas the second one was developed to assess pain in patients suffering from non specific neck pain (The Neck Bournemouth Questionnaire).

A lot of questionnaires which concentrate on pain and disability in patients with low back pain and neck pain already exist. However, since other dimensions are also involved with musculoskeletal pain, the BQ was developed. The development was based on the dimensions of the ICF, which means that, next to the pain and disability, it also takes the affective and cognitive aspects of neck pain and low back pain in account.

Both versions of the questionnaire consist of seven core items, which are: pain intensity, function in activities of daily living, function in social activities, anxiety, depression levels, fear avoidance behavior and locus of control behavior. The only difference between the questionnaire for low back pain and the Neck BQ is the subscript in the item 'activities of daily living'. The items "walking", "climbing stairs" and "getting in/out of bed", described in the Back BQ, where modified to "lifting", "reading" and "driving" in the Neck BQ.

Intended Population

The questionnaire was developed for patients suffering from non specific low back pain or non specific neck pain. Larsen and leboeuf (2005) indicated that the questionnaire is not useful in patients with persistent low back pain.[3]

Method of Use [2]

Both the questionnaires are used in the same way. Completing the test takes apporximately 5 minutes.

The questionnaires consists of 7 questions which contain the different dimensions of the ICF.

Each item is rated on a numeric rating scale (NRS) from 0 to 10:

0 = Much better

5 = no change

10 = much worse.

The score for each measure are added. This can produce a value between a minimum score of 0, and a maximum score of 70. The higher the score reflects the degree of impact on a patient's life.

The BQ has been translated and validated for use in a range of European languages including: French[4], Danish[5], German[6], and Dutch[7].

Evidence

Reliability [1][8]

Homogeneity or internal consistency: It is important for a questionnaire that all the items measure different aspects of the disease; in order to enable computing a total score by summing up all items. The items should all correlate with each other and every item also needs to correlate with the total score. A Chronbach's α of 0.90 was found for both questionnaires, consequently the BQ can be considered a reliable instrument. Furthermore, this indicates that all of the items contribute to the total score.

Test-retest reliability can be tested by using the intra class correlation coefficient (ICC).

This coefficient compares scores on a test that was completed by a person at two different moments.

The ICC in the BQ for back pain patients approached 0,9 for the 3 moments (Pre-, posttreatment and retest), indicating a strong correlation between the total scores in the patients. In the Neck BQ, the ICC amounted 0,65, which indicates a moderate agreement between total scores in these patients.

Validity [1][8]: An instrument is considered to be valid when it measures what it is supposed to measure.

- Content validity: Indicates in which degree a questionnaire covers the aspects of the measured attribute.[9]
- External construct validity: describes the degree in which a measure is related to other measures in a questionnaire. Each of the items can be compared to the items of another questionnaire or against the whole questionnaire. [9]

The BQ for low back pain

To determine the external construct validity, the BQ was tested against:

- Chronic Pain Questionnaire(CPQ)
- Revised Oswestry Disability Questionnaire (RODQ)
- Modified Somatic Pain Questionnaire (MSPQ)
- Fear Avoidance Beliefs Questionnaire (FABQ)
- Pain Locus of Control questionnaire (PLC)

Correlation of BQ with	CPQ	RODQ	**PLC**	**MSPQ**	**FABQ**
Pearson's r	0,77	0,78	0,40	0,36	0,32

The seven items where compared to the CPQ, MSPQ, RODQ, FABQ,zung and PLC.

The comparisation showed a correlation between 0,24 and 0,79. All items showed a significant correlation with their counterpart measure, which means that the test can be considered valid.

The Neck BQ

To determine the external construct validity, the BQ was tested against the CNFDS and the NDI:

	NDI	**CNFDS**
Pretreatment:	0,51	0,63
Posttreatment:	0,71	0,48

The seven items where compared to the NFDS, SF36 and NDI. With a pretreatment correlation between 0,37 - 0,62 and a posttreatment correlation between 0,44 and 0,83. All items showed a good correlation with their counterpart measure.

Responsiveness

The responsiveness or sensitivity is the ability of a questionnaire to detect clinically important changes over time.

The sensitivity to change can be measured by the 'Standardized response mean' (SRM). The SRM calculates the relative magnitude of the mean change compared to the variability of the changes.

A higher SRM indicates a greater sensitivity to change, SRM under the level of 0,5 indicates no sensitivity to change. The Neck BQ showed a SRM of 1,17,which means that the questionnaire had a good sensitivity to changes.[10] The SRM of the BQ for low back pain was 0,78, which means that this questionnaire is less sensitive to changes than the Neck BQ, but can still find significant changes of treatment.[11]

Internal longitudinal construct validity: Internal responsiveness of individual items of the questionnaire. The correlation should be 0,3 or higher to make sure that each item contributes significantly to the total responsiveness of the test.

In the BQ for low back pain all of the 7 items showed a correlation greater than 0,56. In the Neck BQ all of the items obtained a correlation greater than 0,42.[1] [8] This indicates that all the items where significant, which means that each item is individually responsive to clinical significant changes. Furthermore, each item contributes significantly to the change in the total score.

Bolton et al (2004) indicated that an improvement of 13 points on the total score or a percentage change score of 36% was associated with clinically significant improvement. [10]

References

1. Bolton J., Humphreys B., The Bournemouth Questionnaire: a short form comprehensive outcome measure. II. Psychometric properties in neck pain patients. Journal of manupilative andphysiological therapeutics, 2002.(A2)
2. Gay R., Madson T., Cieslak K., Comparison of the neck disability index and the neck Bournemouth questionnaire in a sample of patients with chronic uncomplicated neck pain. Journal of manipulative and physiological therapies, 2007.(B)

3. Larsen K., Leboeuf C., The Bournemouth Questionnaire, Can it be used to monitor and predict treatment outcome in chiropractic patients with persistent low back pain? Journal of manipulative and physiological therapeutics,2005(A2)
4. Hartvigsen J, Lauridsen H, EkströM S, et al. Translation and Validation of the Danish Version of the Bournemouth Questionnaire. Journal of Manipulative and Physiological Therapeutics. 2005:28(6):402– 407. http://www.sciencedirect.com/science/article/pii/S0161475405001739
5. Martel J, Dugas C, Lafond D, et al. Validation de la version française du Questionnaire de Bournemouth. Journal of the Canadian Chiropractic Association. 2009; 53(2):111-120. http://www.ncbi.nlm.nih.gov/pmc/articles/PMC2686031/pdf/jcca-v53-2-102.pdf
6. Soklic M, Peterson C, Humphreys BK. Translation and validation of the German version of the Bournemouth Questionnaire for Neck Pain. Chiropractic & Manual Therapies 2012, 20:2. http://chiromt.com/content/pdf/2045-709X-20-2.pdf.
7. Schmitt MA, de Wijer A, van Genderen FR, et al. The Neck Bournemouth Questionnaire cross-cultural adaptation into Dutch and evaluation of its psychometric properties in a population with subacute and chronic whiplash associated disorders. Spine (Phila Pa 1976). 2009;34(23):2551-61. http://www.ncbi.nlm.nih.gov/pubmed/19927105
8. Bolton J., Humphreys B., The Bournemouth Questionnaire: a short form comprehensive outcome measure. I. Psychometric properties in back pain patients. Journal of manupilative andphysiological therapeutics, 1999.(A2)
9. Liebenson G., Rehabilitation of the spine, Williams and Wilkins, 1996
10. Bolton J., Sensitivity and specificity of outcome measures in patients witch neck pain: Detecting clinically significant improvement. Spine, 2004. (C)
11. Perillo M., Bulbulian R., Responsiveness of the Bournemouth Questionnaire and Oswestry Questionnaire: A prospective pilot study. Journal of manipulative and psychological therapeutics, 2003.(C)

The Bournemouth Questionnaire for Measuring Outcome in Patients with Low Back Pain

Overview: The Bouremouth Questionnaire is a brief comprehensive and easy outcome measure for patients with low back pain. This consists of 7 measures considered important for monitoring patients and is suitable for outpatient practice. The authors are from the Anglo-European College of Chiropractic in Bournemouth England.

Questions – Over the past week:

(1) How would you rate your back pain?

(2) How much has your back pain interfered with your daily activities (housework washing dressing walking climbing stairs getting in/out of bed/chair)?

(3) How much has your back pain interfered with your ability to take part in recreational social and family activities?

(4) How anxious (tense uptight irritable difficulty in concentrating/relaxing) have you been feeling?

(5) How depressed (down-in-the-dumps sad in low spirits pessimistic unhappy) have you been feeling

(6) How have you felt your work (both inside and outside the home) has affected (or would affect) your back pain?

(7) How much have you been able to control (reduce/help) your back pain on your own?

Responses: 11 point numerical rating scale (NRS) Direction of responses: all increasing (a version with both increasing and decreasing response had problems with patients misinterpretation).

	Question	0 Point Response	10 Point Response
1	(back pain)	no pain	worst pain possible
2	(daily activities)	no interference	unable to carry out activity
3	(recreation social activities)	no interference	unable to carry out activity
4	(anxiety)	not at all anxious	extremely anxious
5	(depression)	not at all depressed	extremely depressed
6	(work)	have made it no worse	have made it much worse
7	(control pain on own)	completely control it	no control whatever

Total score = SUM(points for all 7 measures)

Interpretation: •minimum total score: 0

maximum total score: 70

- The higher the score the greater the impact of the back pain on the patient's life.

Performance:

- Good face validity
- High internal consistency (Cronbach alpha 0.9)
- Good test-retest reliability (intraclass correlation coefficient0.95)
- Evaluation of internal longitudinal construct validity indicated responsiveness to clinically significant change.

References: Bolton JE Breen AC. The Bournemouth Questionnaire: A short-form comprehensive outcome measure. I. Psychometric properties in back pain patients. J Manipulative and Physiological Therapeutics. 1999; 22: 503-510

❑❑❑

74

Fibromyalgia Impact Questionnaire (FIQ)

Objective

The FIQ is an assessment and evaluation instrument developed to measure fibromyalgia (FM) patient status, progress and outcomes. [1]

Intended Population

It has been designed to measure the components of health status that are believed to be most affected by FM.

Method of Use

The FIQ is a self administered instrument that takes approximately 5 minutes to complete. The directions are simple and the scoring is self-explanatory.

The FIQ is composed of 10 items. The first item contains 11 questions related to physical functioning – each question is rated on a 4 point Likert type scale. Items 2 and 3 ask the patient to mark the number of days they felt well and the number of days they were unable to work (including housework) because of fibromyalgia symptoms. Items 4 through 10 are horizontal linear scales marked in 10 increments on which the patient rates work difficulty, pain, fatigue, morning tiredness, stiffness, anxiety and depression.

Evidence

This initial assessment indicates that the FIQ has sufficient evidence of reliability and validity to warrant further testing in both research and clinical situations.

References

1. Burckhardt CS1, Clark SR, Bennett RM. The fibromyalgia impact questionnaire: development and validation.J Rheumatol. 1991 May;18(5):728-33.

Fibromyalgia Impact Questionnaire (FIQ)

Name____________________ Date ________________

Directions: For questions 1 through 11, please circle the number that is best describes how you did overall for the past week. If you don't normally do something that is asked, cross the question out

Were you able to:	Always	Most	Occasionally	Never
Do shopping	0	1	2	3
Do laundry with a washer and dryer?	0	1	2	3
Prepare meals?	0	1	2	3
Wash dishes/cooking utensils by hand?	0	1	2	3
Vacuum a rug?	0	1	2	3
Make beds?	0	1	2	3
Walk several blocks?	0	1	2	3
Visit friends or relatives?	0	1	2	3
Do yard work?	0	1	2	3
Drive a car?	0	1	2	3
Climb stairs?	0	1	2	3

Of the 7 days in the past week, how many days did you feel good? 0 ---------- 1 ---------- 2 ---------- 3 ---------- 4 ---------- 5 ---------- 6 ---------- 7
How many days last week did you miss work, including housework, because of fibromyalgia? 0 ---------- 1 ---------- 2 ---------- 3 ---------- 4 ---------- 5 ---------- 6 ---------- 7
When you worked, how much did pain or other symptoms of your fibromyalgia interfere with your ability to do your work, including housework? No problem with work *|---|---|---|---|---|---|---|---|---|---|* Great difficulty with work
How bad has your pain been? No pain *|---|---|---|---|---|---|---|---|---|---|* Very severe pain
How tired have you been? No tiredness *|---|---|---|---|---|---|---|---|---|---|* Very tired
How have you felt when you get up in the morning? Awoke well rested *|---|---|---|---|---|---|---|---|---|---|* Awoke very tired
How bad has your stiffness been? No stiffness *|---|---|---|---|---|---|---|---|---|---|* Very stiff
How nervous or anxious have you felt Not anxious *|---|---|---|---|---|---|---|---|---|---|* Very anxious
How depressed or blue have you felt? Not depressed *|---|---|---|---|---|---|---|---|---|---|* Very depressed

Reference: Burckhardt CS, Clark SR, Bennett RM.The fibromyalgia impact questionnaire: development and validation.J Rheumatol. 1991 May;18(5):728-33.

❑❑❑

75 Revised Fibromyalgia Impact Questionnaire (FIQR)

Objective

The FIQR was developed in response to known deficiencies of the FIQ with the help of a patient focus group.

Intended Population

Patient suffering from Fibromyalgia

Method of Use

The FIQR has the same 3 domains as the FIQ (that is, function, overall impact and symptoms). It differs from the FIQ in having modified function questions and the inclusion of questions on memory, tenderness, balance and environmental sensitivity. All questions are graded on a 0–10 numeric scale.

Evidence: The mean total FIQR score was 56.6 ± 19.9 compared to a total FIQ score of 60.6 ± 17.8 (P < 0.03). The total scores of the FIQR and FIQ were closely correlated (r = 0.88, P < 0.001). Each of the 3 domains of the FIQR correlated well with the 3 related FIQ domains (r = 0.69 to 0.88, P < 0.01). The FIQR showed good correlation with comparable domains in the SF-36, with a multiple regression analysis showing that the three FIQR domain scores predicted the 8 SF-36 subscale scores. The FIQR had good discriminant ability between FM and the 3 other groups; total FIQR scores were HC (12.1 ± 11.6), RA/SLE (28.6 ± 21.2) and MDD (17.3 ± 11.8). The patient completion time was 1.3 minutes; scoring took about 1 minute

Revised Fibromyalgia Impact Questionnaire (FIQR)

Last Name: First Name: Age:

Duration of FM symptoms (years) Time since FM was first diagnosed (years):

Directions: For each of the following 9 questions check the box that best indicates how much your fibromyalgia made it difficult to perform each of the following activities during the past 7 days. If you did not perform a particular activity in the last 7 days, rate the difficulty for the last time you performed the activity. If you can't perform an activity, check the last box

Brush or comb your hair	No difficulty -------------------- Very difficult
Walk continuously for 20 minutes	No difficulty -------------------- Very difficult
Prepare a homemade meal	No difficulty -------------------- Very difficult
Vacuum, scrub or sweep floors	No difficulty -------------------- Very difficult
Lift and carry a bag full of groceries	No difficulty -------------------- Very difficult
Climb one flight of stairs	No difficulty -------------------- Very difficult
Change bed sheets	No difficulty -------------------- Very difficult
Sit in a chair for 45 minutes	No difficulty -------------------- Very difficult
Go shopping for groceries	No difficulty -------------------- Very difficult

Directions: For each of the following 2 questions, check the box that best describes the overall impact of your fibromyalgia over the last 7 days:	
Fibromyalgia prevented me from accomplishing goals for the week	Never -------------------- Always
I was completely overwhelmed by my fibromyalgia symptoms	Never -------------------- Always
Directions: For each of the following 10 questions, select the box that best indicates your intensity of these common fibromyalgia symptoms over the past 7 day	
Please rate your level of pain	No pain -------------------- Unbearable pain
Please rate your level of energy	Lots of energy -------------------- No energy
Please rate your level of stiffness	No stiffness -------------------- Severe stiffness
Please rate the quality of your sleep	Awoke well rested -------------------- Awoke very tired
Please rate your level of depression	No depression -------------------- Very depressed
Please rate your level of memory problems	Good memory -------------------- Very poor memory
Please rate your level of anxiety	Not anxious -------------------- Very anxious
Please rate your level of tenderness to touch	No tenderness -------------------- Very tender
Please rate your level of balance problems	No imbalance -------------------- Severe imbalance
Please rate your level of sensitivity to loud noises, bright lights, odors and cold	No sensitivity -------------------- Extreme sensitivity

Total =

Reference: Bennett RM, Friend R, Jones KD, Ward R, Han BK, Ross RL. The Revised Fibromyalgia Impact Questionnaire (FIQR): validation and psychometric properties. Arthritis Res Ther. 2009;11(4):R120.

❑❑❑

76 Foot and Ankle Disability Index

Objective

The Foot and Ankle Disability Index (FADI)[1][2][3][4] is a region-specific self-report of function, firstly described in 1999 by Martin et al.

The FADI is a former version of the FAAM. The 2 instruments are identical except for an additional 5 items found on the FADI. Four of these items assess pain, and the fifth item evaluates an individual's ability to sleep. These 5 items were subsequently removed from the ADL subscale to improve psychometric properties of the instrument. The sports subscale remained unchanged, resulting in a new instrument, the FAAM.

The Foot and Ankle Disability Index is a 34-item questionnaire divided into two subscales: the Foot and Ankle Disability Index and the Foot and Ankle Disability Index Sport. The FADI has 26 items, and the FADI Sport has 8. The FADI contains 4 pain related items and 22 activity related items. The FADI Sport contains 8 activity related items. It assesses more difficult tasks that are essential to sport. The FADI Sport is unique in that it is a population-specific subscale designed for athletes. It is designed to address this need by detecting deficits in higher functioning subjects.

Intended Population

The foot and ankle disability index was designed to assess functional limitations related to foot and ankle conditions. Hale and Hertel [1] advocate the use of the FADI and FADI Sport self-report instruments in clinical care and research applications in young adults with CAI.

Eechaute et al [2] concluded that the FADI and FAAM were the most appropriate evaluative instruments to quantify functional disabilities in athletes with chronic ankle instability. An advantage of the FADI and FAAM is that they both have a sports subscale in addition to an activities of daily living subscale. The sports subscale may be particularly useful when addressing the limitations of athletes with CAI.

Method of Use

Each of the 34 items is scored on a 5-point Likert scale from 0 (unable to do) to 4 (no difficulty at all). The 4 pain items of the FADI are scored 0 (none) to 4 (unbearable). The FADI has a total point value of 104 points, whereas the FADI Sport has a total point value of 32 points. The FADI and FADI Sport are scored separately as percentages, with 100% representing no dysfunction.[1][2][3]

Evidence

Hale and Hertel [1] examined the reliability and sensitivity of both FADI and FADI Sport and reported that both scales are:

- reliable in detecting functional limitations in subjects with CAI
- sensitive to differences between healthy subjects and subjects with CAI
- responsive to improvements in function after rehabilitation in subjects with CAI.

Reliability

Using Bivariate correlations Hale & Hertel reported a significant relationship between the FADI and the FADI Sport. The correlation for the two scales for the involved ankles was (0.64). contrary to (0.84) which resulted from a combined analysis of the uninvolved extremities of CAI subjects with the matched extremities of healthy subjects. The correlation between the baseline FADI and FADI Sport scores was statistically significant ($P < .0005$) among healthy subjects and subjects with CAI.[1]

Validity

Construct validity of FADI and FADI sport: Significantly lower scores on the involved versus uninvolved side ($p<0.001$)[4]

Validity of FADI and FADI sport was also assessed by Pugia et al through investigating the correlations among both scales , ankle girth measures, weight-bearing status, and the Ankle Osteoarthritis Scale after acute ankle sprains. Moderate to good correlations were noted among the functional measures and between the functional measures and weight-bearing status.[6]

Responsiveness

Subjects scored significantly higher on the FADI and FADI sport after 4 weeks of rehabilitation ($p<0.007$)[2]

FADI: Significant difference after 6 weeks of training: pre training score =87.1% (± 12,1) post training score = 94.4% (± 6,1) ES = 0.52 (n =16)

FADI Sport: Significant difference after 6 weeks of training: pre training score = 78.4% (± 12,9)post training score = 89.5% (± 11,3) ES = 0.71 (n = 16)

References

1. Sheri A. Hale and Jay Hertel†. Reliability and Sensitivity of the Foot and Ankle Disability Index in Subjects With Chronic Ankle Instability. Journal of Athletic Training 2005;40(1):35–40.
2. Eechaute et al. The clinimetric qualities of patient-assessed instruments for measuring chronic ankle instability: A systematic review. BMC Musculoskeletal Disorders 2007, 8:6 doi: 10.1186/1471-2474-8-6.
3. Christopher R. Carcia et al. Validity of the Foot and Ankle Ability Measure in Athletes With Chronic Ankle Instability. Journal of Athletic Training 2008;43(2):179–183.
4. Robroy L. Martin. A survey of self-reported outcome instruments for the foot and ankle. J Orthop Sports Phys Ther 2007;37(2):72-84. doi:10.2519/jospt.2007.2403.
5. Gilani, S. F., & Amin, M. S. (2014). Operative treatment of displaced intra-articular fractures of Calcaneum : Is it worthwhile ? S-162, 64(12), 161–166.
6. Pugia ML, Middel CJ, Seward SW. Comparison of acute swelling and function in subjects with lateral ankle injury. J Orthop Sports Phys Ther. 2001;31:384–388.

The Foot & Ankle Disability Index (FADI) Score

Clinician's name (or ref) Patient's name (or ref)

Please answer every question with one response that most closely describes your condition within the past week. If the activity in question is limited by something other than your foot or ankle, mark N/A

	No difficulty at all	Slight difficulty	Moderate difficulty	Extreme difficulty	Unable to do
1. Standing					
2. Walking on even ground					
3. Walking on even ground without shoes					
4. Walking up hills					
5. Walking down hills					
6. Going up stairs					
7. Going down stairs					
8. Walking on uneven ground					
9. Stepping up and down curves					
10. Squatting					
11. Sleeping					
12. Coming up to your toes					
13. Walking initially					
14. Walking 5 minutes or less					
15. Walking approximately 10 minutes					
16. Walking 15 minutes or greater					
17. Home responsibilities					
18. Activities of daily living					
19. Personal care					
20. Light to moderate work (standing, walking)					
21. Heavy work (push/pulling, climbing, carrying)					
22. Recreational activities					
NO PAIN MILD MODERATE SEVERE UNBEARABLE					
23. General level of pain					
24. Pain at rest					
25. Pain during your normal activity					
26. Pain first thing in the morning					

Thank you very much for completing all the questions in this questionnaire.

❑❑❑

77 Foot Function Index (FFI)

Objective

A Foot Function Index (FFI) was developed in 1991 to measure the impact of foot pathology on function in terms of pain, disability and activity restriction. [1] It is a self-administered index consisting of 23 items divided into 3 sub-scales. Both total and sub-scale scores are produced.

Intended Population: The FFI has been shown to be a reasonable tool for use with low functioning individuals with foot disorders[2] ,patients with rheumatoid arthritis[1] and non-traumatic foot or ankle problems.[3] It can be used in both clinical and research settings. However, it may not be appropriate for individuals who function at or above the level of independence in activities of daily living. [2]

Method of Use: The FFI (questionnaire) consists of 23 self-reported items divided into 3 subcategories on the basis of patient values: pain, disability and activity limitation.[4] The patient has to score each question on a scale from 0 (no pain or difficulty) to 10 (worst pain imaginable or so difficult it requires help), that best describes their foot over the past week.

The pain subcategory consists of 9 items and measures foot pain in different situations, such as walking barefoot versus walking with shoes.

The disability subcategory consists of 9 items and measures difficulty performing various functional activities because of foot problems, such as difficulty climbing stairs.[4] The activity limitation subcategory consists of 5 items and measures limitations in activities because of foot problems, such as staying in bed all day. Recorded on a visual analogue scale (VAS), scores range from 0 to 100 mm, with higher scores indicating worse pain. Both total and subcategory scores are calculated. [1]

Scale	Questions	Scoring
Pain Scale	• Pain in the morning upon taking your first step • Pain standing barefoot • Pain walking barefoot • Pain standing with shoes • Pain walking with shoes • Pain standing with orthotics • Pain walking with orthotics • How is your pain at the end of the day • How severe is your pain at its worst	0/90

Disability Scale	• Difficulty when walking in the house • Difficulty when walking outside • Difficulty when walking four blocks • Difficulty when climbing stairs • Difficulty when descending stairs • Difficulty when getting out of chair • Difficulty when standing tip toe • Difficulty when climbing curbs • Difficulty when running or fast walking	0/90
Activity Limitation	• Stay indoors all day due to feet • Stay in bed all day due to feet • Use an assistive device (stick, walker, crutches, frame) indoors • Use an assistive device outdoors • Limit physical activity	0/50

Evidence

Reliability: Test-retest reliability of the FFI total and subscale scores range from 0.87 to 0.69, while internal consistency ranged from 0.96 to 0.73.[1] It is reported that the FFI is a reliable instrument for patients with rheumatoid arthritis[1] and it has also been recommended as a reliable measurement scale for use in other foot orthopaedic intervention trials. [5]

For the purposes of orthopaedic studies in which one foot serves as an internal control, a study assessed the side-to-side reliability of the seven-question Foot Function Index pain subscale. Internal reliability of the scale was high, with Cronbach's alphas ranging from 0.94 to 0.96, suggesting good left versus right discriminatory abilities. Intraclass correlation coefficients were examined for test-retest reliability (separated by side) and for side-to-side reliability (separated by the day of test). The resultant intraclass correlation coefficients were nearly equivalent, ranging from 0.79 to 0.89. Generalisability analysis yielded similar results. Intraclass correlation coefficients and generalisability analysis demonstrate that the majority of variation is best explained by the differences within subjects or between subjects rather than by test-retest or side-to-side differences. [5]

Validity: The FFI has been validated and determined to be a reliable instrument for patients with rheumatoid arthritis [1]and non-traumatic foot or ankle problems.[3] In the study to examine the construct validity of the FFI there were a total of 87 patients, with rheumatoid arthritis were used. With the exception of two items, factor analysis supported the construct validity of the total index and the sub-scales. Strong correlation between the FFI total and sub-scale scores and clinical measures of foot pathology supported the criterion validity of the index. [1]

Responsiveness: FFI is an instrument that was rated positively (level 3) for responsiveness. [6]

Miscellaneous: FFI-5pt versus original FFI The clinimetric value of the Dutch version of the Foot Function Index (FFI) was assessed in comparison with the original FFI using verbal rating scales (FFI-5pt) rather than visual analogue scales (VAS). The FFI-5pt is a suitable generic measure. Its clinimetric properties are comparable with those of the original FFI. Its administration and data entry are less time-consuming. However, responsiveness has to be more exactly assessed in an intervention study. [7]

There are two versions of the FFI-R: a FFI-R long form (FFI-R L; 4 subscales and 68 items) and the FFI-R short form (FFI-R S; 34 items). Both the FFI short and long from demonstrated good psychometric properties.

FFI-R

Scale	Questions	Scoring
Pain and stiffness	• Before you get up in the morning • First pain standing without shoes • First pain walking without shoes • First pain standing with shoes • First pain walking with shoes • Pain standing with custom shoe inserts • Pain walking with custom shoe inserts • How is your pain at the end of the day • Pain with foot cramps • Pain before sleep • How severe is your pain at its worst • Stiffness before getting up in the morning • Stiffness standing without shoes • Stiffness walking without shoes • Stiffness standing with shoes • Stiffness walking with shoes • Stiffness walking with custom shoe inserts • Stiffness before sleep • Stiffness at worse	Rated 0-6 per item, ranging from No pain Mild pain Moderate pain Severe pain Very severe pain Worst pain imaginable
Difficulty	• Walking around the house • Walking outside on uneven ground • Walking four or more blocks • Climbing stairs • Descending stairs • Getting out of chair • Standing normally • Standing tip toe • Carrying or lifting more than 5 pounds • Running • Fast walking • Walking downhill • Keeping regular walking pace • Walking regular distance • Keeping balance • Keeping foot clean • Walking with assistive devices • Because of hazards at home • Operating vehicle requiring foot to maneuver • Performing daily activities	Rated 0-6 per item, ranging from No difficulty Mild difficulty Moderate difficulty Severe difficulty Very severe difficulty So difficult unable

Activity limitation	• Stay indoors all day due to feet • Stay in bed all day due to feet • Use an assistive device (stick, walker, crutches, frame) indoors • Use an assistive device outdoors • Take extra precautions when walking in crowds for fear of foot injury • Limit outdoor activity • Choose not to use public transportation • Choose not to drive	Rated 0-6 per item, ranging from None of the time A little of the time Some of the time Much of the time Most of the time All of the time
Social issues	• Fear of falling • Embarrassment due to limp • Difficulty finding fashionable footwear • Difficulty finding dress shoes • Embarrassment due to footwear • Depression from foot problems • Difficulty finding suitable footwear • Feeling awful because of foot problem • Limit social activities due to foot problems • Constant aggravation due to managing foot pain • Difficulty participating in social activities due to footwear • Aggravation in performing daily activities • Poor sleep because of foot pain • Burden of taking medication to control pain • Difficulty finding comfortable footwear • Difficulty finding employment • Concern with appearance of feet • Concern about limited work around house • Concern about possible amputation of foot, leg or toes	Rate 0-6 per item, ranging from None of the time A little of the time Some of the time Much of the time Most of the time All of the time

References

1. Budiman-Mak E, Conrad KJ, Roach KE. The Foot Function Index: a measure of foot pain and disability. J Clin Epidemiol. 1991;44:561–570. (level of evidence B)
2. Agel J, Beskin JL, Brage M, Guyton GP, Kadel NJ, Saltzman CL, Sands AK, Sangeorzan BJ, SooHoo NF, Stroud CC, Thordarson DB: Reliability of the foot function index: a report of the AOFAS outcomes committee. Foot Ankle Int 2005, 26:962-967. (level of evidence C)
3. Martin RL, Irrgang JJ. A survey of selfreported outcome instruments for the foot and ankle. J Orthop Sports Phys Ther.2007;37:72–84. (level of evidence A)
4. Kornelia Kulig, Stephen F Reisch I. Nonsurgical Management of Posterior Tibial Tendon Dysfunction With Orthoses and Resistive Exercise: A Randomized Controlled Trial. Physical Therapy, 2009 Jan; 89 (1): 26-37. (Level of evidence 1B)
5. Saag KG, Saltzman CL, Brown CK, Budiman-Mak E: The Foot Function Index for measuring rheumatoid arthritis pain: evaluating side-to-side reliability. Foot Ankle Int 1996, 17:506-510. (level of evidence C)
6. Marike Van Der Leeden, Martijn P.M. Steultjens, Caroline B. Terwee, Dieter Rosenbaum, Debbie Turner, Jim Woodburn and Joost Dekkera. Systematic review of instruments measuring foot

function, foot pain, and foot-related disability in patients with rheumatoid arthritis. Arthritis & Rheumatism (Arthritis Care & Research) Vol. 59, No. 9, September 15, 2008, pp 1257–1269. (level of evidence 1A)

7. Kuyvenhoven MM, Gorter KJ, Zuithoff P, Budiman-Mak E, Conrad KJ, Post MW. The foot function index with verbal rating scales (FFI-5pt): A clinimetric evaluation and comparison with the original FFI. J Rheumatol. 2002 May;29(5):1023-8. (level of evidence C)
8. Budiman-Mak E, Conrad K, Stuck R, Matters M. Theoretical Model and Rasch Analysis to Develop a Revised Foot Function Index. 2006. Foot and Ankle International. (27) 7, 519-527

❑❑❑

78 Fugl-Meyer Assessment of Motor Recovery after Stroke

Objective

The Fugl-Meyer Assessment (FMA) is a stroke-specific, performance-based impairment index. It is designed to assess motor functioning, balance, sensation and joint functioning in patients with post-stroke hemiplegia[1][2]. It is applied clinically and in research to determine disease severity, describe motor recovery, and to plan and assess treatment.

Intended Population

The FMA was designed to be used for patients with post-stroke hemiplegic patients of all ages

Method of Use

Features of the Outcome Measure

Items: The scale is comprised of five domains and there are 155 items in total:

- Motor functioning (in the upper and lower extremities)
- Sensory functioning (evaluates light touch on two surfaces of the arm and leg, and position sense for 8 joints)
- Balance (contains 7 tests, 3 seated and 4 standing)
- Joint range of motion (8 joints)
- Joint pain

The motor domain includes items assessing movement, coordination, and reflex action of the shoulder, elbow, forearm, wrist, hand, hip, knee, and ankle. Items in the motor domain have been derived from Twitchell's 1951[3] description of the natural history of motor recovery following stroke and integrates Brunnstrom's stages of motor recovery [2][4]. Items of the FMA are intended to assess recovery within the context of the motor system. Functional tasks are not incorporated into the evaluation.[5]

Equipment Required: The FMA requires a mat or bed, a few small objects and several different tools for the assessment of sensation, reflexes, and range of motion:

Materials needed;[6]

Scrap of paper	Ball
Cotton ball	Pencil
Reflex hammer	Cylinder (small can or jar)
Goniometer	Stopwatch
Blindfold	Chair
Bedside table	

Scoring: Scoring is based on direct observation of performance. Scale items are scored on the basis of ability to complete the item using a 3-point ordinal scale where 0=cannot perform, 1=performs partially and 2 = performs fully. The total possible scale score is 226.

Points are divided among the domains as follows:

- Motor score: ranges from 0 (hemiplegia) to 100 points (normal motor performance). Divided into 66 points for upper extremity and 34 points for the lower extremity.
- Sensation: ranges from 0 to 24 points. Divided into 8 points for light touch and 16 points for position sense.
- Balance: ranges from 0 to 14 points. Divided into 6 points for sitting and 8 points for standing.
- Joint range of motion: ranges from 0 to 44 points.
- Joint pain: ranges from 0 to 44 points.

Classifications for impairment severity have been proposed based on FMA Total motor scores (out of 100 points):

Fugl-Meyer (1980)	Fugl-Meyer et al. (1975)[1]	Duncan, Goldstein, Horner, Landsman, Samsa, & Matchar (1994)[7]
< 50 = Severe		0-35 = Very Severe
50-84 = Marked	? 84 = Hemiplegia	36-55 = Severe
85-94 = Moderate	85-95 = Hemiparesis	56-79 = Moderate
95-99 = Slight	96-99 = Slight motor dyscoordination	> 79 = Mild

Time to administer: It takes approximately 30-35 minutes to administer the total FMA. Administration of the motor, sensation and balance subscores range from 34 to 110 minutes, with a mean administration time of 58 minutes. When the motor scale is administered on its own, it takes approximately 20 minutes to complete.

Evidence

Reliability

Test-retest Reliability:

General Rehab Sample:

(Platz et al, 2005; n = 37 stroke, 14 MS, and 5 TBI patients; assessed twice within a 7 day interval, General Rehab Sample)[10]

- Excellent Total Motor Score (ICC = 0.97)
- Excellent Sensation (ICC = 0.81)
- Excellent Passive Joint motion (ICC = 0.95)

Interrater/Intrarater Reliability:

Stroke: (Duncan et al, 1983; n = 19; mean age = 56 (13) years; same PT rating on 3 occasions each 3 weeks apart; VA sample, Chronic Stroke) [11]

Interrater Reliability

Rating	Domain	Pearson's r
Excellent	FMA total score	r = 0.98-0.99
Excellent	Upper Extremity	r = 0.995 - 0.996
Excellent	Lower Extremity	r = 0.96
Excellent	Sensation	r = 0.95 - 0.96
Excellent	Joint Range / Pain	r = 0.86 - 0.996
Excellent	Balance	r = 0.89 - 0.98

Validity

Criterion Validity:

Stroke: (Malouin et al, 1994; n = 32; mean age = 60; mean time since stroke = 64.5 days, Acute Stroke) [12]

- Excellent FMA & Motor Assessment Scale (MAS) total score correlations (r = 0.96)
- Poor FMA & MAS sitting balance item correlations (r = -0.10)
- Motor and sensory FMA scores 5 days post-stroke were the strongest predictor of motor recovery 6 months post-stroke (Duncan et al, 1992) [11]

Construct Validity: Stroke:

Acute Stroke:

- Excellent correlation: modified Balance Subscale on FMA and the Barthel Index; r = 0.86 - 0.89 (Mao et al, 2002) [13]
- Excellent correlation: FMA and Functional Independence Measures (FIM) administered to 172 inpatients who had recently had a stoke; r = 0.63 (Shelton et al, 2000) [14]
- FMA effectively distinguished between three levels of self care (Independent, Partly Dependant, and Dependant) in a sample of 109 recent (< 90 days) stroke survivors (Bernspang et al, 1987). [15]
- FMA was a better measure of higher-level recovery than the MAS (Malouin, et al, 1994) [12]

Chronic Stroke: (Dettmann et al, 1987; n = 15; mean age = 64 years; mean time since stroke, 2 years, Chronic Stroke) [16]

- The FMA and the Barthel Index were used to assess a group of 15 participants at an average of 2 years post stroke. Correlations between the measures were excellent (r = 0.67). The strongest correlations were observed in the Balance subscore (r = 0.76) the Upper Extremity subscore of the motor domain (r = 0.75) and FMA Motor total score (r = 0.74)

Responsiveness

Stroke:

(Mao et al, 2002, Acute Stroke) [13]

- Excellent on the modified version of the FMA Balance score
- Between assessments at 14, 30, 90 and 180 days post-stroke

- Responsiveness decreased as the time between stroke and assessments increased

(Hsueh et al, 2009, Chronic Stroke) [17]

- Small to moderate effect sizes were observed on the FMA, the Stroke Rehabilitation Assessment of Movement instrument (STREAM) and each of the measures shortened versions.
- Moderate effect sizes on the shortened version of both measures (0.53 and 0.51)
- Small effect sizes on the long version of the measure (0.045 and 0.38)

References

1. Fugl-Meyer AR, Jääskö L, Leyman I, Olsson S, Steglind S. The post-stroke hemiplegic patient. 1. a method for evaluation of physical performance. Scandinavian journal of rehabilitation medicine. 1975;7(1):13-31.
2. Gladstone DJ, Danells CJ, Black SE. The Fugl-Meyer assessment of motor recovery after stroke: a critical review of its measurement properties. Neurorehabilitation and neural repair. 2002 Sep; 16(3):232-40.
3. Twitchell TE. The restoration of motor function following hemiplegia in man. Brain. 1951 Dec 1;74(4):443-80.
4. Poole JL, Whitney SL. Assessments of motor function post stroke: a review. Physical & Occupational Therapy in Geriatrics. 2001 Jan 1;19(2):1-22.
5. Chae J, Labatia I, Yang G. Upper limb motor function in hemiparesis: concurrent validity of the Arm Motor Ability test. American journal of physical medicine & rehabilitation. 2003 Jan 1;82(1):1-8.
6. Poole JL, Whitney SL. Assessments of motor function post stroke: a review. Physical & Occupational Therapy in Geriatrics. 2001 Jan 1; 19(2):1-22.
7. Duncan PW, Goldstein LB, Horner RD, Landsman PB, Samsa GP, Matchar DB. Similar motor recovery of upper and lower extremities after stroke. Stroke. 1994 Jun 1;25(6):1181-8.
8. Finch E, Brooks D, Stratford P, Mayo N. Physical Rehabilitation Outcome Measures: A guide to Enhanced Clinical. Decision-Making. 2002;2.
9. Khairul Anam. [OCT 463] MedNeuro Ax - Fugl-Meyer Assessment of the Sensorimotor Function. Available from: http://www.youtube.com/watch?v=vvnshSISzjY
10. Platz, T., Pinkowski, C., et al. "Reliability and validity of arm function assessment with standardized guidelines for the Fugl-Meyer Test, Action Research Arm Test and Box and Block Test: a multicentre study." Clin Rehabil 2005 19: 404-411
11. Duncan, P. W., Propst, M., et al. "Reliability of the Fugl-Meyer assessment of sensorimotor recovery following cerebrovascular accident." Phys Ther 1983 63: 1606-1610
12. Malouin, F., Pichard, L., et al. "Evaluating motor recovery early after stroke: comparison of the Fugl-Meyer Assessment and the Motor Assessment Scale." Arch Phys Med Rehabil 1994 75: 1206-1212
13. Mao, H.-F., Hsueh, I. P., et al. "Analysis and comparison of the psychometric properties of three balance measures for stroke patients." Stroke 2002 33: 1022-1027
14. Shelton, F. D., Volpe, B. T., et al. "Motor impairment as a predictor of functional recovery and guide to rehabilitation treatment after stroke." Neurorehabil Neural Repair 2001 15(3): 229-237
15. Bernspang, B., Asplund, K., et al. (1987). "Motor and perceptual impairments in acute stroke patients: effects on self-care ability." Stroke 1987 18: 1081-1086
16. Dettmann, M. A., Linder, M. T., et al. "Relationships among walking performance, postural stability, and functional assessments of the hemiplegic patient." Am J Phys Med 1987 66: 77-90
17. Hsueh, Y. W., Wu, C. Y., et al. (2009). "Responsiveness and validity of three outcome measures of motor function after stroke rehabilitation." Stroke 2009 40(4): 1386-1391

FUGL-MEYER ASSESSMENT UPPER EXTREMITY (FMA-UE) Assessment of sensorimotor function Examiner:

Fugl-Meyer AR, Jaasko L, Leyman I, Olsson S, Steglind S: The post-stroke hemiplegic patient. A method for evaluation of physical performance. Scand J Rehabil Med 1975, 7:13-31.

Name Date

Id Examiner

A. UPPER EXTREMITY, sitting position				
I. Reflex activity		**none**	**can be elicited**	
Flexors: biceps and finger flexors (at least one)		0	2	
Extensors: triceps		0	2	
	Subtotal I (max 4)			
II. Volitional movement within synergies, without gravitational help		**none**	**partial**	**full**
Flexor synergy: Hand from contralateral knee to ipsilateral ear. From extensor synergy (shoulder adduction/ internal rotation, elbow extension, forearm pronation) to flexor synergy (shoulder abduction/ external rotation, elbow flexion, forearm supination).	Shoulder retraction	0	1	2
	elevation	0	1	2
	abduction (90°)	0	1	2
	external rotation	0	1	2
	Elbow Flexion	0	1	2
	Forearm Supination	0	1	2
Extensor synergy: Hand from ipsilateral ear to the contralateral knee	Shoulder adduction/internal	0	1	2
	rotation	0	1	2
	Elbow extension	0	1	2
	Forearm Pronation			
	Subtotal II (max 18)			
III. Volitional movement mixing synergies, without compensation		**none**	**partial**	**full**
Hand to lumbar spine hand on lap	cannot perform or hand in front of ant-sup iliac spine hand behind ant-sup iliac spine (without compensation) hand to lumbar spine (without compensation)	0	1	2
Shoulder flexion 0°- 90° elbow at 0° pronation-supination 0°	immediate abduction or elbow flexion abduction or elbow flexion during movement flexion 90°, no shoulder abduction or elbow flexion	0	1	2
Pronation-supination elbow at 90° shoulder at 0°	no pronation/supination, starting position impossible limited pronation/supination, maintains starting position full pronation/supination, maintains starting position	0	1	2
	Subtotal III (max 6)			
IV. Volitional movement with little or no synergy		**none**	**partial**	**full**
Shoulder abduction 0 - 90° elbow at 0° forearm pronated	0	0	1	2

Shoulder flexion 90° - 180° elbow at 0° pronation-supination 0°	0	0	1	2
Pronation/supination elbow at 0° shoulder at 30°- 90° flexion	0	0	1	2
	Subtotal IV (max 6)			
V. Normal reflex activity assessed only if full score of 6 points is achieved in part IV; compare with the unaffected side		**0 (IV), hype**	**lively**	**normal**
biceps, triceps, finger flexors	2 of 3 reflexes markedly hyperactive or 0 points in part IV 1 reflex markedly hyperactive or at least 2 reflexes lively maximum of 1 reflex lively, non hyperactive	0	1	2
	Subtotal V (max 2)			
	Total A (max 36)			
B. WRIST support may be provided at the elbow to take or hold the starting position, no support at wrist, check the passive range of motion prior testing		**none**	**partial**	**full**
Stability at 15° dorsiflexion elbow at 90°, forearm pronated shoulder at 0°	less than 15° active dorsiflexion dorsiflexion 15°, no resistance tolerated maintains dorsiflexion against resistance	0	1	2
Repeated dorsifexion / volar flexion elbow at 90°, forearm pronated shoulder at 0°, slight finger flexion	cannot perform volitionally limited active range of motion full active range of motion, smoothly	0	1	2
Stability at 15° dorsiflexion elbow at 0°, forearm pronated slight shoulder flexion/abduction	less than 15° active dorsiflexion dorsiflexion 15°, no resistance tolerated maintains dorsiflexion against resistance	0	1	2
Repeated dorsifexion / volar flexion elbow at 0°, forearm pronated slight shoulder flexion/abduction	cannot perform volitionally limited active range of motion full active range of motion, smoothly	0	1	2
Circumduction elbow at 90°, forearm pronated shoulder at 0°	cannot perform volitionally jerky movement or incomplete complete and smooth circumduction	0	1	2
	Total B (max 10)			
C. HAND support may be provided at the elbow to keep 90° flexion, no support at the wrist, compare with unaffected hand, the objects are interposed, active grasp		**none**	**partial**	**full**
Mass flexion from full active or passive extension		0	1	2
Mass extension from full active or passive flexion		0	1	2
GRASP				

a. Hook grasp flexion in PIP and DIP (digits II-V), extension in MCP II-V	cannot be performed can hold position but weak maintains position against resistance	0	1	2
b. Thumb adduction 1-st CMC, MCP, IP at 0°, scrap of paper between thumb and 2-nd MCP joint	cannot be performed can hold paper but not against tug can hold paper against a tug	0	1	2
c. Pincer grasp, opposition pulpa of the thumb against the pulpa of 2-nd finger, pencil, tug upward	cannot be performed can hold pencil but not against tug can hold pencil against a tug	0	1	2
d. Cylinder grasp cylinder shaped object (small can) tug upward, opposition of thumb and fingers	cannot be performed can hold cylinder but not against tug can hold cylinder against a tug	0	1	2
e. Spherical grasp fingers in abduction/ flexion, thumb opposed, tennis ball, tug away	cannot be performed can hold ball but not against tug can hold ball against a tug	0	1	2
	Total C (max 14)			
D. COORDINATION/SPEED, sitting, after one trial with both arms, eyes closed, tip of the index finger from knee to nose, 5 times as fast as possible		**marked**	**slight**	**none**
Tremor	at least 1 completed movement	0	1	2
Dysmetria at least 1 completed movement	pronounced or unsystematic slight and systematic no dysmetria	0	1	2
		≥ 6s	2 - 5s	< 2s
Time start and end with the hand on the knee	at least 6 seconds slower than unaffected side 2-5 seconds slower than unaffected side less than 2 seconds difference	0	1	2
	Total D (max 6)			
	TOTAL A-D (max 66)			
H. SENSATION, upper extremity eyes closed, compared with the unaffected side		**anesthesia**	**hypoesthesia or dysesthesia**	**normal**
Light touch	upper arm, forearm palmary surface of the hand	0 0	1 1	2 2
		less than 3/4 correct or absence	3/4 correct or considerable difference	correct 100%, little or no difference
Position small alterations in the position	shoulder elbow wrist thumb (IP-joint)	0 0 0 0	1 1 1 1	2 2 2 2
	Total H (max12)			

J. PASSIVE JOINT MOTION, upper extremity, sitting position, compare with the unaffected side				J. JOINT PAIN during passive motion, upper extremity		
	only few degrees (less than 10° in shoulder)	**decreased**	**normal**	**pronounced pain during movement or very marked pain at the end of the movement**	**some pain**	**no pain**
Shoulder						
Flexion (0° - 180°)	0	1	2	3	4	5
Abduction (0°-90°)	0	1	2	3	4	5
External rotation	0	1	2	3	4	5
Internal rotation	0	1	2	3	4	5
Elbow						
Flexion	0	1	2	3	4	5
Extension	0	1	2	3	4	5
Forearm						
Pronation	0	1	2	3	4	5
Supination	0	1	2	3	4	5
Wrist						
Flexion	0	1	2	3	4	5
Extension	0	1	2	3	4	5
Fingers						
Flexion	0	1	2	3	4	5
Extension	0	1	2	3	4	5
Total (max 24)				**Total (max 24)**		

A. UPPER EXTREMITY	**/36**
B. WRIST	**/10**
C. HAND	**/14**
D. COORDINATION / SPEED	**/ 6**
TOTAL A-D (motor function)	**/66**
H. SENSATION	**/12**
J. PASSIVE JOINT MOTION	**/24**
J. JOINT PAIN	**/24**

❑❑❑

79 Fullerton Advanced Balance (FAB) Scale

Purpose

The Fullerton Test is mainly intended to identify highly-active older adults who are at an increased risk to experience fall-related injuries due to sensory impairments. The test uses both dynamic and static balance under different situations to identify balance deficits in older adults. The test is mainly performed on the following population:

- breast cancer patients (post-chemotherapy)
- older adults
- Fibromyalgia
- Parkinson's and
- Traumatic brain injuries.

Technique: The test includes the following:

- 10 performance based activities in both static and dynamic phases
- Score of 0-40/40 points possible (higher scores are better)
- Items scored on a 5 point ordinal scale (0-4)

The test is administered for 10-12 mins.

Equipment needed:

- Stopwatch
- Pencil
- 2 and 36 inch rulers
- 6 inch high bench (18'X18' stepping surface)
- Masking tape
- 2 Airex® pads Length of non-slip material between pads if floor is not carpeted
- Metronome

Evidence: Cutt-off scores: Older adults (>=65 years): (Hernandez and Rose, 2008; independently, healthy functioning adults, without fall in previous 12 months, reported falling 2 or more times previous 12 months) Score of 25/40 produces highest sensitivity (74.6%) and specificity (52.6%) in predicting fall risk In 7 out of 10 cases an individual who scores 25 or lower is at a high risk for falls

Test-Retest Reliability:

Excellent test-retest reliability (ICC=0.98) (Rose et al, 2006)

Interrater/Interrater Reliability:

Older Adults: (Rose et al, 2006) : Excellent test re-test reliability (r = 0.96) for total score

Breast cancer (post chemotherapy): (Wampler et al, 2007) (treated with taxane chemotherapy)

Excellent test-retest reliability (ICC=0.98)<u></u>

Internal Consistency:

Older adults: (Rose et al, 2006) : Excellent internal consistency (H coefficients >0.75) for all 10 items

Older adults: (Klein et al, 2010)

Excellent internal consistency (Cronbach's alpha = 0.805)

Content Validity:

Older adults: (Rose et al, 2006) :Established through literature review, administration of test items to 15 older adults, reviewed by 4 experienced physical therapists

References

1. Rose, D. J., Lucchese, N., et al. (2006). "Development of a multidimensional balance scale for use with functionally independent older

adults." Archives of Physical Medicine and Rehabilitation 87(11): 1478-1485.
2. Hernandez, D. and Rose, D. J. (2008). "Predicting which older adults will or will not fall using the Fullerton Advanced Balance scale." Archives of Physical Medicine & Rehabilitation 89(12): 2309-2315
3. Klein, P. J., Fiedler, R. C., et al. (2011). "Rasch Analysis of the Fullerton Advanced Balance (FAB) Scale." Physiother Can 63(1): 115-125
4. Wampler, M. A., Topp, K. S., et al. (2007). "Quantitative and clinical description of postural instability in women with breast cancer treated with taxane chemotherapy." Arch Phys Med Rehabil 88(8): 1002-1008
5. Langley, F. A. and Mackintosh, S. F. H. (2007). "Functional balance assessment of older community dwelling adults: a systematic review of the literature." Internet Journal of Allied Health Sciences & Practice 5
6. https://www.interactivehealthpartner.com/pdf/FAB10.pdf

Fullerton Advanced Balance (FAB) Scale

1. **Stand with feet together and eyes closed**
   0. Unable to obtain the correct standing position independently
   1. Able to obtain the correct standing position independently but unable to maintain the position or keep the eyes closed for more than 10 seconds
   2. Able to maintain the correct standing position with eyes closed for more than 10 seconds but less than 30 seconds
   3. Able to maintain the correct standing position with eyes closed for 30 seconds but requires close supervision
   4. Able to maintain the correct standing position safely with eyes closed for 30 seconds
2. **Reach forward to retrieve an object (pencil) held at shoulder height with outstretched arm**
   0. Unable to reach the pencil without taking more than two steps
   1. Able to reach the pencil but needs to take two steps
   2. Able to reach the pencil but needs to take one step
   3. Can reach the pencil without moving the feet but requires supervision
   4. Can reach the pencil safely and independently without moving the feet
3. **Turn 360 degrees in right and left directions**
   0. Needs manual assistance while turning
   1. Needs close supervision or verbal cueing while turning
   2. Able to turn 360 degrees but takes more than four steps in both directions
   3. Able to turn 360 degrees but unable to complete in four steps or fewer in one direction
   4. Able to turn 360 degrees safely taking four steps or fewer in both directions
4. **Step up onto and over a 6-inch bench**
   0. Unable to step up onto the bench without loss of balance or manual assistance
   1. Able to step up onto the bench with leading leg, but trailing leg contacts the bench or leg swings around the bench during the swing-through phase in both directions
   2. Able to step up onto the bench with leading leg, but trailing leg contacts the bench or swings around the bench during the swing-through phase in one direction
   3. Able to correctly complete the step up and over in both directions but requires close supervision in one or both directions
   4. Able to correctly complete the step up and over in both directions safely and independently
5. **Tandem walk**
   0. Unable to complete 10 steps independently
   1. Able to complete the 10 steps with more than five interruptions
   2. Able to complete the 10 steps with three to five interruptions
   3. Able to complete the 10 steps with one to two interruptions
   4. Able to complete the 10 steps independently and with no interruptions
6. **Stand on one leg**
   0. Unable to try or needs assistance to prevent falling
   1. Able to lift leg independently but unable to maintain position for more than 5 seconds

2. Able to lift leg independently and maintain position for more than 5 but less than 12 seconds
3. Able to lift leg independently and maintain position for 12 or more seconds but less than 20 seconds
4. Able to lift leg independently and maintain position for the full 20 seconds

7. Stand on foam with eyes closed

0. Unable to step onto foam or maintain standing position independently with eyes open
1. Able to step onto foam independently and maintain standing position but unable or unwilling to close eyes
2. Able to step onto foam independently and maintain standing position with eyes closed for 10 seconds or less
3. Able to step onto foam independently and maintain standing position with eyes closed for more than 10 seconds but less than 20 seconds
4. Able to step onto foam independently and maintain standing position with eyes closed for 20 seconds

Do not introduce test item #8 if test item #4 was not performed safely and/or it is contraindicated to perform this test item (review test administration instructions for contraindications). Score a zero and move to next test item.

8. Two-footed jump

0. Unwilling or unable to attempt or attempts to initiate two-footed jump, but one or both feet do not leave the floor
1. Able to initiate two-footed jump, but one foot either leaves the floor or lands before the other
2. Able to perform two-footed jump, but unable to jump farther than the length of their own feet
3. Able to perform two-footed jump and achieve a distance greater than the length of their own feet
4. Able to perform two-footed jump and achieve a distance greater than twice the length of their own feet

9. Walk with head turns

0. Unable to walk 10 steps independently while maintaining 30o head turns at an established pace
1. Able to walk 10 steps independently but unable to complete required number of 30o head turns at an established pace
2. Able to walk 10 steps but veers from a straight line while performing 30o head turns at an established pace
3. Able to walk 10 steps in a straight line while performing 30o head turns at an established pace but head turns less than 30o in one or both directions
4. Able to walk 10 steps in a straight line while performing required number of 30o head turns at established pace

10. Reactive postural control

0. Unable to maintain upright balance; no observable attempt to step; requires manual assistance to restore balance
1. Unable to maintain upright balance; takes two or more steps and requires manual assistance to restore balance
2. Unable to maintain upright balance; takes more than two steps but is able to restore balance independently
3. Unable to maintain upright balance; takes two steps but is able to restore balance independently
4. Unable to maintain upright balance but able to restore balance independently with only one step

TOTAL: 40 POINTS

Evaluating Risk for Falls:

Long Form Fullerton Advanced Balance (FAB) scale Cut-Off Score: ≤ 25/40 Points

Short-Form Fullerton Advanced Balance (FAB) scale Cut-Off Score: ≤ 9/16 Points

❑❑❑

80 Functional Ability Description Tool

About

The challenge of measuring and recording effectiveness of service delivery, particularly for children with long-term disability is a challenge. In NHS Leeds Community Paediatric Physiotherapy Service, we have developed a method of recording Patient Related Outcomes. The outcome recording is used in conjunction with the 'Functional Ability Description Tool for Children with Physical Disabilities.'[1] The service won a "Leading Edge Award for Clinical Service Re-design" in Leeds PCT in July 2008.

Description

1. A simple tool has been designed to describe the functional ability of children with long-term neurological conditions.
2. The clinicians within the paediatric physiotherapy service have combined aspects from well researched validated and reliable assessment tools[2][3]. Eight statements have been produced to describe the children's functional abilities. This is unique to Leeds Community Children's Physiotherapy service.
3. The tool is used in conjunction with Education Leeds to allocate funding and assist in the placement and support for children in the school settings.
4. The tool is easily understood by parents, carers and professionals and therefore a common 'language' can be used when discussing a child's level of physical ability and the resources required to support that child in the school setting.
5. The tool is very simple and quick to use. It has therefore been used in clinical audits and to profile service caseloads. This has resulted in more qualitative information in the management of resources within the service

With a method of describing the caseload validated over three years, a method for recording clinical outcomes was clearly required. McBurney et al [4] used the International Classification of Functional Disability (ICF) framework to theme perception of benefits of muscle strength training. By combining the ICF framework and the 5 principals of Every Child Matters, (ECM) the service developed usable documentation to record the outcomes and measure effectiveness.

By setting 'SMART' objectives in areas of Participation and Activity as well as Body Structure and Function and linking them with ECM, we are able to record measurable objectives that previously we would have not recorded. The historic perception that physiotherapists only have a 'body structures and functions' role can be challenged. The discussions relating to effectiveness and value for money of children's community physiotherapy with commissioners become clearer. This method of recording outcomes has also been piloted in the children's MSK service in LTHT, an acute setting, and results have been encouraging.

Objective

To describe the functional ability of children with long-term neurological conditions.

Intended Population

Children with long-term neurological conditions.

Leeds Community Children's Physiotherapy Service Functional Ability Description Tool for Children with Physical Disabilities

A	Walks in and outdoors and climbs stairs without limitations. Demonstrate some difficulties with more complex gross and fine motor skills due to a reduction in one or more of the following: - Speed, balance, coordination. Independent in self-help skills.
B	Walks in and outdoors and climbs stairs without limitations. Demonstrates difficulties with less complex gross and fine motor skills such as running, jumping and dressing ability.
C	Walks indoors and outdoors and climbs stairs holding onto a rail but experiences limitations when walking on uneven surfaces and inclines and when walking in crowds and confined spaces. Children have at best only minimal ability to perform more complex gross motor skills such as running, jumping. May require some aids and adaptations or physical assistance to perform self-help skills.
D	Walks indoors or outdoors with walking aid. Occasionally requires wheelchair for very long distances. Can sit independently and has good head and trunk control. Will require some assistance with self help skills. Specific postural management equipment may be required.
E	Walks indoors and outdoors on level surfaces with walking aid. More dependent on wheelchair for outdoor mobility and indoors where distance, crowds or other hazards make walking impractical or unsafe. Has independent sitting balance but may require pelvic or trunk support to maximise function and access curriculum. Will require assistance with self-help skills. Specific postural management equipment may be required.
F	No functional walking ability but may use walking as a therapeutic exercise. Can transfer with assistance and may be independently mobile in manual or powered wheelchair. Sitting ability is likely to be limited and postural support required. Will require help in the classroom setting and with all self-help skills. Specific postural management equipment will be required.
G	Unable to walk but may transfer with assistance and equipment. May be independently mobile in powered wheel chair or with assistance in manual wheelchair. Sitting ability is likely to be limited and postural support required. Will require considerable help in the classroom setting and with all self help skills. Specific postural management equipment will be required.
H	Has no independent mobility. Requires assistance for all changes of position. Physical independence in classroom is severely limited. Requires specialist equipment for postural management and is totally dependent for all self-help skills.

Reference

1. PALISANO R,ROSENBAUM P, WALTER S, RUSSELL D, WOOD E, GALUPPI B. (1997) Developmental Medicine and Childhood Neurology 39 pp214-223.
2. POUTNEY T, MULCAHY C, CLARKE S, GREEN E. (2004) Chailey Approach to Postural Management. Active Design Witton Birmingham

Functional Ability DiscriptionTool Outcome Sheet

Child's name: **Date of Birth:** **Physiotherapist:**

Functional Descriptor Band: **Date of objective setting:**

Categories (ICF)	Objective (SMART) Specific, measurable, achievable, realistic, timed.	Outcomes Yes/no	Contextual Factors (societal or environmental that impact on outcome of objectives)
1. Body Functions(Impairment) • Enjoying and achieving • Being Healthy, • Staying safe	1. 2. 3.	1. 2. 3.	
2. Activities(Limitation) • Enjoying and achieving, • Making a positive contribution • Being Healthy • Economic well-being • Staying safe	1. 2. 3.	1. 2. 3.	
3. Participation(Restriction) • Enjoying and achieving • Making a positive contribution • Being healthy • Economic well being • Staying safe	1. 2. 3.	1. 2. 3.	

❑❑❑

81 Functional Ambulation Category

Objective

The Functional Ambulation Categories (FAC) is a 6-point functional walking test that evaluates ambulation ability, determining how much human support the patient requires when walking, regardless of whether or not they use a personal assistive device. The FAC is a quick visual measurement of walking, is simple to use, easy to interpret, and cost-effective because only stairs and 15m of indoor floor are needed to administer the test[1].

Intended Population: It is used in Stroke, Multiple Sclerosis and other neurological conditions to measure their walking ability.

Method of Use

- Clinician- ticked box of walking ability
- 5 min to complete
- Pen and paper needed
- no training requires

Instrument: Scoring and Score Interpretation[2]:

Score	Category	Interpretation
0	Nonfunctional ambulator	
1	Ambulator, dependent on physical assistance – level I	Indicates a patient who requires continuous manual contact to support body weight as well as to maintain balance or to assist coordination.
2	Ambulator, dependent on physical assistance – level II	Indicates a patient who requires intermittent or continuous light touch to assist balance or coordination.
3	Ambulator, dependent on supervision	Indicates a patient who can ambulate on level surface without manual contact of another person but requires standby guarding of one person either for safety or verbal cueing.
4	Ambulator, independent level surface only	Indicates a patient who can ambulate independently on level surface but requires supervision to negotiate (e.g. stairs, inclines, nonlevel surfaces).
5	Ambulator, independent	Indicates a patient who can walk everywhere independently, including stairs.

Evidence

Reliability

- good interrater reliability ($\kappa = .72$)[3]
- excellent test-retest reliability (k = .950)[2]

Validity: Excellent concurrent validity[2]

Responsiveness: moderate to large effect sizes when the FAC was used to evaluate change in ambulation over a period of 6-months[2]

References

1. Wade D.T. Measurement in neurological rehabilitation. Oxford Medical Publications, Oxford. 1992.
2. Mehrholz, J., Wagner, K., Rutte, K., Meiner, D. and Pohl, M. Predictive validity and responsiveness of the Functional Ambulation Category in hemiparetic patients after stroke. Archives of Physical Medicine Rehabilitation, 2007, 88, 1314-1319.
3. Holden M.K., Gill K.M., Magliozzi M.R., Nathan J., Piehl-Baker L. Clinical gait assessment in the neurologically impaired Reliability and meaningfulness. *Phys Ther.* 1984; 64: 35-40

Description of Functional Ambulation Category (FAC)

FAC	Ambulation Description	Definition
0	Nonfunctional ambulation	Subject cannot ambulate, ambulates in parallel bars only, or requires supervision or physical assistance from more than one person to ambulate safely outside of parallel bars
1	Ambulator-Dependent for Physical Assistance Level II	Subject requires manual contacts of no more than one person during ambulation on level surfaces to prevent falling. Manual contacts are continuous and necessary to support body weight as well as maintain balance and/or assist coordination
2	Ambulator-Dependent for Physical Assistance Level I	Subject requires manual contact of no more than one person during ambulation on level surfaces to prevent falling. Manual contact consists of continuous or intermittent light touch to assist balance or coordination
3	Ambulator-Dependent for Supervision	Subject can physically ambulate on level surfaces without manual contact of another person but for safety requires standby guarding on no more than one person because of poor judgment, questionable cardiac status, or the need for verbal cuing to complete the task.
4	Ambulator-Independent Level Surfaces only	Subject can ambulate independently on level surfaces but requires supervision or physical assistance to negotiate any of the following: stairs, inclines, or non-level surfaces
5	Ambulator-Independent	Subject can ambulate independently on nonlevel and level surfaces, stairs, and inclines.

❑❑❑

82

Functional Assessment of Chronic Illness Therapy

Objective

To measure health-related quality of life of people with chronic illnesses. The FACIT questionnaires are some of the more commonly used questionnaires in national and international research settings. Fatigue is one of the most frequent complaints of the elderly and is strongly associated with loss of independence and decreased physical activity and functional decline. Mild depression, anemia, insomnia, and poor nutrition have been associated with fatigue[1]. However, many older persons report complaints of "fatigue" and "exhaustion" even when no underlying medical or psychiatric illness is present[1][2] Thus, the lack of an "underlying illness" makes the impact of unexplained fatigue even more crucial.[1]

Intended Population

Older adults who report fatigue.[1]

Method of Use

Although there are several validated tools for the measurement of fatigue, there is no gold standard[1][3]. One self report questionnaire that has been validated for use with older adults is the Functional Assessment of Chronic Illness Therapy (FACIT)Fatigue Scale (Version 4). The FACIT Fatigue Scale is a short, 13-item, easy to administer tool that measures an individual's level of fatigue during their usual daily activities over the past week. The level of fatigue is measured on a four point Likert scale (4 = not at all fatigued to 0 = very much fatigued)[1]. The FACIT Fatigue Scale is one of many different FACIT scales that are part of a collection of health-related quality of life (HRQOL) questionnaires targeted to the management of chronic illness referred to as The FACIT Measurement System. The group tests newly constructed FACIT subscales on a sample of at least 50 subjects[1]. The FACIT tool has been translated in more than 45 different languages permitting cross-cultural comparisons.

Outcome Measures

Other assessment tools that can be used to measure fatigue includes:

1. Measurement of fatigue in cancer, stroke, and HIV using the Functional Assessment of Chronic Illness Therapy - Fatigue (FACIT-F) scale.[4]
2. Bristol Rheumatoid Arthritis Fatigue Multi-Dimensional Questionnaire (BRAF MDQ) [5]
3. Bristol Rheumatoid Arthritis Fatigue Numerical Rating Scales (BRAF NRS) for severity, effect, and coping[5],
4. Chalder Fatigue Questionnaire (CFQ)[5]
5. Checklist Individual Strength (CIS20R and CIS8R)[5]
6. Fatigue Severity Scale (FSS)[5]
7. Functional Assessment Chronic Illness Therapy (Fatigue) (FACIT-F),[5]
8. Multi-Dimensional Assessment of Fatigue (MAF),[5]
9. Multi-Dimensional Fatigue Inventory (MFI),[5]
10. Pediatric Quality Of Life[5]
11. Multi-Dimensional Fatigue Scale, Profile of Fatigue[5]
12. Short Form 36 Vitality Subscale[5]
13. Visual Analog Scales (VAS).[5]

Evidence

In a 2007 study[6], the FACIT Fatigue Scale was found to have high internal validity (Cronbach's alpha = 0.96) and high test-retest reliability (ICC = 0.95). The correlation between the FACIT and Fatigue Severity Scale (FSS) was -0.79 tool comparison[1]. Thus, the FACIT has demonstrated reliability and sensitivity to change in clients with a variety of chronic health conditions and in the general population and in special populations such as the elderly and those living in rural areas.

References

1. Tennant K. Assessment of fatigue in older adults: the FACIT Fatigue Scale (version 4). Supportive Care in Cancer. 2015;23(5):1355-64.
2. Avlund, K., Pederson, A.N., & Schroll, M. (2003). Functional decline from age 80 to 85: Influence of preceding changes in tiredness in daily activities. Psychosomatic Medicine, 65, 771-777
3. Dittner, A.J., Wessely, S.C., & Brown, R.G. (2004). The assessment of fatigue. A practical guideline for clinicians and researchers. Journal of Psychosomatic Research, 56, 157-170.
4. Butt, Z., Lai, J. S., Rao, D., Heinemann, A. W., Bill, A., & Cella, D. (2013). Measurement of fatigue in cancer, stroke, and HIV using the Functional Assessment of Chronic Illness Therapy - Fatigue (FACIT-F) scale. Journal of psychosomatic research, 74(1), 64–68. doi:10.1016/j.jpsychores.2012.10.011
5. https://onlinelibrary.wiley.com/doi/full/10.1002/acr.20579 Accessed online 17/05/2019
6. Chandran, V., Bhella, S., Schentag, C., & Gladman, D. D. (2007). Functional assessment of chronic illness therapy-fatigue scale is valid in patients with psoriatic arthritis. Annals of the rheumatic diseases, 66(7), 936–939. doi:10.1136/ard.2006.065763

FACIT-F SCORING GUIDELINES (VERSION 4)

Instructions:

1. Record answers in "item response" column. If missing, mark with an X
2. Perform reversals as indicated, and sum individual items to obtain a score.
3. Multiply the sum of the item scores by the number of items in the subscale, then divide by the number of items answered. This produces the subscale score.
4. Add subscale scores to derive total scores (TOI, FACT-G & FACIT-F).
5. **The higher the score, the better the QOL.**

Subscale	**Item Code**	**Reverse item?**		**Item response**		**Item Score**
PHYSICAL	GP1	4	–	________	=	________
WELLBEING	GP2	4	–	________	=	________
(PWB)	GP3	4	–	________	=	________
	GP4	4	–	________	=	________
	GP5	4	–	________	=	________
	GP6	4	–	________	=	________
	GP7	4	–	________	=	________

Sum individual item scores: ________

Multiply by 7: ________

Divide by number of items answered: ________ **=PWB subscale score**

SOCIAL/FAMILY	GS1	0	+	________	=	________
WELLBEING	GS2	0	+	________	=	________
(SWB)	GS3	0	+	________	=	________
	GS4	0	+	________	=	________
	GS5	0	+	________	=	________
	GS6	0	+	________	=	________
	GS7	0	+	________	=	________

Sum individual item scores: ________

Multiply by 7: ________

Divide by number of items answered: ________**=SWB subscale score**

EMOTIONAL	GE1	4	–	________	=________
WELLBEING	GE2	0	+	________	=________
(EWB)	GE3	4	–	________	=________
	GE4	4	–	________	=________
	GE5	4	–	________	=________
	GE6	4	–	________	=________

Sum individual item scores: ________

Multiply by 6: ________

Divide by number of items answered: ________**=EWB subscale score**

FUNCTIONAL	GF1	0	+	________	=________
WELL-BEING	GF2	0	+	________	=________
(FWB)	GF3	0	+	________	=________
	GF4	0	+	________	=________
	GF5	0	+	________	=________
	GF6	0	+	________	=________
	GF7	0	+	________	=________

Sum individual item scores: ________

Multiply by 7: ________

Divide by number of items answered: ________**=FWB subscale score**

FACIT-F SCORING GUIDELINES (VERSION 4) – PAGE 2

Subscale	Item Code	Reverse item?		Item response	Item Score
FATIGUE	HI7	4	—	________	=________
SUBSCALE	HI12	4	—	________	=________
(FS)	An1	4	—	________	=________
	An2	4	—	________	=________
	An3	4	—	________	=________
	An4	4	—	________	=________
	An5	0	+	________	=________
	An7	0	+	________	=________
	An8	4	—	________	=________
	An12	4	—	________	=________
	An14	4	—	________	=________
	An15	4	—	________	=________
	An16	4	—	________	=________

Sum individual item scores:________

Multiply by 13: ________

Divide by number of items answered: ________**=F Subscale score**

To derive a FACIT-F Trial Outcome Index (TOI):

__________ + __________ + __________ =________**=FACIT-F TOI**

(**PWB** score) (**FWB** score) (**FS** score)

To Derive a FACT-G total score:

_________ + _________ + _________ + _________ = ________ **=FACT-G Total score**

(PWB score) **(SWB** score) **(EWB** score) **(FWB** score)

To Derive a FACIT-F total score:

_________ + _________ + _________ + _________ + _________ = ________ **=FACIT-F Total score**

(PWB score) **(SWB** score) **(EWB** score) **(FWB** score) **(FS** score)

*For guidelines on handling missing data and scoring options, please refer to the Administration and Scoring Guidelines in the manual or on-line at www.facit.org.

❑❑❑

83 Functional Assessment of HIV Infection (FAHI)

Objective

The Functional Assessment of HIV Infection (FAHI) is a 47-item disease-specific instrument evaluating Health-Related Quality of Life (HRQL) in human immunodeficiency virus (HIV)-infected patients[1][2][3]. The FAHI is used for measuring quality of life of people living with HIV.[3]

Intended Population

People living with HIV.

Method of Use

The FAHI evaluates physical well-being, functional and global well-being, emotional well-being/living with HIV, social well-being, and cognitive functioning. It yields a total score and individual subscale scores.

Evidence

The FAHI appears to be a reliable and valid measure for assessing quality of life in HIV-positive patients with concurrent drug and alcohol use disorders.[4]

References

1. Cella DF, McCain NL, Peterman AH, Mo F, Wolen D. Development and validation of the Functional Assessment of Human Immunodeficiency Virus Infection (FAHI) quality of life instrument. Quality of Life Research. 1996 Aug 1;5(4):450-63.
2. Peterman AH, Cella D, Mo F, McCain N. Psychometric validation of the revised Functional Assessment of Human Immunodeficiency Virus Infection (FAHI) quality of life instrument. Quality of Life Research. 1997 Nov 1;6(6):572-84.
3. Viala-Danten M, Dubois D, Gilet H, Martin S, Peeters K, Cella D. Psychometric evaluation of the functional assessment of HIV Infection (FAHI) questionnaire and its usefulness in clinical trials. Quality of Life Research. 2010 Oct 1;19(8):1215-27.
4. Byrne S, Petry NM. Reliability and validity of the Functional Assessment of Human Immunodeficiency Virus Infection (FAHI) in patients with drug and alcohol use disorders. AIDS care. 2013 Jan 1;25(1):118-25.

Functional Assessment of HIV Infection (FAHI)

Physical well-being - FAHI [FACIT]

I have a lack of energy

I have nausea

I have pain

I am bothered by side effects of treatment

I am forced to spend time in bed

I have been short of breath

I am bothered by a change in weight

I get tired easily

I feel fatigued

I feel weak all over

I have been coughing

I feel ill

Because of my physical condition, I have trouble meeting the needs of my family

Emotional well-being - living with HIV [FACIT]

I feel sad

I am nervous

I worry about dying

I worry that my condition will get worse
I am unhappy with my appearance
It is hard to tell other people about my infection
I worry about spreading my infection
I am concerned about what the future holds for me
I worry about the effect of stress on my illness
I am embarrassed by my illness
Functional and global well-being [FACIT]
I am able to work (include work at home)
My work (include work at home) is fulfilling
I am able to enjoy life
I have accepted my illness
I am sleeping well
I am enjoying the things I usually do for fun
I am content with the quality of my life right now
I am satisfied with how I am coping with my illness
I am losing hope in the fight against my illness
I feel sexually attractive
I have a good appetite
I feel motivated to do things
I am hopeful about the future
Social well-being [FACIT]
I feel close to my friends
I get emotional support from my family
I get support from my friends
My family has accepted my illness

I am satisfied with family communication about my illness

I felt close to my partner, or the person who is my main support

I have people to help me if I need it

Regardless of your current level of sexual activity, please answer the following question. If you prefer not to answer it, please mark this box and go to the next section.

I am satisfied with my sex life
Cognitive functioning [FACIT]
My thinking is clear
I have trouble concentrating
I have trouble remembering things
Thinking and fatigue [FACIT]
I have a lack of energy
I feel tired
I have trouble starting things because I am tired
I have trouble finishing things because I am tired
I need to rest during the day
I have trouble remembering things
I have trouble concentrating
My thinking is slower than before
I have trouble learning new tasks or directions
Social - family well-being - FAMS [FACIT]
I feel close to my friends
I get emotional support from my family
I get support from my friends
My family has accepted my illness

I am satisfied with family communication about my illness

My family has trouble understanding when my condition gets worse

I feel left out of things
Additional concerns - FAMS [FACIT]
I am bothered by side effects of treatment
I am forced to spend time in bed

I felt close to my partner, or the person who is my main support

I am satisfied with my sex life
I am satisfied with how I am coping with my illness
I am nervous
I worry that my condition will get worse
I am sleeping well
Heat worsens my symptoms
I have trouble controlling my urine
I urinate more frequently than usual
I am bothered by the chills

I am bothered by fevers (episodes of high body temperature)

I am bothered by muscle spasms

84 Functional Gait Assessment

Objective

The Functional Gait Assessment (FGA) is a modification of the Dynamic Gait Index (DGI) that uses higher-level tasks to increase the applicability of the test to people with vestibular disorders and to eliminate the ceiling effect of the original test. Three items were added to the DGI because these were noted to be difficult in people with vestibular disorders. [1]

Intended Population: Adults with Parkinson's Disease, stroke or vestibular disorders [2]

Method of Use [2]

Time to Administer: 5-10 minutes

Number of Test Items: 10

Scoring: Each item is scored on an ordinal scale from 0 - 3, with

- 0 = severe impairment
- 1 = moderate impairment
- 2 = mild impairment
- 3 = normal ambulation

The highest score is 30/30.

Requirements

- A Marked 6-m (20ft) walkways that is marked 20.48cm (12in) in width.
- Stopwatch
- 3. Step or shoe box
- Stairs

Sections and Instructions of the FGA: It is important you keep the instruction the same as described by the test and is the only thing you say as not to influence performance.

1. **Gait on a Level Surface**

   Instruction: Walk at your normal speed from here to the next mark.

   Grading

   3 Normal, walks 6m in less than 5.5 seconds with no adis, in good speed and no evidence of imbalance. Also deviates no more than 15.24cm (6in) outside of the walkway width.

   2 Mild impairment, walks 6m (20 ft) in less than 7 seconds but greater than 5.5 seconds, uses assistive device, slower speed, mild gait deviations, or deviates 15.24–25.4 cm (6–10 in) outside of the walkway width.

   1 Moderate impairment, walks 6 m (20 ft), slow speed, abnormal gait pattern, evidence for imbalance, or deviates 25.4-38.1 cm (10–15 in) outside of the 30.48-cm (12-in) walkway width. Requires more than 7 seconds to ambulate 6 m (20 ft).

   0 Severe impairment, cannot walk 6 m (20 ft) without assistance, severe gait deviations or imbalance, deviates greater than 38.1 cm (15 in) outside of the 30.48-cm (12-in) walkway width or reaches and touches the wall.

2. **Change in Gait Speed**

   Instruction : Begin walking at your normal pace (for 1.5 m [5 ft]). When I tell you "go," walk as fast as you can (for 1.5 m [5 ft]). When I tell you "slow," walk as slowly as you can (for 1.5 m [5 ft]).

   Grading 3 Normal, able to smoothly change walking speed without loss of balance or gait deviation. Shows a significant difference in walking speeds between normal, fast, and slow speeds. Deviates no more than 15.24 cm (6 in) outside of the 30.48-cm (12-in) walkway width.

2 Mild impairment - is able to change speed but demonstrates mild gait deviations, deviates 15.24–25.4 cm (6–10 in) outside of the 30.48-cm (12in) walkway width, or no gait deviations but unable to achieve a significant change in velocity, or uses an assistive device.

1 Moderate impairment , makes only minor adjustments to walking speed, or accomplishes a change in speed with significant gait deviations, deviates 25.4–38.1 cm (10–15 in) outside the 30.48-cm (12-in) walkway width, or changes speed but loses balance but is able to recover and continue walking.

0 Severe impairment, cannot change speeds, deviates greater than 38.1 cm (15 in) outside 30.48-cm (12-in) walkway width,or loses balance and has to reach for wall or be caught.

3. **Gait with Horizontal Head Turns**

Instructions: Walk from here to the next mark 6 m (20 ft) away. Begin walking at your normal pace. Keep walking straight; after 3 steps, turn your head to the right and keep walking straight while looking to the right. After 3 more steps, turn your head to the left and keep walking straight while looking left. Continue alternating looking right and left every 3 steps until you have completed 2 repetitions in each direction.

Grading 3 Normal, performs head turns smoothly with no change in gait. Deviates no more than 15.24 cm (6 in) outside 30.48-cm (12-in) walkway width.

2 Mild impairment, performs head turns smoothly with slight change in gait velocity (eg, minor disruption to smooth gait path), deviates 15.24–25.4 cm (6–10 in) outside 30.48-cm (12-in) walkway width, or uses an assistive device.

1 Moderate impairment—Performs head turns with moderate change in gait velocity, slows down, deviates 25.4–38.1 cm (10–15 in) outside 0.48-cm (12-in) walkway width but recovers, can continue to walk.

0 Severe impairment—Performs task with severe disruption of gait (eg, staggers 38.1 cm [15 in] outside 30.48-cm (12-in) walkway width, loses balance, stops, or reaches for wall).

4. **Gait with Vertical Head Turns**

Instructions: Walk from here to the next mark (6 m [20 ft]). Begin walking at your normal pace. Keep walking straight; after 3 steps, tip your head up and keep walking straight while looking up. After 3 more steps, tip your head down, keep walking straight while looking down. Continue alternating looking up and down every 3 steps until you have completed 2 repetitions in each direction.

Grading 3 Normal, performs head turns with no change in gait. Deviates no more than 15.24 cm (6 in) outside 30.48-cm (12-in) walkway width.

2 Mild impairment, performs task with slight change in gait velocity (eg, minor disruption to smooth gait path), deviates 15.24–25.4 cm (6–10 in) outside 30.48-cm (12-in) walkway width or uses assistive device.

1 Moderate impairment, performs task with moderate change in gait velocity, slows down, deviates 25.4–38.1 cm (10–15 in)outside 30.48-cm (12-in) walkway width but recovers, can continue to walk.

0 Severe impairment, performs task with severe disruption of gait (eg, staggers 38.1 cm [15 in] outside 30.48-cm (12-in) walkway width, loses balance, stops, reaches for wall).

5. **Gait and Pivot Turn**

Instructions: Begin with walking at your normal pace. When I tell you, "turn and stop," turn as quickly as you can to face the opposite direction and stop.

Grading 3 Normal, pivot turns safely within 3 seconds and stops quickly >with no loss of balance.

2 Mild impairment, pivot turns safely in 3 seconds and stops with no loss of balance, or pivot turns safely within 3 seconds and stops with mild imbalance, requires small steps to catch balance.

1 Moderate impairment, turns slowly, requires verbal cueing, or requires several small steps to catch balance following turn and stop.

0 Severe impairment, cannot turn safely, requires assistance to turn and stop.

6. **Step Over Obstacle**

Instructions: Begin walking at your normal speed. When you come to the shoe box, step over it, not around it, and keep walking.

Grading 3 Normal, is able to step over 2 stacked shoe boxes taped together (22.86 cm [9 in] total height) without changing gait speed; no evidence of imbalance.

2 Mild impairment, is able to step over one shoe box (11.43 cm[4.5 in] total height) without changing gait speed; no evidence of imbalance.

1 Moderate impairment, is able to step over one shoe box (11.43 cm [4.5 in] total height) but must slow down and adjust steps to clear box safely. May require verbal cueing.

0 Severe impairment, cannot perform without assistance.

7. **Gait with Narrow Base of Support**

   Instructions: Walk on the floor with arms folded across the chest, feet aligned heel to toe in tandem for a distance of 3.6 m [12 ft]. The number of steps taken in a straight line are counted for a maximum of 10 steps.

   Grading 3 Normal is able to ambulate for 10 steps heel to toe with no staggering.

   2 Mild impairment, ambulates 7–9 steps.

   1 Moderate impairment, ambulates 4–7 steps.

   0 Severe impairment, ambulates less than 4 steps heel to toe or cannot perform without assistance.

8. **Gait with Eyes Closed**

   Instructions: Walk at your normal speed from here to the next mark (6 m [20 ft]) with your eyes closed.

   Grading 3 Normal, walks 6 m (20 ft), no assistive devices, good speed,no evidence of imbalance, normal gait pattern, deviates no more than 15.24 cm (6 in) outside 30.48-cm (12-in) walkway width. Ambulates 6 m (20 ft) in less than 7 seconds.

   2 Mild impairment, walks 6 m (20 ft), uses assistive device,slower speed, mild gait deviations, deviates 15.24–25.4 cm (6–10 in) outside 30.48-cm (12-in) walkway width. Ambulates 6 m (20 ft) in less than 9 seconds but greater than 7 seconds.

   1 Moderate impairment, wWalks 6 m (20 ft), slow speed, abnormal gait pattern, evidence for imbalance, deviates 25.4–38.1 cm (10–15 in) outside 30.48-cm (12-in) walkway width. Requires more than 9seconds to ambulate 6 m (20 ft).

   0 Severe impairment, cannot walk 6 m (20 ft) without assistance,severe gait deviations or imbalance, deviates greater than 38.1cm (15 in) outside 30.48-cm (12-in) walkway width or will not attempt task.

9. **Ambulating Backwards**

   Instructions: Walk backwards until I tell you to stop.

   Grading 3 Normal, walks 6 m (20 ft), no assistive devices, good speed,no evidence for imbalance, normal gait pattern, deviates no more than 15.24 cm (6 in) outside 30.48-cm (12-in) walkway width.

   2 Mild impairment, walks 6 m (20 ft), uses assistive device,slower speed, mild gait deviations, deviates 15.24–25.4 cm (6–10 in) outside 30.48-cm (12-in) walkway width.

   1 Moderate impairment, walks 6 m (20 ft), slow speed, abnormal gait pattern, evidence for imbalance, deviates 25.4–38.1 cm (10–15 in) outside 30.48-cm (12-in) walkway width.

   0 Severe impairment, cannot walk 6 m (20 ft) without assistance,severe gait deviations or imbalance, deviates greater than 38.1 cm (15 in) outside 30.48-cm (12-in) walkway width or will not attempt task.

10. **Steps**

    Instructions: Walk up these stairs as you would at home (ie, using the rail if necessary). At the top turn around and walk down.

    Grading 3 Normal, alternating feet, no rail.

    2 Mild impairment, alternating feet, must use rail.

    1 Moderate impairment, two feet to a stair; must use rail.

    0 Severe impairment, cannot do safely.

Evidence

Reliability: Intrarater reliability of the total FGA: ICC = 0.83 [1] Interrater reliability of the total FGA: ICC = 0.84 [1] Internal Consistency: Cronbach alpha value 0.79 across both trials [1]

Validity: Concurrent Validity - FGA scores were correlated with the following outcome measure scores; [1]

- ABC Scale: r = -.70
- DHI: r = -.064
- PDS: r = -.70
- Number of falls: r = -.66
- TUG: r = -.50
- DGI: r = 0.80

Responsiveness

Miscellaneous: Dynamic Gait Index, the 4-item Dynamic Gait Index, and the Functional Gait Assessment show sufficient validity, responsiveness, and reliability for assessment of walking function in patients with stroke undergoing rehabilitation, but the Functional Gait Assessment is recommended for its psychometric properties[4].

References

1. Wrisley DM, Marchetti GF, Kuharsky DK, Whitney SL. Reliability, Internal Consistency and Validity of Data Obtained with the Functional Gait Assessment. Physical Therapy. 2004; 84(10): 906-918.
2. http://www.rehabmeasures.org/Lists/RehabMeasures/DispForm.aspx?ID=893
3. Julia Krahm. Functional Gait Assessment. Available from: http://www.youtube.com/watch?v=vxzB3ez3y14[last accessed 10/10/14]
4. Lin JH, Hsu MJ, Hsu HW, Wu HC, Hsieh CL. Psychometric Comparisons of 3 Functional Ambulation Measures for Patients With Stroke. Stroke. 2010 Jul 29; online article ahead of print

□□□

85 Functional Independence Measure (FIM)

Objective

The Functional Independence Measure (FIM) is an instrument that was developed as a measure of disability for a variety of populations and is not specific to any diagnosis. The FIM instrument

- Includes measures of independence for self-care, including sphincter control, transfers, locomotion, communication, and social cognition[1].
- Is an 18-item, seven-level, ordinal scale intended to be sensitive to changes over the course of a comprehensive inpatient medical rehabilitation program.
- Uses the level of assistance an individual needs to grade functional status from total independence to total assistance).
- The tool is used to assess a patient's level of disability as well as a change in patient status in response to rehabilitation or medical intervention.[2][3]

Intended Population: Designed to assess areas of dysfunction in activities that commonly occur in subjects with any progressive, reversible or stable neurologic, musculoskeletal, or other disorder ie patients with functional mobility impairments[4]. The FIM is used by healthcare practitioners to assess and grade the functional status of a person based on the level of assistance he or she requires.

Method of Use

Guide for use: Patient function is assessed using the FIM™ instrument at the start of a rehabilitation episode of care and at the end of a rehabilitation episode of care. Admission assessment is collected within 72 hours of the start of a rehabilitation episode. Discharge assessment is collected within 72 hours prior to the end of a rehabilitation episode. FIM™ is comprised of 18 items, grouped into 2 subscales - motor and cognition.

The motor subscale includes:

Eating

Grooming

Bathing

Dressing, upper body

Dressing, lower body

Toileting

Bladder management

Bowel management

Transfers - bed/chair/wheelchair

Transfers – toilet

Transfers - bath/shower

Walk/wheelchair

Stairs

The cognition subscale includes:

Comprehension

Expression

Social interaction

Problem solving

Memory

Each item is scored on a 7 point ordinal scale, ranging from a score of 1 to a score of 7. The higher the score, the more independent the patient is in performing the task associated with that item.[5]

FIM levels

No Helper

- 7. Complete Independence (Timely, Safety)
- 6. Modified Independence (Device)

Helper - Modified Dependence

- 5. Supervision (Subject = 100%)
- 4. Minimal Assistance (Subject = 75% or more)
- 3. Moderate Assistance (Subject = 50% or more)

Helper - Complete Dependence

- 2. Maximal Assistance (Subject = 25% or more)
- 1. Total Assistance or not Testable (Subject less than 25%)

Leave no blanks. Enter 1 if not testable due to risk.[2]

The total score for the FIM

- motor subscale (the sum of the individual motor subscale items) will be a value between 13 and 91.
- cognition subscale (the sum of the individual cognition subscale items) will be a value between 5 and 35.

The total score for the FIM instrument (the sum of the motor and cognition subscale scores) will be a value between 18 and 126.[5]

Reliability and Validity

1. Inter-Rater Reliability of FIM has been established at an acceptable psychometric performance (Intraclass co-relation coefficients ranging from 0.86 to 0.88)
2. The concurrent validity with Barthel Index (ICC > 0.83) have shown strong construct validity between items on Barthel Index and items on the FIM the measure functional limitations[6]

References

1. Cameron MH, Monroe L. Physical Rehabilitation-E-Book: Evidence-based examination, evaluation, and intervention. Elsevier Health Sciences; 2007 Apr 5.Available: https://www.sciencedirect.com/topics/medicine-and-dentistry/functional-independence-measure(accessed 22.5.2021)
2. Linacre JM, Heinemann JW, Wright BD, Granger CV, Hamilton BB. The structure and stability of the functional independence measure. Arch Phys Med Rehabil. 1994. 75: 127-132.
3. Heinemann AW, Linacre JM, Wright BD, Hamilton BB, Granger C. Relationships between impairment and physical disability as measured by the functional independence measure. Arch Phys Med Rehabil. 1993. 74: 566-573.
4. Elia AE, Graziella F, Albanese A. 12 Clinical Trials of Botulinum Toxin in Adult Spasticity. Botulinum Toxin E-Book: Therapeutic Clinical Practice and Science. 2009 Feb 18:148.Available from: https://www.sciencedirect.com/topics/medicine-and-dentistry/functional-independence-measure(accessed 22.5.2021)
5. AIHW FIM Available from:https://meteor.aihw.gov.au/content/index.phtml/itemId/495857 (accessed 22.5.20210
6. Gosman-Hedstrom, G, and Svensson, E: Parallel reliability of the Functional Independence Measure and the Barthel index ADLIndex. Psychiatry 73:188, 2000

Functional Independence Measure (FIM)

ADMISSION DISCHARGE FOLLOW-UP

Self-Car

A. Eating

B. Grooming

C. Bathing

D. Dressing - Upper Body

E. Dressing - Lower Body

F. Toileting

Sphincter Control

G. Bladder Management

H. Bowel Management

Transfers

I. Bed, Chair, Wheelchair

J. Toilet

K. Tub, Shower

Locomotion

L. Walk/Wheelchair

M. Stairs

Motor Subtotal Score

Communication

N. Comprehension

O. Expression

Social Cognition

P. Social Interaction

Q. Problem Solving

R. Memory

Cognitive Subtotal Score

TOTAL FIM Score

❑❑❑

86 Functional Index of Hand Osteoarthritis (FIHOA)

Objective

The FIHOA is a measure to assess hand function in persons with hand osteoarthritis (OA). It is a 10- item questionnaire developed by Dreiser et al in 1995[1][2]. It has been translated in French, Dutch and Argentinian versions. It is targeted towards the functional capacity of hands in OA affected patients[1]. It is also called as Dreiser's index.

Intended Population

The targeted population is Osteoarthritis patients but it can also be used in Rheumatoid arthritis, in patients whose hand functions need to be assessed.

Method of Use

Equipment Required: None. Questionnaire based.

Time to administer: 5-10 mins.

Training Required: None.

Method of Administration: Physician/ physiotherapist administered, self - reported.

Instrument: It contains 10 question with a score range of 0-30[1].

Sr. no.	Question asked	Scoring			
		0	1	2	3
1	Are you able to turn a key in a lock?				
2	Are you able to cut meat with a knife?				
3	Are you able to cut cloth or paper with a pair of scissors?				
4	Are you able to lift a full bottle with the hand?				
5	Are you able to clench your fist?				
6	Are you able to tie a knot?				
7	For women: Are you able to sew? For men: Are you able to use a screwdriver?				
8	Are you able to fasten buttons? 9. 10.				
9	Are you able to write for a long period of time?				
10	Would you accept a handshake without reluctance?				

0 = possible without difficulty, 1 = possible with slight difficulty, 2 = possible with important difficulty, 3 = impossible. Total scores indicate hand function. Lower the scores, better the hand function[1].

Psychometric Properties

Reliability:

1. Interrater: in OA, Cronbach's alpha : 0.90[3][4]. In RA, Cronbach's alpha test :0.94[5]

2. Test- Retest: by administering the FIHOA 2 times 1 week apart gave an ICC of 0.74 and 2 times with a 5-day interval yielded an ICC of 0.96 in OA[3][4]
3. Intra-rater: by testing patients with OA 2 times 1 hour apart. Correlations between the scores were 0.95[3][4]

Validity:

For OA, FIHOA correlated with[4]

1. the Cochin Hand Function Scale (rs = 0.89) and
2. Michigan Hand Outcomes Questionnaire (rs = 0.86),
3. total Australian Canadian Osteoarthritis Hand Index (rs = 0.76)

Thus, it was found reliable, valid for OA.

References

1. Dreiser R, Maheu E, Guillou GB, Caspard H, Grouin JM. Validation of an algofunctional index for osteoarthritis of the hand. Rev Rhum Engl Ed. 1995; 62: 43S– 53S.
2. Dreiser RL, Maheu E, Guillou GB. Sensitivity to change of the functional index for hand osteoarthritis. Osteoarthritis Cartilage 2000; 8: S25– 8.
3. Poole JL, Lucero SL, Mynatt R. Self-reports and performance based tests of hand function in persons with osteoarthritis. Phys Occup Ther Geriatr 2010; 28: 249– 58.
4. Moe R, Garratt A, Slatkowsky-Christensen B, Maheu E, Mowinckel P, Kvien T, et al. Concurrent evaluation of data quality, reliability and validity of the Australian/Canadian Osteoarthritis Hand Index and the Functional Index for Hand Osteoarthritis. Rheumatology (Oxford). 2010; 49: 2327– 36.
5. Bande JM, Caracciolo JÁ, Papasidero SB, Santa Cruz MJ, Medina MA, Klajn DS, Battaglia MG, Giantinoto J, Pelagagge F. Validation of the Functional Index for Hand Osteoarthritis (FIHOA) in Patients with Rheumatoid Arthritis [abstract]. Arthritis Rheumatol. 2018; 70 (suppl 10). Accessed October 24, 2020. https://acrabstracts.org/abstract/validation-of-the-functional-index-for-hand-osteoarthritis-fihoa-in-patients-with-rheumatoid-arthritis/

❑❑❑

87 Functional Movement Screen (FMS)

Objective

The Functional Movement Screen (FMS)[1][2], and later the Selective Functional Movement Assessment (SFMA) [3], was developed to help clinicians and health care professions screen individuals for risk of injury and / or a dysfunctional or performance-limiting movement pattern. The FMS was first presented commercially as a manual for screening athletes and the product line was later expanded to include a range of equipment for performing the screen, certifications for those screening athletes, seminars, books, and videos.[4]

The FMS is a tool used to identify asymmetries which result in functional movement deficiencies. The FMS aims to identify imbalances in mobility and stability during seven fundamental movement patterns. These movement patterns are designed to provide observable performance of basic locomotor, manipulative and stabilising movements by placing an individual in extreme positions where weaknesses and imbalances become noticeable if appropriate mobility and motor control is not utilised. Once these deficiencies have been identified through the FMS, a program of corrective exercises is then developed with the goal of preventing musculoskeletal injuries.

The FMS consists of seven movement patterns which require mobility and stability. The seven following movement patterns are scored from 0-3 points, with the sum creating a score ranging from 0-21 points.

1. Deep Squat
2. Hurdle Step
3. In-line Lunge
4. Active Straight-leg Raise
5. Trunk Stability Push-up
6. Rotary Stability
7. Shoulder Mobility

Intended Population

The FMS was intended to serve as a screen to identify individuals with functional movement deficits that could indicate an increased risk of injury. Use in the literature varies from young, active individuals to middle-aged individuals, elite, collegiate and professional athletes, as well as military and firefighters. A lower FMS scores have been noted to be associated with an increased BMI, increased age, and decreased activity level.[5]

Use

A score of <=14 on the FMS is used as the cut-off score. Individuals who score less than 14 points on the FMS screen have greater odd for sustaining an injury [6]. Research to date is limited and it is not yet clear for which sports or professions the FMS is optimal in predicting injury risk, and whether the original cutoff score of <=14 is valid in different populations [7]. Evidence

Reliability

Multiple studies have demonstrated excellent reliability of the FMS screen.[7][8][9][10] A recent study by Teyhen et al [7] revealed that among novice raters, the FMS demonstrated moderate to good inter-rater and intra-rater reliability, even with minimal training (4 hours).

Validity

Although there is preliminary research by Kiesel et al [6] that suggests that NFL (National Football League) players who score <= 14 on the FMS had a positive likelihood ratio of 5.8 to sustain a time-loss injury. There are concerns remaining regarding the validity of the FMS[10][11]. Moran et al[12] suggest that the strength of association between FMS composite scores and subsequent injury does not support its use as an injury prediction tool. Further more, Alemany et al[13] suggest that pain occurrence may be a stronger indicator of injury risk than a low composite score and provides a simpler method of evaluating injury risk compared to the full FMS.

FMS vs. SFMA

Many clinicians confuse the Functional Movement Screen tool with the Selective Functional Movement Assessment (SFMA). Both tools are a part of the same Functional Movement System created by Cook and colleagues, but their fundamental purposes are quite different. The SFMA is meant to be used in a diagnostic capacity, designed to identify musculoskeletal dysfunction among individuals affected by pain. Whereas the FMS is a screening tool, not intended for diagnosis. The FMS aims to identify imbalances in mobility and stability during functional movements.

References

1. Cook G, Burton L, Fields K, Kiesel K. The Functional Movement Screen. Danville, VA: Athletic Testing Services Inc, 1998.
2. Cook G, Burton L, Hoogenboom BJ, Voight M. Functional movement screening: the use of fundamental movements as an assessment of function-part 2. International journal of sports physical therapy. 2014 Aug;9(4):549-63.
3. Cook G Movement: Functional Movement Systems: Screening, Assessment, and Corrective Strategies. On Target Publications; Santa Cruz, CA: 2010
4. Beardsley C, & Contreras B, The functional movement screen: A review. Strength and Conditioning Journal. 2014; 36(5): 72-80.
5 Mitchell UH, Johnson AW, Vehrs PR, Feland JB, & Hlton SC. Performance on the Functional Movement Screen in older active adults. J Sport & Health Science. 2016; 5(1): 119-125. Doi:[/doi.org/10.1016/j.jshs.2015.04.006 https://doi.org/10.1016/j.jshs.2015.04.006]
6. 4. Kiesel K, Plisky PJ, Voight ML. Can serious injury in professional football be predicted by a preseason functional movement screen? N Am J Sports Phys There. 2007; 2:147-158.
7. 1. Teyhen DS, Shaffer SW, Lorenson CL, Halfpap JP, Donofry DF, Walker MJ, Dugan JL, Childs JD. The functional movement screen: A reliability study. JOSPT. 2012; 42:530-40.
8. 2. Schneiders AG, Davidsson A, Horman E, Sullivan SJ. Functional movement screen normative values in a young, active population. IJSPT. 2011; 6: 75-82
9. 3. Parenteau GE, Gaudreault N, Chambers S, Boisvert C, Grenier A, Gagne G, Balg F. Functional movement screen test: A reliable screening test for young elite ice hockey players. Phys There Sport. 2013.
10. Bonazza NA, Smuin D, Onks CA, Silvis ML, Dhawan A. Reliability, validity, and injury predictive value of the functional movement screen: a systematic review and meta-analysis. The American Journal of Sports Medicine. 2017 Mar;45(3):725-32.
11. Dorrel B, Long T, Shaffer S, Myer GD. The functional movement screen as a predictor of injury in National Collegiate Athletic Association Division II athletes. Journal of athletic training. 2018 Jan;53(1):29-34.
12. Moran RW, Schneiders AG, Mason J, Sullivan SJ. Do Functional Movement Screen (FMS) composite scores predict subsequent injury? A systematic review with meta-analysis. Br J Sports Med. 2017 Dec 1;51(23):1661-9.
13. Alemany JA, Bushman TT, Grier T, Anderson MK, Canham-Chervak M, North WJ, Jones BH. Functional Movement Screen: Pain versus composite score and injury risk. Journal of science and medicine in sport. 2017 Nov 1;20:S40-4.

FUNCTIONAL MOVEMENT SCREEN SCORE SHEET

Name: **Date:** **Dob:** **City,** **State,** **Zip:**
Phone **School/Affiliation:** **Height: Weight:** **Age:**
Gender: **Primary Sport:** **Primary Position:**
Hand/Leg Dominance: **Previous Test Score**

Test	Raw Score		Final Score	Comments
	Left	Right		
Deep Squat				
Hurdle Step				
Inline Lunge				
Shoulder Mobility				
Shoulder Clearing Test				
Active Straight-Leg Raise				
Trunk Stability Pushup				
Extension Clearingtest				
Rotary Stability				
Flexion Clearing Test				
Total Screen Score				

❑❑❑

88 Functional Reach Test (FRT)

Objective

Functional Reach Test (FRT) is a clinical outcome measure and assessment tool for ascertaining dynamic balance in one simple task.

- In standing, measures the distance between the length of an outstretched arm in a maximal forward reach, while maintaining a fixed base of support.
- This information is correlated with risk of falling.
- Measurement Interpretation:
- 10"/25 cm or greater Low risk of falls;
    - 6"/15cm to 10"/25cm Risk of falling is 2x greater than normal;
    - 6"/15cm or less Risk of falling is 4x greater than normal;
    - Unwilling to reach Risk of falling is 8x greater than normal[1][2]
- A number of factors exert a major influence on this evaluation: research revealed that the movement strategy and a reduced spinal flexibility, both affect the reach distance .[3]

Intended Population

- FRT was made to predict fall risk in the elderly and Frail adult[2][4]
- It is one of the 4 tests used in the The Balance Outcome Measure for Elder Rehabilitation (BOOMER)

Method of Use

- The patient is instructed to stand next to, but not touching, a wall and position the arm that is closer to the wall at 90 degrees of shoulder flexion with a closed fist.
- The assessor records the starting position at the 3rd metacarpal head on the yardstick.
- Instruct the patient to "Reach as far as you can forward without taking a step."
- The location of the 3rd metacarpal is recorded.
- Scores are determined by assessing the difference between the start and end position is the reach distance, usually measured in inches.
- Three trials are done and the average of the last two is noted[5]

Criteria to stop the test:

The patient's feet lifted up from the floor or they fell forward. Most patients fall forward with this test. The therapist should guard from the front as that is the direction that you reach forward.

Reduced ability to reach has shown increases in future falls with odds ratios of 8.2 if unable to reach at all and 4 if able to reach < 15.2cm[7]

Evidence

Reliability[2][7]

- The ordinal level tests (supported sitting and standing balance and static tandem standing tests) showed 100% agreement in all aspects of reliability.
- Intra-class correlations for the other tests ranged from 0.93 to 0.99. All the tests showed significant correlations with the appropriate comparator tests ($r=0.32-0.74$ $p\leq0.05$)
- Test-retest reliability $r = 0.89$
- Inter-rater agreement on reach measurement = 0.98

Validity

Eagle et al.[8] found out the following:

- Sensitivity = 76%
- Accuracy = 46%
- Specificity = 34%
- Positive Predictive Value = 33%
- Negative Predictive Value = 77%

Some research found that decreased spinal flexibility and the movement strategy affects the distance reached and also question the ability of FRT to differentiate elderly non-fallers and fallers[9][10]. A research also noted that trunk mobility has a greater contribution to the test than the centre of pressure displacement. [11]

Responsiveness

FRT increased to 28 cm from 18 cm in 22 community-dwelling adults with knee osteoarthritis following a 10weeks aquatic exercise program under physiotherapist lead[12]

References

1. Standardized_Test_Reference_Card_Template Available from:http://functionalpathways.com/intranet-files/Standardized_Test_Reference_Card_Template.pdf (last accessed 16.10.2020)
2. Duncan PW, Weiner DK, Chandler J, Studenski S. Functional reach: a new clinical measure of balance.J Gerontol. 1990;45(6):M192-197.
3. Schenkman M, Morey M, Kuchibhatla M. Spinal flexibility and balance control among community-dwelling adults with and without Parkinson's. J Gerontol A Biol Sci Med Sci. 2000;55(8):M441-445.
4. Weiner DK, Duncan PW, Chandler J, Studenski SA. Functional reach: a marker of physical frailty. J Am Geriatr Soc. 1992;40(3):203-207.
5. FRT Available from:https://www.sralab.org/sites/default/files/2017-06/5Hgjkv-Functional%20Reach%20Test.pdf (last accessed 16.10.2020)
6. SAFA Production. Funtional Reach Test. Available from: http://www.youtube.com/watch?v=yYBmBkbvAyk[last accessed 8/5/2019]
7. Duncan PW, Studenski S, Chandler J, Prescott B. Functional reach: predictive validity in a sample of elderly male veterans. Gerontol. 1992;47(3):M93-98.
8. Eagle JD, Salama S, Whitman D, Evans LA, Ho E, Olde J. Comparison of three instruments in predicting accidental falls in selected inpatients in a general teaching hospital. Journal of Gerontology Nursing. 1999; 25(7): 40-45.
9. Wernick-Robinson M, Krebs DE, Giorgetti MM. Functional reach: Does it really measure dynamic balance? Archives of Physical Medicine and Rehabilitation. 1999; 80(3): 262 - 269
10. Wallmann HW. Comparison of elderly nonfallers and fallers on performance measures of functional reach, sensory organization, and limits of stability.J Gerontol A Biol Sci Med Sci. 2001;56(9):M580-583.
11. Jonsson E, Henriksson M, Hirschfeld H. Does the functional reach test reflect stability limits in elderly people? J Rehabil Med. 2003;35(1):26-30.
12. Lau MC, Lam JK, Siu E, Fung CS, Li KT, Lam MW. Physiotherapist-designed aquatic exercise programme for community-dwelling elders with osteoarthritis of the knee: a Hong Kong pilot study. Hong Kong Med J. 2014;20(1):16-23.

89 Functional Reach Test and Modified Functional Reach Instructions

General Information

The Functional Reach test can be administered while the patient is standing (Functional Reach) or sitting (Modified Functional Reach).

Functional Reach (standing instructions):

- The patient is instructed to next to, but not touching, a wall and position the arm that is closer to the wall at 90 degrees of shoulder flexion with a closed fist.
- The assessor records the starting position at the 3rd metacarpal head on the yardstick.
- Instruct the patient to "Reach as far as you can forward without taking a step."
- The location of the 3rd metacarpal is recorded.
- Scores are determined by assessing the difference between the start and end position is the reach distance, usually measured in inches.
- Three trials are done and the average of the last two is noted.

Modified Functional Reach Test (Adapted for individuals who are unable to stand):

- Performed with a leveled yardstick that has been mounted on the wall at the height of the patient's acromion level in the non-affected arm while sitting in a chair
- Hips, knees and ankles positioned are at 90 degree of flexion, with feet positioned flat on the floor.
- The initial reach is measured with the patient sitting against the back of the chair with the upper-extremity flexed to 90 degrees, measure was taken from the distal end of the third metacarpal along the yardstick.
- Consists of three conditions over three trials
    - Sitting with the unaffected side near the wall and leaning forward
    - Sitting with the back to the wall and leaning right
    - Sitting with the back to the wall leaning left.
- Instructions should include leaning as far as possible in each direction without rotation and without touching the wall
- Record the distance in centimeters covered in each direction
- If the patient is unable to raise the affected arm, the distance covered by the acromion during leaning is recorded
- First trial in each direction is a practice trial and should not included in the final result A 15 second rest break should be allowed between trials

Set-up:

- A yardstick and duck tap will be needed for the assessment.
- The yardstick should be affixed to the wall at the level of the patient's acromion.

References

1. Duncan, P. W., D. K. Weiner, et al. (1990). "Functional reach: a new clinical measure of balance." J Gerontol 45(6): M192-197.
2. Katz-Leurer, M., I. Fisher, et al. (2009). "Reliability and validity of the modified functional reach test at the sub-acute stage post-stroke." Disabil Rehabil 31(3): 243-248.
3. Weiner, D. K., D. R. Bongiorni, et al. (1993). "Does functional reach improve with rehabilitation?" Arch Phys Med Rehabil 74(8): 796-800.
4. Weiner, D. K., P. W. Duncan, et al. (1992). "Functionalreach: amarkerofphysicalfrailty." JAm Geriatr Soc 40(3): 203-207.

Functional Rach Test (FRT)	
Considerations	
Which type of TJA is it appropriate for?	THA and TKA
What part of the TJA continuum is it appropriate for?	Pre-op Post-acute1 Active Living
What domain(s) does it measure within the ICF?	Activity
Who completes it?	Patient and clinician
What does it measure?	Static balance through maximal forward reach from a fixed base of support2
What equipment is required?	Tape measure or pre-measured intervals marked on wall at shoulder level
How long does it take?	~ 5 mins to complete and score
How do I do it?	Instructions available at:2 www.rehabmeasures.org/PDF%20Library/Functional%20Reach%20Test.pdf
How good is it?	Validity: Concurrent – good, correlates with walking speed, tandem walk, and 1-footed stand in community dwelling elderly. 3 Reliability: Inter-rater and test-retest- excellent for adults aged 20 – 87 years.4 Responsiveness: Ability to detect change in TJA or OA population not established. In 22 community-dwelling adults with knee OA, the FRT improved from 20 cm to 28 cm after a 10-week PT-led aquatic exercise program.5 Floor/ceiling effects: Not established in TJA 1
How is it scored? +	Scores are determined by assessing the difference between the start and end position. Three trials are done and average of last two noted.
What do the results mean?	Greater value (distance) = better balance and decreased falls risk. In community dwelling elders, < 17.5 cm suggests limited mobility skills, inability to leave the neighborhood without help, and restriction in ADLs.3 In frail elderly patients, <18.5 cm reach indicates fall risk.6 Based on a Canada-wide sample of 2,305 elderly people, the median FRT distance was 29 cm in cognitively unimpaired subjects.7
Where can I get it?	Available at: www.rehabmeasures.org/PDF%20Library/Functional%20Reach%20Test.pdf Video link: www.youtube.com/watch?v=_aJqJzt-U2s

Developed by the BC Physical Therapy Total Joint Arthroplasty and Outcome Measures Knowledge Translation Task Force: Dr. Marie Westby, Ronda Field, Maureen Duggan, Dolores Langford, Robyn Laytham, Steven Longstaff, Lauren Welch, Alison Hoens. June 2014. A Physical Therapy Knowledge Broker project supported by: UBC Department of Physical Therapy, Physiotherapy Association of BC, Vancouver Coastal Research Institute and Providence Healthcare Research Institute.

❑❑❑

90 Gait and Lower Limb Observation of Pediatrics - (GALLOP)

Introduction

The gait and lower limb observation of paediatrics (GALLOP) is a very new, comprehensive assessment of questions and objective measures developed in 2016. Therefore, very limited research surrounding this proforma exists. Research suggests that children's gait is a frequent concern of parents and therefore they present to podiatrists and physiotherapists with their child regularly for assessment.[1] With this prevalence, Peninsula Health conducted a quality assurance review across Australia, investigating what physiotherapist and podiatrist assessments involved when looking at children's gait and lower limbs. It was found that there was very little consistency amongst professionals, so GALLOP was created as a way of trying to standardise and develop consistency of assessments.[2]

Development

A delphi study was conducted where 50 physiotherapist and podiatrists were invited to participate in the development of the GALLOP, but only 17 participants completed the process. These therapists were selected upon their clinical experience, background, recommendation or involvement in teaching and/or researching within the field of paediatrics in Australia. There were 4 rounds to the delphi study.

Individual assessment outcomes and proformas were collected alongside a literature review of gait and lower limb assessment in paediatrics which were included in the delphi study. The reliability and paediatric norms available on the assessment techniques that reached a consensus or agreement were exacted from the study. This information was then developed into a proforma which could be easily implemented into clinical practice.

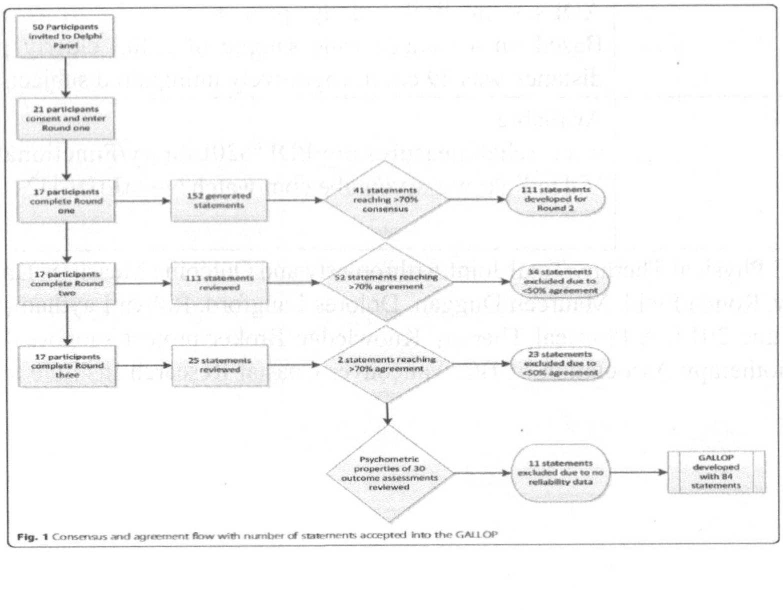

Fig. 1 Consensus and agreement flow with number of statements accepted into the GALLOP

Psychometric Properties

This delphi study, which lead to the production of the GALLOP, highlighted that due to the number of different assessments identified in the process, the only psychometric test that was considered was the reliability, and this was based-on the clinician's opinion only. Due to the lack of formal critique of the psychometric reliability of each individual assessment, a certain degree of caution should be used when implementing into practice. It should also be noted that a formal quality assessment of each of the studies included was not performed, although participants were advised to consider things such as sample size, administration intervals, analysis of data, and population group in relation to the study they were involved. Due to this proforma being such a new tool, no further studies have looked into psychometric properties, therefore it can be concluded that this assessment has face validity only.

Use

The results of the study which produced the GALLOP states that it should be considered by physiotherapists and podiatrists as a systematic approach to collect information and outcome measures related to the foot and lower limb within the paediatric population defined as 0-18 years of age.

References

1. Evans AM, Rome K, Peet L. The foot posture index, ankle lunge test, Beighton scale and the lower limb assessment score in healthy children: a reliability study. Journal of Foot Ankle Research 2012; 5(1)
2. Cranage S, Banwell H, Williams CM. Gait and Lower Limb Observation of Paediatrics (GALLOP): development of a consensus based paediatric podiatry and physiotherapy standardised recording proforma. Journal of Foot and Ankle Research 2016; 9:8

Gait and Lower Limb Observation of Pediatrics - (GALLOP)

Name____________________________ Date of Birth___/__/___ Gender: Male/Female

Vaginal birth: Instrumentation at birth

Spontaneous/Induced Forceps/Ventose

Caesarean: Emergency/Planned

Reason:____________________

Breech: Yes/No

Complications____

____

Other health professionals involved at birth or in first 14 days:______________________

Age of skill acquisition (record in months)

Sitting: ___________ Crawling:__________ Crawl type:__________

Walking: _________ Running:__________ Jumping:____________

History:

Medical/Family____

Previous treatment:____________________________

Previous Pain:___________________________________

Footwear:____

Sport:____

Sensory concerns:________________________________

Weight: ______kg Height: ______cm BMI:

Observation of ability to perform the following appropriate to age (Circle)

Squatting: Yes/No/NA Running: Yes/No/NA Jumping: Yes/No/N/A

Skipping: Yes/No/NA Hopping: Yes/No/NA Single Leg Stance

Left: Yes/No/N/A

Right: Yes/No/N/A

Ability to go up/down stairs:

Yes/No/NA

Observation of functional tasks: ______________________

Quality of body movement: ______________________

Other Observations______________________

Pain

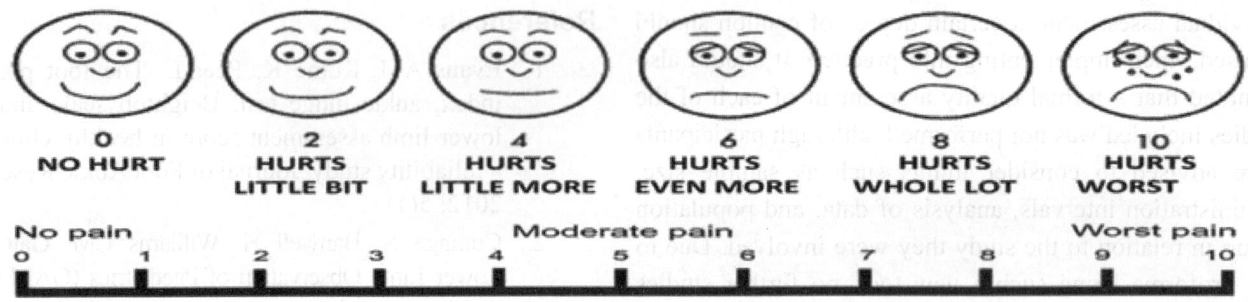

Biomechanical Assessments:

	Left	Right		Left	Right
Hip: Internal ROM			Hip External ROM		
Modified Thomas Test			Hip abduction		
Popliteal angle			Foot thigh angle		
Ankle WBL/NWB Straight			Ankle WBL/NWB Bent		
Foot Posture Index-6			Beighton score _______/9		

Inter-condylar distance: _________cm

Inter-malleoli distance: _________cm

Limb Length Discrepancy*: Left=Right

Left>Right______cm

Left<Right______cm

Other observations of rotation, limb length:______________________

Neurology:

	Left	Right		Left	Right
Patella Reflex (0-4)			Achilles Reflex (0-4)		
Plantar Reflex (Up/down)			Ankle Catch (Yes/No)		
Ankle Clonus (Yes/No)			Gower's Sign		
Dorsiflexion strength (0-5)			Plantarflexion Strength (0-5)		
Inversion strength (0-5)			Eversion strength (0-5)		

Observation of muscle tone or neurological signs:

Gait*

	Left	Right		Left	Right
Head and neck position			Trunk/torso		
Arm swing			Hip		
Knee			Heel contact		
Midstance			Toe-off		
Angle of gait			Base of gait		

Other gait comments:

❑❑❑

91 Galveston Orientation & Amnesia Test

Objective

The Galveston Orientation and Amnesia Test (GOAT) is an instrument originally created by Levin, O'Donnell, and Grossman and first published in 1979. [1] It was developed to evaluate cognition serially during the subacute stage of recovery from a closed head injury (CHI). This practical scale measures orientation to person, place, and time, and memory for events preceding and following the injury. The GOAT assesses post-traumatic amnesia (PTA) and retrograde amnesia (RA) in patients who have had a severe traumatic brain injury (TBI). [2] The GOAT is designed to be a practical, reliable scale that can be used at the bedside or in the emergency room by health service providers of various disciplines. It is important in determining the outcome and prognosis. [2]

Intended Population

The Galveston Orientation and Amnesia Test is primarily used on traumatic brain injury patients with closed head injuries. [2] Modified versions of the GOAT have been designed for use in patient limiting conditions.

Method of Use

Scoring: The 10 items comprising the GOAT are presented orally to the patient in the order as seen in the image to the right. The test form has space for recording the patient's responses in the error score column. Error points which are points to be deducted for an incorrect response, appear in the error score column. [2] Details on how to calculate error scores when listening to the patient's response are provided in the notes column. The total GOAT score is obtained by deducting the sum of the error points from 100. [4]

Variations: There are variations of the GOAT which have been created to address patient limiting conditions.

- Written GOAT is administered to patients who can comprehend the GOAT questions but are unable to communicate due to motor speech impairment. [5]
- Modified GOAT (GOAT-M) was created for patients who can comprehend the GOAT but are unable to communicate due to written impairments. [5]
- COAT is also used for children and adolescents who are in the early stages of recovery from traumatic brain injury. [6]
- A-GOAT Test, it was developed for use with aphasic patients, it is the GOAT administered in a multiple-choice format. The A-GOAT test allows for a comparison of aphasic and non-aphasic patients using the same standard testing. It includes 10 items with a 3-choice response format. [7]

Interpretation

The duration of post-traumatic amnesia (PTA) is defined as the period following a coma in which the GOAT score is <75. PTA is considered to have ended if a score ≥75 is achieved on three consecutive administrations. [8][9][10] A low GOAT score is associated with hospitalization and post-concussion syndrome at early follow-up. [11]

Ranges for the GOAT:

- Score of ≥ 75 for two consecutive days, no longer in the post-traumatic amnesia phase. [4]
- Score between 66 and 75 for two consecutive days, borderline status. [4]
- Score < 66, the patient for two consecutive days, patient still in the post-traumatic amnesia phase. A low GOAT score is associated with hospitalization and post-concussion syndrome at early follow-up. [4]

Relevance to Physical Therapy

In his study, Levin [2] reported that the GOAT is an important measurement of the severity of acute CHI and can be used as a predictor of injury prognosis. Similarly, Bode [12] concluded that the duration of PTA after a TBI provided one of the earliest and best predictors of long-term outcome. Also, it was reported that patients with retrograde amnesia recovered significantly sooner than patients with anterograde amnesia post-TBI and that RA assessment alone had a significant and novel utility in post-TBI assessment. [13]

Multiple studies have shown that health practitioners, including physical therapists, can effectively utilize the GOAT as a predictor of TBI progression and prognosis. Furthermore, using the GOAT to understand a patient's prognosis post-TBI would be essential in determining the patient's suitability for physical therapy and the level of involvement of a physical therapist within the healthcare team. Physical therapists would have more involvement in patients with a positive long-term prognosis in the later stages of recovery, while medical clinicians would likely administer medical treatments for those with a poor prognosis, in the early stages of recovery.

The developers of the Galveston Orientation and Amnesia test determined that the GOAT provided clinicians, including physical therapists with pertinent information regarding on-going treatment and discharge planning.[12] Physical therapists may use the GOAT in combination with other cognitive scales as a means of serial cognitive assessment to monitor the clinical course of neuropsychiatric disorders, including traumatic brain injuries. [2]

Reliability

- The inter-rater reliability of the total GOAT is r=0.98 with an agreement via Kappa coefficient of k=0.73. [4]
- Reliability coefficient for individual items on the GOAT has a Kendall correlation coefficient of 0.99. The research for this is not recent and should be updated. [2]
- The test-retest reliability coefficient for GOAT is predicted to have a low value. [2]

Validity

Looking at construct validity using the Rasch mathematical analysis, researchers found that the constructed item hierarchy for the GOAT confirmed previous research, mostly that the focus should be on the person, that place and time comes before dealing with memories surrounding the injury. [12] GOAT Scores correlated positively with the Glasgow Coma Scale (GSC) scores ($r = 0.456$, $p < 0.002$) as well as with the admission and discharge Functional Independence Measure (FIM) scores ($r = 0.701$ and 0.531, respectively). [8]

When looking at predictive validity, PTA, measured by GOAT scores, is a significant independent predictor of functional outcome ($p = 0.00005$) as assessed by the Disability Rating Scale (DRS) and FIM total, motor, and cognitive scores[10]. The duration of PTA as assessed by GOAT was significantly associated with employment status at one-year post-injury. [14] Performance on the GOAT was also associated with long-term outcome (at least 6 months post-injury) rated by the GOS (Glasgow Outcome Scale) ($p < 0.0001$). [2]

Advantages

- The advantage of GOAT is that it provides an objective rating of early cognitive recovery eliminating the need to utilize ambiguous terms such as "confused". [2]
- Another advantage of the GOAT was from a study conducted by Bode et al. which suggested that a Rasch analysis demonstrated the use of the GOAT for assessing patients with a wide range of cognitive impairments given the items on the test represent a wide range of difficulties. [12]

Limitations

In the GOAT, for items in which partial credit is used, Rasch analysis revealed step disorder. [12] By organizing the response categories to a simple dichotomy (e.g. right versus wrong) it was shown to solve the disorder and allow the construction of an equal interval measure from the GOAT. [12] With modifications in the item scoring of the GOAT, researchers were able to eliminate unreliable differentiation in responses, developing an equal-interval measure of PTA that displayed good reliability and validity.[12] When looking at the GOAT, it is also important to incorporate an age correction factor in order to reduce the possibility of an age effect when comparing younger with older populations.

References

1. Fürbringer e Silva SC, Sousa RM. Galveston Orientation Amnesia Test (GOAT). Revista da Escola de Enfermagem da USP. 2009 Dec; 43 (SPE) : 1027-33.

2. Levin HS, O'Donnell VM, Grossman RG. The Galveston Orientation and Amnesia Test: A practical scale to assess cognition after head injury. Journal of Nervous and Mental Disease. 1979 Nov.
3. Physiopedia. Galveston Orientation & Amnesia Test Assessment. Available from: http://www.youtube.com/watch? v=x88yQNlbIXc[last accessed 30/06/19]
4. Moin P, Khalighinejad N, Yusefi A, Farajzadegan Z, Barekatain M. Converting three general-cognitive function scales into persian and assessment of their validity and reliability. International journal of preventive medicine. 2011 Apr;2(2):82.
5. Transforming Research and Clinical Knowledge in Traumatic Brain Injury. (2016). [ebook p.19. Available at: http://tracktbi.ucsf.edu/sites/tracktbi.ucsf.edu/files/Outcome%20Assessment%20 SOP_edits%20for%20public %20posting.pdf [Accessed 10 May 2018].]
6. Ewing-Cobbs L, Levin HS, Fletcher JM, Miner ME, Eisenberg HM. The Children's Orientation and Amnesia Test: relationship to severity of acute head injury and to recovery of memory. Neurosurgery. 1990 Nov 1;27(5):683-91.
7. Jain N, Layton BS, Murray PK. Are aphasic patients who fail the GOAT in PTA? A modified Galveston Orientation and Amnesia Test for persons with aphasia. The Clinical Neuropsychologist. 2000 Feb 1;14(1):13-7.
8. Novack TA, Bergquist TF, Bennett G, Gouvier WD. Primary caregiver distress following severe head injury. The Journal of Head Trauma Rehabilitation. 1991 Dec.
9. Wade DT. Measurement in neurological rehabilitation. Current opinion in neurology and neurosurgery. 1992 Oct;5(5):682-6.
10. Zafonte RD, Mann NR, Millis SR, Black KL, Wood DL, Hammond F. Posttraumatic amnesia: its relation to functional outcome. Archives of physical medicine and rehabilitation. 1997 Oct 1;78(10):1103-6.
11. Ganti L, Daneshvar Y, Ayala S, Bodhit AN, Peters KR. The value of neurocognitive testing for acute outcomes after mild traumatic brain injury. Military medical research. 2016 Dec;3(1):23.
12. Bode RK, Heinemann AW, Semik P. Measurement properties of the Galveston Orientation and Amnesia Test (GOAT) and improvement patterns during inpatient rehabilitation. The Journal of head trauma rehabilitation. 2000 Feb 1;15(1):637-55.
13. Marshman LA, Hennessy M, Delle Baite L, Britton G. Utility of Retrograde Amnesia Assessment Alone, Compared with Anterograde Amnesia Assessment in Determining Recovery After Traumatic Brain Injury: Prospective Cohort Study. World neurosurgery. 2017 Nov 28.
14. Cifu DX, Keyser-Marcus L, Lopez E, Wehman P, Kreutzer JS, Englander J, High W. Acute predictors of successful return to work 1 year after traumatic brain injury: a multicenter analysis. Archives of physical medicine and rehabilitation. 1997 Feb 1;78(2):125-31

Galveston Orientation & Amnesia Test

Question	Error score	Notes
What is your name?	/ 2	Must give both first name and surname
When were you born?	/ 4	Must give day, month, and year.
Where do you live?	/ 4	Town is sufficient
Where are you now? (a) City (b) Building	/ 5	 (a) Must give actual town. (b) Usually in hospital or rehab center. Actual name necessary
When were you admitted to this hospital?	/ 5	Date.
How did you get here?	/ 5	Mode of transport.
What is the first event you can remember after the injury?	/ 5	Any plausible event is sufficient (record answer)

Can you give some detail?	/ 5	Must give relevant detail.
Can you describe the last event you can recall before the accident?	/ 5	Any plausible event is sufficient (record answer)
What time is it now?	/ 5	1 for each half-hour error, etc.
What day of the week is it?	/ 3	1 for each day error, etc
What day of the month is it? (i.e. the date)	/ 5	1 for each day error, etc.
What is the month?	/ 15	5 for each month error, etc.
What is the year?	/ 30	10 for each year error.
Total Error: 100 - total error		Can be a negative number

6-100 = Normal 66-75 = Borderline < 66 = Impaired

Patient last name: .... Date of birth: . . . / . . . / . . . .

Patient first name: .... Date: . . . / . . . / . . . .

☐☐☐

92 Gartland and Werley Score

Objective and Intended Population

The Gartland & Werley Score is a point-based outcome measure used to evaluate hand and wrist function [1]. The scale, developed in 1951, was initially created for the evaluation of healed Colles fractures. The original scale is based on a "demerit" scoring system involving subjective and objective aspects related to wrist and hand function, residual deformities, range of motion and nerve complications.

Two modified versions of the scale have been implemented:

- The first included measures of pronation and strength [2]
- The second included evaluation of stiffness and reflexes[3].

Method of Use

The score is based on a list of items categorised into four domains namely:

- residual deformity
- subjective evaluation
- objective evaluation
- complications

Each assessed item is evaluated based on a demerit point system. The total score of the four domains is then summed up to construct the final score of the whole test. A final total score of 21 or above refers to "poor" hand function following an "healed" Colles fracture.

The list of items with relative scores and cut-offs is presented below:

Section	Results	Points
1	Residual deformities	
1.1	Prominent ulnar styloid	1
1.2	Residual dorsal tilt	2
1.3	Radial deviation of hand	2 to 3
2	Subjective evaluation	
2.1	No pain, disability or limitation in motion (Excellent)	0
2.2	Occasional pain, slight limitation in motion, no disability (Good)	2
2.3	Occasional pain, some limitation of motion, feeling of weakness in the wrist, no particular disability if careful, activities slightly restricted (Fair).	4
2.4	Pain, limitation of motion, disability, activities more or less markedly restricted (Poor)	6
3	Objective evaluation	
3.1	Loss of dorsiflexion	5
3.2	Loss of ulnar deviation	3
3.3	Loss of supination	2
3.4	Loss of palmar flexion	1
3.5	Loss of radial deviation	1
3.6	Loss of circumduction	1
3.7	Pain in distal radio-ulnar joint	1
4	Complications (Arthritic change)	
4.1	Minimal	1
4.2	Minimal with pain	3
4.3	Moderate	2
4.4	Moderate with pain	4
4.5	Severe	3

4.6	Severe with pain	5
4.7	Nerve complications (Median)	1 to 3
4.8	Poor finger function due to cast	1 to 2

Cut-off scores for end-results point ranges are presented as following:

- 0-2: Excellent
- 3-8: Good
- 9-20: Fair
- 21 or above: Poor

Evidence

This outcome measure is reported to be broadly used by surgeons and in clinical reports [1][4]. However, despite its broad application in the clinical setting, there is, to the date, no evidence concerning reliability, validity or responsiveness of the test.

References

1. Changulani M, Okonkwo U, Keswani T, Kalairajah Y. Outcome evaluation measures for wrist and hand–which one to choose?. International orthopaedics. 2008 Feb 1;32(1):1-6.
2. Sarmiento A, Pratt GW, Berry NC, Sinclair WF. Colles' fractures. Functional bracing in supination. The Journal of bone and joint surgery. American volume. 1975 Apr;57(3):311-7.
3. Lucas GL, Sachtjen KM. An analysis of hand function in patients with Colles' fracture treated by Rush rod fixation. Clinical Orthopaedics and Related Research®. 1981 Mar 1;155:172-9.
4. Dacombe PJ, Amirfeyz R, Davis T. Patient-reported outcome measures for hand and wrist trauma: is there sufficient evidence of reliability, validity, and responsiveness?. Hand. 2016 Mar; 11(1):11-21.

❑❑❑

93 Glasgow Coma Scale

Objective

The Glasgow Coma Scale (GCS) was first created by Graham Teasdale and Bryan Jennett in 1974. It is a clinical scale to assess a patient's "depth and duration of impaired consciousness and coma" following an acute brain injury[1].

Healthcare practitioners can monitor the motor responsiveness, verbal performance, and eye-opening of the patient in the form of a simple chart. The GCS is the most commonly used tool internationally for this assessment and has been translated into 30 languages. It should not, however, be confused with the Glasgow Outcome Scale (GOS), which evaluates persistent disability after brain damage. [2]

Intended Population

The Glasgow Coma Scale was originally developed to help determine the severity of a coma or dysfunction following a traumatic brain injury, but can be useful for any condition leading to impaired consciousness. [3]

Today, it is consistently used for many conditions including:

- stroke (subarachnoid haemorrhage, intracerebral haemorrhage, or ischemic stroke),
- infection,
- seizures,
- brain abscess,
- general traumas and ITU patients
- non-traumatic coma,
- overdose
- poisoning[3]

It can also be administered in a variety of settings such as pre-hospital, arrival at the emergency department and in the hours following admission, giving it the ability to monitor changes and trends in patient consciousness over time.[3]

Modified scales have been developed for use in other populations. The Glasgow Coma Scale - Extended (GCS - E) includes the use of an amnesia scale in order to avoid the premature discharge of patients with mild traumatic brain injury. [4] There have also been modified scales developed for use in the paediatric population.

The motor scale has proved the most useful for assessment in both older children and preverbal children when studying blunt trauma. [5] Research has indicated that using the motor scale alone can simplify the assessment process while maintaining the accuracy of the score. [6]

Method of Use

The GCS Assessment Aid has four steps to the assessment process: Check, observe, stimulate, rate. [7]

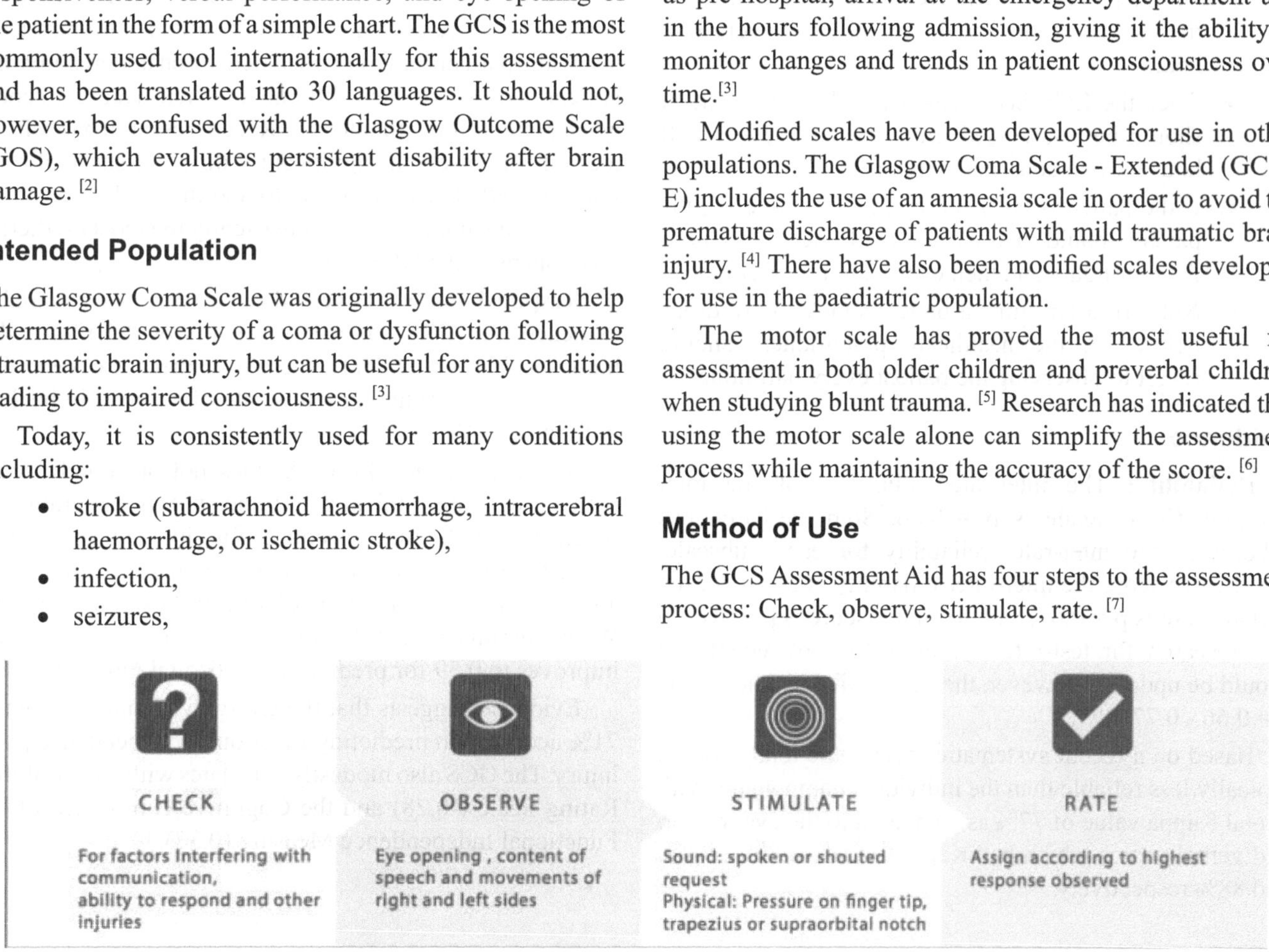

The assessor should evaluate each of the subscales as listed in the Assessment Aid. Each subscale has several components. Based on the level of consciousness, a score is assigned. A higher score indicates a greater level of consciousness.

Eyes	Verbal	Motor
Spontaneous	Oriented	Obey commands
To sound	Confused	Localising
To pressure	Words	Normal Flexion
None	Sounds	Abnormal Flexion
—	None	Extension
—	—	None

The GCS uses three sites for stimulation. This includes fingertip pressure, trapezius pinch and supraorbital notch. When stimulating these areas, health care practitioners should look for one of two responses: an abnormal flexion response or a normal flexion response. [7]

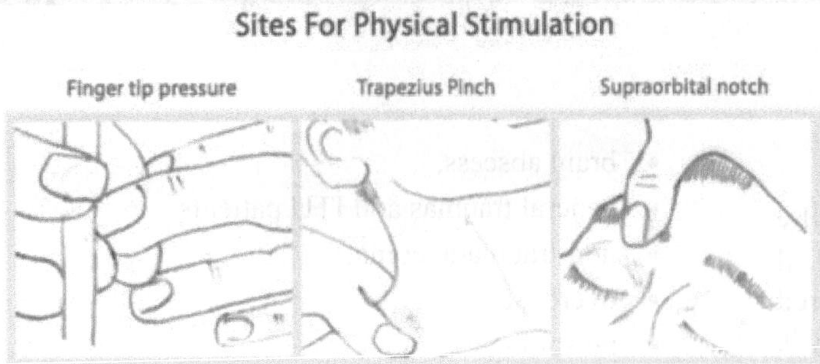

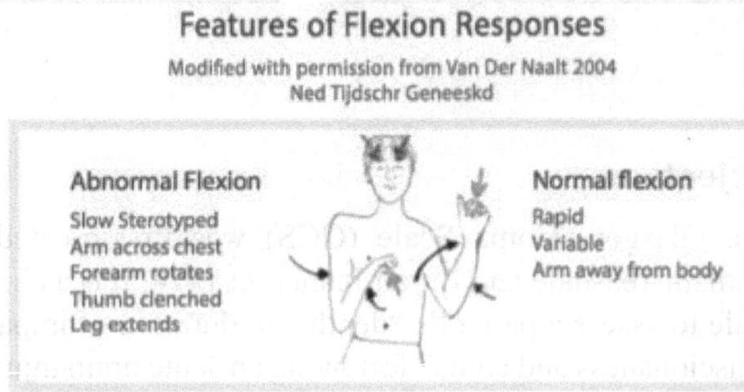

- Until a patient has achieved a GCS score of 15 on the GCS, patients should be observed every half hour.
- Once the GCS Score has reached 15, the patient should be re-assessed using the GCS every half hour for two consecutive hours.
- If the patient's GCS score remains above 15, the patient should then be observed once every hour for four hours and then every 2 hours after that.
- Note: If at any time a patient's GCS score drops below 15, the healthcare practitioners should revert to observing the patient every half hour.[8]

Evidence

Reliability: The inter-rater reliability of the total Glasgow Coma Scale is p = 0.86. Some research has subdivided the inter-rater reliability for each subscale. For the eye score the inter-rater reliability is p = 0.76, the verbal score is p = 0.67, and the motor score is p=0.81. [10] The research for test-retest reliability is not recent and should be updated, however, the best available evidence is k = 0.66 - 0.77. [11]

Based on a recent systematic review, the total score is typically less reliable than the individual components with a total Kappa value of 77% as compared to the eye, motor, and verbal scores which had Kappa values of 89%, 94%, and 88% respectively. [12]

Validity: The validity of the Glasgow Coma Scale comes under fire because a lot of hospitals administer the test while patients have been sedated, often underestimating patient scores. It's also difficult to elicit accurate scores when patients are intubated. [13] Recent research has refuted that intubation elicits significantly different survival rates with the verbal score of r = 0.90 and the total score of r = 0.97. [14] The motor score is consistently the most predictive component of the GCS. [15]

Responsiveness: Given the current best available evidence, the GCS has a low sensitivity (56.1%) and a high specificity (82.2%). Therefore, there are very few false positives predicting a low rate of survival in healthy individuals. [16]

It is argued that the GCS does not accurately score patients who are intubated and does not assess brainstem reflexes, which may account for its low predictive capacity. A GCS administered at 24 hours post-injury has an odds ratio of 0.4 for predicting in-hospital mortality. When administered at 72 hours post-injury, the odds ratio improves to 0.59 for predicting in-hospital mortality. [17]

Evidence suggests that the Glasgow Coma Scale has a 71% accuracy in predicting functional independence post-injury. The GCS also modestly correlates with the Disability Rating Scale (-0.28) and the Cognitive component of the Functional Independence Measure (0.37). [18]

References

1. Teasdale G, Jennett B. Assessment of coma and impaired consciousness: a practical scale. The Lancet. 1974 Jul 13;304(7872):81-4.
2. Frej M, Frej J. The Glasgow Structured Approach to Assessment of the Glasgow Coma Scale: what is GCS - glasgow coma scale. http://www.glasgowcomascale.org/what-is-gcs/ (accessed 7 May 2017).
3. Middleton PM. Practical use of the Glasgow Coma Scale; a comprehensive narrative review of GCS methodology. Australasian Emergency Nursing Journal. 2012 Aug 1;15(3):170-83.
4. Nell V, Yates DW, Kruger J. An extended Glasgow Coma Scale (GCS-E) with enhanced sensitivity to mild brain injury. Archives of physical medicine and rehabilitation. 2000 May 1;81(5):614-7.
5. Holmes JF, Palchak MJ, MacFarlane T, Kuppermann N. Performance of the pediatric Glasgow Coma Scale in children with blunt head trauma. Academic emergency medicine 2005 Sep 1;12(9):814-9. PMID:16141014 (accessed 5 May 2017).
6. Acker SN, Ross JT, Partrick DA, Nadlonek NA, Bronsert M, Bensard DD. Glasgow motor scale alone is equivalent to Glasgow Coma Scale at identifying children at risk for serious traumatic brain injury. Journal of trauma and acute care surgery. 2014 Aug 1;77(2):304-9.
7. Institute of Neurological Sciences NHS Greater Glasgow and Clyde. Glasgow Coma Scale: do it this way [Internet]. Sir Graham Teasdale; 2015 [cited 2017 May 7]. Available from: http://www.glasgowcomascale.org/downloads/GCS-Assessment-Aid-English.pdf?v=3
8. National Institute for Health and Care Excellence. Head Injury: assessment and early management [Internet]. https://www.nice.org.uk/guidance/cg176/resources/head-injury-assessment-and-early-management-pdf-35109755592901 (accessed 7 May 2017).
9. GCS at 40. Glasgow Coma Scale at 40 | The new approach to Glasgow Coma Scale assessment. Available from: https://www.youtube.com/watch?v=v6qpEQxJQO4 [last accessed 05/07/17]
10. Gill M, Reiley D, Green S. Interrater reliability of Glasgow Coma Scale scores in the emergency department. Annals of Emergency Medicine 2004;43(2):215-223. https://doi.org/10.1016/S0196-0644(03)00814-X (accessed 6 May 2017).
11. Brott T, Adams H, Olinger C, Marler J, Barsan W, Biller J et al. Measurements of acute cerebral infarction: a clinical examination scale. Stroke 1989;20(7):864-870. PMID: 2749846 (accessed 6 May 2017).
12. Reith F, Synnot A, van den Brande R, Gruen R, Maas A. Factors influencing the reliability of the Glasgow Coma Scale: a systematic review. Neurosurgery 2017;42:3-15. PMID: 28327922 (accessed 7 May 2017).
13. Marion D, Carlier P. Problems with initial Glasgow Coma Scale assessment caused by prehospital treatment of patients with head injuries. The Journal of Trauma: Injury, Infection, and Critical Care 1994;36(1):89-95. PMID: 8295256 (accessed 6 May 2017).
14. Meredith W, Rutledge R, Fakhry S, Emery S, Kromhout-Schiro S. The conundrum of the Glasgow Coma Scale in intubated patients. The Journal of Trauma: Injury, Infection, and Critical Care 1998;44(5):839-845. PMID: 9603086 (accessed 7 May 2017).
15. Lesko M, Jenks T, Perel P, O'Brien S, Childs C, Bouamra O et al. Models of mortality probability in severe traumatic brain injury: results of the modeling by the UK Trauma Registry. Journal of Neurotrauma 2013;30(24):2021-2030. PMID: 23865489 (accessed 6 May 2017).
16. Grote S, Böcker W, Mutschler W, Bouillon B, Lefering R. Diagnostic value of the Glasgow Coma Scale for traumatic brain injury in 18,002 patients with severe multiple injuries. Journal of Neurotrauma 2011;28(4):527-534. PMID: 21265592 (accessed 6 May 2017).
17. McNett M, Amato S, Gianakis A, Grimm D, Philippbar S, Belle J et al. The FOUR Score and GCS as predictors of outcome after traumatic brain injury. Neurocritical Care 2014;21(1):52-57. doi:10.1007/s12028-013-9947-6 (accessed 5 May 2017).
18. McNett M. A review of the predictive ability of Glasgow Coma Scale scores in head-injured patients. Journal of Neuroscience Nursing 2007; 39(2):68-75. PMID: 17477220 (accessed 6 May 2017).

19. Jennett B. Assessment of outcome after severe brain damage: a practical scale. The Lancet 1975; 305(7905):480-484. http://www.sciencedirect.com/science/article/pii/S0140673675928305?via%3Dihub (accessed 7 May 2017).

Glasgow Coma Scale

Eye Opening Response

- Spontaneous--open with blinking at baseline 4 points
- To verbal stimuli, command, speech 3 points
- To pain only (not applied to face) 2 points
- No response 1 point

Verbal Response

- Oriented 5 points
- Confused conversation, but able to answer questions 4 points
- Inappropriate words 3 points
- Incomprehensible speech 2 points
- No response 1 point

Motor Response

- Obeys commands for movement 6 points
- Purposeful movement to painful stimulus 5 points
- Withdraws in response to pain 4 points
- Flexion in response to pain (decorticate posturing) 3 points
- Extension response in response to pain (decerebrate posturing) 2 points
- No response 1 point

References

1. Teasdale G, Jennett B. Assessment of coma and impaired consciousness. Lancet 1974; 81-84. Teasdale G, Jennett B. Assessment and prognosis of coma after head injury. Acta Neurochir 1976; 34:45-55.

2. Categorization:

   Coma: No eye opening, no ability to follow commands, no word verbalizations (3-8)

   Head Injury Classification:

   Severe Head Injury----GCS score of 8 or less
   Moderate Head Injury----GCS score of 9 to 12
   Mild Head Injury----GCS score of 13 to 15

   (Adapted from: Advanced Trauma Life Support: Course for Physicians, American College of Surgeons, 1993).

❑❑❑

94 Gross Motor Function Measure

Introduction

The Gross Motor Function Measure (GMFM) is an observational clinical tool designed to evaluate change in gross motor function in children with cerebral palsy. There are two versions of the GMFM - the original 88-item measure (GMFM-88) and the more recent 66-item GMFM (GMFM-66) [1].

Objective

The objective of Gross Motor Function Measure is to evaluate the gross motor functions in children with Cerebral Palsy (CP). The evaluation of motor function is essential to monitor and adjust therapies to optimize the effect of rehabilitation of children with cerebral palsy (CP).

Intended Population

Children with Cerebral Palsy (CP) aged between 5 months to 16 years whose motor skills is delayed compared to those of the same age. Although the GMFM-88 has been developed for children with CP, it is also validated for other populations, such as children with Down Syndrome and acquired brain damage. Whereas the GMFM-66 is so far only validated in children with CP [2] .

Method of Use

The GMFM-88 item scores can be summed to calculate raw and percent scores for each of the five GMFM dimensions of interest, selected goal areas and a total GMFM-88 score. For the GMFM-66 a free computer program, the Gross Motor Ability Estimator (GMAE), is required to calculate total scores.

GMFM Scores

The scoring system of the GMFM is a four-point scale that consists of 66 items divided into five dimensions of gross motor function:(a) lying and rolling, (b) sitting, (c) crawling and kneeling, (d) standing, and (e) walking, running and jumping [3]. Specific descriptors for scoring items are detailed in the administration and scoring guidelines. A 5-year old child without motor disabilities is able to reach the maximum score [1] .

Time Administer

Administering the GMFM-88 may take approximately 45 to 60 minutes for someone familiar with the measure, depending on the skill of the assessor, the ability of the child and the child's level of the cooperation and understanding. The GMFM-66 should take less time to administer as there are fewer items [1] .

Required Qualifications

The GMFM was designed for use by pediatric therapists who are familiar with assessing motor skills in children. Users should familiarize themselves with the GMFM guidelines and score sheet prior to assessing children.

Equipment Needed

Physiotherapy Department (e.g mat, bench, toys).Access to stairs (with at least 5 steps) is also necessary .

Evidence

The GMFM show sufficient validity, responsiveness, and reliability for assessment of motor skills of children with Cerebral Palsy undergoing rehabilitation [4]. Therefore, for young children and children with severe motor disabilities the GMFM-88 gives a more detailed description of their abilities and limitations. Additionally, the GMFM-88 can be administrated with shoes, ambulatory aids and/or orthoses, whereas the GMFM-66 must be administrated barefoot without aids [2].

Reliability & Validity

Reliability refers to dependability, consistency, and stability of scores on an assessment tool. Both versions of GMFM were shown to be highly reliable, with the intraclass correlation coefficient (ICC)s of greater than .98 (95% confidence interval=0.965-0.994) and both of them can be used in clinical practice or research.

Validity and Responsiveness: Validity includes responsiveness, which is defined as the ability to differentiate clinically important differences. Both versions of GMFM also demonstrated high levels of validity, with an intraclass correlation coefficient (ICC) of .99 (95% confidence interval=0.972-0.997), reflecting associations with the GMFM-66.

Miscellaneous

Evaluating child abilities and the level of difficulty using the GMFM can be useful in identifying the impairments in motor skills and in evaluating the improvement as a result of intervention thereby providing much more information to assist with realistic goal setting [4].

Reference

1. Ko J, Kim M. Reliability and responsiveness of the gross motor function measure-88 in children with cerebral palsy. Physical therapy. 2013 Mar 1;93(3):393-400.
2. Beckers LW, Bastiaenen CH. Application of the Gross Motor Function Measure-66 (GMFM-66) in Dutch clinical practice: a survey study. BMC pediatrics. 2015 Dec;15(1):1-10.
3. Vaščáková T, Kudláček M, Barrett U. Halliwick concept of swimming and its influence on motoric competencies of children with severe disabilities. European Journal of Adapted Physical Activity. 2015;8(2).
4. Russell DJ, Rosenbaum P, Wright M, Avery LM. Gross motor function measure (GMFM-66 & GMFM-88) users manual. Mac keith press; 2002.

ROSS MOTOR FUNCTION MEASURE (GMFM) SCORE SHEET (GMFM-88 and GMFM-66 scoring)

Child's Name: ID#:

Assessment Date:

GMFCS Level1: 1 / 2 / 3 / 4 / 5

Date of Birth:

Chronological Age:

Evaluator's Name:

Testing Condition (e.g., room, clothing, time, others present):

The GMFM is a standardized observational instrument designed and validated to measure change in gross motor function over time in children with cerebral palsy. The scoring key is meant to be a general guideline. However, most of the items have specific descriptors for each score. It is imperative that the guidelines contained in the manual be used for scoring each item.

SCORING KEY

- 0 = does not initiate
- 1 = initiates
- 2 = partially completes
- 3 = completes
- 9 (or leave blank) = not tested (NT) [used for the GMAE-2 scoring*]

It is important to differentiate a true score of "0" (child does not initiate) from an item which is Not Tested (NT) if you are interested in using the GMFM-66 Ability Estimator (GMAE) Software.

	A: LYING & ROLLING	Score				
		0	1	2	3	NT
	1. Sup, Head in Midline: Turns Head With Extremities Symmetrical 2. Sup: Brings Hands to Midline, Fingers One With The Other 3. Sup: Lifts Head 45° 4. Sup: Flexes R Hip & Knee Through Full Range 5. Sup: Flexes L Hip & Knee Through Full Range 6. Sup: Reaches Out With R Arm, Hand Crosses Midline Toward Toy 7. Sup: Reaches Out With L Arm, Hand Crosses Midline Toward Toy 8. Sup: Rolls to Pr Over R Side 9. Sup: Rolls to Pr Over L Side 10. Pr: Lifts Head Upright 11. Pr On Forearms: Lifts Head Upright, Elbows Ext., Chest Raised 12. Pr On Forearms: Weight on R Forearm, Fully Extends Opposite Arm Forward 13. Pr On Forearms: Weight on L Forearm, Fully Extends Opposite Arm Forward 14. Pr: Rolls to Sup Over R Side 15. Pr: Rolls to Sup Over L Side 16. Pr: Pivots to R 90° Using Extremities 17. Pr: Pivots to L 90° Using Extremities					
	Total A					

	B: SITTING	Score				
		0	1	2	3	NT
	18. Sup, Hands Grasped By Examiner: Pulls Self To Sitting With Head Control 19. Sup: Rolls To R Side, Attains Sitting 20. Sup: Rolls To L Side, Attains Sitting 21. Sit On Mat, Supported At Thorax By Therapist: Lifts Head Upright, Maintains 3 Seconds 22. Sit On Mat, Supported At Thorax By Therapist: Lifts Head Midline, Maintains 10 Seconds 23. Sit On Mat, Arm(S) Propping: Maintains, 5 Seconds 24. Sit On Mat: Maintain, Arms Free, 3 Seconds 25. Sit On Mat With Small Toy In Front: Leans Forward, Touchestoy, Re-Erects Without Arm Propping 26. Sit On Mat: Touches Toy Placed 45° Behind Child's R Side, Returns To Start 27. Sit On Mat: Touches Toy Placed 45° Behind Child's L Side, Returns To Start 28. R Side Sit: Maintains, Arms Free, 5 Seconds 29. L Side Sit: Maintains, Arms Free, 5 Seconds 30. Sit On Mat: Lowers To Pr With Control 31. Sit On Mat With Feet In Front: Attains 4 Point Over R Side 32. Sit On Mat With Feet In Front: Attains 4 Point Over L Side 33. Sit On Mat: Pivots 90°, Without Arms Assisting 34. Sit On Bench: Maintains, Arms And Feet Free, 10 Seconds 35. Std: Attains Sit On Small Bench 36. On The Floor: Attains Sit On Small Bench 37. On The Floor: Attains Sit On Large Bench					
	Total B					

	C: CRAWLING & KNEELING	Score				
		0	1	2	3	NT
	38. Pr: Creeps Forward 1.8M (6') 39. 4 Point: Maintains, Weight On Hands And Knees, 10 Seconds 40. 4 Point: Attains Sit Arms Free 41. Pr: Attains 4 Point, Weight On Hands And Knees 42. 4 Point: Reaches Forward With R Arm, Hand Above Shoulder Level 43. 4 Point: Reaches Forward With L Arm, Hand Above Shoulder Level 44.4 Point: Crawls Or Hitches Forward 1.8M(6') 45. 4 Point: Crawls Reciprocally Forward1.8m (6') 46. 4 Point: Crawls Up 4 Steps On Hands And Knees/Feet 47. 4 Point: Crawls Backwards Down 4 Steps On Hands And Knees/Feet 48. Sit On Mat: Attains High Kn Using Arms, Maintains, Arms Free, 10 Seconds 49. High Kn: Attains Half Kn On R Knee Using Arms, Maintains, Arms Free, 10 Seconds 50. High Kn: Attains Half Kn On L Knee Using Arms, Maintains, Arms Free, 10 Seconds 51. High Kn: Kn Walks Forward 10 Steps, Arms Free					
	Total C					
	D: STANDING	**Score**				
		0	1	2	3	NT
	52. On The Floor: Pulls To Std At Large Bench 53. Std: Maintains, Arms Free, 3 Seconds 54. Std: Holding On To Large Bench With One Hand, Lifts R Foot, 3 Seconds 55. Std: Holding On To Large Bench With One Hand, Lifts L Foot, 3 Seconds 56. Std: Maintains, Arms Free, 20 Seconds 57. Std: Lifts L Foot, Arms Free, 10 Seconds 58. Std: Lifts R Foot, Arms Free, 10 Seconds 59. Sit On Small Bench: Attains Std Without Using Arms 60. High Kn: Attains Std Through Half Kn On R Knee, Without Using Arms 61. High Kn: Attains Std Through Half Kn On L Knee, Without Using Arms 62. Std: Lowers To Sit On Floor With Control, Arms Free 63. Std: Attains Squat, Arms Free 64. Std: Picks Up Object From Floor, Arms Free, Returns To Stand					

	E: WALKING, RUNNING & JUMPING	Score				
		0	1	2	3	NT
	65. Std, 2 Hands On Large Bench: Cruises 5 Steps To R 66. Std, 2 Hands On Large Bench: Cruises 5 Steps To L 67. Std, 2 Hands Held: Walks Forward 10 Steps 68. Std, 1 Hand Held: Walks Forward 10 Steps 69. Std: Walks Forward 10 Steps 70. Std: Walks Forward 10 Steps, Stops, Turns 180°, Returns 71. Std: Walks Backward 10 Steps 72. Std: Walks Forward 10 Steps, Carrying A Large Object With 2 Hands 73. Std: Walks Forward 10 Consecutive Steps Between Parallel Lines 20Cm (8") Apart 74. Std: Walks Forward 10 Consecutive Steps On A Straight Line 2Cm (3/4") Wide 75. Std: Steps Over Stick At Knee Level, R Foot Leading 76. Std: Steps Over Stick At Knee Level, L Foot Leading0£ 1£ 2£ 3£ 76. 77. Std: Runs 4.5M (15'), Stops & Returns 78. Std: Kicks Ball With R Foot 79. Std: Kicks Ball With L Foot 80. Std: Jumps 30Cm (12") High, Both Feet Simultaneously 81. Std: Jumps Forward 30 Cm (12"), Both Feet Simultaneously 82. Std On R Foot: Hops On R Foot 10 Times Within A 60Cm (24") Circle 83. Std On L Foot: Hops On L Foot 10 Times Within A 60Cm (24") Circle 84. Std, Holding 1 Rail: Walks Up 4 Steps, Holding 1 Rail, Alternating Feet 85. Std, Holding 1 Rail: Walks Down 4 Steps, Holding 1 Rail, Alternating Feet 86. Std: Walks Up 4 Steps, Alternating Feet 87. Std: Walks Down 4 Steps, Alternating Feet 88. Std On 15Cm (6") Step: Jumps Off, Both Feet Simultaneously .					
	Total E					

GMFM-88 SUMMARY SCORE

Dimension	**Calculation of Dimension % Scores**	**Goal Area (indicated with check)**
A. Lying & Rolling	Total Dimension A /51 = ----- / 51 × 100 = ----- %	A
B. Sitting Total Dimension	Total Dimension B /60 = ----- / 60 × 100 = ----- %	B
C. Crawling & Kneeling	Total Dimension C /42 = ----- / 42 × 100 = ----- %	C
D. Standing	Total Dimension D /39 = ----- / 39 × 100 = ----- %	D
E. Walking, Running & jumping	Total Dimension E /72 = ----- / 72 × 100 = ----- %	E

TOTAL SCORE = (%A + %B + %C + %D + %E) / Total # of Dimensions = ---- /5 = ------- = ------- %

GOAL

TOTAL = (Sum of % scores for each dimension identified as a goal area) / # of Goal areas = ------ = -------%

SCORE

TESTING WITH AIDS/ORTHOSES USING THE GMFM-88

Indicate below with a check (4) which aid/orthosis was used and what dimension it was first applied. (There may be more than one).

AID	Dimension	Orthosis	Dimension
Rollator/pusher		Hip Control	
Walker		Knee	
H Frame crutches		Ankle-foot Control	
Crutches		Foot Control	
Quad Cane		Shoes	
Cane		None	
None		Other (please specify)	
Other (please specify)			

GMFM-88 SUMMARY SCORE USING AIDS/ORTHOSES

Dimension	Calculation of Dimension % Scores	Goal Area (Indicated With Check)
F. Lying & Rolling	Total Dimension A /51 = ----- / 51 × 100 = ----- %	A
G. Sitting	Total Dimension B /60 = ----- / 60 × 100 = ----- %	B
H. Crawling & Kneeling	Total Dimension C /42 = ----- / 42 × 100 = ----- %	C
I. Standing	Total Dimension D /39 = ----- / 39 × 100 = ----- %	D
J. Walking, Running & Jumping	Total Dimension E /72 = ----- / 72 × 100 = ----- %	E

TOTAL SCORE = (%A + %B + %C + %D + %E) / Total # of Dimensions = ---- /5 = ------- = ------- %

GOAL

TOTAL = (Sum of % scores for each dimension identified as a goal area) / # of Goal areas = ------ = -------%

SCORE

Reference:https://canchild.ca/system/tenon/assets/attachments/000/000/218/original/gmfm88_and_66_scoresheet.pdf

❑❑❑

95

Harris Hip Score

Objective

The Harris Hip Scale (HHS) was developed for the assessment of the results of hip surgery, and is intended to evaluate various hip disabilities and methods of treatment in an adult population. The original version was published 1969[1]. The HHS is an outcome measure administered by a qualified health care professional, such as a physician or a physical therapist.

Intended Population

People with a total hip replacement (THR), femoral neck fractures or osteoarthritis[2].

Method of Use

No training is required to administer the HHS and it requires very little time or equipment (goniometer, plinth) to complete. There are ten items covering four domains. The domains are pain, function, absence of deformity, and range of motion[2].

The pain domain measures pain severity and its effect on activities and need for pain medication. The function domain is divided into daily activities and gait. The deformity domains observes hip flexion, adduction, internal rotation, and extremity length discrepancy while the range of motion domain asses hip ROM.

The HHS is divided into three sections. The first section are questions about pain and its impact which are answered by the patient or client. The second and third sections require the physiotherapist to assess the patient or client's hip joint and function.

The HHS is a measure of dysfunction so the higher the score, the better the outcome for the individual. Results can be recorded and calculated online. The maximum score possible is 100. Results can be interpreted with the following[1]: <70 = poor result; 70–80 = fair, 80–90 = good, and 90–100 = excellent.

Evidence

Reliability: Test-retest reliability is "excellent" for both physicians ($r = 0.94$) and physiotherapists ($r = 0.95$)[3] with an interval of three to for weeks.

One study[3] reported the inter-rater correlation as good to excellent (0.74–1.0) for the domain scores, as did a study by Kirmit et al[4].

Validity: In terms of content validity, The HHS has demonstrated no major differences when tested against the Western Ontario and McMaster Universities Osteoarthritis Index (WOMAC), and the Short Form 36 (SF-36)[3].

When assessing for construct validity, the pain and function domains in HHS have been shown to correlate with similar domains in the WOMAC[3][5], Nottingham Health Profile[5][6], and the SF-36[3][5], particularly the physical (but not mental) domains of the SF-36[7].

Responsiveness: Wamper et al[8] report unacceptable ceiling effects in 31 of 59 studies. Pooled data across the studies included ($n = 6,667$ patients) suggested ceiling effects of 20% (95% confidence interval 18–22).

In a study of 335 THRs, Shi et al[9] found the HHS was responsive to pain and function at six months post-operatively but week at the two year follow up.

References

1. Harris WH. Traumatic arthritis of the hip after dislocation and acetabular fractures: treatment by mold arthroplasty. An end-result study using a new method of result evaluation. J Bone Joint Surg Am 1969; 51:737–55.

2. Nilsdotter A, Bremander A. Measures of hip function and symptoms: Harris Hip Score (HHS), Hip Disability and Osteoarthritis Outcome Score (HOOS), Oxford Hip Score (OHS), Lequesne Index of Severity for Osteoarthritis of the Hip (LISOH), and American Academy of Orthopedic Surgeons (AAOS) Hip and Knee Questionnaire. Arthritis Care Res. 2011. 63; S11 Supplement: Special Outcomes: S200-S207. Accessed 21 June 2019.
3. Söderman P, Malchau H. Is the Harris hip score system useful to study the outcome of total hip replacement? Clin Orthop Relat Res. 2001 Mar;(384):189-97. Accessed 21 June 2019.
4. Kirmit L, Karatosun V, Unver B, Bakirhan S, Sen A, Gocen Z. The reliability of hip scoring systems for total hip arthroplasty candidates: assessment by physical therapists. Clin Rehabil. 2005 Sep;19 (6):659-61. Accessed 21 June 2019.
5. Soderman P, Malchau H, Herberts P.Outcome of total hip replacement: a comparison of different measurement methods. Clin Orthop Relat Res 2001; 390:163–72.
6. Garellick G, Malchau H, Herberts P.Specific or general health outcome measures in the evaluation of total hip replacement: a comparison between the Harris Hip Score and the Nottingham Health Profile. J Bone Joint Surg Br 1998; 80: 600–6.
7. Lieberman JR, Dorey F, Shekelle P,Schumacher L, Kilgus DJ, Thomas BJ, et al.Outcome after total hip arthroplasty: comparison of a traditional disease-specific and a quality-of-life measurement of outcome. J Arthroplasty 1997; 12: 639–45.
8. Wamper KE, Sierevelt IN, Poolman RW, Bhandari M, Haverkamp D. The Harris hip score: Do ceiling effects limit its usefulness in orthopedics? Acta Orthop. 2010 Dec;81 (6):703-7. Accessed 21 June 2019.
9. Shi HY, Mau LW, Chang JK, Wang JW,Chiu HC. Responsiveness of the Harris Hip Score and the SF-36: five years after total hip arthroplasty. Qual Life Res 2009; 18:1053–60. Accessed 22 June 2019.

Harris Hip Score

Section 1

	Pain		Support
☐	None, or ignores it	☐	None
☐	Slight, occasional, no compromise in activity	☐	Cane/Walking stick for long walks
☐	Mild pain, no effect on average activities, rarely moderate pain with unusual activity, may take aspirin	☐	Cane/Walking stick most of the time
☐	Moderate pain, tolerable but makes concessions to pain. Some limitations of ordinary activity or work. May require occasional pain medication stronger than aspirin	☐	One crutch
☐	Marked pain, serious limitation of activities	☐	Two Canes/Walking sticks
☐	Totally disabled, crippled, pain in bed, bedridden	☐	Two crutches or not able to walk

	Distance walked		Limp
☐	Unlimited	☐	None
☐	Six blocks (30 minutes)	☐	Slight
☐	Two or three blocks (10 - 15 minutes)	☐	Moderate

☐	Indoors only	☐	Severe or unable to walk
☐	Bed and chair only		

Activities - shoes, socks		**Stairs**	
☐	With ease	☐	Normally without using a railing
☐	With difficulty	☐	Normally using a railing
☐	Unable to fit or tie	☐	In any manner
		☐	Unable to do stairs

Public transportation		**Sitting**	
☐	Able to use transportation (bus)	☐	Comfortably, ordinary chair for one hour
☐	Unable to use public transportation (bus)	☐	On a high chair for 30 minutes
		☐	Unable to sit comfortably on any chair

To score this section all four must be 'yes', then get 4 points. Nb. Not 1 point for each four or nothing.

Section 2	
Does your patient have ALL of the following: -	
☐ yes ☐ no	Less than 30degrees of fixed flexion Less than 10 degrees of fixed int rotation in extension Less than 10 degrees of fixed adduction Limb length discrepancy less than 3.2 cm (1.5 inches)

Section 3 - Motion			
Total degrees of Flexion		**Total degrees of Abduction**	
☐	None	☐	None
☐	0 >8	☐	0 > 5
☐	8 > 16	☐	5 > 10
☐	16 > 24	☐	10 > 15
☐	24 > 32	☐	15 > 20
☐	32 > 40	**Total degrees of Ext Rotation**	
☐	40 > 45	☐	None

☐	45 > 55	☐	0 > 5
☐	55 > 65	☐	5 > 10
☐	65 > 70	☐	10 > 15
☐	70 > 75	**Total degrees of Adduction**	
☐	75 > 80	☐	None
☐	80 > 90	☐	0 > 5
☐	90 > 100	☐	5 > 10
☐	100 > 110	☐	10 > 15

Reference for Score: Harris WH. Traumatic arthritis of the hip after dislocation and acetabular fractures: treatment by mold arthroplasty. An end-result study using a new method of result evaluation. J Bone Joint Surg Am. 1969 Jun;51(4):737-55

Reference for grading: Marchetti P, Binazzi R, Vaccari V, Girolami M, Morici F, Impallomeni C, Commessatti M, Silvello L. Long-term results with cementless Fitek (or Fitmore) cups. J Arthroplasty. 2005 Sep;20(6): 730-7.

❑❑❑

96 Oxford Knee Score

Objective

The Oxford Knee Score (OKS) was developed in 1998 and validated to measure pain and function after total knee replacement[1].

Intended Population

The OKS was originally developed and validated for use with individuals undergoing knee arthroplasty but has also been used to measure outcomes in pharmacological treatments, after osteotomies, following rehabilitation or with fractures[2]. It is a primary outcome measure of choice for national audits of knee replacements[3]. It has also been used to predict revisions six months after replacement[4].

Method of Use

The OKS is a patient reported outcome measure that consists of 12 questions obout an individual's activities of daily living and how they have been affected by pain over the preceding four weeks.

Questions

The patient is first asked to date their questionnaire and confirm which side/leg they are receiving treatment for. If both knees are involved, a questionnaire is done for each leg[5].

From Dawson et al 1998[1] and Oxford University Innovation[5]	
Questions	Scoring
How would you describe the pain you usually have from your knee?	None Very mild Mild Moderate Severe
2. Have you had any trouble with washing and drying yourself (all over) because of your knee?	No trouble Very little trouble Moderate trouble Extreme difficulty Impossible to do
3. Have you had any trouble getting in and out of a car or using public transport because of your knee? (whichever you tend to use)	No trouble Very little trouble Moderate trouble Extreme difficulty Impossible to do

4. For how long have you been able to walk before the pain from your knee becomes severe (with or without a stick)	No pain/more than 30 minutes 16 to 30 minutes 5 to 15 minutes Around the house only Not at all/pain severe when walking
5. After a meal (sat at a table), how painful has it been for you to stand up from a chair because of your knee?	Not at all painful Slightly painful Moderately painful Very painful Unbearable
6. Have you been limping when walking, because of your knee?	Rarely/ never Sometimes, or just at first Often,not just at first Most of the time All of the time
7. Could you kneel down and get up again afterwards?	Yes, easily With little difficulty With moderate difficulty With extreme difficulty No, impossible
8. Have you been troubled by pain from your knee in bed at night?	No nights Only 1 or 2 nights Some nights Most nights Every night
9. How much has pain from your knee interfered with your usual work (including housework)?	Not at all A little bit Moderately Greatly Totally
10. Have you felt that your knee might suddenly "give way" or let you down?	Rarely/ never Sometimes, or just at first Often, not just at first Most of the time All of the time
11. Could you do the household shopping on your own?	Yes, easily With little difficulty With moderate difficulty With extreme difficulty No, impossible
12. Could you walk down a flight of stairs?	Yes, easily With little difficulty With moderate difficulty With extreme difficulty No, impossible

Scoring

When the OKS was originally developed, it was designed to be as simple as possible in order to promote use. The original scoring system was a 1-5 where one represented the best outcome[5]. However, clinicians found this confusing in practice and adaptations began to appear so the original authors developed a new scoring system from 0-4 where four is the best outcome and total scores range from 0 (worst outcome) to 48 (best outcome)[5].

If there are more than two missing answers, it is recommended that the overall score should not be calculated. In the event one or two questions are unanswered, it is recommended that clinicians put in a mean answer from the patient's other answer, If a question has more than one answer, the worst response i.e. smallest number is used for calculations[5].

Equipment: Pen and paper, or online calculator.

Reference: Original article by Dawson et al 1998

Evidence

Reliability: The OKS has demonstrated strong test-retest reliability in its original testing[1]. A 2016 systematic review of 23 studies found good evidence of its reproducibility[6].

Validity: OKS shows significant correlation with similar measures (American Knee Society Score, SF-36, Health Assessment Questionnaire), particularly the pain and physical function domains[1]. A 2016 systematic review (23 studies) found good evidence for its internal consistency and construct validity[6].

Responsiveness: Research suggests the OKS is responsive to change post operatively [1][6] and a change of four or more points represents "real" change for an individual while a change of seven or more points represents "clinically relevant"[7].

Miscellaneous: Research[8] suggests that the OKS should not be used to decide whether or not an individual should have surgery because it can be biased in regards to gender, older age and to individuals reporting worse symptoms in order to meet criteria for surgery. Instead, the individual's pain symptoms should be used to determine surgery.

References

1. Dawson J, Fitzpatrick R, Murray D, Carr A. Questionnaire on the perceptions of patients about total knee replacement surgery. J. Bone Joint Surg 1998; 80-B:63-69. Accessed 15 January 2020.
2. Murray D, Rogers K, Pandit H, Beard D, Carr A, Dawson, J. The use of the Oxford Hip and Knee Scores. The Journal of Bone and Joint Surgery. 2007. 89; 8: 1010-4. Accessed 2 December 2019.
3. Browne J, Lewsey L, Van Der Muelen J, Black N. Report to the Department of Health. London, UK: London School of Hygiene & Tropical Medicine; 2007. Patient Reported Outcome Measures (PROMS) in Elective Surgery.
4. Rothwell A, Hooper G, Hobbs A, Frampton C. An analysis of the Oxford hip and knee scores and their relationship to early joint revision in the New Zealand Joint Registry. J Bone Joint Surg Br. 2010 Mar;92(3):413-8. Accessed 15 January 2020.
5. Oxford University Innovation. The Oxford Knee Score (OKS). 2016. Accessed online from https://innovation.ox.ac.uk/outcome-measures/oxford-knee-score-oks/ on 15 January 2020.
6. Harris K, Dawson J, Gibbons E, Lim C, Beard D, Fitzpatrick R, Price A. Systematic review of measurement properties of patient-reported outcome measures used in patients undergoing hip and knee arthroplasty. Patient Relat Outcome Meas. 2016; 7: 101–108. Published online 2016 Jul 25. doi: 10.2147/PROM.S97774. Accessed 15 January 2020.
7. Beard D, Harris K, Dawson J, Doll H, Murray DW, Carr AJ, Price AJ. Meaningful changes for the Oxford hip and knee scores after joint replacement surgery. J Clin Epidemiol. 2015 Jan;68(1):73-9. doi: 10.1016/j.jclinepi.2014.08.009. Epub 2014 Oct 31. Accessed 15 January 2020.
8. Robb C, McBryde C, Caddy S, Thomas A, Pynser P. Oxford scores as a triage tool for lower limb arthroplasty lead to discrimination and health inequalities. Ann R Coll Surg Engl (Suppl) 2013; 95. Accessed 15 January 2020.

❑❑❑

97

Oxford Hip Score

Introduction

The Oxford Hip Score (OHS) is a joint-specific, patient-reported outcome measure tool designed to assess disability in patients undergoing total hip replacement (THR)[1]. It was developed in 1996[2] to be simple to administer in order to facilitate use[2], with new scoring introduced in 2007[3].

Objective

Its primary goal during development was to assess pain and function in patients undergoing joint replacement surgery. Apart from it's utility in evaluating THR patients, the OHS is also used to assess patients after alternative non-surgical interventions. This includes physical therapy, joint supplements, and anti-inflammatory medications.

The OHS is used for studies, trials and national registers[4].

Method of Use

The OHS is a short 12-item survey that can be done with pen and paper, or online. Patients are asked to reflect on their pain and functional ability over the previous four weeks. There are two domains (pain and function) with six items or questions in each. Each item has five possible responses. In the original scoring[2] responses were from 1 = least difficult to 5= most difficult. Item scores are summed to give a total score from anywhere between 12 and 60. The lower the score, the better the outcome.

In a 2007 update, due to confusion and variability in the clinical setting, the original authors recommended using the following scoring: Responses range from 0 to 4 where 0 represents the worst outcome and 4 represents the best, In this use, 48 is the maximum (and best) score achievable[3]. A guide to the new scoring can be found here. A minimum clinically important difference of 3-5 points has been suggested by not verified[3].

Regardless of which scoring system is used, it should be clearly documented which one is used[3].

Score Interpretation

The scores for the 0-48 scale can be interpreted as follows[5]:

Score 0 to 19 May indicate severe hip arthritis. It is highly likely that you may well require some form of surgical intervention, contact your family physician for a consult with an orthopaedic surgeon.

Score 20 to 29 May indicate moderate to severe hip arthritis. See your family physician for an assessment and x-ray. Consider a consult with an orthopaedic surgeon.

Score 30 to 39 May indicate mild to moderate hip arthritis. Consider seeing your family physician for an assessment and possible x-ray. You may benefit from non-surgical treatment, such as exercise, weight loss, and/ or anti-inflammatory medication.

Score 40 to 48 May indicate satisfactory joint function. May not require any formal treatment.

Validity and Reliability

One review[4] of the OHS alongside other similar outcome measures noted the OHS has "excellent psychometric properties" although issues to look out for were double-barrelled questions and a lack of questions regarding medication and aids.

Nilsdotter et al[4] reported that the OHS more responsive than both generic measures, such as the Short Form 36 and EuroQol 5-domain, and the disease-specific measures the Western Ontario and McMaster Universities Osteoarthritis Index and the Arthritis Impact Measurement Scales.

A review of the validity of this score has shown a strong correlation, practicable, reliable, and valid for self assessment of pain and function in German-speaking patients with hip osteoarthritis[6]. The OHS has also been translated to Dutch[7], Japanese[8] and French[9].

References

1. Wylde V, Learmonth ID, Cavendish VJ. The Oxford hip score: the patient's perspective. Health and quality of life outcomes. 2005 Dec;3(1):66. Accessed 24 June 2019.
2. Dawson J, Fitzpatrick R, Carr A, Murray D. Questionnaire on the perceptions of patients about total hip replacement. J Bone Joint Surg Br 1996; 78: 185–90. Accessed 24 June 2019.
3. Murray DW, Fitzpatrick R, Rogers K,Pandit H, Beard DJ, Carr AJ, et al. The use of the Oxford Hip and Knee Scores. J Bone Joint Surg Br 2007; 89: 1010–4. Accessed 24 June 2019.
4. Nilsdotter A, Bremander A. Measures of hip function and symptoms: Harris Hip Score (HHS), Hip Disability and Osteoarthritis Outcome Score (HOOS), Oxford Hip Score (OHS), Lequesne Index of Severity for Osteoarthritis of the Hip (LISOH), and American Academy of Orthopedic Surgeons (AAOS) Hip and Knee Questionnaire. Arthritis Care Res. 2011. 63; S11 Supplement: Special Outcomes: S200-S207. Accessed 21 June 2019.
5. MEDICI Medical Practice, 2019. Accessed 24 June 2019. Available from: http://www.medicipractice.co.uk/navigator/oxford-hip-score/
6. Florian D, Marc S, Franco M, Fabian VK, Anne F, Micheal L. Reliability and Validity of the cross-culturally Adapted German Oxford Hip Score. Clin Orthop Relat Res. 2009;467(4):952-957. Accessed 24 June 2019.
7. Gosens T, Hoefnagels NH, de Vet RC,Dhert WJ, van Langelaan EJ, Bulstra SK, et al.The "Oxford Heup Score": the translation and validation of a questionnaire into Dutch to evaluate the results of total hip arthroplasty. Acta Orthop 2005; 76: 204–11.
8. Uesugi Y, Makimoto K, Fujita K, Nishii T,Sakai T, Sugano N. Validity and responsiveness of the Oxford Hip Score in a prospective study with Japanese total hip arthroplasty patients. J Orthop Sci 2009; 14:35–9.
9. Delaunay C, Epinette JA, Dawson J,Murray D, Jolles BM. Cross-cultural adaptations of the Oxford-12 Hip score to the French speaking population. Orthop Traumatol Surg Res 2009; 95: 89–99.

Oxford Hip Score

During the past 4 weeks......

1. How would you describe the pain you usually have in your hip?		**7. Have you been able to put on a pair of socks, stockings or tights?**	
☐	None	☐	Yes, easily
☐	Very mild	☐	With little difficulty
☐	Mild	☐	With moderate difficulty
☐	Moderate	☐	With extreme difficulty
☐	Severe	☐	No, impossible

2. Have you been troubled by pain from your hip in bed at night?	
☐	No nights
☐	Only 1 or 2 nights
☐	Some nights
☐	Most nights
☐	Every night

3. Have you had any sudden, severe pain (shooting, stabbing, or spasms) from your affected hip?	
☐	No days
☐	Only 1 or 2 days
☐	Some days
☐	Most days
☐	Every day

4. Have you been limping when walking because of your hip?	
☐	Rarely/never
☐	Sometimes or just at first
☐	Often, not just at first
☐	Most of the time
☐	All of the time

8. After a meal (sat at a table), how painful has it been for you to stand up from a chair because of your hip?	
☐	Not at all painful
☐	Slightly painful
☐	Moderately painful
☐	Very painful
☐	Unbearable

9. Have you had any trouble getting in and out of a car or using public transportation because of your hip?	
☐	No trouble at all
☐	Very little trouble
☐	Moderate trouble
☐	Extreme difficulty
☐	Impossible to do

10. Have you had any trouble with washing and drying yourself (all over) because of your hip?	
☐	No trouble at all
☐	Very little trouble
☐	Moderate trouble
☐	Extreme difficulty
☐	Impossible to do

	5. For how long have you been able to walk before the pain in your hip becomes severe (with or without a walking aid)?
☐	No pain for 30 minutes or more
☐	16 to 30 minutes
☐	5 to 15 minutes
☐	Around the house only
☐	Not at all

	6. Have you been able to climb a flight of stairs?
☐	Yes, easily
☐	With little difficulty
☐	With moderate difficulty
☐	With extreme difficulty
☐	No, impossible

	11. Could you do the household shopping on your own?
☐	Yes, easily
☐	With little difficulty
☐	With moderate difficulty
☐	With extreme difficulty
☐	No, impossible

	12. How much has pain from your hip interfered with your usual work, including housework?
☐	Not at all
☐	A little bit
☐	Moderately
☐	Greatly
☐	Totally

Grading for the Oxford Hip Score	
Score 0 to 19	May indicate severe hip arthritis. It is highly likely that you may well require some form of surgical intervention, contact your family physician for a consult with an Orthopaedic Surgeon.
Score 20 to 29	May indicate moderate to severe hip arthritis. See your family physician for an assessment and x-ray. Consider a consult with an Orthopaedic Surgeon.
Score 30 to 39	May indicate mild to moderate hip arthritis. Consider seeing you family physician for an assessment and possible x-ray. You may benefit from non-surgical treatment, such as exercise, weight loss, and / or anti-inflammatory medication
Score 40 to 48	May indicate satisfactory joint function. May not require any formal treatment.

Reference for Score: Dawson J, Fitzpatrick R, Carr A, Murray D. Questionnaire on the perceptions of patients about total hip replacement. J Bone Joint Surg Br. 1996 Mar;78(2):185-90.

❑❑❑

98 Headache Disability Index

NAME: **Age** **DATE:**

Score Total = ---- / 100 : E ---- / (52s) : F ---- / (48)

INSTRUCTIONS: Please CIRCLE the correct response:

1. I have headaches: [1] I per month [2] more than I but less than 4 per month [3] more than one per week
2. My headache is: [1] mild [2] moderate [3] severe

Instructions: (Please read carefully): The purpose of the scale is to identify difficulties that you may be experiencing because of your headache. Please check off "YES", *SOMETIMES', OR'NO" to each item. Answer each question as it pertains to your headache only.

	Yes	Some times	No
El. Because of my headaches I feel handicapped.			
F2. Because of my headaches I feel restricted in performing my routine daily activities.			
E3. No one understands the effect my headaches have on my life.			
F4. I restrict my recreational activities (e.g. sports, hobbies) because of my headaches.			
E5. My headaches make me angry.			
E6. Sometimes I feel that I am going to lose control because of my headaches.			
F7 . Because of my headaches I am less likely to sociaLize.			
E8. My spouse (significant other), or family and friends have no idea what I am going through because of my headaches.			
E9. My headaches are so bad that I feel I am going to go insane.			
E10. My outlook on the world is affected by my headaches.			
Ell. I am afraid to go outside when I feel that a headache is starting.			
E12. I feel desperute because of my headaches.			
F13. I am conceryed that I am paying penalties at work or at home because ofmy headaches.			
E14. My headaches place stess on my relationships with familv or friends.			
F15. I avoid being around people when I have a headache.			
F16. I believe my headaches are making it difficult for me to achieve my goalsin life.			
Fl7. I am unable to think clearly because of my headaches.			
F18. I get tense (e.g. muscle tension) because of my headaches.			
F19. I do not enioy social gatherings because of my headaches.			
E20. I feel irritable because of my headaches.			

Fzl. I avoid traveling because of my headaches.			
822. My headaches make me feel confused.			
F;23. My headaches make me feel frushated.			
F24. I find it difficult to read because of my headaches.			
F25. I find it diffrcult to focus my attention away from my headaches and on other things.			

Jacobson Gary P., Ramadan NM, et al., The Henry Ford Hospital headache disability inventory GIDD. Neurology 1994;44:837-842.

❑❑❑

99 The Migraine Disability Assessment Test

The MIDAS (Migraine Disability Assessment) questionnaire was put together to help you measure the impact your headaches have on your life. The information on this questionnaire is also helpful for your primary care provider to determine the level of pain and disability caused by your headaches and to find the best treatment for you.

INSTRUCTIONS

Please answer the following questions about ALL of the headaches you have had over the last 3 months. Select your answer in the box next to each question. Select zero if you did not have the activity in the last 3 months. Please take the completed form to your healthcare professional.

1. On how many days in the last 3 months did you miss work or school because of your headaches?
2. How many days in the last 3 months was your productivityatworkorschoolreducedbyhalformore because of your headaches? (Do not include days you counted in question 1 where you missed work or school.)
3. On how many days in the last 3 months did you not do household work (such as housework, home repairs and maintenance, shopping, caring for children and relatives) because of your headaches?
4. How many days in the last 3 months was your productivity in household work reduced by half of more because of your headaches? (Do not include days you counted in question 3 where you did not do household work.)
5. On how many days in the last 3 months did you miss family, social or leisure activities because of your headaches?

Total (Questions 1-5)

What your Physician will need to know about your headache:

A. On how many days in the last 3 months did you have a headache? (If a headache lasted more than 1 day, count each day.)

B. On a scale of 0 - 10, on average how painful were these headaches? (where 0=no pain at all, and 10= pain as bad as it can be.)

Scoring: After you have filled out this questionnaire, add the total number of days from questions 1-5 (ignore A and B).

MIDAS Grade	Definition	MIDAS Score
I	Little or No Disability	0-5
II	Mild Disability	6-10
III	Moderate Disability	11-20
IV	Severe Disability	21+

If Your MIDAS Score is 6 or more, please discuss this with your doctor.

❑❑❑

100 High Level Mobility and Assessment Tool (HiMAT)

Objective

The High Level Mobility and Assessment tool (HiMAT) is a standardised outcome measure used to quantify motor performance in individuals with high-level balance and mobility deficits. It was created by Gavin Williams in 2005 to address a gap in uni-dimensional tools for recording high-level motor function in people with traumatic brain injury (TBI). The HiMAT is scored over 13 items which were derived from the opinions' of expert clinicians and from existing multi-dimensional mobility scales.[1][2]

Intended Population

Although designed for use with patients with TBI, the HiMAT can be used for a number of other neurological and musculoskeletal conditions that result in vestibular and motor deficits. For example, in stroke victims and Parkinson's patients - particularly in young adults[3]. As per the tool instructions, those being assessed using the HiMAT must at least have the ability to walk greater than 20 meters independently without gait aids and with or without orthoses.

Method of Use

Equipment Required

- at least 20m even surface walkway
- 1 house brick
- access to a flight of 14 stairs
- stopwatch
- tape measure
- pen and a copy of the HiMAT tool

Preparation of Environment

- Measure and mark a 20m walkway to count the middle 10m

Instructions

- Patients are permitted 1 practice trial per item
- Patients are to perform each task at the maximum safe speed except for bounding and stair items
- All items (except stairs) are timed or counted in the middle 10m of the 20m walkway
- The items to be scored are: {| class="wikitable" !HiMAT TASKS |- |walk |- |walk backwards |- |walk on toes |- |walk over obstacle |- |run |- |skip |- |hop forward (affected) |- |bound (affected) |- |bound (less affected) |- |up stairs dependent (rail OR not reciprocal; if not score 5 and rate below) |- |up stairs independent (no rail AND reciprocal: if not score 0 and rate above) |- |down stairs dependent (rail OR not reciprocal; if not score 5 and rate below) |- |down stairs independent (no rail AND reciprocal: if not score 0 and rate above) |}

Scoring

- Each item is categorised into points 1 being the lowest score and 4 being the highest
- The faster the task is completed OR the greater the distance achieved, the higher the score
- Total score is out of 54

Evaluation

In January 2013, the Traumatic Brain Injury Evidence Database to Guide Effectiveness (TBIEDGE) task force presented a compilation of outcome measure recommendations for clinicians working with TBI patients. Below is a table showing their final recommendations; the conclusion being that the HiMAT is highly recommended in the outpatient setting as a standardised outcome measure.[5

References

1. Williams G, Robertson V, Greenwood K, Goldie P & Morris, M. The high-level mobility assessment tool (HiMAT) for traumatic brain injury. Part 1: Item Generation, Brain Injury, 2005;19(11): 925-932.https://www.tandfonline.com/doi/abs/10.1080/02699050500058687 (accessed 10/06/18).
2. Williams, G. The High Level Mobility Assessment Tool. The Center for Outcome Measurement in Brain Injury. 2006. (accessed August 26, 2019).
3. Williams G, Robertson V, Greenwood K, Goldie P & Morris M. The high-level mobility assessment tool (HiMAT) for traumatic brain injury. Part 2: Content validity and discriminability, Brain Injury, 2009;19(10):833-843https://www.tandfonline.com/doi/abs/10.1080/02699050500058687
4. Carl Peterson. Neuro #3, Outcome Measure: High Level Mobility Assessment Tool. Available from https://www.youtube.com/watch?v=IdkfvcxYjh0 [last accessed 15/06/2018]
5. McCulloch K, De Joya A, Donnelly E, Kayes K, Johnson T, Nirider C, Roth H, Saliga S, Ward I. TBIEDGE Task Force

HiMAT: HIGH LEVEL MOBILITY ASSESSMENT TOOL

Date...................................... Date Of Accident................. Diagnosis............................. Affected Side Left / Right

Patient Id Label

			Score					
Item	**Performance**		**0**	**1**	**2**	**3**	**4**	**5**
Walk		sec	X	> 6.6	5.4-6.6	4.3-5.3	< 4.3	X
Walk Backward		sec		> 13.3	8.1-13.3	5.8-8.0	< 5.8	X
Walk on Toes		sec		> 8.9	7.0-8.9	5.4-6.9	< 5.4	X
Walk Over Obstacle		sec		> 7.1	5.4-7.1	4.5-5.3	< 4.5	X
Run		sec		> 2.7	2.0-2.7	1.7-1.9	< 1.7	X
Skip		sec		> 4.0	3.5-4.0	3.0-3.4	< 3.0	X
Hop Forward (Affected)		sec		> 7.0	5.3-7.0	4.1-5.2	< 4.1	X
Bounded (Affected)	(1) (2) (3)	cm cm cm		< 8.0	80-103	104-132	>132	X
Bounded (Less-Affected)	(1) (2) (3)	cm cm cm		< 8.2	82-105	106-129	>129	X
UP Stairs Dependent (Rail OR not reciprocal: if not, score 5 and rate below)		sec		> 22.8	14.6-22.8	12.3-14.5	>12.3	
UP Stairs Independent (No rail AND reciprocal: if not score 0 and rate above)		sec		> 9.1	7.6-9.1	6.8-7.5	<6.8	X
Down Stairs Dependent (Rail OR not reciprocal: if not score 5 and rate below)		sec		> 24.3	17.6-24.3	12.8-17.5	<12.8	
Down Stairs Independent (No rail AND reciprocal: if not score 0 and rate above)		sec		> 8.4	6.6-8.4	5.8-6.5	<5.8	X
		Subtotal						

❑❑❑

101 Hip Disability and Osteoarthritis Outcome Score

Objective

The hip disability and osteoarthritis outcome score (HOOS) is a questionnaire intended to be used to assess the patient's opinion about their hip and associated problems and to evaluate symptoms and functional limitations related to the hip during a therapeutic process [1][2]. Other questionnaires that can be presented are the Western Ontario and McMaster Universities Osteoarthritis Index (WOMAC), the Algo Functional Index (AFI) and the Intermittent and Constant Osteoarthritis Pain Index (ICOAP) [3].

Intended Population

This measuring instrument, judging functions and anatomical qualities combined with activities and participation, is recommended when there is talk of hip disability with or without osteoarthritis (OA). Hip osteoarthritis is a common and chronic musculoskeletal condition and a cause of pain, functional disability and reduced quality of life [4]. The HOOS is meant to be used over short and long-term intervals to assess changes induced by treatment (medication, physical therapy, operation) or over years due to the primary injury or post-traumatic osteoarthritis [2].

Method of Use

The HOOS questionnaire is self explanatory, user-friendly, patient-administered and takes 7 to 10 minutes to complete. The outcome score consists of 40 items assessing 5 subscales. The 5 separate patient-relevant dimensions are Pain (P), Symptoms (S), Activity limitations daily living (ADL), Function in sport and recreation (SP) and hip related quality of life (QOL). Pain (P) includes 10 items with a total score of 40 points, Symptoms (S) includes 5 items with a total score of 20, Activity limitations daily living (ADL) includes 17 items with a total score of 68 and finally Function in sport and recreation (SP) and hip related quality of life both include 4 items with a total score of 16 each.

To answer the questions, standardized answer options are given in 5 Likert-boxes with scores from 0 to 4 (no, mild, moderate, severe and extreme).

To interpret the score, the outcome measure is transformed in a worst to best scale from 0 to 100, with 100 indicating no symptoms and 0 indicating extreme symptoms.

To calculate the total HOOS score the subscales need to be summed up, using following formula for all dimension.

100 – [(patient's score of the subscale x 100)/(total score of the subscale)]

The subscales can be plotted as a HOOS profile, by connecting the mean scores for all 5 dimensions with a line[1][2].

Evidence

Reliability

The Dutch hip disability and osteoarthritis outcome score questionnaire has a good internal consistency and reliability [5]. The HOOS score is entirely based on self-report of functional status and performance. This may be a disadvantage in comparison to instruments that include objective physical examination findings or an assessment of symptoms. It is recommended to use the HOOS score as a tool to complete additional information [6].

Validity

The construct validity is good with absence of floor and ceiling effects [5]. The hip osteoarthritis outcome score is valid in a sample of subject at a mean of 3 years after hip arthroscopy and for patients with different stadia of hip OA [5][6].

Responsiveness

Thanks to the addition of two subscales, sport and recreation function (SP) and hip related quality of life (QOL), the HOOC shows a higher sensitivity and responsiveness, compared to the Western Ontario and McMaster Universities osteoarthritis index (WOMAC). Patients younger than 66 years report higher responsiveness in all five subscales than patients older than 66 years [1].

References

1. NILSDOTTER A.K., LOHMANDER L.S., KLÄSSBO M., ROOS E.M., Hip disability and osteoarthritis outcome score (HOOS) – validity and responsiveness in total hip replacement, BMC Musculoskeletal Disord., May 2003, level of quality C
2. Pain symptoms ADL, Hip disability and osteoarthritis outcome score (HOOS). www.koos.nu (accessed 23 October)
3. KNGF-guidline, osteoarthritis of the hip and knee. https://www.kngfrichtlijnen.nl/downloads/Osteoarthritis_of_the_hip_and_knee_V06-2010_PRL_ENG.pdf (accessed 23 October)
4. POULSEN E., Conservative treatment of hip osteoarthritis: effect of manual therapy and hip school on pain, function and quality of life – a single-blind randomized controlled trial (abstract), December 2009
5. DE GROOT I.B., REIJMAN M., TERWEE C.B., BEIRMA-ZEINSTRA S.M.A., FAVEJEE M., ROOS E.M., VERHAAR J., Validation of the Dutch version of the hip disability and osteoarthritis outcome score, Osteoarthritis and cartilage, vol. 15 nr. 1, 2007, page. 104-109, level of quality C
6. MARTIN R.L., PHILIPPON M.J., Evidence of validity for the hip outcome score in hip arthroscopy, The journal of arthroscopic and related surgery, vol. 23 nr. 8, August 2007, page. 822-826, level of quality B

Hip Disability and Osteoarthritis Outcome Score

Symptoms: These questions should be answered thinking of your hip symptoms during the **last week.**

S1. Do you feel grinding, hear clicking or any other type of noise from you hip?

(1) Never (2) Rarely
(3) Sometimes (4) Often
(5) Always

S2. Difficulties spreading legs wide apart

(1) None (2) Mild
(3) Moderate (4) Severe
(5) Extreme

S3. Difficulties to stride out when walking

(1) None (2) Mild
(3) Moderate (4) Severe
(5) Extreme

Stiffness: The following questions concern the amount of joint stiffness you have experienced during the last week in your hip. Stiffness is a sensation of restriction or slowness in the ease with which you move your hip joint.

S4. How severe is your hip joint stiffness after first wakening in the morning?

(1) None (2) Mild
(3) Moderate (4) Severe
(5) Extreme

S5. How severe is your hip stiffness after sitting, lying or resting later in the day?

(1) None (2) Mild
(3) Moderate (4) Severe
(5) Extreme

Subtotal:

Pain

P1. How often is your hip painful?

(1) Never (2) Monthly
(3) Weekly (4) Daily
(5) Always

What amount of hip pain have you experienced the last week during the following activities?

P2. Straightening your hip fully

(1) None (2) Mild
(3) Moderate (4) Severe
(5) Extreme

P3. Bending your hip fully

(1) None (2) Mild
(3) Moderate (4) Severe
(5) Extreme

P4. Walking on flat surface
(1) None (2) Mild
(3) Moderate (4) Severe
(5) Extreme

P5. Going up or down stairs
(1) None (2) Mild
(3) Moderate (4) Severe
(5) Extreme

P6. At night while in bed
(1) None (2) Mild
(3) Moderate (4) Severe
(5) Extreme

P7. Sitting or lying
(1) None (2) Mild
(3) Moderate (4) Severe
(5) Extreme

P8. Standing upright
(1) None (2) Mild
(3) Moderate (4) Severe
(5) Extreme

P9. Walking on a hard surface (asphalt, concrete, etc)
(1) None (2) Mild
(3) Moderate (4) Severe
(5) Extreme

P10. Walking on an uneven surface
(1) None (2) Mild
(3) Moderate (4) Severe
(5) Extreme

Subtotal:

Function, daily living: The following questions concern your physical function. By this we mean your ability to move around and to look after yourself. For each of the following activities please indicate the degree of difficulty you have experienced in the last week due to your hip.

Al. Descending stairs
(1) None (2) Mild
(3) Moderate (4) Severe
(5) Extreme

A2. Ascending stairs
(1) None (2) Mild
(3) Moderate (4) Severe
(5) Extreme

A3. Rising from sitting
(1) None (2) Mild
(3) Moderate (4) Severe
(5) Extreme

A4. Standing
(1) None (2) Mild
(3) Moderate (4) Severe
(5) Extreme

A5. Bending to floor/pick up an object
(1) None (2) Mild
(3) Moderate (4) Severe
(5) Extreme

A6. Walking on flat surface
(1) None (2) Mild
(3) Moderate (4) Severe
(5) Extreme

A7. Getting in/out of car
(1) None (2) Mild
(3) Moderate (4) Severe
(5) Extreme

A8. Going shopping
(1) None (2) Mild
(3) Moderate (4) Severe
(5) Extreme

A9. Putting on socks/stockings
(1) None (2) Mild
(3) Moderate (4) Severe
(5) Extreme

A10. Rising from bed
(1) None (2) Mild
(3) Moderate (4) Severe
(5) Extreme

A11. Taking off socks/stockings
(1) None (2) Mild
(3) Moderate (4) Severe
(5) Extreme

A12. Lying in bed (turning over, maintaining hip position)
(1) None (2) Mild
(3) Moderate (4) Severe
(5) Extreme

A13. Getting in/out of bath

(1) None (2) Mild
(3) Moderate (4) Severe
(5) Extreme

A14. Sitting

(1) None (2) Mild
(3) Moderate (4) Severe
(5) Extreme

A15. Getting on/off toilet

(1) None (2) Mild
(3) Moderate (4) Severe
(5) Extreme

A16. Heavy domestic duties (moving heavy boxes, scrubbing floors, etc)

(1) None (2) Mild
(3) Moderate (4) Severe
(5) Extreme

A17. Light domestic duties (cooking, dusting, etc)

(1) None (2) Mild
(3) Moderate (4) Severe
(5) Extreme

Subtotal:

Function, sports and recreational activities: The following questions concern your physical function when being active on a higher level. The questions should be answered thinking of what degree of difficulty you have experienced during the last week due to your hip.

SP1. Squatting

(1) None (2) Mild
(3) Moderate (4) Severe
(5) Extreme

SP2. Running

(1) None (2) Mild
(3) Moderate (4) Severe
(5) Extreme

SP3. Twisting/pivoting on your injured knee

(1) None (2) Mild
(3) Moderate (4) Severe
(5) Extreme

SP4. Walking on uneven surface

(1) None (2) Mild
(3) Moderate (4) Severe
(5) Extreme

Subtotal:

Quality of Life

Q1. How often are you aware of your hip problem?

(1) Never (2) Monthly
(3) Weekly (4) Daily
(5) Constantly

Q2. Have you modified your life style to avoid potentially damaging activities to your hip?

(1) Not at all (2) Mildly
(3) Moderately (4) Severely
(5) Totally

Q3. How much are you troubled with lack of confidence in your hip?

(1) Not at all (2) Mildly
(3) Moderately (4) Severely
(5) Extremely

Q4. In general, how much difficulty do you have with your hip?

(1) None (2) Mild
(3) Moderate (4) Severe
(5) Extreme

Subtotal:

❑❑❑

102 Non-Arthritic Hip Score

- The Following five questions concern the amount of pain you are currently experiencing in the hip that you are having evaluated today.
- For each situation, please circle the response that most accurately reflects the amount of pain experienced in the past 48 hours.
- Please circle one answer that best describes your situation.

Question-: how much pain you have –

1. Walking on a flat surface?
   4 = none 3 = mild
   2 = moderate 1 = severe
   0 = extreme
2. Going up or down stairs?
   4 = none 3 = mild
   2 = moderate 1 = severe
   0 = extreme
3. At night while in bed?
   4 = none 3 = mild
   2 = moderate 1 = severe
   0 = extreme
4. Sitting or lying?
   4 = none 3 = mild
   2 = moderate 1 = severe
   0 = extreme
5. Standing upright?
   4 = none 3 = mild
   2 = moderate 1 = severe
   0 = extreme

The Following four questions concern the symptoms that you are currently experiencing in the hip that you are having evaluated today.

- For each situation, please circle the response that most accurately reflects the amount of pain experienced in the past 48 hours.
- Please circle one answer that best describes your situation.

Question- how trouble do you have with –

1. Catching or locking of your hip?
   4 = none 3 = mild
   2 = moderate 1 = severe
   0 = extreme
2. Your hip giving way on you?
   4 = none 3 = mild
   2 = moderate 1 = severe
   0 = extreme
3. Stiffness in your hip?
   4 = none 3 = mild
   2 = moderate 1 = severe
   0 = extreme
4. Decreased movement in your hip?
   4 = none 3 = mild
   2 = moderate 1 = severe
   0 = extreme

- The Following five questions concern your physical function.
- For each of the following activities, please circle the response that most accurately reflects the difficulty you have experienced in the past 48 hours because of your hip pain.
- Please circle one answer that best describes your situation.

Question- what degree of difficulty do you have with –

1. Descending stairs?
   4 = none 3 = mild
   2 = moderate 1 = severe
   0 = extreme
2. Ascending stairs?
   4 = none 3 = mild
   2 = moderate 1 = severe
   0 = extreme
3. Rising from sitting?
   4 = none 3 = mild
   2 = moderate 1 = severe
   0 = extreme
4. Putting on socks / stockings?
   4 = none 3 = mild
   2 = moderate 1 = severe
   0 = extreme
5. Rising from bed?
   4 = none 3 = mild
   2 = moderate 1 = severe
   0 = extreme

The Following six questions concern your ability to participate in certain types of activities.

- For each of the following activities, please circle the response that most accurately reflects the difficulty you have experienced in the last month because of your hip pain.
- If you do not participate in a certain type of activity, please estimate how much trouble your hip would have caused if you had to perform that type of activity
- Please circle one answer that best describes your situation

Question- how much pain do you have –

1. High demand sports involving sprinting or cutting (eg football, basket ball, tennis & exercise aerobics)?
   4 = none 3 = mild
   2 = moderate 1 = severe
   0 = extreme
2. Low- demand sports (eg golf / bowling)?
   4 = none 3 = mild
   2 = moderate 1 = severe
   0 = extreme
3. Jogging for exercise?
   4 = none 3 = mild
   2 = moderate 1 = severe
   0 = extreme
4. Walking for exercise?
   4 = none 3 = mild
   2 = moderate 1 = severe
   0 = extreme
5. Heavy household duties (eg lifting firewood / moving furniture)?
   4 = none 3 = mild
   2 = moderate 1 = severe
   0 = extreme
6. Light household duties (eg cooking, dusting, vacuuming & laundry)?
   4 = none 3 = mild
   2 = moderate 1 = severe
   0 = extreme

TOTAL SCORE =

❑❑❑

103 Hoehn and Yahr Scale

Introduction

Hoehn and Yahr was originally published in 1967 in the journal *Neurology* by Margaret Hoehn and Melvin Yahr and included stages 1 through 5[1]. In 1983 Larsen et al. [2] published an article entitled "Theoretical and practical issues in assessment of deficits and therapy in Parkinsonism," wherein they included a modification of the original Hoehn and Yahr scale. They added some minor alterations which did not substantially change the basic classification published in 1967. This scale is used along with Unified Parkinson's Disease Rating Scale for a better assessment of Parkinson's disease.

Purpose

The scale has been used for the staging of the functional disability associated with Parkinson's disease. It helps in describing the progression of the disease through various stages, thus allowing us to measure the severity of the case.

Technique

The assessment requires a medical examination and according to the history given by the patients and their caregivers, the scoring is done.

Stage	Hoehn and Yahr Scale	Modified Hoehn and Yahr Scale
1	Unilateral involvement only usually with minimal or no functional disability	Unilateral involvement only
1.5	—	Unilateral and axial involvement
2	Bilateral or midline involvement without impairment of balance	Bilateral involvement without impairment of balance
2.5	—	Mild bilateral disease with recovery on pull test
3	Bilateral disease: mild to moderate disability with impaired postural reflexes; physically independent	Mild to moderate bilateral disease; some postural instability; physically independent
4	Severely disabling disease; still able to walk or stand unassisted	Severe disability; still able to walk or stand unassisted
5	Confinement to bed or wheelchair unless aided	Wheelchair bound or bedridden unless aided

Evidence

In a review of the use of Hoehn and Yahr staging, the Movement Disorder Society concluded that the modified scale should not be used due to a lack of clinimetric testing, and that the broad categories of the original scale do not allow for detection of effective interventions[3]. For these reasons, the scale is used in clinical trials to define inclusion and exclusion criteria, but not typically as an outcome measure.

References

1. Hoehn MM, Yahr MD. Parkinsonism: onset, progression, and mortality. Neurology. 1998 Feb 1;50(2):318-.

2. Larsen TA, LeWitt PA, Calne DB. Theoretical and practical issues in assessment of deficits and therapy in parkinsonism. Lisuride and other dopamine agonists. 1983:363-73.
3. Goetz CG, Poewe W, Rascol O, Sampaio C, Stebbins GT, Counsell C, Giladi N, Holloway RG, Moore CG, Wenning GK, Yahr MD. Movement Disorder Society Task Force report on the Hoehn and Yahr staging scale: status and recommendations the Movement Disorder Society Task Force on rating scales for Parkinson's disease. Movement disorders. 2004 Sep;19(9):1020-8.

Stage	Hoehn and Yahr Scale	Modified Hoehn and Yahr Scale
1	Unilateral involvement only usually with minimal or no functional disability	Unilateral involvement only
1.5	-	Unilateral and axial involvement
2	Bilateral or midline involvement without impairment of balance	Bilateral involvement without impairment of balance
2.5	-	Mild bilateral disease with recovery on pull test
3	Bilateral disease: mild to moderate disability with impaired postural reflexes; physically independent	Mild to moderate bilateral disease; some postural instability; physically independent
4	Severely disabling disease; still able to walk or stand unassisted	Severe disability; still able to walk or stand unassisted
5	Confinement to bed or wheelchair unless aided	Wheelchair bound or bedridden unless aided

❑❑❑

104 Houghton Scale

Introduction

The Houghton Scale was developed by a team of British researchers, led by a vascular surgeon named A.D. Houghton, MD. They were out to determine the rate of successful rehabilitation among individuals with lower-limb amputations of vascular etiologies. The scale quantifies functional outcomes among people with lower-limb amputations. Devin et al[1] proposed Houghton Scale parallels Medicare K-level classifications. They implied a score > 9 on the Houghton scale indicative of satisfactory rehabilitation corresponds to the K3 functional level (the ability to walk at variable cadence and negotiate most environmental obstacles for prosthesis use beyond simple locomotion) while Houghton score > 6 indicative of mobility on the prosthesis around the house corresponds to the K2 functional level (ability to walk outdoors and negotiate low environmental barriers-curbs and stairs)and Houghton Scale scores < 6 are suggested as corresponding to the K1 functional level (ability to walk on level, indoor surfaces)[2]

Objective

The Houghton scale[3] is a 4-item instrument that accesses prosthetic use in people with lower extremity amputations. It reflects a person's perception of prosthetic use. It's self-administered and easy to score.

Intended Population

The scale is intended for use by individuals with lower limb amputation

Method of Use

The first 3 items are scored on a 4-point scale and it attempts to capture prosthetic wearing habits whilst the fourth question has 3 dichotomous (yes/no) items that assess a patient's comfort level when negotiating different outdoor surfaces. Results are reported as a total score out of 12, with higher scores indicating greater performance and greater comfort.

Houghton Score Categories

It defines community and household walking ability.

- Houghton Scale score ≥ 9- independent community
- Houghton Scale scores 6–8- household and limited community
- Houghton Scale score ≤ 5- limited household

Evidence

Miller et al[4] compared the Houghton Scale with the Prosthesis Evaluation Questionnaire (PEQ) and the Locomotor Capabilities Index of the Prosthetic Profile of the Amputee (PPA) and concluded that Houghton Scale had modest internal consistency, good test retest reliability, and was the only scale tested that could discriminate between people with transfemoral and transtibial amputations.

Reliability

Devlin et al[1] found the reliability of the Houghton Scale to be high .Intraclass correlation coefficient = 0.96 n=49

Validity

Internal consistency moderate at discharge (Cronbach α=.71) and follow-up (Cronbach α=.70)[1]

Significant but moderate correlation between the Houghton Scale and the physical composite score of the Medical Outcomes Study 36-Item Short-Form Health

Survey (r =.393, P <.01) and the 2-minute walk test at admission (r= .620, P <.01) and discharge (r =.653, P <.01)

Responsiveness

Significantly increased scores at 3 months follow up (P<.001) [1]

Mean ± standard deviation of 6.14±2.40 at discharge to 7.70±2.62 at 3 months follow up

References

1. Devlin, M., T. Pauley, K. Head, and S. Garfinkel. 2004. Houghton Scale of prosthetic use in people with lower extremity amputations: Reliability, validity, and responsiveness to change. Archives of Physical Medicine and Rehabilitation 85 (8):1339-44.
2. Wong, C. K., W. Gibbs, and E. S. Chen. 2016. Use of the Houghton scale to classify community and household walking ability in people with lower-limb amputation: Criterion-related validity. Archives of Physical Medicine and Rehabilitation 97 (7):1130-6.
3. Houghton AD, Taylor PR, Thurlow S, Rootes E, McColl I. Success rates for rehabilitation of vascular amputees: implications for preoperative assessment and amputation level. Br J Surg 1992;79:753-5
4. Miller WC, Deathe AB, Speechley M. Lower extremity prosthetic mobility: a comparison of 3 self-report scales. Arch Phys Med Rehabil 2001;84:1432-40.

Houghton Scale

1. Do you wear your prosthesis:
   0-Less than 25% of waking hours(1–3 hours)
   1-Between 25% and 50% of walking hours (4–8 hours)
   2-ore than 50% of waking hours (more than 8 hours)
   3-All waking hours (12–16 hours)
2. Do you use your prosthesis to walk:
   0-Just when visiting the doctor or limb-fitting center
   1-At home but not to go outside
   2-Outside the home on occasion
   3-Inside and outside all the time
3. When going outside wearing your prosthesis, do you:
   0-Use a wheelchair
   1-Use two crutches, two canes, or a walker
   2-Use one cane
   3-Use nothing
4. When walking with your prosthesis outside, do you feel unstable when:
   4a. Walking on a flat surface
   0-Yes 1-No
   4b. Walking on slopes
   0-Yes 1-No
   4c. Walking on rough ground
   0-Yes 1-No

❑❑❑

105 Ibadan Knee/Hip Osteoarthritis Outcome Measure (IKHOAM)

Outcome measures often reflect the environment and culture of the people they were originally developed for. Some of the existing osteoarthritis (OA) outcome measures include few items that may not be readily understood by Nigerian especially those with low educational attainments. Almost all existing OA outcome measures exclude activities that are important to many patients seen in Nigerian clinics. The need to develop an appropriate outcome measure for knee and hip OA for the Nigerian environment was identified [1].

Objective

To assess end results of care in patients with knee and/or hip OA.

Intended Population

Patients with knee and/or hip OA.

Description

The Ibadan Knee/Hip Osteoarthritis Outcome Measure (IKHOAM) is a 3-domain/part, 33- item instrument.

The domains are:

1. **Activity limitations domain (part 1)** - comprises 25 items/activities of daily living that are being performed by individuals with knee/hip osteoarthritis. The degree of difficulty and assistance required in carrying out the activities are rated on a 5 point (0-4) ordinal scale.
2. **Participation restrictions domain (part 2)** – comprises 3 items/activities in societal participation due to knee/hip osteoarthritis. The restrictions experienced in carrying out the activities are rated on a 4 point (0-3) ordinal scale.
3. **Physical performance tests domain (part 3)** – includes 5 tests that are rated by the clinician. These tests are:
   - 250m walk test rated on a 6 point (0-5) ordinal scale.
   - One leg stance test rated on a 6 point (0-5) ordinal scale.
   - Stairs climbing test rated on a 5 point (0-4) ordinal scale.
   - Squat test rated on a 5 point (0-4) ordinal scale.
   - Balance test rated on a 6 point (0-5) ordinal scale.

Parts 1 and 2 are patient reported, which may be completed by the patient (self) or through an interview.

Scoring:

Part one: Maximum obtainable score of 200. Degree of difficulty and nature of assistance required for each of 25 items were scored between 0 and 4 each.

Part two: Extent of participation in performing the three items was scored between 0 and 3 giving a maximum obtainable score of 9.

Part three: Maximum obtainable score of 23 (5 for 250m walk test, 5 for one leg stance test, 4 for stairs climbing test, 4 for squat test, 5 for balance test).

The maximum obtainable score on IKHOAM is 232 (200 + 9 + 23). The score for a subject was calculated in percentage as Subject's score/Total possible score × 100

Low score on IKHOAM implies low level of physical functioning ability and high level means high level of physical functioning ability.

Duration for Completion

About 15 minutes.

Scoring

1. **Part 1 rates** 25 disability attributes on a 5-point ordinal scale for degree of difficulty experienced and nature of assistance required (maximum obtainable score of 200)
2. **Part 2 rates** 3 attributes of participation restrictions on a 4-point ordinal scale(maximum obtainable score of 9)
3. **Part 3 rates** 5 items (maximum obtainable score of 23) maximum obtainable score on IKHOAM is 232(200 + 9 + 23)

Score for a subject can be calculated as subject's score × 100

Validity

Akinpelu AO, Odole AC, Adegoke BOA, Adeniyi AF (2007) Development and Initial Validation of Ibadan Knee/Hip Osteoarthritis Outcome Measure (IKHOAM). South African Journal of Physiotherapy Vol. 63:3-8

Reliability

Akinpelu AO, Akinwola MO, Odole AC, Gbiri CA (2011) The Reliability of the English version of Ibadan Knee/Hip Osteoarthritis Outcome Measure (IKHOAM). Physical and Occupational Therapy in Geriatrics Early online: 1-8 DOI: 10.3109/02/02703181.2011.589566

References

1. Odole AC, Akinpelu AO, Bamgboye EA (2006): Validity and Internal Consistency of a Yoruba version of the Ibadan Knee/Hip Osteoarthritis Outcome Measure (Yoruba IKHOAM). African Journal of Medicine and Medical Science. Vol. 35: 349-357.
2. Akinpelu AO, Odole AC, Adegoke BOA, Adeniyi AF (2007) Development and Initial Validation of Ibadan Knee/Hip Osteoarthritis Outcome Measure (IKHOAM). South African Journal of Physiotherapy Vol. 63:3-8
3. Odole AC, Akinpelu AO (2008): Validity and internal consistency of a Hausa version of the Ibadan Knee/Hip Osteoarthritis Outcome Measure. Health and Quality of Life Outcomes Vol.6: 86
4. Odole AC, Akinpelu AO (2010): Translation of the Ibadan Knee/Hip Osteoarthritis Outcome Measure into Igbo language. African Journal of Biomedical Research 13, 169-175
5. Akinpelu AO, Akinwola MO, Odole AC, Gbiri CA (2011) The Reliability of the English version of Ibadan Knee/Hip Osteoarthritis Outcome Measure (IKHOAM). Physical and Occupational Therapy in Geriatrics Early online: 1-8 DOI: 10.3109/02/02703181.2011.589566

IBADAN KNEE/HIP OSTEOARTHRITIS OUTCOME MEASURE (IKHOAM)

Part I: Indicate the extent of limitations you experience in carrying out the following activities using these scales:

Degree of difficulty: 4 = no difficulty; 3 = mild difficulty; 2 = moderate difficulty; 1 = severe difficulty; 0 = inability to carry out the activity.

Nature of Assistance: 4 = requires no assistance; 3= requires use of aid(s)/device(s) only; 2 = requires assistance of one person only; 1 = requires assistance of one person and the use of aid(s); 0 - unable to perform the activity.

	Difficulty	Assistance
1. Washing all body parts during shower.		
2. Walking within the house		
3. Sweeping with a short broom		
4. Walking outside the house for 15-20 minutes		
5. Putting on under clothes		
6. Getting in and out of a salon car		
7. Hand washing of clothes at floor/low level		
8. Rising from bed/mat		
9. Rising from high chair (dining/office chair)		
10. Putting on/lacing shoes or buckling sandals		
11. Rising from an easy chair or sofa		
12. Sweeping with a long brush/broom or using mop stick		
13. Participating in coitus		
14. Incomplete kneeling/prostrating to show courtesy/greet elders		
15. Getting on/off water closet toilet		
16. Getting in and out of a bus/high vehicle		
17. Standing for at least 15 minutes (waiting at bus stop/working in a modern kitchen with high cooker)		
18. Manũal grass cutting/hoeing/gardening		
19. Sitting on the heels (Islamic praying posture)		
20. Climbing stairs		
21. Picking things from floor/low level (kitchen cabinet)		
22. Kneeling (Christian praying posture)		
23. Sitting on a very low stool (e.g. when cooking on a low stove or firewood at floor level)		
24. Descending stairs		
25. Using pit/Asiatic toilet		

Part II: Indicate the extent of restriction you experience participating in the following life situations using the scale below Extent of restriction: 3-full participation, 2- at risk full participation, 1-participation with restriction, 0-no participation

	Extent
1. Performing duties at work (office or at home.	
2. Travelling for one hour or more	
3. Participation in social gatherings (e.g. wedding, naming, funeral, birthday parties)	

Part III: Physical performance tests

250m Walk Test

5 - able to walk 250m or more at one stretch

4 - able to walk 200-<250m at one stretch

3 - able to walk 150-<200m at one stretch

2 - able to walk 100-<150m at one stretch

1 - able to walk 50-<100m at one stretch

0 - able to walk <50m at one stretch

Squat Test

4 - ≥100 degree knee flexion

3 - 70-99 degree knee flexion

2 - 40-69 degree knee flexion

1 - 10-39 degree knee flexion

0 - < 10 degree knee flexion

One leg Stance Test

5 - can be maintained for 4 minutes or more

4 – can be maintained for 3-<4 minutes

3 - can be maintained for 2-<3 minutes

2 - can be maintained for 1-<2 minutes

1 - can be maintained for <1 minute

0 - unable to perform the test

Stairs Climbing Test

4 - can climb with no difficulty and no assistance

3 - can climb with mild difficulty (one railing)

2 - can climb with moderate difficulty (two railings)

1 - can climb with severe difficulty (two railings and help)

0 - unable to climb.

Balance Test on a Balance Board

5 - can balance for 45 seconds or more

4 - can balance for 30-<45 seconds

3 - can balance for 20-<30 seconds

2 - can balance for 10-<20 seconds

1 - can balance for <10 second

0 - unable to balance at all.

❑❑❑

106 ICU Mobility Scale

Objective

- To record the patient's highest level of mobility in the Intensive Care Unit (ICU)[1][2]

Intended Population

- The patient's admitted in ICU [2]

Method of Use

Health professionals working in the ICU setting can easily use the outcome tool in the patient to check the highest mobility level of the patient.[1]

There is a total of 11 categories on this scale and the maximum score obtained is 10. The scoring is done based on the mobility achieved by the patient. the classified mobility stages are, nothing (lying on the bed), sitting in bed and exercising in bed, passively moved to the chair (no standing), sitting over the edge of the bed, standing, transferring bed to chair, marching on the spot at bedside. walking with the assistance of 2 or more person, walking with the assistance of 1 person, walking independently with gait aid, walking independently without gait aid. If the patient is unable to move and lying in bed, it is scored as 0 and when the patient is able to walk independently without gait aid, it is scored as 10.

Evidence

Reliability

- Intraclass correlation: 0.80 (0.75-0.84)[1]
- Interrater reliability with kappa score: 0.84 for senior and junior physiotherapists, 0.77 for senior physiotherapists and nurses and 0.90 for junior physiotherapists and nurses[1].

Validity

Construct validity

- The convergent validity was assessed by finding the correlation between ICU mobility scale and muscle strength and was found to be moderate($r=0.64$, $P<0.001$)[3]
- The divergent validity was assessed by finding the correlation between weight and gender of the patient and no correlation was found.[3]

Predictive validity

- The mobility score was associated with survival of patient to 90 days with OR, 1.38; 95% CI, 1.14–1.66[3]
- The mobility score was associated with a discharge home (OR, 1.16; 95% CI, 1.02–1.32). Patients who score high in the ICU mobility scale were discharged directly at home rather than in any rehabilitation center or other centers.[3]
- The mobility score wasn't associated with return to work at 6months. [3]

Responsiveness

- The effect size for the change in score from admission to discharge from ICU to 6 months follow up was large i.e, 0.8 between each time point
- Around 86% of survivors had improved in the ICU score between the start and discharge from ICU and 92% had shown improvement between discharge and 6 months follow up.[3]

Floor and ceiling effect

- It was calculated by assessing the number and percentage of participants scoring the lowest value (0) and the highest value (10) initially and at ICU discharge. If the value was less than 15%, it was considered acceptable.
- ICU mobility scale has acceptable floor and ceiling effect. 14% of patient scored 0(means acceptable floor) and 4% scored 10 (means acceptable ceiling)at the time of discharge and 96% scored 0 at the time of admission when the patient was deeply sedated. [3]

References

1. Hodgson C, Needham D, Haines K, Bailey M, Ward A, Harrold M, Young P, Zanni J, Buhr H, Higgins A, Presneill J. Feasibility and inter-rater reliability of the ICU Mobility Scale. Heart & Lung. 2014 Jan 1;43(1):19-24.
2. Tipping CJ, Holland AE, Harrold M, Crawford T, Halliburton N, Hodgson CL. The minimal important difference of the ICU mobility scale Heart & Lung. 2018 Sep 1;47(5):497-501 Tipping CJ, Holland AE, Harrold M, Crawford T, Halliburton N, Hodgson CL. The minimal important difference of the ICU mobility scale. Heart & Lung. 2018 Sep 1;47(5):497-501.
3. Tipping CJ, Bailey MJ, Bellomo R, Berney S, Buhr H, Denehy L, Harrold M, Holland A, Higgins AM, Iwashyna TJ, Needham D. The ICU mobility scale has construct and predictive validity and is responsive. A multicenter observational study. Annals of the American Thoracic Society. 2016 Jun;13(6):887-93.

ICU Mobility Scale

	Classification	Definition
0	Nothing (lying in bed)	Passively rolled or passively exercised by staff, but not actively moving.
1	Sitting in bed, exercises in bed	Any activity in bed, including rolling, bridging, active exercises, cycle ergometry and active assisted exercises; not moving out of bed or over the edge of the bed
2	Passively moved to chair (no standing).	Hoist, passive lift or slide transfer to the chair, with no 3standing or sitting o4n the edge of the bed.
3	Sitting over edge of bed	May be assisted by staff, but involves actively sitting over the side of the bed with some trunk control
4	Standing	Weight bearing through the feet in the standing position, with or without assistance. This may include use of a standing lifter device or tilt table
5	Transferring bed to chair	Able to step or shuffle through standing to the chair. This involves actively transferring weight from one leg to another to move to the chair. If the patient has been stood with the assistance of a medical device, they must step to the chair (not included if the patient is wheeled in a standing lifter device)
6	Marching on spot (at bedside).	Able to walk on the spot by lifting alternate feet (must be able to step at least 4 times, twice on each foot), with or without assistance
7	Walking with assistance of 2 or more people	Walking away from the bed/chair by at least 5 metres (5 yards) assisted by 2 or more people.
8	Walking with assistance of 1 person	Walking away from the bed/chair by at least 5 metres (5 yards) assisted by 1 person
9	Walking independently with a gait aid	Walking away from the bed/chair by at least 5 metres (5 yards) with a gait aid, but no assistance from another person. In a wheelchair bound person, this activity level includes wheeling the chair independently 5 metres (5 yards) away from the bed/chair.
10	Walking independently without a gait aid	Walking away from the bed/chair by at least 5 metres (5 yards) without a gait aid or assistance from another person.

Reference: Carol Hodgson, Dale Needham, Michael Bailey, Paul Young, Heidi Buhr, Alisa Higgins, Jeff Presneill and Sue Berney, and was originally published in Heart and Lung 2014:43;19-24.DOI: http://dx.doi.org/10.1016/j.hrtlng.2013.11.003

❑❑❑

107 Jebsen-Taylor Hand Function Test

The Jebsen-Taylor Hand Function Test (JTHFT) is a standardized and objective measure of fine and gross motor hand function using simulated activities of daily living (ADL). [1][2] The JTHFT has seven subsets which are writing, simulated page-turning, lifting small objects, simulated feeding, stacking, and lifting large, lightweight, and heavy objects. [1] JTHFT finds easy applicability in clinical settings since it can be administered in a short time by using readily available materials. [3]

Intended Population: A number of studies report that the JTHFT is a valid assessment tool for the measurement of hand dysfunctions from a variety of patient populations. [4][5][6][7] The JTHFT has been widely used in the clinical and research settings as well as in different patient populations such as those with Spinal cord injury stroke Cerebral palsy Multiple sclerosis Hand and wrist fractures osteoarthritis Rheumatoid arthritis[8][9][10][11][12][13]

Method of Use: To evaluate hand function using the JTHFT, each of its subset is timed and can be compared with the established norms. [1] The JTHFT includes a series of seven subtests representing fine motor, non-weighted and weighted hand function in ADL, which includes:

1. Printing a 24-letter, third grade reading difficulty sentence
2. Turning over 7.6×12.7 cm (3×5-inch) cards (simulated page turning)
3. Picking up small, common objects (e.g. pennies, paper clips, bottle caps) and placing them in a container
4. Stacking checkers (test of eye-hand co-ordination)
5. Simulated feeding
6. Moving large empty cans
7. Moving large weighted [0.45 kg (1 lb)] cans.

The subtests are scored by recording the number of seconds required to complete each test.

Time Required: Length: 15-45 minutes to complete the JTHFT.

Scoring: Total score is the sum of time taken for each sub-test, which are rounded to the nearest second. Shorter times indicate better performance.

Equipment: Stopwatch Chair (18" seat height) Desk/ table (30" high) 4 sheets of unruled
white paper Clipboard -Sentences typed in upper case centered on a 5 × 8" index card on a bookstand
5 index cards (ruled on one side only) Empty 1 pound coffee can 2 paper clips 2 regular sized bottle caps 2 U.S. pennies 5 kidney beans (~5/8" long) 1 regular teaspoon

Wooden board (41 ½" long, 11 ¼" wide, ¾" thick)

"C" clamp -Plywood (20" long, 2" wide, ½" thick) glued to the board

4 standard size (1 ¼" diameter) red wooden checkers
5 No. 303 cans

A test kit can be obtained which includes all instructions, items required for all sub tests, a carrying bag, and blank record forms.

Procedure: A detailed procedure of the JTHFT is available in this document.

Evidence: Studies have shown that the JTHFT is a valid assessment tool for the measurement of hand dysfunction from a variety of patient populations.[4][5][6][7] Test–retest reliability was established from the original JTHFT, wherein results were found to be fairly to moderately consistent over time.[2] Several studies also demonstrated that the JTHFT had moderate to high test–retest reliability and excellent intrarater reliability ($r=0.84$ and 0.85, $P<0.05$) with absent practice effect ($P<0.05$).[2]

References

1. Jebsen R, Taylor N, Trieschmann R, Trotter M, Howard L. An objective and standardized test of hand function. Arch Phys Med Rehabil 1969; 50:311–319.
2. Takla MK, Mahmoud EA, Abd El-Latif N. Jebsen Taylor Hand Function test: Gender, dominance, and age differences in healthy Egyptian population. Bulletin of Faculty of Physical Therapy. 2018 Jul 1;23(2):85.
3. Sears E, Chung K. Validity and responsiveness of the Jebsen-Taylor Hand Function Test. J Hand Surg Am 2010; 35:30–37.
4. Bovend'Eerdt H, Dawes H, Johansen-Berg H, Wade T. Evaluation of the Modified Jebsen Test of Hand Function and the University of Maryland Arm Questionnaire for Stroke. Clin Rehabil 2004; 18:195–202
5. Feys P, Duportail M, Kos D, van Asch P, Ketelaer P. Validity of the TEMPA for the measurement of upper limb function in multiple sclerosis. Clin Rehabil 2002; 16:166–173.
6. Vliet Vieland TP, van der Wijk TP, Jolie IM, Zwinderman AH. Determinants of hand function in patients with rheumatoid arthritis. J Rheumatol 1996;23:835–840.
7. Sharma S, Schumacher HR, McLellan AT. Evaluation of the Jebsen Hand Function Test for use in patients with rheumatoid arthritis. Arthritis Care Res 1994; 7:16–19.
8. Beekhuizen S, Field-Fote C. Massed practice versus massed practice with stimulation: effects on upper extremity function and cortical plasticity in individuals with incomplete cervical spinal cord injury. Neurorehabil Neural Repair 2005; 19:33–45
9. Alon G, Sunnerhagen S, Geurts H, Ohry A. A home-based, selfadministered stimulation program to improve selected hand functions of chronic stroke. NeuroRehabilitation 2003; 18:215–225
10. Charles R, Wolf L, Schneider A, Gordon M. Efficacy of a child-friendly form of constraint-induced movement therapy in hemiplegic cerebral palsy: a randomized control trial. Dev Med Child Neurol 2006; 48:635–642.
11. Feys P, Duportail M, Kos D, van Asch P, Ketelaer P. Validity of the TEMPA for the measurement of upper limb function in multiple sclerosis. Clin Rehabil 2002; 16:166–173.
12. Kreder J, Agel J, McKee D, Schemitsch H, Stephen D, Hanel P. A randomized, controlled trial of distal radius fractures with metaphyseal displacement but without joint incongruity: closed reduction and casting versus closed reduction, spanning external fixation, and optional percutaneous K-wires. J Orthop Trauma 2006; 20:115–121.
13. Rettig A, Luca L, Murphy S. Silicone implant arthroplasty in patients with idiopathic osteoarthritis of the metacarpophalangeal joint. J Hand Surg Am 2005; 30:667–672
14. Davis Sears E, Chung KC. Validity and responsiveness of the Jebsen-Taylor Hand Function Test. J Hand Surg Am 2010;35(1):30–7
15. Jebsen Taylor Hand Function Test, Jennifer Nichole.

Jebsen Hand Function Test

Adapted from Jebsen RH et al. An Objective and Standardized Test of Hand Function, Arch Phys Med Rehabil, 50 (6): 311-318, 1969; Methods. Used with permission from Elsevier Publishing.

The Jebsen Hand Function Test was designed to provide a short, objective test of hand function for activities of daily living. It has 7 items and takes approximately 15-45 minutes to administer.

7 items include: writing, turning over 3-by-5 inch cards, picking up small common objects, simulated feeding, stacking checkers, picking up large light objects and picking up large heavy objects. The results are measured by timing the time taken to accomplish each task. The tests are always presented in the same order and are performed with the non-dominant hand first.

Item 1: Writing

The examiner has a small index card with the blank side facing the subject propped up so the subject can easily read it. The index card has a sentence of third-grade reading difficulty ,with 24 letters.

The subject is seated and given a pen and several sheets of white paper attached to a clipboard. The subject is instructed to begin copying the sentence from the index card onto the sheet when the examiner flips the index card and says "go".

Record the time taken from "go" until the subject lifts their pen off the page after finishing the sentence.

Repeat with the dominant hand using a new sentence.

Verbal Instructions:

"Do you require glasses for reading? If so, put them on. Take this pen in your left hand and arrange everything so that it is comfortable for you to write with your left hand. On the other side of this card (indicate) is a sentence. When I turn the card over and say 'Go', write the sentence as quickly and as clearly as you can using your left hand. Write, do not print. Do you understand? Ready? Go."

For the dominant hand – "All right, now repeat the same thing, only this time using your right hand. I've given you a different sentence. Are you ready? Go."

Item 2: Card Turning

Place 5 index cards (3x5 in) in a horizontal row 2 in apart on a desk in front of the subject. Each card should be placed 5 inches from the front edge of the desk (indicate this with tape).

Record the time from "go" until the subject turns the last card over. The cards do not have to be in the same placement after turning.

Repeat with the dominant hand.

Verbal Instructions:

"Place your left hand on the table please. When I say "go". Use your left hand to turn these cards over one at a time as quickly as you can, beginning with this one (indicate card to extreme right). You may turn them over in any way that you wish and they need not be in a neat pattern when you finish. Do you understand? Ready? Go."

For the dominant hand – "Now the same thing with the right hand beginning with this one (indicate extreme left card). Ready? Go."

Item 3: Small Common Objects

Place an empty 1-pound coffee can in front of the subject, 5 inches from the front edge of the desk. Next, place 2 United States pennies (closest to coffee can), 2 bottle caps with the inside facing up and 2 one-inch paper clips (farthest from coffee can) to the left, each of these items should be separated by 2 inches.

Record the time from "go" until the last item is placed inside the coffee can.

Repeat with the dominant hand – with the layout as a mirror image of the non-dominant setup.

Verbal instructions:

"Place your left hand on the table please. When I say "go", use your left hand to pick up these objects one at a time and place them in the can as fast as you can beginning with this one (indicate paper clip on the extreme left). Do you understand? Ready? Go."

For the dominant hand – "Now the same thing with the right hand beginning here (indicate paper clip now on the extreme right). Ready? Go."

Item 4: Simulated feeding

Place 5 kidney beans and an empty coffee can on a board clamped to the desk in front of the subject, 5 inches from the front edge of the desk. The beans should be oriented to the left of center, parallel to and touching the upright of the board 2 inches apart, the coffee can should be in the center. Give the subject a teaspoon. Record the time from the word "go" until the last bean hits the bottom of the coffee can.

Repeat with the dominant hand – placing the beans on the right side of the can if right hand, left side of the can if left hand.

Verbal instructions:

"Take the teaspoon in your left hand please. When I say "go", use your left hand to pick up these beans one at a time with the teaspoon and place them in this can as fast as you can beginning with this one (indicate bean on the extreme left). Do you understand? Ready? Go."

For the dominant hand – "now the same thing with the right hand beginning here (indicate bean on extreme right). Ready? Go."

Item 5: Checkers

Place 4 standard sized (1.25 inch diameter) wooden checkers in front of a board clamped to the desk in front of the subject, 5 inches from the front edge of the desk. The checkers should be placed 4 in a row, 2 on each side of the center. Record the time from the word "go" until the fourth checker makes contact with the third checker (subject is stacking the checkers one on top of another).

Repeat with the dominant hand.

Verbal instructions:

"Place your left hand on the table please. When I say "go", use your left hand to stack these checkers on the board in front of you as fast as you can like this, one on top of the other (demonstrate). You may begin with any checker. Do you understand? Ready? Go."

For the dominant hand – "Now the same thing with the right hand. Ready? Go."

Item 6: Large Light Object

Place 5 empty cans in front of a board clamped to the desk, 5 inches from the front edge of the desk, in front of the subject. Space the cans 2 inches apart with the open end of the can facing down. The subject is to place each can onto the board in front of the cans. Record the time from the word "go" until the subject releases the fifth can.

Repeat with the dominant hand.

Verbal instructions:

"Place your left hand on the table please. When I say 'Go', use your left hand to stand these cans on the board in front of you like this (demonstrate). Begin with this one (indicate can on extreme left). Do you understand? Ready? Go."

Dominant hand – "Now the same thing with the right hand beginning here (indicate extreme right can). Ready? Go."

Item 7: Large Heavy Objects

Place 5 full (1 pound) cans in front of a board clamped to the desk in front of the subject, 5 inches from the front edge of the desk. Space the cans 2 inches apart with the open end of the can facing down. The subject is to place each can onto the board in front of the cans. Record the time from the word "go" until the subject releases the fifth can.

Repeat with the dominant hand.

Verbal instructions:

"Now do the same thing with these heavier cans. Place your left hand on the table. When I say "Go", use your left hand to stand these cans on the board as fast as you can. Begin here (indicate can on extreme left). Do you understand? Ready? Go."

For the dominant hand – "Now the same thing with your right hand beginning here (indicate can on far right). Ready? Go."

Jebsen Hand Function Test Worksheet:

Patient Name: ____________________

Date: ____________________

The tests are performed with the non-dominant hand first.

The results are measured by timing the time taken to accomplish each task.

Writing: ____________ seconds

Card turning: ____________ seconds

Small common object: ____________ seconds

Simulated feeding: ____________ seconds

Checkers: ____________ seconds

Large light object: ____________ seconds

Large heavy object: ____________ seconds

❑❑❑

108 Katz ADL

Objective

The purpose of the Index of ADL, or KATZ ADL, is to monitor the prognosis and treatment of older adults and chronically ill people[1]. In particular, the KATZ ADL measures a person's independence in common activities of daily living (ADL).

Age-related changes and health problems frequently show themselves as declines in the functional status of older adults. This decline often places the older adult on a downwards health spiral. An effective way to evaluate the health status of older adults is through their functional ability. An objective assessment which provides objective data helps indicate decline or improvement in health status, allowing the physiotherapist to plan and intervene appropriately[2].

Intended Population

Older adults and individuals with chronic diseases.

Method of Use

The Katz ADL, is an appropriate tool to assess functional status when measuring the client's ability to perform activities of daily living independently. It takes less than five minutes to perform and requires training[4].

Physiotherapists use the tool when assessing function and detect problems in performing ADL and formulate a plan care. The Index ranks adequacy of performance in six functions: bathing, dressing, toileting, transferring, continence, and feeding. One point means the person is independent; zero points means the person requires supervision, direction, personal assistance or total care.

The following is referenced from McCabe[2].

BATHING

Points: __________

1 POINT: Bathes self completely or needs help in bathing only a single part of the body such as the back, genital area or disabled extremity.

0 POINTS: Need help with bathing more than one part of the body, getting in or out of the tub or shower. Requires total bathing.

DRESSING

Points: __________

1 POINT: Get clothes from closets and drawers and puts on clothes and outer garments complete with fasteners. May have help tying shoes.

0 POINTS: Needs help with dressing self or needs to be completely dressed.

TOILETING

Points: __________

1 POINT: Goes to toilet, gets on and off, arranges clothes, cleans genital area without help.

0 POINTS: Needs help transferring to the toilet, cleaning self or uses bedpan or commode.

TRANSFERRING

Points: __________

1 POINT: Moves in and out of bed or chair unassisted. Mechanical transfer aids are acceptable.

0 POINTS: Needs help in moving from bed to chair or requires a complete transfer.

CONTINENCE

Points: __________

1 POINT: Exercises complete self control over urination and defecation.

0 POINTS: Is partially or totally incontinent of bowel or bladder.

FEEDING

Points: __________

1 POINT: Gets food from plate into mouth without help. Preparation of food may be done by another person.

0 POINTS: Needs partial or total help with feeding or requires parenteral feeding.

TOTAL POINTS: ________ SCORING: 6 = High (patient independent) 0 = Low (patient very dependent)

Evidence

Validity

Construct Validity

Scores on the Katz ADL Index are correlated with scores on the Barthel Index[2].

Predictive Validity

There is an indication the KATZ may have a predictive quality in regards to living situation and mortality[5], as well as stroke prognosis[6].

Turkish[7] and Spanish[8] versions have been translated and assessed for validity.

Responsiveness

The KATZ has a significant floor effect, i.e. it is unable to detect change at low levels of disability[9].

This occurs as it does not assess more advanced activities of daily living and it is limited in its ability to measure small increments of change seen in the rehabilitation of older adults. A comprehensive geriatric assessment should follow when appropriate.

References

1. Katz S, Ford AB, Moskowitz RW, Jackson BA, Jaffe MW. Studies of Illness in the Aged: The Index of ADL: A Standardized Measure of Biological and Psychosocial Function JAMA. 1963;185(12):914–919.
2. McCabe D. Katz Index of Independence in Activities of Daily Living (ADL). Best Practices in Nursing Care to Older Adults. 2019. 2. Accessed 24 June 2019.
3. Describing occupation. Katz ADL Available from: https://www.youtube.com watch? v = ekwu49fH5QM (last accessed 5.5.2019)
4. Katz P. Measures of Adult General Functional Status. Arthritis Care Res (Hoboken). 2003. 49; 5S: S15–S27. Accessed 24 June 2019.
5. Brorsson B, Asberg KH. Katz index of independence in ADL. Reliability and validity in short-term care. Scand J Rehabil Med. 1984;16(3):125-32.
6. Asberg KH, Nydevik I. Early prognosis of stroke outcome by means of Katz Index of activities of daily living. Scand J Rehabil Med. 1991;23(4):187-91.
7. Arika G, Varana, HD, Yavuza BB, Karabulutb E, Karaa O, Kilica MK. Validation of Katz index of independence in activities of daily living in Turkish older adults. Arch Gerontol Geriatr. 2015. 61: 344–350. Accessed 24 June 2019.
8. Cabañero-Martínez MJ, Cabrero-García J, Richart-Martínez M, Muñoz-Mendoza CL. The Spanish versions of the Barthel index (BI) and the Katz index (KI) of activities of daily living (ADL): a structured review. Arch Gerontol Geriatr. 2009 Jul-Aug;49(1):e77-84. doi: 10.1016/j.archger.2008.09.006. Epub 2008 Nov 5.
9. McDowell I, Newell C. Measuring health: a guide to rating scales and questionnaires. 2nd Ed. New York: Oxford University Press; 1996. p. 63–7. Accessed 24 June 2019.

❑❑❑

109 Knee Injury and Osteoarthritis Outcome Score

Introduction

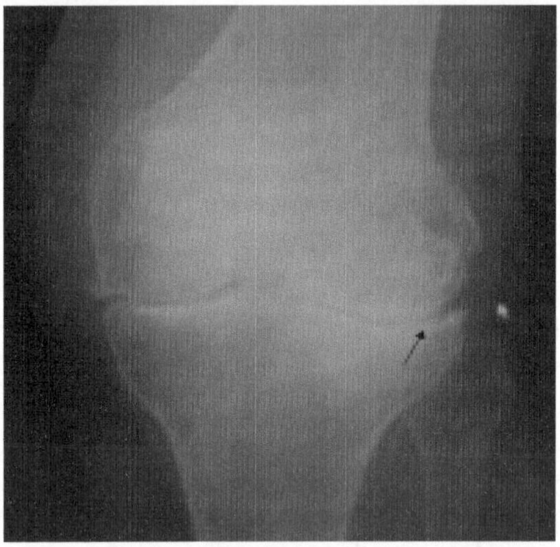

The Knee Injury and Osteoarthritis Outcome Score (KOOS) is a knee-specific instrument, developed to assess the patients' opinion about their knee and associated problems. The KOOS evaluates both short-term and long-term consequences of knee injury. It holds 42 items in 5 separately scored subscales; Pain, other Symptoms, Function in daily living (ADL), Function in Sport and Recreation (Sport/Rec), and knee-related Quality of Life (QOL).It is an extension of the WOMAC Osteoarthritis Index[1].The Knee injury and Osteoarthritis Outcome Score (KOOS) is self-administered.The KOOS proved reliable, responsive to surgery and physical therapy, and valid for patients undergoing anterior cruciate ligament reconstruction. The KOOS meets basic criteria of outcome measures and can be used to evaluate the course of knee injury and treatment outcomes[2].

Development

The KOOS questionnaire was developed in the 1990s as an instrument to assess the patient's opinion about their knee and associated problems. Since the first publication in 1998, the psychometric properties of the KOOS have been assessed in more than twenty individual studies from all over the world. Furthermore, KOOS has been evaluated and compared to other instruments in several reviews[1][3][4][5]

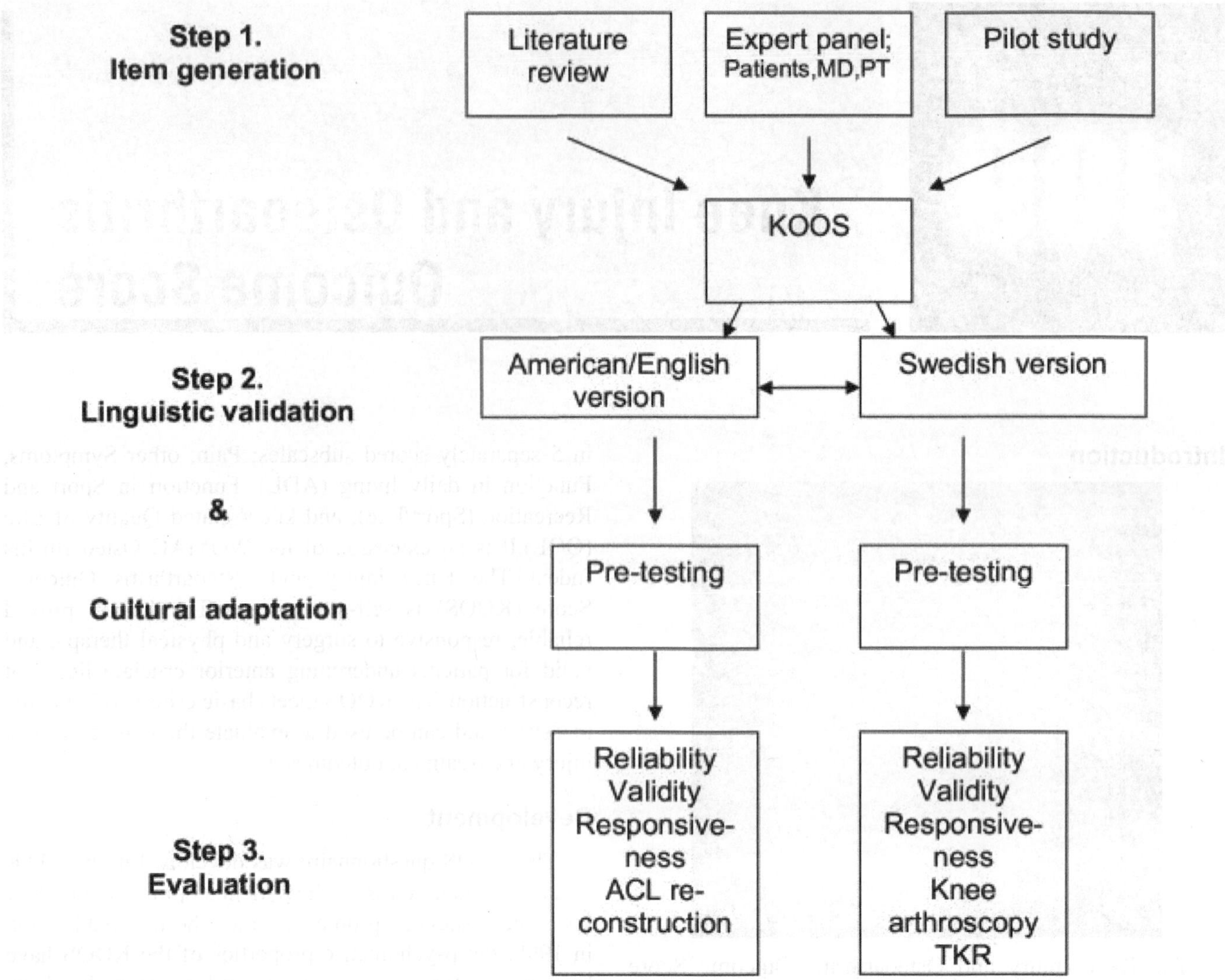

Validation

The KOOS has been validated in several different populations having surgical procedures due to knee complaints. To ensure the instrument being valid for both short-term and long-term consequences, validations have been carried out in different populations with varying diseases and durations and at varying ages and activity levels. Firstly, the American-English version was validated in subjects (age range 18–46) undergoing surgical reconstruction of the ACL[6].Secondly, the Swedish version was validated in subjects (age range 16–79) undergoing knee arthroscopy.[7]. Thirdly, the KOOS was compared to the WOMAC in subjects meniscectomized 16 years previously (age range 38–76) with and without OA[8]. Fourthly, a validation study was carried out in subjects (age range 43–86) treated with total knee replacement for OA[9]. For patients on the waiting-list for total knee replacement for OA, content validity was assessed before surgery by asking the patients to rate the importance of improvement in each of the five KOOS subscales on a 5-point Likert-scale as extremely important, very important, moderately important, somewhat important, or not important at all. For each subscale examples of questions within the subscale were given. Over 90% reported that improvement in the four subscales Pain, Symptoms, Activities of Daily Living, and knee-related Quality of Life was extremely or very important when deciding to have their knee operated on. 51% reported that improvement in functions included in the subscale Sport and Recreation Function such as squatting, kneeling, jumping, turning/twisting and running was extremely or very important when deciding to have their knee operated on. Postoperatively, patients tended to start doing physical functions they did not do prior to the operation.

Convergent and divergent construct validity was determined in comparison to the SF-36[10], and when applicable also to the Lysholm knee scoring scale[11]

Uses

- KOOS is intended to be used for:
- knee injury that can result in post traumatic osteoarthritis (OA)
- ACL (anterior cruciate ligament) injury
- Meniscus injury
- Chondral injury
- Ankle and foot problems (FAOS)
- Hip problem (HOOS)
- Rheumatoid arthritis and other inflammatory joint diseases (RAOS)

Advantages of the KOOS

- Inclusion of two different subscales of physical function relating to daily life, and sport and recreation. This enhances the instrument's validity for patients with a wide range of current and expected physical activity levels.
- Short- and long-term time intervals
- Assess changes from week to week induced by treatment (medication, operation, physical therapy) or over years following a primary injury or OA.
- Used in research to assess groups and to monitor individuals.

Scoring

The five patient-relevant subscales of KOOS are scored separately:

- Pain (nine items)
- Symptoms (seven items)
- ADL Function (17 items)
- Sport and Recreation Function (five items)
- Quality of Life (four items)

A Likert scale is used and all items have five possible answer options scored from 0 (No Problems) to 4 (Extreme Problems) and each of the five scores is calculated as the sum of the items included. Scores are transformed to a 0–100 scale, with zero representing extreme knee problems and 100 representing no knee problems as common in orthopaedic assessment scales and generic measures. Scores between 0 and 100 represent the percentage of total possible score achieved. An aggregate score is not calculated since it is regarded desirable to analyze and interpret the five dimensions separately.

The score is a percentage score from 0 to 100, 0 representing extreme problems and 100 representing no problems. This direction, 100 indicating no problems, is common in orthopaedic instruments and generic measures like the SF-36. In measures developed by rheumatologists, like the WOMAC, 100 usually represents worst possible result.

References

1. Roos EM, Lohmander LS. Knee injury and Osteoarthritis Outcome Score (KOOS): from joint injury to osteoarthritis. Health Qual Life Outcomes 2003;1:64.
2. Roos EM1, Roos HP, Lohmander LS, Ekdahl C, Beynnon BD.Knee Injury and Osteoarthritis Outcome Score (KOOS)--development of a self-administered outcome measure.J Orthop Sports Phys Ther. 1998 Aug;28(2):88-96.
3. Rodriguez-Merchan EC. Knee instruments and rating scales designed to measure outcomes. Journal of orthopaedics and traumatology : official journal of the Italian Society of Orthopaedics and Traumatology 2012;13:1-6.
4. Collins NJ, Misra D, Felson DT, Crossley KM, Roos EM. Measures of knee function: International Knee Documentation Committee (IKDC) Subjective Knee Evaluation Form, Knee Injury and Osteoarthritis Outcome Score (KOOS), Knee Injury and Osteoarthritis Outcome Score Physical Function Short Form (KOOS-PS), Knee Outcome Survey Activities of Daily Living Scale (KOS-ADL), Lysholm Knee Scoring Scale, Oxford Knee Score (OKS), Western Ontario and McMaster Universities Osteoarthritis Index (WOMAC), Activity Rating Scale (ARS), and Tegner Activity Score (TAS). Arthritis care & research 2011;63 Suppl 11:S208-28.
5. Alviar MJ, Olver J, Brand C, Hale T, Khan F. Do patient-reported outcome measures used in assessing outcomes in rehabilitation after hip and knee arthroplasty capture issues relevant to patients? Results of a systematic review and

ICF linking process. Journal of rehabilitation medicine : official journal of the UEMS European Board of Physical and Rehabilitation Medicine 2011;43:374-81.

6. Roos EM, Roos HP, Lohmander LS, Ekdahl C, Beynnon BD: Knee Injury and Osteoarthritis Outcome Score (KOOS)--development of a self-administered outcome measure. J Orthop Sports Phys Ther 1998, 28:88-96.
7. Roos EM, Roos HP, Ekdahl C, Lohmander LS: Knee injury and Osteoarthritis Outcome Score (KOOS)--validation of a Swedish version. Scand J Med Sci Sports 1998, 8:439-448
8. Roos EM, Roos HP, Lohmander LS: WOMAC Osteoarthritis Index--additional dimensions for use in subjects with post-traumatic osteoarthritis of the knee. Western Ontario and MacMaster Universities.Osteoarthritis Cartilage 1999, 7:216-221
9. Roos EM, Toksvig-Larsen S: Knee injury and Osteoarthritis Outcome Score (KOOS) - validation and comparison to the WOMAC in total knee replacement.Health Qual Life Outcomes 2003, 1:17.
10. Ware J. E., Jr., Sherbourne CD: The MOS 36-item short-form health survey (SF-36). I. Conceptual framework and item selection.Med Care 1992, 30:473-483
11. Tegner Y, Lysholm J: Rating systems in the evaluation of knee ligament injuries.Clin Orthop 1985, 43-49.

KOOS KNEE SURVEY

Today's date: ____/____/________

Date of birth: ____/____/________

Name: ______________________

INSTRUCTIONS:

This survey asks for your view about your knee. This information will help us keep track of how you feel about your knee and how well you are able to perform your usual activities. Answer every question by ticking the appropriate box, only one box for each question. If you are unsure about how to answer a question, please give the best answer you can.

Symptoms

These questions should be answered thinking of your knee symptoms during the last week.

S1. Do you have swelling in your knee?

Never Rarely Sometimes
Often Always

S2. Do you feel grinding, hear clicking or any other type of noise when your knee moves?

Never Rarely Sometimes
Often Always

S3. Does your knee catch or hang up when moving?

Never Rarely Sometimes
Often Always

S4. Can you straighten your knee fully?

Always Often Sometimes
Rarely Never

S5. Can you bend your knee fully?

Always Often Sometimes
Rarely Never

Stiffness The following questions concern the amount of joint stiffness you have experienced during the last week in your knee. Stiffness is a sensation of restriction or slowness in the ease with which you move your knee joint.

S6. How severe is your knee joint stiffness after first wakening in the morning?

None Mild Moderate
Severe Extreme

S7. How severe is your knee stiffness after sitting, lying or resting later in the day?

None Mild Moderate
Severe Extreme

Pain

P1. How often do you experience knee pain?

Never Monthly Weekly
Daily Always

What amount of knee pain have you experienced the last week during the following activities?

P2. Twisting/pivoting on your knee

None Mild Moderate
Severe Extreme

P3. Straightening knee fully

None Mild Moderate
Severe Extreme

P4. Bending knee fully

None Mild Moderate
Severe Extreme

P5. Walking on flat surface

None Mild Moderate

Severe Extreme

P6. Going up or down

None Mild Moderate

Severe Extreme

P7. At night while in bed

None Mild Moderate

Severe Extreme

P8. Sitting or lying

None Mild Moderate

Severe Extreme

P9. Standing

None Mild Moderate

Severe Extreme

Function, daily living: The following questions concern your physical function. By this we mean your ability to move around and to look after yourself. For each of the following activities please indicate the degree of difficulty you have experienced in the last week due to your knee.

A1. Descending

None Mild Moderate

Severe Extreme

A2. Ascending

None Mild Moderate

Severe Extreme

For each of the following activities please indicate the degree of difficulty you have experienced in the last week due to your knee.

A3. Rising from sitting

None Mild Moderate

Severe Extreme

A4. Standing

None Mild Moderate

Severe Extreme

A5. Bending to floor/pick up an object

None Mild Moderate

Severe Extreme

A6. Walking on flat surface

None Mild Moderate

Severe Extreme

A7. Getting in/out of car

None Mild Moderate

Severe Extreme

A8. Going shopping

None Mild Moderate

Severe Extreme

A9. Putting on socks/stockings

None Mild Moderate

Severe Extreme

A10. Rising from bed

None Mild Moderate

Severe Extreme

A11. Taking off socks/stockings

None Mild Moderate

Severe Extreme

A12. Lying in bed (turning over, maintaining knee position)

None Mild Moderate

Severe Extreme

A13. Getting in/out of bath

None Mild Moderate

Severe Extreme

A14. Sitting

None Mild Moderate

Severe Extreme

A15. Getting on/off toilet

None Mild Moderate

Severe Extreme

For each of the following activities please indicate the degree of difficulty you have experienced in the last week due to your knee.

A16. Heavy domestic duties (moving heavy boxes, scrubbing floors, etc)

None Mild Moderate

Severe Extreme

A17. Light domestic duties (cooking, dusting, etc)

None Mild Moderate

Severe Extreme

Function, sports and recreational activities

The following questions concern your physical function when being active on a higher level. The questions should be answered thinking of what degree of difficulty you have experienced during the last week due to your knee.

SP1. Squatting

None Mild Moderate

Severe Extreme

SP2. Running

None Mild Moderate

Severe Extreme

SP3. Jumping

None Mild Moderate

Severe Extreme

SP4. Twisting/pivoting on your injured knee

None Mild Moderate

Severe Extreme

SP5. Kneeling

None Mild Moderate

Severe Extreme

Quality of Life

Q1. How often are you aware of your knee problem?

Never Monthly Weekly

Daily Constantly

Q2. Have you modified your life style to avoid potentially damaging activities to your knee?

Not at all Mildly Moderately

Severely Totally

Q3. How much are you troubled with lack of confidence in your knee?

Not at all Mildly Moderately

Severely Extremely

Q4. In general, how much difficulty do you have with your knee?

Not at all Mildly Moderately

Severely Extremely

Thank you very much for completing all the questions in this questionnaire.

❑❑❑

110 Knee Injury and Osteoarthritis Outcome Score – Child

The knee injury osteoarthritis score (KOOS) is an adult outcome measure used for assessing the patients' perspectives of their knee pain and disability. This tool was developed initially to use on adults. The KOOS psychometric properties have shown high reliability and validity, and is responsive to change in subjects with knee degeneration or knee injury.[1]

Development

Historically it was known that there were no specific paediatric outcome measures for knee pain, therefore the KOOS for adults was being used on children. It was not until 2012 when a group of researchers decided to look at the use of the adult KOOS with children.[2] They conducted cognitive interviews with 34 Swedish children between the ages of 10 and 16 years old. Cognitive interviewing has been found to be the gold standard methodology for assessing flaws in surveys due to lack of comprehension of the subjects. [3][4][5]

It was highlighted form this study that children who had undergone knee surgery or physiotherapy had a greater understanding of the medical terminology than those who had not. As such. they had a better comprehension of the KOOS for adults. It was recommended that due to this lack of comprehension in those who were not familiar with the terminology or younger children that the KOOS would need to be modified for them. This study did not identify a cut-off age for which the KOOS adult should be used, but recommended that comprehension was limited in younger children.[6]

The development of the KOOS - Child has lead to 5 sections with 39 questions in total. These categories are split into:

- Knee problems
- How painful
- Difficulty during daily activities
- Difficulty during sport and playing
- How has your injury affected your life

Within these categories there are:

- 7 questions on symptoms
- 8 questions on pain
- 11 questions on activities
- 7 questions on sports and play, and
- 6 questions on quality of life

Psychometric Properties[7]

After the development of the KOOS - Child, the psychometric properties were evaluated in 2014. This study looked at children who were seeking medical attention for knee symptoms between the ages of 7-16 years old.[6] These authors attempted to evaluate:

- Construct validity - All of the hypothesis were confirmed therefore this indicated that there was excellent construct validity.
- Test-retest reliability - found that all test-retest's were excellent for all sub-scale except the symptoms scale which was slightly lower reliability.
- Responsiveness - a hypothesis of a correlation of $\geq$ 0.3 between the KOOS Child sub-scale scores and the Global Perceived Effect (GPE) was confirmed therefore confirming the responsiveness of the KOOS Child.
- Interperability - there were no floor to ceiling effects found. Minimal important changes (MIC) were found to complement the 95% Confidence Intervals (CI), and the MIC were better than the smallest detectable change (SDC) for subjects

who reported they were 'better' and 'much better'

Overall, the KOOS-Child shows excellent psychometric properties in all areas except internal consistency where the category 'symptoms' showed lower homogeneity, similar to the KOOS - Adult, and was thought to be due to patients being able to experience a wide variety of symptoms with knee conditions.

Uses

Unlike the KOOS - Adult where certain conditions are recommended for its use, the KOOS - Child can be used in a broad population of children with different knee disorders.[6]

Scoring

Each question has 5 possible answers, with each score ranging from 0-4. The least severe answer is scored as a 0, with the most seere being scored as a 4. For example:

1. During the past month, how often have you experienced knee pain?
    - Never = 0
    - Rarely = 1
    - Sometimes = 2
    - Often = 3
    - Always = 4

Calculating the Score

Each subcategory is then added together. For example, all questions relating to pain are numbered P1, P2, P3, all questions relating to symptoms are numbered S1, S2, S3, etc.

The following is the manual calculation. This resultant score is the KOOS-Child subscale estimate for that particular cross-sectional assessment of the individual patient:

1. PAIN $100 - \frac{\text{Mean Score (P1} - \text{P9)} \times 100}{4}$
   = ROOS child Pain
2. SYMPTOMS $100 - \frac{\text{Mean Score (S1} - \text{S9)} \times 100}{4}$
   = KOOS – child Symptoms
3. ADL $100 - \frac{\text{Mean Score (A1} - \text{A17)} \times 100}{4}$
   = KOOS – child ADL
4. SPORT/PLAY $100 - \frac{\text{Mean Score (SP1} - \text{SP 7)} \times 100}{4}$
   = KOOS child Sport/Play
5. QOL $100 - \frac{\text{Mean Score (Q1} - \text{QN 6)} \times 100}{4}$
   = KOOS – child QOL

References

1. Roos E M, Roos H P, Ekdahl C, Lohmander L S. Knee injury and Osteoarthritis Outcome Score (KOOS)—validation of a Swedish version. Scandinavian Journal of Medical Science and Sports 1998; 8:439-48.
2. Örtqvist M1, Roos EM, Broström EW, Janarv PM, Iversen MD. Development of the Knee Injury and Osteoarthritis Outcome Score for children (KOOS-Child):Comprehensibility and content validity. Acta Orthopaedica 2012; 83(6): 666–673
3. Willis G B, Royston P, Bercini D. The use of verbal report methods in the development and testing of survey questionnaires. Applied cognitive Psychology 1991; 5: 251-67.
4. Willis G B. Cognitive interviewing: A tool for improving questionnaire design. Sage Publications, Thousand Oaks 2005
5. Tourangeau R, Rips L J, Rasinski K. The psychology of survey response. Cambridge University Press, Cambridge 2002
6. Örtqvist M1, Roos EM, Broström EW, Janarv PM, Iversen MD. Development of the Knee Injury and Osteoarthritis Outcome Score for children (KOOS-Child):Comprehensibility and content validity. Acta Orthopaedica 2012; 83(6): 666–673
7. Örtqvist M, Iversen MD, Janarv P-M, Broström EW, Roos EM. Psychometric properties of the Knee injury and Osteoarthritis Outcome Score for Children (KOOS-Child) in children with knee disorders. British Journal of Sports Medicine 2014; 48:1437–1446

KOOS-Child KNEE SURVEY

Today's date: ________________

Date of birth: ________________

Name: ______________________

INSTRUCTIONS

These questions collect information about how your injured knee affects you. Answer every question by ticking the appropriate box, only one box for each question. If you are unsure about how to answer a question, please select the best answer you can.

KNEE PROBLEMS

S1. During the past 7 days, how often has your knee been swollen?

Never Rarely Sometimes
Often Always

S2. During the past 7 days, how often has your knee made any noise/sounds

Never Rarely Sometimes
Often Always

S3. During the past 7 days, how often did your knee get stuck

Never Rarely Sometimes
Often Always

S4. During the past 7 days, how often have you been able to fully straighten your knee on your own?

Always Often Sometimes
Rarely Never

S5. During the past 7, days how often have you been able to fully bend your knee on your own?

Always Often Sometimes
Rarely Never

S6. During the past 7 days, how much difficulty have you had moving your knee just after waking up in the morning?

No difficulty A little Some
A lot Extreme difficulty

S7. During the past 7 days, how much difficulty have you had later in the day moving your knee after being sedentary for a while?

None A little Some
A lot Extreme

P1. During the past month, how often have you experienced knee pain?

Never Rarely Sometimes
Often All the time

HOW PAINFUL

How much knee pain have you experienced in the past 7 days during the following activities? Check the best answer for each item

	No pain	A little pain	Some pain	A lot of pain	Extreme pain
P2. Twisting/pivoting on your injured knee when walking/standing/running					
P3. Fully straightening your injured knee					
P4. Fully bending your injured knee					
P6a. Walking up stairs					
P6b. Walking down stairs					
P8a. Sitting with your injured knee bent					
P9. Standing upright on both legs for any amount of time					

DIFFICULTY DURING DAILY ACTIVITIES

A1. During the past 7 days, how much difficulty have you had walking down stairs?

No difficulty A little Some
A lot Extreme difficulty

A2. During the past 7 days, how much difficulty have you had walking up stairs?

No difficulty A little Some
A lot Extreme difficulty

A3. During the past 7 days, how much difficulty have you had standing up from a chair?

No difficulty A little Some
A lot Extreme difficulty

A5. During the past 7 days, how much difficulty have you had to bend down and pick

No difficulty A little Some
A lot Extreme difficulty

A7. During the past 7 days, how much difficulty have you had getting in to/out of a car?

No difficulty A little Some

A lot Extreme difficulty

A10. During the past 7 days, how much difficulty have you had to get out of bed?

No difficulty A little Some

A lot Extreme difficulty

A12. During the past 7 days, how much difficulty have you had to change knee position when lying in bed?

No difficulty A little Some

A lot Extreme difficulty

A13. During the past 7 days, how much difficulty have you had getting in to/out of the bathtub/shower?

No difficulty A little Some

A lot Extreme difficulty

A14. During the past 7 days, how much difficulty have you had to sit in a chair with your injured knee bent?

No difficulty A little Some

A lot Extreme difficulty

A16. During the past 7 days, how much difficulty have you had to carry heavy bags /backpacks etc?

No difficulty A little Some

A lot Extreme difficulty

A17. During the past 7 days, how much difficulty have you had to do light chores such as cleaning your room, filling/emptying the dishwasher, making your bed, etc?

No difficulty A little Some

A lot Extreme difficulty

DIFFICULTY DURING SPORTS AND PLAYING

SP1. During the past 7 days, how much difficulty have you had to squat down during play or sports activities?

No difficulty A little Some

A lot Extreme difficulty

SP2. During the past 7 days, how much difficulty have you had to run during play or sports activities?

No difficulty A little Some

A lot Extreme difficulty

SP3. During the past 7 days, how much difficulty have you had to jump during play or sports activities?

No difficulty A little Some

A lot Extreme difficulty

SP4. During the past 7 days, how much difficulty have you had to twist/pivot because of your injured knee during play or sports activities?

No difficulty A little Some

A lot Extreme difficulty

SP5. During the past 7 days, how much difficulty have you had to kneel because of your injured knee?

No difficulty A little Some

A lot Extreme difficulty

SPN6. During the past 7 days, how much difficulty have you had to keep your balance when walking /running on uneven ground?

No difficulty A little Some

A lot Extreme difficulty

SPN7. During the past 7 days, how much difficulty have you had playing sports because of your injured knee?

No difficulty A little Some

A lot Extreme difficulty

HOW HAS YOUR INJURY AFFECTED YOUR LIFE?

Q1. How often do you think about your knee problem?

Never Rarely Sometimes

Often All the time

Q2. How much have you changed your lifestyle because of your injured knee?

Not at all A little Some

A lot Very much

Q3. How much do you trust your injured knee?

Completely A lot Some

A little Not at all

Q4. Overall, how much difficulty do you have with your injured knee?

No difficulty A little Some

A lot Extreme difficulty

QN5. How much difficulty have you had getting to school or walking around in school (climbing stairs, opening doors, carrying books, participating during recess) because of your injured knee?

No difficulty A little Some

A lot Extreme difficulty

QN6. How much difficulty have you had to do things with friends because of your injured knee?

No difficulty A little Some

A lot Extreme difficulty

Thank you very much for completing all the questions in this questionnaire!

❑❑❑

111

The L test

Definition:

The L Test of Functional Mobility (L Test) is a performance-based measure that can be used to assess physical function, including dynamic balance ability.The test is a modification of the Timed Up and Go (TUG) designed to overcome the ceiling effect of the TUG found in higher-functioning patients.[1]

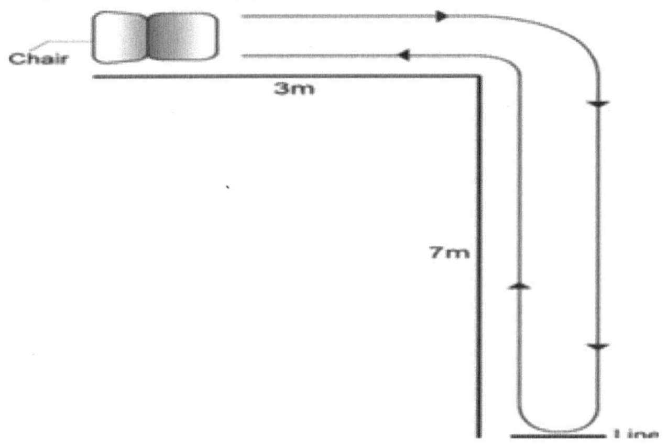

Description:

Participants completed two timed trials of both outcome measurements, with a 1-minute rest between trials and a 2-minute rest between measurements. This was performed on two occasions, seven days apart, to establish test–retest reliability. In order to control medication effects, the trials were completed at approximately the same time of day. Participants completed the TUG and L-test in a randomised order, which was kept consistent between the two occasions. Participants were instructed to walk at their comfortable walking speed, with or without any of their usual walking aids. Prior to participation, the participants received a standardized demonstration and explanation of both outcome measurements. For participant safety, chairs were placed in close proximity to the testing area. In addition, one of the researchers walked in close proximity to the participant without providing any encouragement or trying to set the walking pace. The mean times of both trials were used for data analysis.[2]

Technique:

Equipment:

- Standard chair without armrests; 1
- Lines on the floor indicating the 3-meter mark and the 7-meter mark as shown in the Figure;
- Stopwatch;
- Assistive device.

Test Set-Up: Have patient sit on the chair with his or her back against the chair, arms resting on the chair's arms, and if applicable, assistive device at hand.

Patient Instructions[3]: On the word 'go,' stand up from the chair, walk to the first line, turn 90 degrees, and walk to the 2nd line, then turn 180 degrees, and return to sit in the chair.

Clinician Instructions : Start the timer on the word "go" and stop the timer when the patient's buttocks first hits the seat surface when they return. The patient may use an assistive device if needed. Allow 1 practice and then time and record at least 1 trial. The patient walks at their comfortable walking speed.

Scoring:

1. Objective Scoring = test time taken (generally average score of 3 test trials)
2. Subjective Scoring = observational information regarding the quality of gait.

Clinical relevance:

The L Test of Functional Mobility (L Test) can be used to assess physical function in patients with a lower-limb amputation who are using a prosthesis[4], in people with Parkinson's[5].

The L-test provides an assessment of walking over a longer walking distance and involves turning in two directions.

References

1. Kim, J.S., Chu, D.Y., Jeon, H.S. Reliability and validity of the L test in participants with chronic stroke.Physiotherapy. 2015;101:161–165
2. Death BA, Miller WC. The L test of functional mobility: measurement properties of a modified version of the timed up and go test designed for people with lower-limb amputations. Phys Ther 2005;85(7):626-35
3. 3Resnik, L., Borgia, M. Reliability of Outcome Measures for People with Lower-Limb Amputations: Distinguishing True Change from Statistical Error. Phys Ther. 2011:91:555-565
4. Deathe, A.B., Miller, W.C. The L Test of Functional Mobility: Measurement Properties of a Modified Version of the Timed "Up & Go" Test Designed for People with LowerLimb Amputations. Phys Ther. 2005:85:626-635
5. M Sinha, N Hamdani (PT) Measurement Properties of L Test for Functional Mobility in Stroke Patient International Journal of Scientific Research, Vol : 4, Issue : 7 July 2015

❑❑❑

112 Locomotor Capabilities Index-5

The original Locomotor Capabilities Index (LCI) was developed in Canada in 1993 as part of the Prosthetic Profile of the Amputee questionnaire[1]. According to its developers the LCI "computes the global, basic, and advanced locomotor skills of the lower limb amputee with the prosthesis and assesses level of independence"[2][3]. The new LCI version with a 5-point ordinal scale presents similar general psychometric properties to the original LCI, a lower ceiling effect and a larger effect size[4].

Objective

The LCI is a disease-specific, self-administered instrument for assessing locomotor abilities generally considered essential for basic and advanced ADLs of people with lower-limb amputation and an enabling factor associated with long-term prosthetic use[5]. It is easily administered and quickly completed[4].

It is composed of 14 questions (phrased as "Would you say that you are able to do the following activities with your prosthesis on?") about different locomotor activities and selected primarily from the locomotor disabilities classification of the World Health Organization[6]. A 4-level ordinal scale (0–3 points; ranging from "not able" to "able to accomplish the activity alone") scores the degree of a person's perceived independence in performing each of the 14 activities while wearing the prosthesis.The LCI-5 splits the upper ordinal level of each item, "Yes, able to accomplish the activity alone" into "Yes, . . . alone with ambulation aids" (score: 3 points) and "Yes, . . . alone without ambulation aids" (score: 4 points), with a possible maximum score of 56. The LCI can be divided into two 7-item subscales that cover basic (items 1, 4, 5, 8–11) and advanced (items 2, 3, 6, 7,12–14) activities, respectively. Higher scores reflect greater locomotor capabilities with the prosthesis and less dependence on assistance[4].

Evidence

The construct validity of LCI and LCI-5 was analyzed by correlation with the Rivermead Mobility Index, a timed walking test, and the FIM instrument. The item-to-total correlations (Spearman) ranged from .50 to .87 (P<.0001 for all). Both the LCI and LCI-5 correlated with all criterion measures (p range, .61–.76), with the LCI-5 showing a larger effect size and a lower ceiling effect. The test-retest reliability, both the LCI and LCI-5 showed a high degree of correspondence and agreement (ICC values) between their total scores, and the Bland-Altman plot confirmed the good reproducibility of both the versions[4].

al Locomotor Capabilities Index (LCI) was developed in Canada in 1993 as part of the Prosthetic Profile of the Amputee questionnaire[1]. According to its developers the LCI "computes the global, basic, and advanced locomotor skills of the lower limb amputee with the prosthesis and assesses level of independence"[2][3]. The new LCI version with a 5-point ordinal scale presents similar general psychometric properties to the original LCI, a lower ceiling effect and a larger effect size[4].

References

1. Grise MC, Gauthier-Gagnon C, Martineau GG: Prosthetic profile of people with lower extremity amputation: conception and design of a follow-up questionnaire. Arch Phys Med Rehabil 1993, 74:862-870.
2. Gauthier-Gagnon C, Grise MC: Tools to measure outcome of people with lower limb amputation; Update on the PPA and LCI. J Prosthet Orthot 2006, 18:61-69.
3. Larsson, B., Johannesson, A., Andersson, I. H., & Atroshi, I. (2009). The Locomotor Capabilities

Index ; validity and reliability of the Swedish version in adults with lower limb amputation, 9, 1–9. https://doi.org/10.1186/1477-7525-7-44

4. Franchignoni, F., Orlandini, D., Ferriero, G., & Moscato, T. A. (2004). Reliability , Validity , and Responsiveness of the Locomotor Capabilities Index in Adults With Lower-Limb Amputation. https://doi.org/10.1016/j.apmr.2003.06.010

5. Gauthier-Gagnon C, Grise MC, Potvin D. Enabling factors related to prosthetic use by people with transtibial and transfemoral amputation. Arch Phys Med Rehabil 1999;80:706-13.

6. Gauthier-Gagnon C, Grise MC, Lepage Y. The Locomotor Capabilities Index: content validity. J Rehabil Outcomes Meas 1998; 2:40-6.

Locomotor Capabilities Index-5

	No (0)	Yes, If Someone Helps Me (1)	Yes, If Someone Is Near Me (2)	Yes, Alone, With Ambulation Aids (3)	Yes, Alone, Without Ambulation Aids (4)
1. Get up from a chair					
2. Pick up an object from the floor when you are standing up with your prosthesis					
3. Get up from the floor (eg, if you fell)					
4. Walk in the house					
5. Walk outside on even ground					
6. Walk outside on uneven ground (eg, grass, gravel, slope)					
7. Walk outside in inclement weather (eg, snow, rain, ice)					
8. Go up the stairs with a hand-rail					
9. Go down the stairs with a hand-rail					
10. Step up a sidewalk curb					
11. Step down a sidewalk curb					
12. Go up a few steps (stairs) without a hand-rail					
13. Go down a few steps (stairs) without a hand-rail					
14. Walk while carrying an object					

❑❑❑

113 Upper Extremity Functional Index

The Upper Extremity Functional Index (UEFI) is a patient reported outcome measure used to assess the functional impairment in individuals with musculoskeletal upper limb dysfunction.[1] The original UEFI consists of 20 questions on a 5- point rating scale assessing level of difficulty in performing activities of daily living using the upper extremities including household and work activities, hobbies, lifting a bag of groceries, washing your scalp, pushing up on your hands, driving etc.

There are currently two versions of the upper extremity functional index; UEFI 20-item and UEFI 15-item. The 15-item was developed to fit the Rasch analysis and it has been recommended because it's unidimensional. The effect of arm dominance on the positive minimal clinically important difference (pMCID) has not been determined for both versions of UEFI.

The UEFI has been adapted into other languages including Turkish, French Canadian and Spanish.

Intended Population

The UEFI is intended for use in individuals with upper extremity (including the shoulder, elbow, wrist and hand) dysfunction of musculoskeletal origin. A study by Binkley et al[2] supported the use of UEFI in patients after breast cancer surgery.

Method of Use

The UEFI is easy to administer as it is a self-reported questionnaire. Patients respond to each item by circling a number that best describes their level of difficulty. Item scores range from 0 to 4, 0 indicates extreme difficulty while 4 indicates no difficulty with a task and the total score is a total of the item scores. Possible range on the UEFI 20-item from 0 – 80 with 0 indicating lowest functional status and 80 indicating highest functional status. The minimum amount of change that is considered to be clinically significant is 9 points[3]

However, the UEFI-15 item is scored 0-59 and converted to give an interval level total score 0-100 with 0 indicating worst state and 100 best state.

The 20 tasks in the UEFI include:

1. Any of your usual work, housework, or school activities
2. Your usual hobbies, recreational or sporting activities
3. Lifting a bag of groceries to waist level
4. Lifting a bag of groceries above your head
5. Grooming your hair
6. Pushing up on your hands (eg, from bathtub or chair)
7. Preparing food (eg, peeling, cutting)
8. Driving
9. Vacuuming, sweeping or raking
10. Dressing
11. Doing up buttons
12. Using tools or appliances
13. Opening doors
14. Cleaning
15. Tying or lacing shoes
16. Sleeping
17. Laundering clothes (eg, washing, ironing, folding)
18. Opening a jar
19. Throwing a ball
20. Carrying a small suitcase with your affected limb

Evidence

Reliability

In a study by Chesworth et al[4], reliability for the UEFI-20 and UEFI-15 was the same (ICC=0.94 for both measures). MDC values were 9.4/80 for the UEFI-20 and 8.8/100 for the UEFI-15. Positive minimal clinically important difference values were 8/80 for the UEFI-20 and 6.7/100 for the UEFI-15; pMCID was higher for people whose non-dominant arm was affected.

Validity

In a study by Stratford et al[1], comparing Upper Extremity Functional Index (UEFI 20- item) and the Upper Extremity Functional Scale (UEFS), the discriminant cross-sectional validity of the UEFI was found to be 6.65 with p = .003 while the convergent cross-sectional validity coefficient between the UEFI and the UEFS was 0.82. In the same study, the longitudinal validity coefficient between the UEFI and the UEFS was 0.74. This study concluded that the longitudinal validity of the Upper Extremity Functional Index was superior to the Upper Extremity Functional Scale.

References

1. Stratford PW, Binkley JM, Stratford DM. Development and initial validation of the upper extremity functional index. Physiotherapy Can. 2001;53:259–67
2. Jill M. Binkley, Paul Stratford, Stephanie Kirkpatrick,Clara R. Farley, Joel Okoli, Sheryl Gabram Estimating the Reliability and Validity of the Upper Extremity Functional Index in Women After Breast Cancer Surgery. 2018 Clinical Breast Cancer, Vol. 18, No. 6, e1261-7.
3. Liebenson, C. (2007). Rehabilitation of the spine: A practitioner's manual. Baltimore, MD: Lippincott Williams & Wilkins.
4. Chesworth BM, Hamilton CB, Walton DM, et al. Reliability and validity of two versions of the upper extremity functional index. *Physiother Can.* 2014;66(3):243–253

UPPER EXTREMITY FUNCTIONAL INDEX

We are interested in knowing whether you are having any difficulty at all with the activities listed below because of your upper limb problem for which you are currently seeking attention. Please provide an answer for each activity. Today, do you or would you have any difficulty at all with: (Circle one number on each line)

	Extreme Difficulty	Quite a bit of Difficulty	Moderate Difficulty	A Little bit of Difficulty	No Difficulty
a. Any of your usual work, housework or school activities					
b. Your usual hobbies, recreational or sporting activities					
c. Lifting a bag of groceries to waist level					
d. Placing an object onto, or removing it from an overhead shelf					
e. Washing your hair or scalp					
f. Pushing up on your hands (e.g., from bathtub or chair)					
g. Preparing food (e.g., peeling, cutting)					
h. Driving					
I. Vacuuming, sweeping, or raking					
j. Dressing					
k. Doing up buttons					

l. Using tools or appliances					
m. Opening doors					
n. Cleaning					
o. Tying or lacing shoes					
p. Sleeping					
q. Laundering clothes. (e.g., washing, ironing, folding)					
r. Opening a jar					
s. Throwing a ball					
t. Carrying a small suitcase with your affected limb					
Column Totals:					
Column Totals:					

Score: / 80

❑❑❑

114 Lower Extremity Functional Scale (LEFS)

The lower extremity functional scale (LEFS) is a valid patient-rated outcome measure (PROM) for the measurement of lower extremity function. It was first developed by Binkley et al. (1999) in a group of patients with various musculoskeletal conditions.[1] The scale is originally developed in English language and according to western culture.

Objective

The objective of the Lower Extremity Functional Scale (LEFS) is to measure "patients' initial function, ongoing progress, and outcome" for a wide range of lower-extremity conditions.[1][2][3]

Intended Population

The LEFS is intended for use with adults, with lower extremity conditions.[1][2]

Method of Use

The LEFS is a self-report questionnaire. Patients answer the question "Today, do you or would you have any difficulty at all with:" in regards to twenty different everyday activities.[1][2]

Patients select an answer from the following scale for each activity listed:

1. Extreme Difficulty or Unable to Perform Activity
2. Quite a Bit of Difficulty
3. Moderate Difficulty
4. A Little Bit of Difficulty
5. No Difficulty

The patient's score is tallied at the bottom of the page. The maximum possible score is 80 points, indicating very high function. The minimum possible score is 0 points, indicating very low function.

Evidence

Reliability

Internal reliability for the LEFS is excellent (α=0.96). Test-retest reliability estimates were R=.86 (95% lower limit CI=.80) for the entire sample (n=98) and R=.94 (95% lower limit CI=.89) for the subset of patients with more chronic conditions (n=31).[1]

Validity

The LEFS is a valid tool as compared to the SF-36.[1]

Responsiveness

The minimum detectable change (MDC) for the LEFS is 9 points. That is, a change of more than 9 points represents a true change in the patient's condition.[1]

The minimum clinically important difference (MCID) for the LEFS is 9 points. That is, "Clinicians can be reasonably confident that a change of greater than 9 points is... a clinically meaningful functional change."[1]

The capacity of the LEFS to detect change in lower-extremity function appears to be superior to that of the SF-36 physical function subscale, as indicated by higher correlations with an external prognostic rating of change.[1]

The LEFS has good measurement properties--namely test-retest reliability and cross-sectional construct validity--and it could be an alternative to WOMAC-PF. [5]

Miscellaneous

The LEFS has an error of +/- 5 points. That is, the

tabulated score is within 5 points of a patient's "true" score.[1]

References

1. Binkley JM, Stratford PW, Lott SA, Riddle DL. The lower extremity functional scale (LEFS): scale development, measurement properties, and clinical application. Phys Ther 1999;79:371-383.
2. Rehabilitation Measures Database Lower Extremity Functional Scale http://www.rehabmeasures.org/Lists/RehabMeasures/DispForm.aspx?ID=1113 (accessed 24 Mar 2015).
3. Lower extremity functional scale https://www.researchgate.net/figure/Source-originale-Binkley-JM-Stratford-PW-Lott-SA-Riddle-DL-The-Lower-Extremity_fig1_221874838 (accessed on 29 August 2018)
4. Fillechaud. Scoring the LEFS. Available from: https://www.youtube.com watch? v = 4CDhRMZCWQ4 [last accessed 24/03/2015]
5. Pua YH, Cowan SM, Wrigley TV, Bennell KL. The Lower Extremity Functional Scale could be an alternative to the Western Ontario and McMaster Universities Osteoarthritis Index physical function scale. Journal of Clinical Epidemiology. 2009 Oct;62(10):1103-1111. DOI: 10.1016/j.jclinepi.2008.11.011.

The Lower Extremity Functional Scale

We are interested in knowing whether you are having any difficulty at all with the activities listed below because of your lower limb problem for which you are currently seeking attention. Please provide an answer for each activity. Today, do you or would you have any difficulty at all with:

Activities	Extreme Difficulty or Unable to Perform Activity (0)	Quite a Bit of Difficulty (1)	Moderate Difficulty (2)	A Little Bit of Difficulty (3)	No Difficulty (4)
1. Any of your usual work, housework, or school activities.					
2. Your usual hobbies, recreational or sporting activities.					
3. Getting into or out of the bath.					
4. Walking between rooms.					
5. Putting on your shoes or socks					
6. Squatting.					
7. Lifting an object, like a bag of groceries from the floor.					
8. Performing light activities around your home					
9. Performing heavy activities around your home.					
10. Getting into or out of a car.					
11. Walking 2 blocks.					
12. Walking a mile					
13. Going up or down 10 stairs (about 1 flight of stairs).					

14. Standing for 1 hour.					
15. Sitting for 1 hour					
16. Running on even ground.					
17. Running on uneven ground.					
18. Making sharp turns while running fast.					
19. Hopping.					
20. Rolling over in bed					
Column Totals					

Minimum Level of Detectable Change (90% Confidence): 9 points

SCORE: ____ **/ 80** (fill in the blank with the sum of your responses)

Source: Binkley et al (1999): The Lower Extremity Functional Scale (LEFS): Scale development, measurement properties, and clinical application. Physical Therapy. 79:371-383.

❑❑❑

115 Patient Specific Functional Scale

Objective

Patient Specific Functional Scale was developed by Stratford et al 1995 as a self-report outcome measure of function that could be used in patients with varying levels of independence.[1] The aim of PSFS is to provide clinicians with a valid, reliable, responsive and efficient outcome measure that would be easy to use and applicable to a large number of clinical presentations.[2]

Intended Population

The PSFS is a self-reported valid, reliable, and responsive outcome measure for patients with back, neck, knee and upper extremity problems[3][4]. It has also been shown to have a high test-retest reliability in both generic lower back pain and knee dysfunction issues.[5][1] It is also clinically responsive to changes over time with chronic pain patients[6]

Method of Use

1. Patients are asked to identify up to five important activities they are unable to perform or are having difficulty with as a result of their problem eg putting socks on, shopping.
2. Patients are asked to rate (on an 11-point scale) the current level of difficulty associated with each activity.
3. Following the intervention, patients are asked again to rate the activities previously identified (and are given the chance to nominate new problematic activities that might have arisen during that time).
4. "0" represents "unable to perform" and "10" represents "able to perform at prior level"
5. Patients select a value that best describes their current level of ability on each activity assessed.

Advantages

- Gives the patient positive re-enforcement that the intervention is effective[7]
- Keeps therapy goal orientated
- Quick to complete
- Relatively easy for patients to complete
- Helpful to redirect subjective assessment to function as opposed to pain
- Can be used on a wide variety of musculoskeletal and neurological conditions[8]

Disadvantages

- Not obtaining a final PSFS score. For example if a patient cancels their final appointment it is not always possible to ask for the score completion.[7]
- Some patients can find rating their activities on a numerical scale difficult
- Not specific to condition
- May require further outcome measures specific to condition to be completed[4]

Evidence

The PSFS is a valid, reliable, and responsive outcome measure for patients with back, neck, knee and upper extremity problems[3][4]. It has also been shown to have a high test-retest reliability in both generic lower back pain and knee dysfunction issues.[5]

Reliability

A study into cervical radiculopathy found the test-retest reliability of the PSFS to be high (Intraclass correlation coefficient = 0.82; 95% Confidence interval= 0.54–0.93) in comparison with the Neck Disability Index.[9]

Moderate to good reliability for patient with upper extremity musculoskeletal problems ICC = 0,713.[10]

Poor reliability exhibited in patient with cervical radiculopathy.[11]

Validity

PSFS is a valid tool (p<.001) in detecting patient with upper extremity problem.[10]

Responsiveness

Adequate responsiveness in patient with cervical radiculopathy (3.3) while the clinically important difference is 2.2.[11]

References

1. Horn KK, Jennings S, Richardson G, Van Vliet D, Hefford C, Abbott JH. The patient-specific functional scale: psychometrics, clinimetrics, and application as a clinical outcome measure. journal of orthopaedic & sports physical therapy. 2012 Jan;42(1):30-D17.
2. Stratford P, Gill C, Westaway M, Binkley J. Assessing disability and change on individual patients: a report of a patient specific measure. Physiotherapy canada. 1995 Oct;47(4):258-63.
3. Hefford C, Abbott JH, Arnold R, Baxter GD. The patient-specific functional scale: validity, reliability, and responsiveness in patients with upper extremity musculoskeletal problems. journal of orthopaedic & sports physical therapy. 2012 Feb;42(2):56-65.
4. Westaway MD, Stratford PW, Binkley JM. The patient-specific functional scale: validation of its use in persons with neck dysfunction. Journal of Orthopaedic & Sports Physical Therapy. 1998 May;27(5):331-8.
5. Chatman AB, Hyams SP, Neel JM, Binkley JM, Stratford PW, Schomberg A, Stabler M. The Patient-Specific Functional Scale: measurement properties in patients with knee dysfunction. Physical therapy. 1997 Aug 1;77(8):820-9.
6. Maughan EF, Lewis JS. Outcome measures in chronic low back pain. European Spine Journal. 2010 Sep 1;19(9):1484-94.
7. Nicholas P, Hefford C, Tumilty S. The use of the Patient-Specific Functional Scale to measure rehabilitative progress in a physiotherapy setting. Journal of Manual & Manipulative Therapy. 2012 Aug 1;20(3):147-52.
8. Maughan EF, Lewis JS. Outcome measures in chronic low back pain. European Spine Journal. 2010 Sep 1;19(9):1484-94.
9. Cleland JA, Fritz JM, Whitman JM, Palmer JA. The reliability and construct validity of the Neck Disability Index and patient specific functional scale in patients with cervical radiculopathy. Spine. 2006 Mar 1;31(5):598-602.
10. The Patient-Specific Functional Scale: Validity, Reliability, and Responsiveness in Patients With Upper Extremity Musculoskeletal Problems
11. Reliability, Construct Validity, and Responsiveness of the Neck Disability Index, Patient-Specific Functional Scale, and Numeric Pain Rating Scale in Patients with Cervical Radiculopathy

The Patient-Specific Functional Scale

Initial Assessment:

I am going to ask you to identify up to three important activities that you are unable to do or are having difficulty with as a result of your ________________ problem. Today, are there any activities that you are unable to do or having difficulty with because of your ____________ problem? (Clinician: show scale to patient and have the patient rate each activity).

Follow-up Assessments:

When I assessed you on (state previous assessment date), you told me that you had difficulty with (read all activities from list at a time). Today, do you still have difficulty with: (read and have patient score each item in the list)?

Patient-specific activity scoring scheme (Point to one number):

0	1	2	3	4	5	6	7	8	9	10
Unable to perform activity										Able to perform activity at the same level as before injury or problem

(Date and Score)

Activity	Initial					
1						
2						
3						
4						
5						
Additional						
Additional						

Total score = sum of the activity scores/number of activities

Minimum detectable change (90%CI) for average score = 2 points

Minimum detectable change (90%CI) for single activity score = 3 points

Resource: Stratford, P., Gill, C., Westaway, M., & Binkley, J. (1995). Assessing disability and change on individual patients: a report of a patient specific measure. Physiotherapy Canada, 47, 258-263.

❏❏❏

116

Manchester–Oxford Foot Questionnaire (MOFQ)

Foot and ankle surgery accounts for approximately one fifth of orthopaedic practice and has a high level of patient dissatisfaction. The Manchester-Oxford Foot Questionnaire's (MOXFQ's) are 16-item Patient Reported Outcome (PRO) measures developed and validated for use in clinical trials involving foot surgery. These self-administered PROs assesses how foot problems impair health-related quality of life can be completed before and after surgery.

The original MOXFQ (foot) PRO was developed as an outcome measure of hallux valgus (bunions) corrective surgery and has recently been slightly amended and validated for use among patients with a variety of foot or ankle problems. The MOXFQ (foot) and the MOXFQ (foot and ankle) PROs are available for license through iOutcomes.

The MOXFQ PROs were developed by researchers in the University of Oxford using interviews with patients and partially drawing on a pain related foot disability measure, the Manchester Foot Pain and Disability Index (MFPDI), as a template for item generation and content. The MFPDI is also available through iOutcomes.

Intended Population

Originally proven for use in hallux valgus corrective surgery[1][2], and more recently proven for use with patients receiving surgery for a variety of foot or ankle problems[3][4].

Method of Use

16 item questionnaire consisting of three domains/scales: 'Walking/standing' (seven items), 'Pain' (five items) and 'Social interaction' (four items) each having good measurement properties.

Evidence

Reliability

The MOXFQ PROs exhibit good internal consistency. The MOXFQ (foot and Ankle) has also demonstrated good test-retest reliability within different foot and ankle surgical subgroups at baseline assessment.

Validity

The MOXFQ PROs have been rigorously tested to demonstrate good content and construct validity.

Acceptability

Pre-testing and high completion rates suggest the PROs are easy to complete and acceptable within the test population.

The PROs (Patient Reported Outcome)

The MOXFQ PROs are self-administered, paper based measures consisting of 16-items. The PROs measure three domains:

Walking/standing (7 items)

Pain (5 items)

Social interaction (4 items)

Response options consist of a 5 point Likert scale ranging from no limitation to maximum limitation.

Developers' of the PROs recommend using the MOXFQ (foot) questionnaire for clinical trials that are specifically investigating outcomes of interventions for hallux valgus correction and use of the MOXFQ (foot and ankle) in all other instances. For example, trials of surgery or audits of outcomes involving all other foot or ankle condition (this may include people with hallux valgus).

Scoring System:

Scores for each domain are calculated by summing the responses to each item within a given domain. Raw scores can be converted to a 0-100 metric where 100=most severe. As mentioned above, the domains can also be summed to give a Summary Index score.

Development:

The MOFOX PROs were developed in a multistage process consistent with industry best practice:

References

1. Jill Dawson, Jane Coffey, Helen Doll, Grahame Lavis, Paul Cooke, Mark Herron and Crispin Jenkinson. A patient-based questionnaire to assess outcomes of foot surgery: Validation in the context of surgery for hallux valgus. 2006. Quality of Life Research, Volume 15, Number 7:1211-1222.
2. Dawson J, Doll H, Coffey J, Jenkinson C; Oxford and Birmingham Foot and Ankle Clinical Research Group. Responsiveness and minimally important change for the Manchester-Oxford foot questionnaire (MOXFQ) compared with AOFAS and SF-36 assessments following surgery for hallux valgus. Osteoarthritis Cartilage. 2007 Aug;15(8):918-31. Epub 2007 Mar 26.
3. J. Dawson, I. Boller, H. Doll, G. Lavis, R. Sharp, P. Cooke, C. Jenkinson. The MOXFQ patient-reported questionnaire: Assessment of data quality, reliability and validity in relation to foot and ankle surgery. The FootfckLRVolume 21, Issue 2 , Pages 92-102, June 2011
4. Dawson, J., Boller, I., Doll, H., Lavis, G., Sharp, R., Cooke, P., Jenkinson, C. Responsiveness of the Manchester-Oxford foot questionnaire (MOXFQ) compared with AOFAS, SF-36 and EQ-5D assessments following foot or ankle surgery. 2011, Journal of Bone and Joint Surgery,February 2012, vol. 94-B no. 2:205-209

Manchester–Oxford Foot Questionnaire (MOFQ)

Circle as appropriate: RIGHT / LEFT During the past 4 weeks this has applied to me:	**None of the time**	**Rarely**	**Some of the time**	**Most of the time**	**All of the time**
1. I have pain in my foot/ankle					
2. I avoid walking long distances because of pain in my foot/ankle					
3. I change the way I walk due to pain in my foot/ankle					
4. I walk slowly because of pain in my foot/ankle					
5. I have to stop and rest my foot/ankle because of pain					
6. I avoid some hard or rough surfaces because of pain in my foot/ankle					
7. I avoid standing for a long time because of pain in my foot/ankle					
8. I catch the bus or use the car instead of walking, because of pain in my foot/ankle					
9. I feel self-conscious about my foot/ankle					
10. I feel self-conscious about the shoes I have to wear					

11. The pain in my foot/ankle is more painful in the evening					
12. I get shooting pains in my foot/ankle					
13. The pain in my foot/ankle prevents me from carrying out my work/everyday activity					
14. I am unable to do all my social or recreational activities because of pain in my foot/ankle					
15. During the past 4 weeks how would you describe the pain you usually have in your foot/ankle?	None	Very mild	Mild	Moderate	Severe
16. During the past 4 weeks have you been troubled by pain from your foot/ankle in bed at night?	No nights	Only 1 or 2nights	Some nights	Most nights	Every night
Finally, please check that you have answered every question Thank you very much					
MOXFQ v2 University of Oxford, Department of Public Health (HSRU), Old Road Campus, Oxford OX37LF, UK					

❑❑❑

117 Manual Assessment of Respiratory Motion (MARM)

Objective

The MARM is a palpatory procedure based on the examiners interpretation and estimation of motion perceived by their hands at the posterior and lateral lower rib cage. The examiner using the MARM can gauge various aspects of breathing such as rate, regularity, but its particular utility is for assessing breathing pattern and the relative distribution of breathing motion between upper rib cage and lower rib cage and abdomen.

Intended Population

Subjects with Dysfunctional Breathing or Altered Breathing

Method of Use

The MARM also takes into account the form of the spinal column, whose extended or flexed form constitutes a third degree of freedom of breathing movement (Smith and Mead 1986). Extension of the spinal column increases the distance between the pubic symphysis and xiphoid process, elevates the ribcage, facilitating upward motion of the sternum/upper thorax (pump-handle motion) as well as abdominal expansion. Thus, it facilitates inhalation in a vertical direction ('length breathing'). By contrast, a slumped posture inhibits the vertical movement of inhalation, increases pressure of abdominal contents to increase diaphragm length and promotes lateral expansion and sideways elevation of the lower ribs or bucket-handle movement. Thus, it facilitates inhalation in a horizontal direction ('width breathing').

TheMARM is able to differentiate between these breathing patterns and assess asymmetry between the two sides of the body. In case of scoliosis or sideways distortion of the spinal column there is a marked difference in breathing movement between the left and right sides of the body and this can be registered clearly by the examiners two hands. Such asymmetry adds even more degrees of freedom of breathing movement.

An assumption of the MARM procedure is that breathing is a global movement of expansion (inhalation) and contraction (exhalation) of the body. From the manual assessment of motion at the lower ribs the examiner constructs a mental picture of global breathing motion, represented by an upper line and a lower line, originating from the centre of a circle or ellipse, together creating a slice in a pie chart, which represents the area of expansion. Specific features of the global change in form that can be estimated are: the degree that the sternum and upper thorax are lifted upwards, the degree that the lower ribs lift and expand sideways and the degree that diaphragmatic descent expands the abdomen outwards. The predominance of motion in either the upper rib cage/sternum or the lower rib cage/abdomen determines the direction of the global change with inhalation, as either predominantly in an upward or downward direction and the shape as either elongation or widening. Individuals may differ in their breathing response to postural change. For example when the spine is extended inspiration may result in a general increase in breathing motion with greater involvement of both upper thorax and abdomen or result in upward elevation of the chest with little increase or paradoxical decrease in abdominal motion.

With the MARM, having the subject intentionally breathe in different ways, the examiner can test the functionality of breathing. [1]

Evidence

Reliability& Validity

The MARM appears to be a valid and reliable clinical and research tool for assessing breathing movement with good inter-examiner and a greater ability to distinguish vertical ribcage motion. Further studies to confirm its clinical utility are warranted.

References

1. Rosalba Courtney, Jan van Dixhoorn,fckLRMarc Cohen; Evaluation of Breathing Pattern: Comparison of a Manual Assessment of Respiratory Motion(MARM) and Respiratory Induction Plethysmography. Appl Psychophysiol Biofeedback (2008) 33:91–100
2. Rosalba Courtney, Jan van Dixhoorn,fckLRMarc Cohen; Evaluation of Breathing Pattern: Comparison of a Manual Assessment of Respiratory Motion(MARM) and Respiratory Induction Plethysmography. Appl Psychophysiol Biofeedback (2008) 33:91–100

□□□

118 Assessment of Breathing Pattern Disorders

Introduction

Breathing Pattern Disorders (BPD) or Dysfunctional Breathing are abnormal respiratory patterns, specifically related to over-breathing. They range from simple upper chest breathing to, at the extreme end of the scale, hyperventilation (HVS).[1]

Dysfunctional breathing (DB) is defined as chronic or recurrent changes in the breathing pattern that cannot be attributed to a specific medical diagnosis, causing respiratory and non-respiratory complaints.[1] It is not a disease process, but rather alterations in breathing patterns that interfere with normal respiratory processes. BPD can, however, co-exist with diseases such as COPD or heart disease.[2][3] This page addresses the Assessment of Breathing Pattern Disorders. Read the Physiopedia page on Breathing Pattern Disorders for in-depth knowledge on the anatomy, aetiology, classification, etc.

Diagnostic Procedures

Capnography

Capnography is a reliable diagnostic tool for BPDs. It measures the average CO_2 partial pressure at the end of exhalation (End Tidal CO_2).[4][5]

Nijmegen Questionnaire

High scores on the Nijmegen questionnaire have been shown to be both sensitive and specific for detecting people with tendencies consistent with breathing pattern disorders. The sensitivity of the Nijmegen questionnaire in relation to the clinical diagnosis was 91% and the specificity 95%.[6] However, a 2020 study by Pauwen and colleagues found that in a primary care setting, the Nijmegen questionnaire might have lower predictive properties than anticipated.[7] Thus, the authors have suggested that the Hyperventilation Provocation Test is used to confirm a positive Nijmegen.[7]

Physical Assessment

Assessment of Breathing Patterns

When assessing breathing patterns, it is important to understand what normal breathing looks like. The resting respiratory rate changes throughout the lifespan:[8]

- Babies breathe 35 - 58 times per minute
- Toddlers 15-22 times per minute
- Adolescents 12-16 times per minute
- Once lungs stop growing at around 22 years of age, adults adopt a respiratory rate of 10-14 breaths per minute

At rest, a normal pattern will be nose / abdominal. Exhalation should be slightly longer than inhalation, with an approximate ratio of 1:2 (inhalation to exhalation). There should be a slight pause at the end of exhalation. This pattern is vital to maintain homeostasis and pH.[8]

Important assessment tests include:

- **Breath Holding** – Ask the patient to exhale and then hold his/her breath. People are usually able to hold their breath for 25 to 30 seconds.[9] If a patient holds less than 15 seconds, it may indicate low tolerance to carbon dioxide.
- **Breathing Hi-Low Test** - Patient is either seated or supine – Place your hands on the patient's chest and stomach. Ask the patient to exhale fully and then inhale normally. Observe where the movement initiates and where the most movement occurs. Look specifically for lateral expansion and upward hand pivot.[9]

- **Breathing Wave** – Patient lies prone. Ask him/her to breathe normally. The spine should move in a wave-like pattern towards the head. Segments that rise as a group may represent thoracic restrictions.[9]
- **Seated Lateral Expansion** – Place hands on lower thorax and monitor motion while breathing. Looking for symmetrical lateral expansion.[9]
- **Manual Assessment of Respiratory Motion (MARM)** - Assess and quantify breathing pattern, in particular, the distribution of breathing motion between the upper and lower parts of the rib cage and abdomen under various conditions. It is a manual technique that once acquired is practical, quick and inexpensive.[10]
- **Sniff Test** - Assesses bilateral diaphragm function. It is useful in assessing for upper or lower chest pattern dominance. The therapist places his/her hand 3 fingers below the patients xiphoid process. The patient performs a quick sniff. The therapist should feel an outward movement of the abdominal wall. This indicates that both hemi-diaphragms are working. Upper chest breathers usually have no diaphragmatic excursion or they may in-draw their abdominal wall.[9]
- **Respiratory Induction Plethysmography (RIP) and Magnetometry**: consists of two sinusoid wires coils insulated and placed one around thoracic (placed around the rib cage under the armpits) and the second(placed around the abdomen at the level of the umbilicus). The frequency from these wires coils converted to digital respiration wave form that is an indicator for inspired breath volume.

Assessment of the Musculoskeletal System

- Observe for elevated and depressed ribs and clavicle with rib palpation techniques.
- Check for muscle tone and length especially in the psoas, quadratus lumborum, latissimus dorsi, upper trapezius, scalene, and sternocleidomastoid.
- Assess for alterations in the mobility of the thoracic and rib articulations.

Assessment of Respiratory Function

- Oximetry - to measure oxygen saturation (SpO_2)
- Capnography - to measure end-tidal CO_2 levels in exhaled air (as described above)
- Peak expiratory flow rate - the highest flow of air out of the lungs from peak inspiration in a fast single forced breath out
- Manual Assessment of Respiratory Motion (MARM)

Outcome Measures

- Nijmegen Questionnaire
- Rowley Breathing Self-Efficacy Scale (RoBE)[12]
- Self Evaluation of Breathing Questionnaire) SEBQ)[13]
- Hospital Anxiety and Depression Questionnaire (HAD)[14]

Differential Diagnosis

BPDs can often mimic more serious conditions such as cardiac, neurological and gastrointestinal conditions. These must all be ruled out by the medical team.

References

1. Lum LC. Hyperventilation syndromes in medicine and psychiatry: a review. Journal of the Royal Society of Medicine. 1987 Apr;80(4):229-31..
2. Sueda S et al. 2004 Clinical impact of selective spasm provocation tests Coron Artery Dis 15(8):491–497
3. Ajani AE, Yan BP. The mystery of coronary artery spasm. Heart, Lung and circulation. 2007 Feb 1;16(1):10-5.
4. Bradley H, Esformes J. Breathing pattern disorders and functional movement. Int J Sports Phys Ther. 2014 Feb;9(1):28-39.
5. McLaughlin L. Breathing evaluation and retraining in manual therapy. Journal of Bodywork and Movement Therapies. 2009 Jul 1;13(3):276-82.
6. Van Dixhoorn J, Duivenvoorden HJ. Efficacy of Nijmegen Questionnaire in recognition of the hyperventilation syndrome. J Psychosom Res. 1985;29(2):199-206.
7. Pauwen N, Colot T, Boucharessas F, Sergysels R, Bertuit J, Ninane V et al. Validity of the Nijmegen questionnaire for screening hyperventilation syndrome in primary care. European Respiratory Journal. 2020;56(suppl 64):2697.
8. Clifton-Smith T. The Science of Breathing Well Course. Physioplus. 2020.

9. Chaitow, L. Dysfunctional Breathing Course Videos. Physioplus 2019. https://members.physio-pedia.com/2014/04/01/breathing-disorders/#resource
10. Rosalba Courtney, Jan van Dixhoorn, Marc Cohen; Evaluation of Breathing Pattern: Comparison of a Manual Assessment of Respiratory Motion(MARM) and Respiratory Induction Plethysmography. Appl Psychophysiol Biofeedback (2008) 33:91–100
11. UFGATEP2014. DrWest seated lateral rib expansion. Available from: http://www.youtube.com/watch?v=by45ML3QMXA[last accessed 16/4/2020]
12. Rowley J, Nicholls DA. Development of the RoBE self-efficacy scale for people with breathing pattern disorders.
13. Rosalba Courtney, Kenneth Mark Greenwood, Marc Cohen. Relationships between measures of dysfunctional breathing in a population with concerns about their breathing. Journal of Bodywork & Movement Therapies (2011) 15, 24-34
14. http://www.svri.org/documents/health-and-well-being (Accessed 16th September, 2017)

❑❑❑

119 Nijmegen Questionnaire

Objective

The Nijmegen Questionnaire (NQ) gives a broad view of symptoms associated with dysfunctional breathing patterns. The Nijmegen Questionnaire was introduced over 30 years ago as a screening tool to detect patients with hyperventilation complaints that could benefit from breathing regulation through capnographic feedback.

Intended Population

Mostly used for people with hyperventilation syndrome.

Method of Use

The NQ consists of 16 items to be answered on a five-point scale ranging from 'never' counted as zero to 'very often' counted as 4. The total score ranges from 0-64. Completion of the questionnaire only takes a few minutes.

A score of over 19 denotes the presence of respiratory distress and dysfunction. The higher the score the more distress is present. Values below 20 are considered within the normal and functional domain.[1]

Evidence

162 Greek asthma out-patients (86 with mild and 76 moderate asthma) participated in the study. Hyperventilation was assessed using NQ and clinical measures such as breath holding time (BHT), respiratory rate (RR) and end-tidal CO2 (ETCO2). Construct validity was tested through factor analysis and cross-sectional validity through correlations of the NQ score with BHT, ETCO2 and RR (Pearson's r correlation coefficient).

Validity

The sensitivity of the Nijmegen Questionnaire in relation to the clinical diagnosis was 91% and the specificity 95%.[3] However, a 2020 study by Pauwen and colleagues found that in a primary care setting, the Nijmegen questionnaire might have lower predictive properties than anticipated.[4] Thus, the authors have suggested that the Hyperventilation Provocation Test is used to confirm a positive Nijmegen.[4]

Responsiveness

The advantage of the NQ is that it is short and responsive to treatment.[1] Thus, it can be used repeatedly over a course of treatment to measure progress.

References

1. Courtney, R. and Dixhoorn, J. Questionnaires and manual methods for assessing breathing dysfunction. Chapter 6.5 in: Chaitow, L., Bradley, D., and Gilbert, C. Recognizing and treating breathing disorders. 20014, Elsevier
2. http://www.heartofengland.nhs.uk/wp-content/uploads/Nijmegen_Questionnaire.pdf
3. an Dixhoorn J, Duivenvoorden HJ. Efficacy of Nijmegen Questionnaire in recognition of the hyperventilation syndrome. J Psychosom Res. 1985;29(2):199-206
4. Pauwen N, Colot T, Boucharessas F, Sergysels R, Bertuit J, Ninane V et al. Validity of the Nijmegen questionnaire for screening hyperventilation syndrome in primary care. European Respiratory Journal. 2020;56(suppl 64):2697.

The Nijmegen Questionnaire

The Nijmegen questionnaire gives a broad view of symptoms associated with dysfunctional breathing patterns.

It is only a preliminary guide to breathing training.

Please ring the score that best describes the frequency with which you experienced the symptoms listed

Symptom	Never (0)	Seldom (1)	Some-times (2)	Often (3)	Very often(4)
1.Chest pain 2.Blurred vision Dizziness 3.Confusion or loss of touch with reality 4.Fast or deep breathing 5.Shortness of breath 6.Tightness across chest 6.Bloated sensation in stomach Tingling in fingers and hands 7.Difficulty breathing or taking deep breaths 8.Stiffness or cramps in fingers and hands Tightness around the mouth 9.Cold hands or fee 10.Palpitations in the chest 11.Anxiety **Totals**					

A grand total score of over 20 indicates significant hyperventilation.

A grand total score of between 10 and 20 suggests mild hyperventilation.

If your score is under 10 your breathing may not be causing you any serious health problems.

However with any score over zero you should do the other checks on your breathing.

❑❑❑

120 Hospital Anxiety and Depression Scale (HADS)

Tick the box beside the reply that is closest to how you have been feeling in the past week. Don't take too long over you replies: your immediate is best.

D	A		D	A	
		I feel tense or 'wound up':			**I feel as if I am slowed down:**
	0	Most of the time	0		Nearly all the time
	1	A lot of the time	1		Very often
	2	From time to time, occasionally	2		Sometimes
	3	Not at all	3		Not at all
		I still enjoy the things I used to enjoy			**I get a sort of frightened feeling like**
					'butterflies' in the stomach:
0		Definitely as much		0	Not at all
1		Not quite so much		1	Occasionally
2		Only a little		2	Quite Often
3		Hardly at all		3	Very Often
		I get a sort of frightened feeling as if something			**I have lost interest in my appearance**:
		awful is about to happen:			
	0	Very definitely and quite badly	0		Definitely
	1	Yes, but not too badly	1		I don't take as much care as I should
	2	A little, but it doesn't worry me	2		I may not take quite as much care
	3	Not at all	3		I take just as much care as ever
		I can laugh and see the funny side of things:			**I feel restless as I have to be on the move**:
0		As much as I always could		0	Very much indeed
1		Not quite so much now		1	Quite a lot
2		Definitely not so much now		2	Not very much
3		Not at all		3	Not at all
		Worrying thoughts go through my			**I look forward with enjoyment to things**:
		mind:	0		As much as I ever did
0		A great deal of the time	1		Rather less than I used to
1		A lot of the time	2		Definitely less than I used to
2		From time to time, but not too often	3		Hardly at all
3		Only occasionally			**I get sudden feelings of panic**:
		I feel cheerful:		0	Very often indeed
	0	Not at all		1	Quite often
	1	Not often		2	Not very often
	2	Sometimes		3	Not at all
	3	Most of the time			

		I can sit at ease and feel relaxed:			**I can enjoy a good book or radio or TV program:**
	0	Definitely	**0**		Often
	1	Usually Not	**1**		Sometimes
	2	Often	**2**		Not often
	3	Not at all	**3**		Very seldom

Scoring:

Total score: Depression (D) __________ Anxiety (A) ____________

0-7 = Normal

8-10 = Borderline abnormal (borderline case)

11-21 = Abnormal (case)

❑❑❑

121 Mayo Elbow Performance Index

Introduction

The Mayo Elbow Performance score (MEPS) or Mayo Elbow Performance Index[1] (MEPI) is an instrument used to test the limitations, caused by pathology, of the elbow during activities of daily living (ADL) . This specific test uses 4 subscales:

1. Pain,
2. Range of Motion (arc of motion of the art. humeroulnaris)
3. Stability
4. Daily Function

MEPS can be used to measure which treatment work best for different conditions, An example would be when deciding the best post-operative treatment for example: the difference in prognosis between open and closed fractures when operated.

Clinically Relevant Anatomy

The elbow is an articulation between the humerus in the upper arm and the radius and ulna in the lower arm. The art. humeroulnaris connects the humerus and the ulna and allows flexion and extension in the elbow. Assessing movement is a key factor in the MEPI and has its own subscale.

Muscles responsible for movement at the elbow and the forearm can be divided into four groups: the flexors, the extensors, the pronators and the supinators.

- Flexors: Biceps, Coracobrachialis, Brachioradials, Brachialis, Pronator Teres, flexors of the wrist
- Extensors: Triceps, Anconeus, Supinator
- Pronators: Pronator Teres,Pronator Quadratus, Brachioradialis
- Supinators: Supinator, Brachioradialis, Biceps

Technique

MEPS is a 4 part test where clinical information is rated based on a 100 points scale[1].

- <60 - poor
- 60-74 – fair
- 75-89 - good
- 90-100 – excellent

Part 1: Pain

The therapist asks the patient how severe the pain is and in how frequent the pain appears.

- 45 points are for patients who do not have pain,
- 30 points are given to patients who have mild pain,
- moderate pain results in 15 points,
- patients with severe pain get 0 points.

Part 2: Range of motion

The patient starts with his elbow fully extended and then tries to flex the elbow.

- 20 points are given when the arm reaches more than 100° flexion,
- 15 points If the angle is between 100°-50°
- 5 Points when the elbow bends 50° or less

Part 3: Stability

- When the elbow is considered stable 10 points are given.
- A mildly unstable elbow results in 5 points.
- An unstable elbow does not receive points (0).

Part 4: ADL

Based on 5 ADL's who are each given 5 points an image

is sketched how well the patient is able to participate in the daily life. The activities are:

- Combing your hair
- Performing personal hygiene
- Eating
- Putting on shirt and shoes.

Variations of the Index

Mayo elbow performance index has 2 variants[1]. The first one excludes function and ADLs; it has just 3 criteria pain, range of motion and stability and is used for comparison between pre – and postoperative results with patients who had a Kudo elbow prosthesis. The prosthesis was placed as a treatment for rheumatic arthritis[2]. The points are added up and put on a 100 points scale with norms equal to the standard test.

In the second variant[1] of the MEPI the the ADL is removed and replaced with a strength category. The following adaptions are also made:

- The factor pain is rated at a scale of 40 with 40 no pain and 0 for greatest pain ever, the way rating is the same as for normal test.
- Both stability and arc of motion are rated equal to the standard MEPI.
- The strength is measured on clinical rating scale
  - 20 for normal strength over
  - 14 for mild loss of strength
  - 7 for moderate loss of strength
  - 0 for marked loss of strength.

The results are graded with a maximum of 100 points and categorised into 4 groups:

- 91- 100: excellent
- 90 – 81: good
- 80 – 71: fair
- <70: poor

Evidence

Turchin et al[3]. described the MEPS a: "The Mayo elbow-performance index as having a clear format. The associated costs were low because only a goniometer was necessary. Little training was needed, and the system was suitable for use in a clinic. Neither strength nor deformity was included in the content of the scale, and motion was assessed only in terms of flexion and extension. The scaling was ordinal and seemed appropriate. Function and motion were weighted less heavily than pain."

Mayo Elbow Performance Index often appears in scientific documentation as a golden standard for questionnaires[4], to measure improvement after surgery, to compare treatments or conditions and as an indication for therapy. Nevertheless Longo et al[1]. concluded that further research is necessary to document validity and sensitivity of a lot of elbow tests including the MEPS and only one study was found where MEPS was really tested[5]. This study showed that the correlation with the other tests (Broberg and Morrey, Ewald et al, The Hospital for Special Surgery and Pritchard) was high but the correlation with a visual analogue scale was only moderate[5]. A study in 2014 concluded that MEPS has strong reliability when assessed at different times and when compared with a validated elbow outcomes instrument, although the study was small and had only 42 participants[6].

References

1. Longo UG, Franceschi F, Loppini M, Maffulli N, Denaro V. Rating systems for evaluation of the elbow. British medical bulletin. 2008 Jun 6;87(1):131-61.
2. Morrey BF, Bryan RS. Revision total elbow arthroplasty. The Journal of bone and joint surgery. American volume. 1987 Apr;69(4):523-32.
3. Turchin DC, Beaton DE, Richards RR. Validity of observer-based aggregate scoring systems as descriptors of elbow pain, function, and disability. JBJS. 1998 Feb 1;80(2):154-62.
4. Eygendaal D, Jolie IM, Hazes JM, Rozing PM. Clinical reliability and validity of elbow functional assessment in rheumatoid arthritis. The Journal of rheumatology. 1999 Sep;26(9):1909-17.
5. The B, Reininga IH, El Moumni M, Eygendaal D. Elbow-specific clinical rating systems: extent of established validity, reliability, and responsiveness. Journal of shoulder and elbow surgery. 2013 Oct 1;22(10):1380-94.
6. Cusick MC, Bonnaig NS, Azar FM, Mauck BM, Smith RA, Throckmorton TW. Accuracy and reliability of the Mayo elbow performance score. The Journal of hand surgery. 2014 Jun 1;39(6):1146-50.

Mayo Elbow Performance Index

Section 1 - Pain Intensity

None	Mild
Moderate	Severe

Section 2 -Motion

Arc of motion greater than 100 degrees

Arc of motion between 50 and 100 degrees

Arc of motion less than 50 degrees

Section 3 Stability

Stable Moderate

Stable Grossly Stable

Section 4 – Function (Tick as many as able)

Can comb hair Can Eat

Can perform hygiene Can do shirt

Can do shoe

122 McGill Pain Questionnaire

Objective

The McGill Pain Questionnaire (MPQ) is a self-reporting measure of pain used for patients with a number of diagnoses. It assesses both quality and intensity of subjective pain.

Intended Population

Validated for patients with Cancer, Chronic Pelvic Pain, Fibromyalgia, Headaches, Herniated intervertebral discs, Ischemic muscular pain, Low back pain, Lumbago-sciatica, Orthodontics/Dental pain, Postoperative complications, Rheumatic pain, Trigeminal neuralgia and atypical facial pain, Vulvar pain

Method of Use

The MPQ is composed of 78 words, of which respondents choose those that best describe their experience of pain. Seven words are selected from the following categories: dimension 1 to 10 (pain descriptors), three words; dimensions 11 to 15 (affective components of pain), dimension 16 (evaluation of pain) one word, and dimension 17 to 20 (miscellaneous) one word. Scores are tabulated by summing values associated with each word; scores range from 0 (no pain) to 78 (severe pain). Qualitative differences in pain may be reflected in respondent's word choice [1]

Reference

Evidence

Reliability

Test-retest Reliability:

(Ferraz et al., 1990; n = 91 (66 literate & 25 illiterate) [2]
Excellent test-retest reliability (literate) r = 0.96
Excellent test-retest reliability (illiterate) r = 0.95

Validity

Criterion Validity:

Lung, Head or Neck, and Prostate Cancer: (Fisher et al., 2010; n = 302; mean age = 60.5 (11.5) years; all patients undergoing radiation treatment) [3]

Concurrent validity: number of words chosen predicted by (using standardized regression coefficients, Beta):

- State Anxiety (Beta = 0.06)
- Depression (Beta = 0.07)
- Greater number of coping strategies used (Beta = 0.16)

Construct Validity:

Low Back Pain:

(Byrne et al, 1982; n = 98 (63 female, 35 male); mean age 41.7 (male); 48.1 (female) years; mean duration of back pain 5.5 and 7.7 years respectively) [4]

- Factor analyses was used, loadings were compared to prior research (e.g. Prieto et al., 1980[5]). Comparisons suggest a similar pattern of factor loadings.

Content Validity:

Literature Review:

(Melzack, 1975; measure development) [6]

- Subject Matter Experts classified 102 words

gleaned from the extant literature.

- Words were categorized into 3 classes and 16 subclasses, these include:

Sensory qualities: temporal, spatial, pressure, thermal and "other" properties of pain.

Affective qualities: tension fear and automatic properties of pain.

Evaluative terms: a subjective assessment of overall pain intensity.

- Groups of doctors, patients and students then assigned numeric intensity values to each word
- High levels of agreement were observed despite difference in cultural, socio-economic and educational levels

Responsiveness

Not established

References

1. Melzack, R. "The McGill Pain Questionnaire: major properties and scoring methods." Pain 1975 1(3): 277-299
2. Ferraz, M. B., Quaresma, M. R., et al. "Reliability of pain scales in the assessment of literate and illiterate patients with rheumatoid arthritis." J Rheumatol 1990 17(8): 1022-1024
3. Fischer, D. J., Villines, D., et al. "Anxiety, depression, and pain: differences by primary cancer." Support Care Cancer 2010 18(7): 801-810
4. Byrne, M., Troy, A., et al. "Cross-validation of the factor structure of the McGill Pain Questionnaire." Pain 13(2): 193-201Byrne, M., Troy, A., et al. (1982). "Cross-validation of the factor structure of the McGill Pain Questionnaire." Pain 1982 13(2): 193-201
5. Prieto, E. J., Hopson, L., et al. "The language of low back pain: factor structure of the McGill pain questionnaire." Pain 8(1): 11-19.Prieto, E. J., Hopson, L., et al. (1980). "The language of low back pain: factor structure of the McGill pain questionnaire." Pain 1980 8(1): 11-19.
6. Melzack, R. "The McGill Pain Questionnaire: major properties and scoring methods." Pain 1975 1(3): 277-299

The McGill Pain Questionnaire

Overview: The McGill Pain Questionnaire can be used to evaluate a person experiencing significant pain. It can be used to monitor the pain over time and to determine the effectiveness of any intervention. It was developed at by Dr. Melzack at McGill University in Montreal Canada and has been translated into several languages.

Sections:

1. What Does Your Pain Feel Like?
2. How Does Your Pain Change with Time?
3. How Strong is Your Pain?

What Does Your Pain Feel Like?

Statement: Some of the following words below describe your present pain. Circle ONLY those words that best describe it. Leave out any category that is not suitable. Use only a single word in each appropriate category - the one that applies best.

Group	Descriptor	Points
1 (temporal)	flickering	1
	quivering	2
	pulsing	3
	throbbing	4
	beating	5
	pounding	6
2 (spatial)	jumping	1
	flashing	2
	shooting	3
3 (punctate pressure)	pricking	1
	boring	2
	drilling	3
	stabbing	4
	lancinating	5
4 (incisive pressure)	sharp	1
	cutting	2
	lacerating	3
5 (constrictive pressure)	pinching	1
	pressing	2
	gnawing	3
	cramping	4
	crushing	5
6 (traction pressure)	tugging	1
	pulling	2
	wrenching	3
7 (thermal)	hot	1
	boring	2
	scalding	3
	searing	4

8 (brightness)	tingling	1
	itchy	2
	smarting	3
	stinging	4
9 (dullness)	dull	1
	sore	2
	hurting	3
	aching	4
	heavy	5
10 (sensory miscellaneous)	tender	1
	taut	2
	rasping	3
	splitting	4
11 (tension)	tiring	1
	exhausting	2
12 (autonomic)	sickening	1
	suffocating	2
13 (fear)	fearful	1
	frightful	2
	terrifying	3
14 (punishment)	punishing	1
	gruelling	2
	cruel	3
	vicious	4
	killing	5
15 (affective-evaluative-sensory: miscellaneous)	wretched	1
	blinding	2
16 (evaluative)	annoying	1
	troublesome	2
	miserable	3
	intense	4
	unbearable	5
17 (sensory: miscellaneous)	spreading	1
	radiating	2
	penetrating	3
	piercing	4
18 (sensory: miscellaneous)	tight	1
	numb	2
	drawing	3
	squeezing	4
	tearing	5
19 (sensory)	cool	1
	cold	2
	freezing	3
20 (affective-evaluative: miscellaneous)	nagging	1
	nauseating	2
	agonizing	3
	dreadful	4
	torturing	5

pain score = SUM (points for applicable descriptors)

How Does Your Pain Change with Time?

Question	Response	Points
Which word or words would you use to describe the pattern of your pain?	**a)** continuous steady constant	1
	b) rhythmic periodic intermittent	2
	c) brief momentary transient	3

Do the following items increase or decrease your pain?

1. liquor
2. stimulants such as coffee
3. eating
4. heat
5. cold
6. damp
7. weather changes
8. massage or use of a vibrator
9. pressure
10. no movement
11. movement
12. sleep or rest
13. lying down
14. distraction (TV reading etc.)
15. urination or defecation
16. tension
17. bright lights
18. loud noises
19. going to work
20. intercourse
21. mild exercise
22. fatigue

How Strong is Your Pain?

Statement: People agree that the following 5 words (mild discomforting distressing horrible excruciating represent pain of increasing intensity. To answer each question below write the number of the most appropriate word in the space beside the question.

Question	Response	Points
Which word describes your pain right now?	mild	1
	discomforting	2
	distressing	3

	horrible	4
	excruciating	5
Which word describes it at its worst?	mild	1
	discomforting	2
	distressing	3
	horrible	4
	excruciating	5
Which word describes it when it is least?	mild	1
	discomforting	2
	distressing	3
	horrible	4
	excruciating	5
Which word describes the worst toothache you ever had?	mild	1
	discomforting	2
	distressing	3
	horrible	4
	excruciating	5
Which word describes the worst headache	mild	1
	discomforting	2
	distressing	3
	horrible	4
	excruciating	5
Which word describes the worst stomach-ache you ever had?	mild	1
	discomforting	2
	distressing	3
	horrible	4
	excruciating	5

Interpretation:

- **minimum pain score: 0** (would not be seen in a person with true pain)
- **maximum pain score: 78**
- **The higher the pain score the greater the pain.**

References: Melzack R. The McGill Pain Questionnaire: Major properties and scoring methods. Pain. 1975; 1: 277-299. Stein C Mendl G. The German counterpart to McGill Pain Questionnaire. Pain. 1988; 32: 251-255.

❑❑❑

123 Mental Health Outcome Measures for Physiotherapists in Clinical Practice

Introduction

Strong mental health is fundamental to the well-being of individuals, families and communities alike.[1] Mental health is defined as "a state of well-being in which every individual realizes his or her own potential, can cope with the normal stresses of life, can work productively and fruitfully, and is able to make a contribution to her or his community".[2] Poor mental health has been identified as one of the largest causes of disability, poor quality of life and reduced productivity among adults.[3]

The correlations between poor mental health and an increased prevalence of chronic and preventable diseases, musculoskeletal conditions and multi-regional pain emphasizes the need for an effective and holistic multidisciplinary approach to the management of this condition.[4] Through a multidisciplinary approach, physiotherapists can address the physical well-being of individuals with mental health conditions from across their lifespan. Improvements to physical well-being can improve mental well-being and prevent the development of mental health conditions, such as depression which are often associated with other physiological conditions.[5]

As physiotherapists working within these dimensions, there is a need to evaluate clinical outcomes, receive feedback and engender new approaches. Outcome measures play a key role in achieving these feats. There are several mental health outcome measures in use and there are ongoing projects for the development of more. Below you will find mental health outcome measures that can be used by physiotherapists in clinical practice.

Mental Health Outcome Measures for Clinical Physiotherapists

An outcome measure in mental health care can be defined as a tool used to measure the effect on a person's mental health as a result of health care intervention, plus any additional extra-therapeutic influences.[6] Specifically, outcome measures are quantitative indicators used at two or more points in time: baseline, post intervention, discharge, or follow-ups.[7] To be useful, mental health outcome measures must be valid and reliable, sensitive to change, comparable across relevant client groups and service types, and meaningful to both clients and clinicians.[8]

Furthermore, outcome measures need to be meaningful to clients and relevant to the areas in which they have treatment goals. Research with mental health service consumers shows that many measures are not particularly relevant to their situations and do not capture outcomes that are personally meaningful.[9] Determining an outcome measure that is applicable in both clinical work and service evaluation is challenging.[10] Mental health is a broad construct that comprises a number of different measurement domains.[11] These include measures that cover recovery, cognitive performance and emotional experience, quality of life, ability to undertake daily activities and maintain interpersonal relationships consistent with development stage, and general life satisfaction and wellbeing.[12][13] The Physiotherapist is concerned about these measures and would work in improving and assessing them.

Outcome Measures

Health of the Nation Outcome Scales[14] (HoNOS)

Health of the Nation Outcomes Scales (HoNOS) as developed during the early 90s by the Royal College of Psychiatrists as a measure of the health and social functioning of people with severe mental illness. The scales contain 12 items measuring behaviour, impairment, symptoms and social functioning. The scales are completed after routine clinical assessments in any setting.[15]

Global Assessment of Functioning[16] (GAF) Scale

The GAF is a clinician-rated scale giving a measure of overall psychiatric disturbance integrating three dimensions of functioning: psychological, social and occupational. It is a single-item measure on a 100-point scale divided into 10-point intervals.[17] It has shown good construct and concurrent validity, but questions have been raised over its content validity. Inter-rater reliability can be low, particularly in routine clinical use.[13] It is sensitive to change when correlated with change in the Positive and Negative Syndrome Scale (PANSS).[18] The GAF is brief, easy to use and reliability can be increased with minimal training, which makes it more acceptable in routine clinical settings.[13]

Short Form 36[19] (SF -36)

SF-36 is a set of generic, coherent, and easily administered quality-of-life measures. These measures rely upon patient self-reporting and are now widely utilized by managed care organizations and by Medicare for routine monitoring and assessment of care outcomes in adult patients. The physical functioning (PF) domain of the established and widely used SF-36 questionnaire asks about limitations on ten aspects of everyday life. It is freely available online. File:Sf 36.pdf

Patient – Clinician Dialogue Interaction [21]

It is an outcomes measure to support structured conversation between patients and clinician focusing on the patients' views of quality of life, needs for care and treatment satisfaction.

Questions include:

1. How satisfied are you with your mental health?
2. How satisfied are you with your physical health?
3. How satisfied are you with your job situation?
4. How satisfied are you with your accommodation?
5. How satisfied are you with your leisure activities?
6. How satisfied are you with your friendships?
7. How satisfied are you with your partner/family?
8. How satisfied are you with your personal safety?
9. How satisfied are you with your medication?
10. How satisfied are you with the practical help you receive?
11. How satisfied are you with consultations with mental health professionals?

The rating for each item is:

1. Couldn't be worse
2. Displeased
3. Mostly dissatisfied
4. Mixed
5. Mostly satisfied
6. Pleased
7. Couldn't be better
8. No response

Additional help needed: Yes/No

Mini Mental State Examination (MMSE)[22]

MMSE is a tool that can be used to systematically and thoroughly assess mental status. It is an 11-question measure that tests five areas of cognitive function: orientation, registration, attention and calculation, recall, and language. The maximum score is 30. A score of 23 or lower is indicative of cognitive impairment. The MMSE takes only 5-10 minutes to administer and is therefore practical to use repeatedly and routinely.

The MMSE is effective as a screening tool for cognitive impairment with older, community dwelling, hospitalized and institutionalized adults. Assessment of an older adult's cognitive function is best achieved when it is done routinely, systematically and thoroughly.

Since its creation in 1975, the MMSE has been validated and extensively used in both clinical practice and research. The MMSE is effective as a screening instrument to separate patients with cognitive impairment from those without it. In addition, when used repeatedly the instrument is able to measure changes in cognitive status that may benefit from intervention. However, the tool is not able to diagnose the case for changes in cognitive function and should not replace a complete clinical assessment of mental status.

Brief Psychiatric Rating Scale (BPRS)

The BPRS is a rating scale which a clinician or researcher may use to measure psychiatric symptoms such as depression, anxiety, hallucinations and unusual behaviour.[23] Each symptom is rated 1-7 and depending on the version between a total of 18-24 symptoms are scored. The scale is one of the oldest, most widely used scales to measure psychotic symptoms and was first published in 1962.

References

1. Department of Health and Ageing (2008). National

Mental Health Policy. Department of Health and Ageing, Canberra.

2. World Health Organization. Mental health: a state of well-being 2014.
3. Mental Health and Physiotherapy (2011) .Australian Physiotherapy Association. http://www.physiotherapy.asn.au/
4. Gureje, O., Ademola, A. & Olley, B. O. (2008) Depression and Disability: Comparisons with Common Physical Conditions in the Ibadan Study of Aging. Journal of the American Geriatrics Society 56: 2033-38.
5. Australian Institute of Health and Welfare (2010) When Musculoskeletal Conditions and Mental Disorders Occur Together. Cat. No. AUS 129. Canberra: AIHW.
6. Slade M. What outcomes to measure in routine mental health services, and how to assess them: a systematic review. Aust N Z J Psychiatry. 2002;36(6): 743–53.
7. Batty MJ, Moldavsky M, Foroushani PS, Pass S, Marriott M, Sayal K, et al. Implementing routine outcome measures in child and adolescent mental health services: from present to future practice. Child Adolesc Mental Health. 2013;18(2):82–7. doi:10.1111/j.1475-3588.2012.00658.x.
8. Happell B. The value of routine outcome measurement for consumers of mental health services: master or servant? Int J Soc Psychiatry. 2008;54(4): 317–27
9. Crawford MJ, Robotham D, Thana L, Patterson S, Weaver T, Barber R et al. Selecting outcome measures in mental health: the views of service users. Journal of Mental Health. 2011;20(4):336–46. doi:doi:10.3109/09638237.2011. 577114.
10. Wolpert M. Uses and Abuses of Patient Reported Outcome Measures (PROMs): Potential Iatrogenic Impact of PROMs Implementation and How It Can Be Mitigated. Adm Policy Ment Health. 2014;41(2):141–5. doi:10.1007/ s10488-013-0509-1.
11. Wolpert M, Cheng H, Deighton J. Measurement Issues: Review of four patient reported outcome measures: SDQ, RCADS, C/ORS and GBO–their strengths and limitations for clinical use and service evaluation. Child Adolesc Mental Health. 2015;20(1):63–70. doi:10.1111/camh. 12065.
12. Australia AMHOaCNaCMH. National Community Managed Organisation (CMO) Outcome Measurement Project: Final Report to the Mental Health Information Strategy Standing Committee 1.1. Sydney, NSW2013.
13. Fossey EM, Harvey CA. A conceptual review of functioning: implications for the development of consumer outcome measures. Aust N Z J Psychiatry. 2001;35(1):91–8. doi:10.1046/j.1440-1614.2001.00846.x.
14. Australian mental health outcomes and classification network.https://www.amhocn.org/publications/health-nation-outcome-scales-honos
15. https://mentalhealthpartnerships.com/resource/health-of-the-nation-outcome-scales-honos/
16. https://www.albany.edu/counseling_center/docs/GAF.pdf
17. Startup M, Jackson MC, Bendix S. The concurrent validity of the Global Assessment of Functioning (GAF). Br J Clin Psychol. 2002;41(4):417–22. doi:10.1348/014466502760387533.
18. Barber CC, Neese DT, Coyne L, Fultz J, Fonagy P. The Target Symptom Rating: a brief clinical measure of acute psychiatric symptoms in children and adolescents. J Clin Child Adolesc Psychol. 2002;31(2):181–92.
19. https://www.rand.org/health/surveys_tools/mos/36-item-short-form.html
20. https://clinmedjournals.org/articles/jmdt/jmdt-2-023-figure-1.pdf
21. Priebe, S., McCabe, R., et al (2007) Structured patient–clinician communication and 1-year outcome in community mental healthcare: Cluster randomised controlled trial.
22. https://www.mountsinai.on.ca/care/psych/on-call-resources/on-call-resources/mmse.pdf
23. Overall JE, Gorham DR (1962). The brief psychiatric rating scale. Psychological Reports 1962 vol. 10, pp799-812
24. https://www.public-health.uiowa.edu/icmha/outreach/documents/BPRS_expanded.PDF

❑❑❑

124 Health of the Nation Outcome Scale

Introduction:

The Health of the Nation Outcome Scales (HoNOS) is a clinician rated instrument comprising 12 simple scales measuring behaviour, impairment, symptoms and social functioning for those in the 18 - 64 years old age group[1].

Health of The Nation Outcome Scale (HoNOS) rating guidelines

- Rate items in order from 1 to 12.
- Use all available information in making your rating.
- Do not include information already rated in an earlier item.
- Consider both the degree of distress the problem causes and the effect it has on behavior
- Rate the most severe problem that occurred in the period rated.
- The rating period is generally the preceding two weeks, except at discharge from inpatient care, when it is the previous three days.
- Each item is rated on a five-point item of severity (0 to 4) as follows:

0 No problem.

1 Minor problem requiring no formal action.

2 Mild problem.

3 Problem of moderate severity.

4 Severe to very severe problem.

9 Not known or not applicable.

- As far as possible, the use of rating point 9 should be avoided, because missing data make scores less comparable over time or between settings.
- Specific information on how to rate each point on each item is provided in the Glossary.

HoNOS glossary

1. Overactive, aggressive, disruptive or agitated behaviour

Include such behaviour due to any cause, eg, drugs, alcohol, dementia, psychosis, depression, etc. Do not include bizarre behaviour, rated at Scale 6.

0 No problems of this kind during the period rated.

1 Irritability, quarrels, restlessness etc. Not requiring action.

2 Includes aggressive gestures, pushing or pestering others; threats or verbal aggression; lesser damage to property (eg, broken cup or window); marked over-activity or agitation.

3 Physically aggressive to others or animals (short of rating 4); threatening manner; more serious over, activity or destruction of property.

4 At least one serious physical attack on others or on animals; destruction of property (e.g., fire-setting); serious intimidation or obscene behaviour.

2. Non-accidental self-injury

Do not include accidental self-injury (due eg, to dementia or severe learning disability); the cognitive problem is rated at Scale 4 and the injury at Scale 5.

Do not include illness or injury as a direct consequence of drug or alcohol use rated at Scale 3, (eg, cirrhosis of the liver or injury resulting from drunk driving are rated at Scale 5).

0 No problem of this kind during the period rated.

1 Fleeting thoughts about ending it all, but little risk during the period rated; no self-harm.

2 Mild risk during period; includes non-hazardous

self-harm eg, wrist– scratching.

3 Moderate to serious risk of deliberate self-harm during the period rated; includes preparatory acts eg, collecting tablets.

4 Serious suicidal attempt or serious deliberate self-injury during the period rated.

3. Problem drinking or drug-taking

Do not include aggressive or destructive behaviour due to alcohol or drug use, rated at Scale 1. Do not include physical illness or disability due to alcohol or drug use, rated at Scale 5.

0 No problem of this kind during the period rated.

1 Some over-indulgence, but within social norm.

2 Loss of control of drinking or drug-taking; but not seriously addicted.

3 Marked craving or dependence on alcohol or drugs with frequent loss of control, risk taking under the influence, etc.

4 Incapacitated by alcohol or drug problems.

4. Cognitive problems

Include problems of memory, orientation and understanding associated with any disorder: learning disability, dementia, schizophrenia, etc. Do not include temporary problems (eg, hangovers) resulting from drug or alcohol use, rated at Scale 3.

0 No problem of this kind during the period rated.

1 Minor problems with memory or understanding eg, forgets names occasionally.

2 Mild but definite problems, eg, has lost way in a familiar place or failed to recognise a familiar person; sometimes mixed up about simple decisions.

3 Marked disorientation in time, place or person, bewildered by everyday events; speech is sometimes incoherent, mental slowing.

4 Severe disorientation, eg, unable to recognise relatives, at risk of accidents, speech incomprehensible, clouding or stupor.

5. Physical illness or disability problems

Include illness or disability from any cause that limits or prevents movement, or impairs sight or hearing, or otherwise interferes with personal functioning. Include side-effects from medication; effects of drug/alcohol use; physical disabilities resulting from accidents or self-harm associated with cognitive problems, drunk driving etc. Do not include mental or behavioural problems rated at Scale 4.

0 No physical health problem during the period rated.

1 Minor health problem during the period (eg, cold, non-serious fall, etc).

2 Physical health problem imposes mild restriction on mobility and activity.

3 Moderate degree of restriction on activity due to physical health problem.

4 Severe or complete incapacity due to physical health problem.

6. Problems associated with hallucinations and delusions

Include hallucinations and delusions irrespective of diagnosis. Include odd and bizarre behaviour associated with hallucinations or delusions. Do not include aggressive, destructive or overactive behaviours attributed to hallucinations or delusions, rated at Scale 1.

0 No evidence of hallucinations or delusions during the period rated.

1 Somewhat odd or eccentric beliefs not in keeping with cultural norms.

2 Delusions or hallucinations (eg, voices, visions) are present, but there is little distress to patient or manifestation in bizarre behaviour, that is, moderately severe clinical problem.

3 Marked preoccupations with delusions or hallucinations, causing much distress and/or manifested in obviously bizarre behaviour, that is, moderately severe clinical problem.

4 Mental state and behaviour is seriously and adversely affected by delusions or hallucinations, with severe impact on patient.

7. Problems with depressed mood

Do not include over-activity or agitation, rated at Scale 1. Do not include suicidal ideation or attempts, rated at Scale 2. Do not include delusions or hallucinations, rated at Scale 6.

0 No problems associated with depressed mood during the period rated.

1 Gloomy; or minor changes in mood.

2 Mild but definite depression and distress: eg, feelings of guilt; loss of selfesteem.

3 Depression with inappropriate self-blame, preoccupied with feelings of guilt.

4 Severe or very severe depression, with guilt or self-accusation.

8. Other mental and behavioural problems

Rate only the most severe clinical problem not considered at items 6 and 7 as follows: specify the type of problem by entering the appropriate letter: A phobic: B anxiety; C obsessive-compulsive; D stress; E dissociative; F somatoform; G eating; H sleep; I sexual; J other, specify.

0 No evidence of any of these problems during period rated.

1 Minor non-clinical problems.

2 A problem is clinically present at a mild level, eg, patient/client has a degree of control.

3 Occasional severe attack or distress, with loss of control eg, has to avoid anxiety provoking situations altogether, call in a neighbour to help, etc., that is, a moderately severe level of problem. 4 Severe problem dominates most activities.

9. Problems with relationships

Rate the patient's most severe problem associated with active or passive withdrawal from social relationships, and/or non-supportive, destructive or selfdamaging relationships.

0 No significant problems during the period.

1 Minor non-clinical problems.

2 Definite problems in making or sustaining supportive relationships: patient complains and/or problems are evident to others.

3 Persisting major problems due to active or passive withdrawal from social relationships, and/or to relationships that provide little or no comfort or support.

4 Severe and distressing social isolation due to inability to communicate socially and/or withdrawal from social relationships.

10. Problems with activities of daily living

Rate the overall level of functioning in activities of daily living (ADL): eg, problems with basic activities of self-care such as eating, washing, dressing, toilet; also complex skills such as budgeting, organising where to live, occupation and recreation, mobility and use of transport, shopping, self-development, etc. Include any lack of motivation for using self-help opportunities, since this contributes to a lower overall level of functioning. Do not include lack of opportunities for exercising intact abilities and skills, rated at Scale 11 and Scale 12.

0 No problems during period rated; good ability to function in all areas.

1 Minor problems only eg, untidy, disorganised.

2 Self-care adequate, but major lack of performance of one or more complex skills (see above).

3 Major problems in one or more areas of self-care (eating, washing, dressing, toilet) as well as major inability to perform several complex skills.

4 Severe disability or incapacity in all or nearly all areas of self-care and complex skills.

11. Problems with living conditions

Rate the overall severity of problems with the quality of living conditions and daily domestic routine. Are the basic necessities met (heat, light, hygiene)? If so, is there help to cope with disabilities and a choice of opportunities to use skills and develop new ones? Do not rate the level of functional disability itself, rated at Scale 10. NB: Rate patient's usual accommodation. If in acute ward, rate the home accommodation. If information not obtainable, rate 9.

0 Accommodation and living conditions are acceptable; helpful in keeping any disability rated at Scale 10 to the lowest level possible, and supportive of self-help.

1 Accommodation is reasonably acceptable although there are minor or transient problems (eg, not ideal location, not preferred option, doesn't like food, etc).

2 Significant problems with one or more aspects of the accommodation and/or regime (eg, restricted choice; staff or household have little understanding of how to limit disability, or how to help develop new or intact skills).

3 Distressing multiple problems with accommodation (eg, some basic necessities absent); housing environment has minimal or no facilities to improve patient's independence.

4 Accommodation is unacceptable (eg, lack of basic necessities, patient is at risk of eviction, or 'roofless', or living conditions are otherwise intolerable making patient's problems worse).

12. Problems with occupation and activities

Rate the overall level of problems with quality of day–time environment. Is there help to cope with disabilities, and opportunities for maintaining or improving occupational and recreational skills and activities? Consider factors such as stigma, lack of qualified staff, access to supportive facilities, eg, staffing and equipment of day centres, workshops, social clubs, etc. Do not rate the level of functional disability itself, rated at Scale 10. NB: Rate the patient's usual situation. If in acute ward, rate activities during period before admission. If information not available, rate 9.

0 Patient's day–time environment is acceptable; helpful in keeping any disability rated at Scale 10 to the lowest level possible, and supportive of self-help.

1 Minor or temporary problems, eg, late pension cheques, reasonable facilities available but not always at desired times etc.

2 Limited choice of activities, eg, there is a lack of reasonable tolerance (eg, unfairly refused entry to public library or baths etc.); or handicapped by lack of a permanent address; or insufficient carer or professional support; or helpful day setting available but for very limited hours.

3 Marked deficiency in skilled services available to help minimise level of existing disability; no opportunities to use intact skills or add new ones; unskilled care difficult to access.

4 Lack of any opportunity for daytime activities makes patient's problem worse.

References

1. AMHOCM HoNOS Available from: https://www.amhocn.org/publications/health-nation-outcome-scales-honos(accessed9.4.2021)

❑❑❑

125 Global Assessment of Functioning Scale

Consider psychological, social, and occupational functioning on a hypothetical continuum of mental health-illness. Do not include impairment in functioning due to physical (or environmental) limitations

Code (Note: Use intermediate codes when appropriate, e.g., 45, 68, 72.)

100 | 91: Superior functioning in a wide range of activities, life's problems never seem to get out of hand, is sought out by others because of his or her many positive qualities. No symptoms.

90 | 81: Absent or minimal symptoms (e.g., mild anxiety before an exam), good functioning in all areas, interested and involved in a wide range of activities. socially effective, generally satisfied with life, no more than everyday problems or concerns (e.g. an occasional argument with family members).

80 | 71: If symptoms are present, they are transient and expectable reactions to psychosocial stressors (e.g., difficulty concentrating after family argument); no more than slight impairment in social, occupational or school functioning (e.g., temporarily failing behind in schoolwork).

70 | 61: Some mild symptoms (e.g.depressed mood and mild insomnia) OR some difficulty in social, occupational, or school functioning (e.g., occasional truancy, or theft within the household), but generally functioning pretty well, has some meaningful interpersonal relationships.

60 | 51: Moderate symptoms (e.g., flat affect and circumstantial speech, occasional panic attacks) OR moderate difficulty in social, occupational, or school functioning (e.g..few friends, conflicts with peers or co-workers).

50 | 41: Serious symptoms (e.g.suicidal ideation, severe obsessional rituals, frequent shoplifting) OR any serious impairment in social, occupational, or school functioning (e.g., no friends, unable to keep a job).

40 | 31: Some impairment in reality testing or communication (e.g., speech is at times illogical, obscure, or irrelevant) OR major impairment in several areas, such as work or school, family relations, judgment, thinking, or mood (e.g., depressed man avoids friends, neglects family, and is unable to work; child frequently beats up younger children, is defiant at home, and is failing at school).

30 | 21: Behavior is considerably influenced by delusions or hallucinations OR serious impairment in communication or judgment (e.g., sometimes incoherent, acts grossly inappropriately, suicidal preoccupation) OR inability to function in almost all areas (e.g., stays in bed all day; no job, home, or friends).

20 | 11: Some danger of hurting self or others (e.g., suicide attempts without clear expectation of death; frequently violent; manic excitement) OR occasionally fails to maintain minimal personal hygiene (e.g., smears feces) OR gross impairment in communication (e.g., largely incoherent or mute).

10 | 1: Persistent danger of severely hurting self or others (e.g., recurrent violence) OR persistent inability to maintain minimal personal hygiene OR serious suicidal act with clear expectation of death. 0 Inadequate information.

0 Inadequate information

❑❑❑

126 Mini-Mental State Examination

The Mini-mental state examination is used to measure cognitive impairment in older adults. According to Folstein et al, it can be used to screen for cognitive impairment, to estimate the severity of cognitive impairment at a given point in time, to follow the course of cognitive changes in an individual over time, and to document an individual's response to treatment.[1] It assesses different subset of cognitive status including attention, language, memory, orientation, visuospatial proficiency. It has also been recommended for the screening of cognition in depressed patients[2] The mini-mental state examination is proprietary and takes about 10-15 minutes to administer. According to some studies, patients with Alzheimer's disease score significantly lower on orientation to time and place, and recall compared to patients with dementia with Lewy bodies, vascular dementia and Parkinson's dementia.[3][4][5] However, it should not be used to exclusively diagnose or differentiate the different types of dementia.[6][7] The Mini-Cog and revised Addenbrooke's Cognitive Examination are preferred alternatives to the Mini-Mental State Examination for dementia screening, and the Montreal Cognitive Assessment is a preferred alternative to detect mild cognitive impairment.[8]

Scoring and Interpretation of Scores: The Mini-mental state examination is scored on a scale of 0-30 with scores > 25 interpreted as normal cognitive status.

(a) Severe cognitive impairment: 0-17
(b) Mild cognitive impairment: 18-23
(c) No cognitive impairment: 24-30

Interpretation of the mental status examination must take into account the patient's native language, education level, and culture as these factors can affect perfromance.[9]

Validity:

In 14 studies, the MMSE had a sensitivity of 88.3% (95% confidence interval [CI], 81.3% to 92.9%) and a specificity of 86.2% (95% CI, 81.8% to 89.7%) for dementia, with a score cutoff of 23 to 25 indicating significant impairment.[8] A more recent meta-analysis of 108 cohort studies found a sensitivity of 81% (95% CI, 78% to 84%) and specificity of 89% (95% CI, 87% to 91%)

References

1. Folstein MF, Folstein SE, McHugh PR "Mini-mental state". A practical method for grading the cognitive state of patients for the clinician. J Psychiatr Res. 1975 Nov; 12(3):189-98.
2. Special Report, Expert Consensus Guideline Series, Postgraduate Medicine, October 2001.
3. Ala, TA; Hughes, LF; Kyrouac, GA; Ghobrial, MW; Elble, RJ. "The Mini-Mental Status exam may help in the differentiation of dementia with Lewy bodies and Alzheimer's disease". International Journal of Geriatric Psychiatry. June 2002;17 (6): 503–9.
4. Jefferson, AL; Cosentino, SA; Ball, SK; Bogdanoff, B; Leopold, N; Kaplan, E; Libon, DJ. "Errors produced on the mini-mental status examination and neuropsychological test performance in Alzheimer's disease, ischemic vascular dementia, and Parkinson's". The Journal of Neuropsychiatry and Clinical Neurosciences. 2002;14 (3): 311–20.
5. Palmqvist, S; Hansson, O; Minthon, L; Londos, E. "Practical suggestions on how to differentiate dementia with Lewy bodies from Alzheimer's disease with common cognitive

tests". International Journal of Geriatric Psychiatry. December 2009;24 (12): 1405–12.

6. Arevalo-Rodriguez I.; Smailagic N.; Ciapponi A.; Sanchez-Perez E.; Giannakou A.; Figuls M.; Cullum S. "Mini-Mental Status Examination (MMSE) for the detection of Alzheimer's disease and other dementias in people with mild cognitive impairment (MCI)". 2015.
7. Creavin ST, Wisniewski S, Noel-Storr AH, et al. Mini-Mental State Examination (MMSE) for the detection of dementia in clinically unevaluated people aged 65 and over in community and primary care populations. Cochrane Database Syst Rev. 2016;(1):CD011145.
8. Tsoi KK, Chan JY, Hirai HW, Wong SY, Kwok TC. Cognitive tests to detect dementia: a systematic review and meta-analysis. JAMA Intern Med. 2015;175(9):1450–1458.
9. Faber RA. The neuropsychiatric mental status examination. Semin Neurol. 2009;29(3):185–193. Level of evidence C

Mini-Mental State Examination (SMMSE)

Please see accompanying guidelines for administration and scoring instructions

Say: I am going to ask you some questions and give you some problems to solve. Please try to answer as best you can.

1. Allow ten seconds for each reply. **Say**:

(a) What year is this? (accept exact answer only) /1

(b) What season is this? (during the last week of the old season or first week of a new season, accept either) /1

(c) What month is this? (on the first day of a new month or the last day of the previous month, accept either) /1

d) What is today's date? (accept previous or next date) /1

(e) What day of the week is this? (accept exact answer only) /1

2. Allow ten seconds for each reply. Say:

(a) What country are we in? (accept exact answer only) /1

(b) What state are we in? (accept exact answer only) /1

(c) What city/town are we in? (accept exact answer only) /1

(d) <At home> What is the street address of this house? (accept street name and house number or equivalent in rural areas) /1

<In facility> What is the name of this building? (accept exact name of institution only) /1

(e) <At home> What room are we in? (accept exact answer only) /1

<In facility> What floor of the building are we on? (accept exact answer only) /1

3. **Say**: I am going to name three objects. When I am finished, I want you to repeat them. Remember what they are because I am going to ask you to name them again in a few minutes (say slowly at approximately one-second intervals).

Ball Car Man

For repeated use: Bell, jar, fan; bill, tar, can; bull, bar, pan

Say: Please repeat the three items for me (score one point for each correct reply on the first attempt) /3

Allow 20 seconds for reply; if the person did not repeat all three, repeat until they are learned or up to a maximum of five times (but only score first attempt)

4. Say: Spell the word WORLD (you may help the person to spell the word correctly). Say: Now spell it backwards please (allow 30 seconds; if the person cannot spell world even with assistance, score zero). Refer to accompanying guide for scoring instructions (score on reverse of this sheet) /5

5. Say: Now what were the three objects I asked you to remember? /3

(score one point for each correct answer regardless of order; allow ten seconds)

6. Show wristwatch. **Ask**: What is this called? /1

score one point for correct response; accept 'wristwatch' or 'watch'; do not accept 'clock' or 'time', etc.; allow ten seconds)

7. Show pencil. Ask: What is this called? /1

(score one point for correct response; accept 'pencil' only; score zero for pen; allow ten seconds for reply)

8. Say: I would like you to repeat a phrase after me: No ifs, ands, or buts /1

(allow ten seconds for response. Score one point for a correct repetition. Must be exact, e.g. no ifs or buts, score zero)

9. Say: Read the words on this page and then do what it

says /1

Then, hand the person the sheet with CLOSE YOUR EYES (score on reverse of this sheet) on it. If the subject just reads and does not close eyes, you may repeat: Read the words on this page and then do what it says, a maximum of three times. See point number three in Directions for Administration section of accompanying guidelines. Allow ten seconds; score one point only if the person closes their eyes. The person does not have to read aloud.

10. Hand the person a pencil and paper. **Say**: Write any complete sentence on that piece of paper (allow 30 seconds. Score one point. The sentence must make sense. Ignore spelling errors). /1

11. Place design (see page 3), pencil, eraser and paper in front of the person. Say: Copy this design please. Allow multiple tries. /1

Wait until the person is finished and hands it back. Score one point for a correctly copied diagram. The person must have drawn a four-sided figure between two five-sided figures. Maximum time: one minute.

12. Ask the person if he is right or left handed. **Take** a piece of paper, hold it up in front of the person and **say** the following: Take this paper in your right/left hand (whichever is non-dominant), fold the paper in half once with both hands and put the paper down on the floor.

Takes paper in correct hand__________ /1
Folds it in half___________ /1
Puts it on the floor________ /1

TOTAL TEST SCORE: /30
ADJUSTED SCORE: /

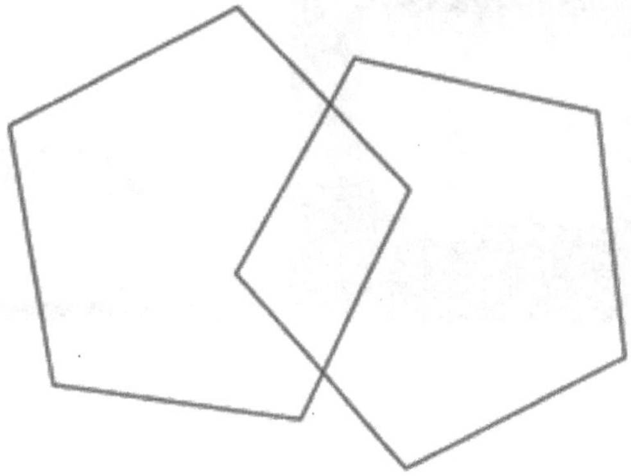

Molloy DW, Alemayehu E, Roberts R. Reliability of a standardized Mini-Mental State Examination compared with the traditional Mini-Mental state Examination. American Journal of Psychiatry, Vol. 14, 1991a, pp.102-105

❑❑❑

127 Brief Psychiatric Rating Scale (BPRS)

Response Categories:

Not present
Very Mild
Mild
Moderate
Moderately Severe
Severe
Extremely Severe

This form consists of 24 symptom constructs, each to be rated in a 7-point scale of severity ranging from 'not present' to 'extremely severe' If a specific symptom is not rated, mark 'NA' (not assessed). Circle the number headed by the term that best describes the patient's present condition.

1 Somatic concern	NA	1	2	3	4	5	6	7
2 Anxiety	NA	1	2	3	4	5	6	7
3 Depression	NA	1	2	3	4	5	6	7
4 Suicidality	NA	1	2	3	4	5	6	7
5 Guilt	NA	1	2	3	4	5	6	7
6 Hostility	NA	1	2	3	4	5	6	7
7 Elated Mood	NA	1	2	3	4	5	6	7
8 Grandiosity	NA	1	2	3	4	5	6	7
9 Suspiciousness	NA	1	2	3	4	5	6	7
10 Hallucinations	NA	1	2	3	4	5	6	7
11 Unusual thought content	NA	1	2	3	4	5	6	7
12 Bizarre behavior	NA	1	2	3	4	5	6	7
13 Self-neglect	NA	1	2	3	4	5	6	7
14 Disorientation	NA	1	2	3	4	5	6	7
15 Conceptual disorganization	NA	1	2	3	4	5	6	7
16 Blunted affect	NA	1	2	3	4	5	6	7
17 Emotional withdrawal	NA	1	2	3	4	5	6	7
18 Motor retardation	NA	1	2	3	4	5	6	7
19 Tension	NA	1	2	3	4	5	6	7
20 Uncooperativeness	NA	1	2	3	4	5	6	7
21 Excitement	NA	1	2	3	4	5	6	7
22 Distractibility	NA	1	2	3	4	5	6	7
23 Motor hyperactivity	NA	1	2	3	4	5	6	7
24 Mannerisms and posturing	NA	1	2	3	4	5	6	7

The following consists of four of the above constructs being measured:

For the following selected items, rate items based on patient's self-report.

(#4) Suicidality: Expressed desire, intent or actions to harm or kill self.

Have you felt that life wasn't worth living? Have you thought about harming or killing yourself? Have you felt tired of living or as though you would be better off dead? Have you ever felt like ending it all?

[If patient reports suicidal ideation, ask the following:]

How often have you thought about [use patient's description]?

Did you [Do you] have a specific plan?

2 Very Mild

Occasional feelings of being tired of living. Not overt suicidal thoughts

3 Mild

Occasional suicidal thoughts without intent or specific

plan OR he/she feels they would be better off dead.

4 Moderate

Suicidal thoughts frequent without intent or plan

5 Moderately Severe

Many fantasies of suicide by various methods. May seriously consider making an attempt with specific time and plan OR impulsive suicide attempt using non-lethal method or in full view of potential saviors.

6 Severe

Clearly wants to kill self. Searches for appropriate means and time, OR potentially serious suicide attempt with patient knowledge of possible rescue.

7 Extremely Severe

Specific suicidal plan and intent (e.g., "as soon as _______. I will do it by doing X"), OR suicide attempt characterized by plan patient thought was lethal or attempt in secluded environment.

(#10) Hallucinations: Reports of perceptual experiences in the absence of relevant external stimuli. When rating degree to which functioning is disrupted by hallucinations, include preoccupation with the content and experience of the hallucinations, as well as functioning disrupted by acting out on the hallucinatory content (e.g., engaging in deviant behavior due to command hallucinations). Include thoughts aloud ("gedankenlautwerden") or pseudohallucinations (e.g., hears a voice inside heard) if a voice quality is present.

Do you ever seem to hear your name being called?

Have you heard any sounds or people talking to you or about you when there has been nobody around? [If hears voices:] What does the voice/voices say? Did it have a voice quality?

Do you ever have visions or see things that others do not see? What about smell odors that others do not smell?

[If the patient reports hallucinations, ask the following]:

Have these experiences interfered with your ability to perform your usual activities/work? How do you explain them? How often do they occur?

2 Very Mild

While resting or going to sleep, sees visions, smells odors, or hears voices, sounds or whispers in the absence of external stimulation, but no impairment in functioning.

3 Mild

While in a clear state of consciousness, hears a voice calling the subject's name, experiences non-verbal auditory hallucinations (e.g., sounds or whispers), formless visual hallucinations, or has sensory experiences in the presence of a modality-relevant stimulus (e.g., visual illusions) infrequently (e.g., 1-2 times per week) and with no functional impairment.

4 Moderate

Occasional verbal, visual, gustatory, olfactory, or tactile hallucinations with no functional impairment OR non-verbal auditory hallucinations/visual illusions more than infrequently or impairment.

5 Moderately Severe

Experiences daily hallucinations OR some areas of functioning are disrupted by hallucinations.

6 Severe

Experiences verbal or visual hallucinations several times a day OR many areas of functioning are disrupted by these hallucinations.

7 Extremely Severe

Persistent verbal or visual hallucinations throughout the day OR most areas of functioning are disrupted by these hallucinations.

(#11) Unusual Thought Content: Unusual, odd, strange or bizarre thought content. Rate the degree of unusualness, not the degree of disorganization of speech. Delusions are patently absurb, clearly false or bizarre ideas that are expressed with partial or full conviction. Consider the patient to have full conviction if he/she has acted as though the delusional belief were true. Ideas of reference/ persecution can be differentiated from delusions in that ideas are expressed with much doubt and contain more elements of reality. Include thought insertion, withdrawal and broadcast. Include grandiose, somatic and persecutory delusions even if rated elsewhere.

Have you been receiving any special messages from people or from the way things are arranged around you? Have you seen any reference to yourself on TV or in the newspaper?

Can anyone read your mind?

Do you have a special relationship with God?

Is anything like electricity, X-rays, or radio waves affecting you?

Are thoughts put into your head that are not your own?

Have you felt that you were under the control of another person or force?

[If patient reports any odd ideas/delusions, ask the following]:

How often do you think about [use patient's description]?

Have you told anyone about these experiences? How do

you explain the things that have been happening [specific]?

2 Very Mild

Ideas of references (people may stare or may laugh at him), ideas of persecution (people may mistreat him). Unusual beliefs in psychic powers, spirits, UFO's, or unrealistic beliefs in one's own abilities. Not strongly held. Some doubt.

3 Mild

Same as 2, but degree of reality distortion is more severe as indicated by highly unusual ideas or greater conviction. Content may be typical of delusions (even bizarre), but without full conviction. The delusion does not seem to have fully formed, but is considered as one possible explanation for an unusual experience.

4 Moderate

Delusion present but no preoccupation or functional impairment. May be an encapsulated delusion or a firmly endorsed absurd belief about past delusional circumstances.

5 Moderately Severe

Full delusion(s) present with some preoccupation OR some areas of functioning disrupted by delusional thinking.

6 Severe

Full delusion(s) present with much preoccupation OR many areas of functioning are discrupted by delusional thinking.

7 Extremely Severe

Full delusion(s) present with almost total preoccupation OR most areas of functioning are disrupted by delusional thinking.

(#12) Bizarre Behavior: Reports of behaviors which are odd, unusual, or psychotically criminal. Not limited to interview period. Include inappropriate sexual behavior and inappropriate affect.

Have you done anything that has attracted the attention of others?

Have you done anything that could have gotten you into trouble with the police?

Have you done anything that seemed unusual or disturbing to others?

2 Very Mild

Slightly odd or eccentric public behavior, e.g., occasionally giggles to self, fails to make appropriate eye contact, that does not seem to attract the attention of others OR unusual behavior conducted in private, e.g., innocuous rituals that would not attract the attention of others.

3 Mild

Noticeably peculiar public behavior, e.g., inappropriately loud talking, makes inappropriate eye contact, OR private behavior that occasionally, but not always, attracts the attention of others, e.g., hoards food, conducts unusual rituals, wears gloves indoors.

4 Moderate

Clearly bizarre behavior that attracts or would attract (if done privately) the attention or concern of others, but with no corrective intervention necessary. Behavior occurs occasionally, e.g., fixated staring into space for several minutes, talks back to voices once, inappropriate giggling/laughter on 1-2 occasions, talking loudly to self.

5 Moderately Severe

Clearly bizarre behavior that attracts or would attract (if done privately) the attention of others or the authorities, e.g., fixated staring in a socially disruptive way, frequent inappropriate giggling/laughter, occasionally responds to voices, or eats non-foods.

6 Severe

Bizarre behavior that attracts attention of others and intervention by authorities, e.g., directing traffic, public nudity, staring into space for long periods, carrying on a conversation with hallucinations, frequent inappropriate giggling/laughter.

7 Extremely Severe

Serious crimes committed in a bizarre way that attract the attention of others and the control of authorities, e.g., sets fires and stares at flames

OR almost constant bizarre behavior, e.g., inappropriate giggling/laughter, responds only to hallucinations

❑❑❑

128 Michigan Hand Outcomes Questionnaire

Scoring Mechanism

The Michigan Hand Questionnarire (MHQ) contains 6 scales: (1) overall hand function, (2) activities of daily living, (3) work performance, (4) pain, (5) aesthetics,and (6) satisfaction with hand function.In the pain scale,high scores indicate greater pain;in the other 5 scales,high scores denote better hand performance.

The raw scale score for each of the 6 scales is the sum of the responses of each scales item.The raw score is converted to a score range from 0 to 100.The scoring equation for each of the scales is listed below.

The score for the affrected hand is obtained by selecting either the right- or left-hend score.If both hands are affected(eg,rheumatoid patients),the right- and left-hand scale scores are averaged to get the score.

Missing values in each scales may affect the validity of the scores.If 50% or more of the items in a scale are missing,then that particular scale cannot be scored.For scales with less than 50% missing,the average of the existing scale items may be imputed for the missing items.An overall MHQ score can be obtained by summing the scores for all 6 scales and divide by 6. If scores for more than 2 scales are missing, an overall MHQ score cannot be computed.

Scoring Algorithm Scale	Recode†	Raw Score Range‡	Normalization§
Overall hand function	None	5to25	-(raw score-25)/20 ＊ 100
Activities of daily living	None	5to25 7to35 2-handed Overall ADL	1-handed =-(raw score-25) 20＊100 =-(raw score-35) 28＊100 =(1-handed+2-handed)/2
Work	None	5to25	(raw score-5)/20＊100
Pain	Question 2 (1=5)(2=4) (4=2)(5=1)	5to25	If question1=5,then pain score =0; if question 1≠5,then - (raw score-25)/20＊100
Aesthetics	Question 1: (1=5)(2=4) (4=2)(5=1)	4to16	(raw score-4)/16＊100
Satisfaction	None	6to30 -	(raw score-30)/24＊100

＊ The scoring algorithm is from the authors in SAS program

† The response categories for some of the questions are reversed and are recoded

‡ Sum of the responses for each scale

§ For the pain scale, higher scores indicate more pain. For the other 5 scales, higher scores indicate better hand performance. The scores are normalized to a range of 0to 100.

Michigan Hand Outcomes Questionnaire

Instructions: This survey asks for your views about your hands and your health. This information will help keep track of how you feel and how well you are able to do your usual activities. Answer everyquestion by marking the answer as indicated. If you are unsure about how to answer a question, please give the best answer you can.

I. The following questions refer to the function of your hand(s)/wrist(s) during the past week. (Please circle 1 answer for each question.)

	Very Good	Good	Fair	Poor	Very Poor
A. The following questions refer to your right hand/wrist.					
1. Overall, how well did your right hand work?	1	2	3	4	5
2. How well did your right fingers move?	1	2	3	4	5
3. How well did your right wrist move?	1	2	3	4	5
4. How was the strength in your right hand?	1	2	3	4	5
5. How was the sensation (feeling) in your right hand?	1	2	3	4	5
B. The following questions refer to your left hand/wrist					
1. Overall, how well did your left hand work?	1	2	3	4	5
2. How well did your left fingers move?	1	2	3	4	5
3. How well did your left wrist move?	1	2	3	4	5
4. How was the strength in your left hand?	1	2	3	4	5
5. How was the sensation (feeling) in your left hand?	1	2	3	4	5

II. The following questions refer to the ability of your hand(s) to do certain tasks during the past week.(Please circle 1 answer for each question.)

	Not at All Difficult	A Little Difficult	Somewhat Difficult	Moderately Difficult	Very Difficult
A. How difficult was it for you to perform the following activities using your right hand?					
1. Turn a door knob	1	2	3	4	5
2. Pick up a coin	1	2	3	4	5
3. Hold a glass of water	1	2	3	4	5
4. Turn a key in a lock	1	2	3	4	5
5. Hold a flying pan	1	2	3	4	5
B. How difficult was it for you to perform the following activities using your left hand?					
1. Turn a door knob	1	2	3	4	5
2. Pick up a coin	1	2	3	4	5
3. Hold a glass of water	1	2	3	4	5
4. Turn a key in a lock	1	2	3	4	5
5. Hold a flying pan	1	2	3	4	5

C. How difficult was it for you to perform the following activities using both of your hands?					
1. Open a jar	1	2	3	4	5
2. Button a shirt/blouse	1	2	3	4	5
3. Eat with a knife/fork	1	2	3	4	5
4. Carry a grocery bag	1	2	3	4	5
5. Wash dishes	1	2	3	4	5
6. Wash your hair	1	2	3	4	5
7. Tie shoelaces/knots	1	2	3	4	5

III. The following questions refer to how you did in your normal work (including both housework and school work) during the past 4 week. (Please circle 1 answer for each question.)

	Always	**Often**	**Sometimes**	**Rarely**	**Never**
1. How often were you unable to do your work because of problem with your hand(s)/wrist(s)?	1	2	3	4	5
2. How often did you have to shorten your work day because of problems with your hand(s)/wrist(s)?	1	2	3	4	5
3. How often did you have to take it easy at your work because of problems with your hand(s)/wrist(s)?	1	2	3	4	5
4. How often did you accomplish less in your work because of problems with your hand(s)/wrist(s)?	1	2	3	4	5
5. How often did you take longer to do the tasks in your work because of problem with your hand(s)/wrist(s)?	1	2	3	4	5

IV. The following questions refer to how much pain you had in your hand(s)/wrist(s) during the past week. (Please circle 1 answer for each question.)

1. How often did you have pain in your hand(s)/wrist(s)?

   1. Always 2. Often 3. Sometimes 4. Rarely 5. Never

If you answered never to question IV-I- above, please skip the following question and go to the next page.

2. Please describe the pain you have in your hand(s)/wrist(s).

   1. Very mild 2. Mild 3. Moderate 4. Severe 5. Very severe

	Always	**Often**	**Sometimes**	**Rarely**	**Never**
3. How often did the pain in your hand(s)/wrist(s) interfere with your sleep?	1	2	3	4	5
4. How often did the pain in your hand(s) s/wrist(interfere with your daily activities (such as eating or bathing)?	1	2	3	4	5
5. How often did the pain in your hand (s)/wrist(s) make you unhappy?	1	2	3	4	5

	Strongly Agree	Agree	Neither Agree Nor Disagree	Disagree	Strongly Disagree

V.A. The following questions refer to the appearance (look) of your right hand during the past week. (Please circle I answer for each question.)

	Strongly Agree	Agree	Neither Agree Nor Disagree	Disagree	Strongly Disagree
1. I was satisfied with the appearance (look) of my right hand.	1	2	3	4	5
2. The appearance (look) of my right hand sometimes made me uncomfortable in public.	1	2	3	4	5
3. The appearance (look) of my right hand made me depressed.	1	2	3	4	5
4. The appearance (look) of my right hand interfered with my normal social activities.	1	2	3	4	5

B. The following questions refer to the appearance (look) of your left hand during the past week. (Please circle 1 answer for each question.)

	Strongly Agree	Agree	Neither Agree Nor Disagree	Disagree	Strongly Disagree
1. I was satisfied with the appearance (look) of my left hand.	1	2	3	4	5
2. The appearance (look) of my left hand sometimes made me uncomfortable in public.	1	2	3	4	5
3. The appearance (look) of my left hand made me depressed.	1	2	3	4	5
4. The appearance (look) of my left hand interfered with my normal social activities.	1	2	3	4	5

VI.A. The following questions refer to your satisfaction with your right hand/wrist during the past week. (Please circle 1 answer for each question.)

	Very Satisfied	Somewhat Satisfied	Neither Satisfied Nor Dissatisfied	Somewhat Satisfied Somewhat Dissatisfied	Very Dissatisfied
1. Overall function of your right hand	1	2	3	4	5
2. Motion of the fingers in your right hand	1	2	3	4	5
3. Motion of your right wrist	1	2	3	4	5
4. Strength of your right hand	1	2	3	4	5
5. Pain level of your right hand	1	2	3	4	5
6. Sensation (feeling)	1	2	3	4	5

of your right hand

B. The following questions refer to your satisfaction with your left hand/wrist during the past week. (Please circle 1 answer for each question.)

1. Overall function of your left hand	1	2	3	4	5
2. Motion of the fingers in your left hand	1	2	3	4	5
3. Motion of your left wrist	1	2	3	4	5
4. Strength of your left hand	1	2	3	4	5
5. Pain level of your left hand	1	2	3	4	5
6. Sensation (feeling) of your left hand	1	2	3	4	5

Please provide the following information about yourself. (Please circle 1 answer for each question.)

1. Are you right-handed or left-handed?
   a. Right-handed b. Left-handed c. Both
2. Which hand gives you the most problem?
   a. Right hand b. Left hand c. Both
3. Have you changed your job since you had problem with your hand(s)?
   a. Yes b. No

Please describe the type of job you did before you had problem with your hand(s).

Please describe the type of job you are doing now.

4. What is your gender?
   a. Male b. Female
5. What is your ethnic background?
   a. White
   b. Black
   c. Hispanic
   d. Asian or Pacific Islander
   e. American Indian or Alaskan Native
   f. Other (please specify)
6. What is the highest level of education you received?
   a. Less than high school graduate
   b. High school graduate
   c. Some college
   d. College graduate
   e. Professional or graduate school
7. What is your approximate family income, including wages, disability payment, retirement income, and welfare?
   a. <$10.00
   b. $10.000-$19.999
   c. $20.000-$29.999
   d. $30.000-$39.999
   e. $40.000-$49.999
   f. $50.000-$59.999
   g. $60.000-$6.999
   h. >$70.000
8. Is your injury covered by Worke's Compensation?
   a. Yes b. No

Kevin C. Chung,MD , et al . Reliablity and Validity Testing of the Michigan Hand Outcomes Questionnarire. The Journal of Hand Surgery 1998 Vol.23A

❑❑❑

129 Modified Ashworth Scale

Objective

Modified Ashworth Scale (MAS) is used to assess spasticity.[1]

Intended Population

Modified Ashworth Scale (MAS) have been utilized in the following populations: stroke, spinal cord injury, multiple sclerosis, cerebral palsy, traumatic brain injury, pediatric hypertonia and central nervous system lesions[2]

Method of Use

Description: Its performed by extending the patients limb first from a position of maximal possible flexion to maximal possible extension (the point at which the first soft resistance is met). Afterwards, the modified Ashworth scale is assessed while moving from extension to flexion[3]

Scoring

0 No increase in tone

1 slight increase in tone giving a catch when slight increase in muscle tone, manifested by the limb was moved in flexion or extension.

1+ slight increase in muscle tone, manifested by a catch followed by minimal resistance throughout (ROM)

2 more marked increase in tone but more marked increased in muscle tone through most limb easily flexed

3 considerable increase in tone, passive movement difficult

4 limb rigid in flexion or extension

Evidence

Studies that have investigated the reliability of the modified Ashworth Scale as measures of spasticity[4]

Reference	Study details	Relevant results
Bohannon and Smith (1987)13	Inter-rater reliability of the MAS. Muscles tested: elbow flexors in the impaired arm. Ns = 30 [MS (1), HI (5), CVA (24)] Na = 2 [physiotherapist] The assessors independently assessed each subject once	86.7% agreement between assessors (Kendall's $\tau = 0.847$; $p < 0.001$) Cohen's κ was calculated as 0.826a
Bodin and Morris (1991)48	Inter-rater reliability of the MAS. Muscle tested: wrist flexors. Ns = 18 [CVA] Na = 2 [physiotherapist] The assessors independently assessed each subject under three different conditions (immediately after positioning, after a 90 s stretch of the flexors and after a 90 s stretch of the extensors).	76% agreement between assessors (Kendall's τ of 0.857) Cohen's κ was calculated as 0.745a
Sloan et al. (1992)49	Inter-rater reliability of the MAS. Muscles tested: elbow flexors and extensors, and knee flexors. Measurements taken bilaterally. Ns = 34 [hemiplegia] Na = 4 [physiotherapist (2), doctor (2)] The assessors serially assessed each subject	Spearman's ρ varied from 0.56 and 0.90 at the elbow and between 0.26 and 0.62 at the knee

Allison et al. (1996)50	Inter- and Intra-rater reliability of the MAS. Muscles tested: ankle plantar flexors. Measurements were taken bilaterally. Day-1 of testing Ns = 30 [HI] Na = 2 [physiotherapist] Both testers assessed all subjects independently. Day-2 of testing Tester 1 assessed Ns = 21 subjects.	Day-1 Inter-rater reliability tester 1 and tester 2: 55% agreement ($\rho = 0.727$; $\tau = 0.647$; $\kappa = 0.397$) Intra-rater reliability of tester 1: 53% agreement ($\rho = 0.741$; $\tau = 0.674$; $\kappa = 0.694$) Intra-rater reliability of tester 2: 48% agreement ($\rho = 0.550$; $\tau = 0.478$; $\kappa = 0.286$) Day-2 Intra-rater reliability of tester 1: 58% agreement ($\rho = 0.821$; $\tau = 0.739$; κ 0.422)

Reliability

Interrater/Intrarater Reliability:

muscle tested; Elbow flexor and extensor and knee flexor in Hemiplegia patients

49 Measurements taken bilaterally. Ns = 34 [hemiplegia] Na = 4 [physiotherapist (2), doctor (2)] The assessors serially assessed each subject)[5]

- Spearman's ρ varied from 0.56 and 0.90 at the elbow and between 0.26 and 0.62 at the knee

In daily practice the use of the Modified Ash-worth Scale procedure is quick and easy and is a common tool in the measurement of spasticity. Additionally,the Modified Ashworth Scale is widely used in research, In different patient groups such as stroke,multiple sclerosis and spinal cord injury, moderate to good intra-rater reliability and poor to moderate inter-rater reliability of the scale was found.[6]

Validity

Criterion Validity: 35 have shown good correlations between the modified Ashworth scores and EMG parameters derived from simultaneous surface EMG recordings from the muscles tested,[7]

- It is not possible to draw unequivocal support for the modified Ashworth score being a valid and ordinal measure of spasticity due to one key methodological inconsistency.
- The actual time to grade spasticity (by passively moving the limb) was reported to be between 0.25 and 0.33 s, however, many of the derived EMG parameters were poorly referenced to this time window[4]

Construct Validity: 13 modified the original scale by adding an additional category, a 1+ falling between 1 and 2, with the aim of increasing its sensitivity. Both scales have since been used as measures of spasticity for clinical and research purposes. A clinical rating of spasticity on the Ashworth Scales is made after an assessor tests the resistance to passive movement about a joint.Both scales describe the resistance perceived while moving a joint through its full range of movement – except in grade '4[8]

Content Validity: he Ashworth Scale was initially developed as a simple clinical tool to test the efficacy of an anti-spastic drug in patients with multiple sclerosis, Ashworth Scales are measures of spasticity

References

1. Charalambous CP. Interrater reliability of a modified Ashworth scale of muscle spasticity. InClassic papers in orthopaedics 2014 (pp. 415-417). Springer, London.
2. Morris S. Ashworth and Tardieu Scales: Their clinical relevance for measuring spasticity in adult and paediatric neurological populations. Physical Therapy Reviews. 2002 Mar 1;7(1):53-62.
3. Rw B, Smith MB. Interrater reliability of a modified Ashworth scale of muscle spasticity. Phys ther. 1987;67(2):206-7.
4. Ad P, Johnson GR. Price CiM, Curless RH, Barnes MP, Rodgers H. A review of the properties and limitations of the Ashworth and modified Ashworth Scales as measures of spasticity. Clin Rehabil. 1999;13(5):373-83.
5. Pandyan AD, Johnson GR, Price CI, Curless RH, Barnes MP, Rodgers H. A review of the properties and limitations of the Ashworth and modified Ashworth Scales as measures of spasticity. Clinical rehabilitation. 1999 Oct;13(5):373-83.
6. Mehrholz J, Wagner K, Meißner D, Grundmann K, Zange C, Koch R, Pohl M. Reliability of the Modified Tardieu Scale and the Modified Ashworth Scale in adult patients with severe brain injury: a comparison study. Clinical rehabilitation. 2005 Nov;19(7):751-9.
7. Ansari NN, Naghdi S, Younesian P, Shayeghan M. Inter-and intrarater reliability of the Modified Modified Ashworth Scale in patients with knee extensor poststroke spasticity. Physiotherapy theory and practice. 2008 Jan 1;24(3):205-13.
8. Bohannon RW, Smith MB. Assessment of strength deficits in eight paretic upper extremity muscle groups of stroke patients with hemiplegia. Physical therapy. 1987 Apr 1;67(4):522-5.

❑❑❑

130 Pediatric Balance Scale

Objective

The Pediatric Balance Scale is a modified version of the Berg Balance Scale that is used to assess functional balance skills in school-aged children. The scale consists of 14 items that are scored from 0 points (lowest function) to 4 points (highest function) with a maximum score of 56 points.[1]

Intended Population

The Pediatric Balance Scale is intended for use with school-aged children with mild to moderate motor impairments. Pilot testing was performed on children aged 5 to 15 years.[1]

Method of Use

Equipment

The equipment used is[1]:

- Adjustable height bench
- Chair with back support and arm rests
- Stopwatch or watch with a second hand
- Masking tape (1 inch wide)
- Step stool 6 inches in height
- Chalkboard eraser
- Ruler or yardstick
- Small level

Optional equipment that may be helpful includes: 2 child size footprints, blindfold, brightly colored object at least 2 inches in size, flash cards, 2 inches of adhesive-backed hook Velcro, two 1 foot strips of loop Velcro.

Item Descriptions

1. Sitting to standing
2. Standing to sitting
3. Transfers
4. Standing unsupported
5. Sitting unsupported
6. Standing with eyes closed
7. Standing with feet together
8. Standing with one foot in front
9. Standing on one foot
10. Turning 360 degrees
11. Turning to look behind
12. Retrieving object from floor
13. Placing alternate foot on stool
14. Reaching forward with outstretched arm

Evidence

Reliability

Reliability testing performed with a sample of 20 children ages 5-15 years old with mild to moderate motor impairments showed good test-retest reliability (ICC=0.998) and good interrater reliability (ICC=0.997).[1]

Validity

Validity testing performed with a sample of 30 children ages 4-10 years old with spastic cerebral palsy in GMFCS Levels I-III showed a strong correlation between the Pediatric Balance Scale and the self-care ($r=0.73, p<0.001$) and mobility ($r=0.82, p<0.001$) dimensions of the Pediatric Disability Evaluation Inventory (PEDI).[2]

Validity testing performed with a sample of 23 children ages 6-15 years old with spastic cerebral palsy (hemiplegia or diplegia) showed a strong correlation ($r=0.797, p<0.05$) between the Pediatric Balance Scale and the Selective

Control Assessment of Lower Extremity (Scale).[3]

References

1. Franjoine MR, Gunther JS, Taylor MJ. Pediatric balance scale: a modified version of the berg balance scale for the school-age child with mild to moderate motor impairment. Pediatr Phys Ther 2003;15(2):114-28.
2. Duarte Nde A, Grecco LA, Franco RC, Zanon N, Oliveira CS. Correlation between pediatric balance scale and functional test in children with cerebral palsy. J Phys Ther Sci 2014;26(6):849-53.
3. Lim H. Correlation between the selective control assessment of lower extremity and pediatric balance scale scores in children with spastic cerebral palsy. J Phys Ther Sci 2015;27(12):3645-49.

Pediatric Balance Scale

1. Sitting to Standing (best of three trials)

- ☐ Able to stand without using hands and stabilize independently (+4)
- ☐ Able to stand independently using hands (+3)
- ☐ Able to stand using hands after several tries (+2)
- ☐ Needs minimal assist to stand or to stabilize (+1)
- ☐ Needs moderate or maximal assist to stand (0)

2. Standing to Sitting (best of three trials)

- ☐ Sits safely with minimal use of hands (+4)
- ☐ Controls descent by using hands (+3)
- ☐ Uses back of legs against chair to control decent (+2)
- ☐ Sits independently, but has uncontrolled descent (+1)
- ☐ Needs assistance to sit (0)

3. Transfers (best of three trials)

- ☐ Able to transfer safely, with minor use of hands (+4)
- ☐ Able to transfer safely; definite need of hands (+3)
- ☐ Able to transfer with verbal cueing and/or supervision (spotting) (+2)
- ☐ Needs one person to assist (+1)
- ☐ Needs two people to assist or supervise (close guard) to be safe (0)

4. Standing Unsupported

- ☐ Able to stand safely 30 seconds (+4)
- ☐ Able to stand 30 seconds with supervision (spotting) (+3)
- ☐ Able to stand 15 seconds unsupported (+2)
- ☐ Needs several tries to stand 10 seconds unsupported (+1)
- ☐ Unable to stand 10 seconds unassisted (0)

4.1. Optional (if you wish to record)

5. Sitting with Back Unsupported and Feet Supported on the Floor

- ☐ Able to sit safely and securely 30 seconds (+4)
- ☐ Able to sit 30 seconds under supervision (spotting) or may require definite use of upper extremities to maintain sitting position (+3)
- ☐ Able to sit 15 seconds (+2)
- ☐ Able to sit 10 seconds (+1)
- ☐ Unable to sit 10 seconds without support (0)

5.1. Optional (if you wish to record)

6. Standing Unsupported with Eyes Closed (best of three trials)

- ☐ Able to stand 10 seconds safely (+4)
- ☐ Able to stand 10 seconds with supervision (spotting) (+3)
- ☐ Able to stand 3 seconds (+2)
- ☐ Unable to keep eyes closed 3 seconds but stays steady (+1)
- ☐ Need help to keep from falling (0)

6.1. Optional (if you wish to record)

7. Standing Unsupported with Feet Together (best of three trials)

- ☐ Able to place feet together independently and stand 30 seconds safely (+4)

- ☐ Able to place feet together independently and stand for 30 seconds with supervision (spotting) (+3)
- ☐ Able to place feet together independently but unable to hold for 30 seconds (+2)
- ☐ Needs help to attain position but able to stand 30 seconds with feet together (+1)
- ☐ Needs help to attain position and/or unable to hold for 30 seconds (0)

7.1. Optional (if you wish to record)

8. Standing Unsupported One Foot in Front (best of three trials)

- ☐ Able to place feet tandem independently and hold 30 seconds (+4)
- ☐ Able to place foot ahead of other independently and hold 30 seconds (Note: The length of the step must exceed the length of the stationary foot and the width of the stance should approximate the subject's normal stride width) (+3)
- ☐ Able to take small step independently and hold 30 seconds, or requires assistance to place foot in front, but can stand for 30 seconds (+2)
- ☐ Needs help to step, but can hold 15 seconds (+1)
- ☐ Loses balance while stepping or standing (0)

8.1. Optional (if you wish to record)

9. Standing On One Leg (3 trials average score)

- ☐ Able to lift leg independently and hold 10 seconds (+4)
- ☐ Able to lift leg independently and hold 5 to 9 seconds (+3)
- ☐ Able to lift leg independently and hold 3 to 4 seconds (+2)
- ☐ Tries to lift leg; unable to hold 3 seconds but remains standing (+1)
- ☐ Unable to try or needs assist to prevent fall (0)

9.1. Optional (if you wish to record)

10. Turn 360 Degrees

- ☐ Able to turn 360 degrees safely in 4 seconds or less each way (total of less than eight seconds) (+4)
- ☐ Able to turn 360 degrees safely in one direction only in 4 seconds or less, complete turn in other direction requires more than four seconds (+3)
- ☐ Able to turn 360 degrees safely but slowly (+2)
- ☐ Needs close supervision (spotting) or constant verbal cueing (+1)
- ☐ Needs assistance while turning (0)

10.1. Optional (if you wish to record)

11. Turning to Look Behind Left & Right Shoulders While Standing Still

- ☐ Looks behind/over each shoulder; weight shifts while trunk rotation (+4)
- ☐ Looks behind/over one shoulder with trunk rotations; weight shift in the opposite direction is to the level of the shoulder; no trunk rotation (+3)
- ☐ Turns head to look to level of shoulder; no trunk rotation (+2)
- ☐ Needs supervision (spotting) when turning; the chin moves greater than half the distance to the shoulder (+1)
- ☐ Needs assistance to keep from losing balance or falling; movement of the chin is less than half the distance to the shoulder (0)

12. Pick Up Object from the Floor from a Standing Position

- ☐ Able to pick up an eraser safely and easily (+4)
- ☐ Able to pick up eraser but needs supervision (spotting) (+3)
- ☐ Unable to pick up eraser but reaches 1 to 2 inches from eraser and keeps balance independently (+2)
- ☐ Unable to pick up eraser; needs supervision (spotting) while attempting (+1)
- ☐ Unable to try, needs assistance to keep from losing balance or falling (0)

13. Placing Alternate Foot on Step Stool while Standing Unsupported

- ☐ Stands independently and safely and completes 8 steps in 20 seconds (+4)
- ☐ Able to stand independently and complete 8 steps >20 seconds (+3)
- ☐ Able to complete 4 steps without assistance, but requires close supervision (spotting) (+2)
- ☐ Able to complete 2 steps; needs minimal assistance (+1)
- ☐ Needs assistance to maintain balance or keep from falling, unable to try (0)

13.1. Optional (if you wish to record)

14. Reaching Forward with Outstretched Arm while Standing (3 trials average results)

- ☐ Can reach forward confidently >10 inches (+4)
- ☐ Can reach forward >5 inches, safely (+3)
- ☐ Can reach forward >2 inches, safely (+2)
- ☐ Reaches forward but needs supervision (spotting) (+1)
- ☐ Loses balance while trying, requires external support (0)

❑❑❑

131 Moss Attention Rating Scale

Objective

The Moss Attention Rating Scale (MARS) is an observational rating scale of attention-related behaviors, useful in assessing people with moderate to severe TBI, particularly those undergoing acute inpatient rehabilitation. It was developed by Whyte and Hart at Moss Rehabilitation Research Institute[1].

Intended Population

Patients with brain injury at Rancho level IV or higher[2].

I	No response to all stimulus	Total assist
II	Generalised response	Total assist
III	Localised response	Total assist
IV	Confused agitated inappropriate response	Max assist
V	Confused non-agitation inappropriate response	Max assist
VI	Confused appropriate response	Mod-Max assist
VII	Automatic appropriate robot-like response	Mod assist
VIII	Purposeful appropriate response - may display depression - abstract reasoning ability decreased	Min assist / stand by assist
IX	Purposeful appropriate response - difficulty with reasoning, judgement & social appropriateness	Stand by assist
X	Purposeful appropriate response - uses compensatory strategies where needed	Modified independent / independent

Method of Use

The scale is a 22 item measure to be administered manually by clinicians, Each item is a behavioral descriptor rated on a five-point Likert-type scale according to how well that behavior describes the patient, ranging from "definitely true" to "definitely false."

The Scale is free of cost and requires no special training.

Scoring ranges from 22-110, higher scores showing better attention.

Instrument

The questionnaire consists of 22 items which the clinician has to score on observation[1]:

1. Is restless or fidgety when unoccupied
2. Sustains conversation without interjecting irrelevant or off-topic comments
3. Persists at a task or conversation for several minutes without stopping or "drifting off"
4. Stops performing a task when given something else to do or to think about
5. Misses materials needed for tasks even though they are within sight and reach
6. Performance is best early in the day or after a rest
7. Initiates communication with others
8. Fails to return to a task after an interruption unless prompted to do so
9. Looks toward people approaching
10. Persists with an activity or response after being told to stop
11. Has no difficulty stopping one task or step in order to begin the next one
12. Attends to nearby conversations rather than the current task or conversation
13. Tends not to initiate tasks which are within his/her capabilities
14. Speed or accuracy deteriorates over several minutes on a task, but improves after a break
15. Performance of comparable activities is inconsistent from one day to the next
16. Fails to notice situations affecting current performance, e.g., wheelchair hitting against table
17. Perseverates on previous topics of conversation or previous actions
18. Detects errors in his/ her own performance
19. Initiates activity (whether appropriate or not) without cuing
20. Reacts to objects being directed toward him /her
21. Performs better on tasks when directions are given slowly
22. Begins to touch or manipulate nearby objects not related to task

Scoring:

1 = Definitely false

2 = False, for the most part

3 = Sometimes true, sometimes false

4 = True, for the most part

5 = Definitely true

Evidence

Reliability

- Excellent inter-rater and intra-rater reliability(r=0.64)[3]

Validity

- strongly correlated to concurrent measures thought to assess attention (e.g., (Digit Span)
- were more strongly correlated to Cognitive than Motor FIM scores
- predicted 1-year outcomes of TBI (Disability Rating Scale scores) better than a battery of psychometric measures of attention administered concurrently with the MARS[4].

Responsiveness

- Studies have showed MARS score increases during rehabilitation showing good responsiveness[1].

References

1. Whyte J, Hart T, Ellis CA, Chervoneva I. The Moss Attention Rating Scale for traumatic brain injury: Further explorations of reliability and sensitivity to change. Archives of physical medicine and rehabilitation. 2008 May 1;89(5):966-73.
2. Hart T, Whyte J, Millis S, Bode R, Malec J, Richardson RN, Hammond F. Dimensions of disordered attention in traumatic brain injury: further validation of the Moss Attention Rating Scale. Archives of physical medicine and rehabilitation. 2006 May 1;87(5):647-55.
3. Hart T, Whyte J, Ellis C, Chervoneva I. Construct validity of an attention rating scale for

traumatic brain injury. Neuropsychology. 2009 Nov;23(6):729.
4. Whyte J, Hart T, Bode RK, Malec JF. The Moss Attention Rating Scale for traumatic brain injury: initial psychometric assessment. Archives of physical medicine and rehabilitation. 2003 Feb 1;84(2):268-76.

Moss Attention Rating Scale

Subject's name ________________

ID#________________

Person doing rating ________________

Discipline: OT / PT / Sp / Nursing (circle) Other: ________

Complete the ratings based on two of the following three days of observations:

__________,______ __________,______ ________,______(*Note: If you have worked with the patient all three days, base your ratings on the second & third day.)

Write the 2 dates on which your ratings are based on here. ________&________.

Did any of the observations you made over the 2 days involve co-treatment with another rater?

Y / N (circle)..

Using the number key below, please indicate to what degree each descriptor applies to the person you are rating. If any of your sessions during the 2 days were done in co-treatment with another rater, please note this above, and please make sure that you don't discuss the rating scale at all with your co-rater until both of you have filled it out independently.

Please don't leave any items blank. If you are not sure how to answer, just make your best guess.

1 = Definitely false
2 = False, for the most part
3 = Sometimes true, sometimes false
4 = True, for the most part
5 = Definitely true

1. ________ Is restless or fidgety when unoccupied
2. ________ Sustains conversation without interjecting irrelevant or off-topic comments
3. ________ Persists at a task or conversation for several minutes without stopping or"drifting off"
4. ________ Stops performing a task when given something else to do or to think about
5. ________ Misses materials needed for tasks even though they are within sight and reach
6. ________ Performance is best early in the day or after a rest
7. ________ Initiates communication with others
8. ________ Fails to return to a task after an interruption unless prompted to do so
9. ________ Looks toward people approaching
10. ________ Persists with an activity or response after being told to stop
11. ________ Has no difficulty stopping one task or step in order to begin the next one
12. ________ Attends to nearby conversations rather than the current task or conversation
13. ________ Tends not to initiate tasks which are within his/her capabilities
14. ________ Speed or accuracy deteriorates over several minutes on a task, but improves after a break
15. ________ Performance of comparable activities is inconsistent from one day to the next
16. ________ Fails to notice situations affecting current performance, e.g., wheelchair hitting against table
17. ________ Perseverates on previous topics of conversation or previous actions
18. ________ Detects errors in his/ her own performance
19. ________ Initiates activity (whether appropriate or not) without cuing
20. ________ Reacts to objects being directed toward him /her
21. ________ Performs better on tasks when directions are given slowly
22. ________ Begins to touch or manipulate nearby objects not related to task

132 Neck Disability Index

Definition:

The Neck Disability Index (NDI) (modification of the Oswestry Low Back Pain Disability Index).

- Patient-completed, condition-specific functional status questionnaire with 10 items including pain, personal care, lifting, reading, headaches, concentration, work, driving, sleeping and recreation.
- The NDI has sufficient support and usefulness to retain its current status as the most commonly used self-report measure for neck pain [1].
- The NDI is translated in many languages (Greek, German, Dutch, Korean, Spanish, French) each has its own validity and reliability outcomes.
- The NDI can be used to evaluate the patients status presence and to evaluate the evolution during the therapy

Intended Population

- Chronic neck or upper back pain
- Musculoskeletal neck pain
- Whiplash injuries and whiplash associated disorders
- Cervical radiculopathy and Thoracic Disc Syndrome[1]

NDI Questionnaire

Below is the questionnaire.

This questionnaire has been designed to give us information as to how your neck pain has affected your ability to manage in everyday life. Please answer every section and mark in each section only the one box that applies to you. We realise you may consider that two or more statements in any one section relate to you, but please just mark the box that most closely describes your problem.

Section 1: Pain Intensity

- I have no pain at the moment
- The pain is very mild at the moment
- The pain is moderate at the moment
- The pain is fairly severe at the moment
- The pain is very severe at the moment
- The pain is the worst imaginable at the moment

Section 2: Personal Care (Washing, Dressing, etc.)

- I can look after myself normally without causing extra pain
- I can look after myself normally but it causes extra pain
- It is painful to look after myself and I am slow and careful
- I need some help but can manage most of my personal care
- I need help every day in most aspects of self care
- I do not get dressed, I wash with difficulty and stay in bed

Section 3: Lifting

- I can lift hcavy weights without extra pain
- I can lift heavy weights but it gives extra pain
- Pain prevents me lifting heavy weights off the floor, but I can manage if they are conveniently placed, for example on a table
- Pain prevents me from lifting heavy weights but I can manage light to medium weights if they are

conveniently positioned
- I can only lift very light weights
- I cannot lift or carry anything

Section 4: Reading

- I can read as much as I want to with no pain in my neck
- I can read as much as I want to with slight pain in my neck
- I can read as much as I want with moderate pain in my neck
- I can't read as much as I want because of moderate pain in my neck
- I can hardly read at all because of severe pain in my neck
- I cannot read at all

Section 5: Headaches

- I have no headaches at all
- I have slight headaches, which come infrequently
- I have moderate headaches, which come infrequently
- I have moderate headaches, which come frequently
- I have severe headaches, which come frequently
- I have headaches almost all the time

Section 6: Concentration

- I can concentrate fully when I want to with no difficulty
- I can concentrate fully when I want to with slight difficulty
- I have a fair degree of difficulty in concentrating when I want to
- I have a lot of difficulty in concentrating when I want to
- I have a great deal of difficulty in concentrating when I want to
- I cannot concentrate at all

Section 7: Work

- I can do as much work as I want to
- I can only do my usual work, but no more
- I can do most of my usual work, but no more
- I cannot do my usual work
- I can hardly do any work at all
- I can't do any work at all

Section 8: Driving

- I can drive my car without any neck pain
- I can drive my car as long as I want with slight pain in my neck
- I can drive my car as long as I want with moderate pain in my neck
- I can't drive my car as long as I want because of moderate pain in my neck
- I can hardly drive at all because of severe pain in my neck
- I can't drive my car at all

Section 9: Sleeping

- I have no trouble sleeping
- My sleep is slightly disturbed (less than 1 hr sleepless)
- My sleep is mildly disturbed (1-2 hrs sleepless)
- My sleep is moderately disturbed (2-3 hrs sleepless)
- My sleep is greatly disturbed (3-5 hrs sleepless)
- My sleep is completely disturbed (5-7 hrs sleepless)

Section 10: Recreation

- I am able to engage in all my recreation activities with no neck pain at all
- I am able to engage in all my recreation activities, with some pain in my neck
- I am able to engage in most, but not all of my usual recreation activities because of pain in my neck
- I am able to engage in a few of my usual recreation activities because of pain in my neck
- I can hardly do any recreation activities because of pain in my neck
- I can't do any recreation activities at all

Score: /50 Transform to percentage score x 100 = %points

Scoring: For each section the total possible score is 5: if the first statement is marked the section score = 0, if the last statement is marked it = 5. If all ten sections are completed the score is calculated

Minimum Detectable Change (90% confidence): 5 points or 10 %points[2]

Method of Use

The NDI can be scored as a raw score [3]or doubled and expressed as a percent [4].

- Each section is scored on a 0 to 5 rating scale, in which zero means 'No pain' and 5 means 'Worst imaginable pain'.
- Points summed to a total score.
- The test can be interpreted as a raw score, with a maximum score of 50, or as a percentage.
- 0 points or 0% means : no activity limitations ,
- 50 points or 100% means complete activity limitation.
- A higher score indicates more patient-rated disability. There is no statement in the original literature on how to handle missing data. To use the NDI for patient decisions, a clinically important change was calculated as 5 points, with a sensitivity of 0.78 and a specificity of 0.80[5].
- Mean duration of the test: 3 to 7.8 minutes [1]

Some benchmarks can be found in literature [1]

- 0-4points (0-8%) no disability,
- 5-14points (10 – 28%) mild disability,
- 15-24points (30-48%) moderate disability,
- 25-34points (50- 64%) severe disability,
- 35-50points (70-100%) complete disability

Evidence

Reliability

The NDI has a fair to moderate test-retest reliability in patients with mechanical neck pain but also for patients with cervical radiculopathy . [6],[7]. although intra class correlations can change between 0,50 and 0,98 . These difference may occur because some studies do not separate chronic or acute neck pain or due to the fact that the study only used patients with acute neck pain and the retestinterval was 72 hours [1].

Validity

- Validity is tested in different trails by comparing NDI with different instruments: eg VAS, Patient-specific Functional Scale, The Disability Rating Index.
- They all had strong correlation coefficients suggesting their content is highly comparable: The NDI has a good construct validity.[3][8][7]
- The NDI is seen as a valid tool to measure neck pain and disabilities in patients with neck pain due to acute or chronic conditions as well as in patients suffering from musculoskeletal dysfunctions, whiplash - associated disorders and cervical radiculopathy. [5][1]

Responsiveness

The NDI

Good responsiveness in measuring neck pain and disabilities in patients with neck pain due to acute or chronic conditions as well as patients suffering from musculoskeletal dysfunctions, whiplash associated disorders and cervical radiculopathy [1]

Demonstrate adequate responsiveness in patients with neck pain and concomitant upper extremity referred symptoms. Young et al suggest that a 10-point change should be used as the minimum clinically important difference.[9].

Identified problems

Does not include

- Psychosocial aspects
- Emotional aspects

Very common in:

- Chronic neck pain
- Whiplash associated disorders
- Cervical Radiculopathy

References

1. Macdermid JC, Walton DM, Avery S, Blanchard A, Etruw E, McAlpine C, Goldsmith CH. Measurement properties of the neck disability index a sustematic review Journal of Orthopedic and Sports Physical Therapy. 2009 May;39(5):400-17.
2. NDI developed by: Vernon, H. & Mior, S. (1991). The Neck Disability Index: https://www.sralab.org/rehabilitation-measures/neck-disability-index. Journal of Manipulative and Physiological Therapeutics. 14, 409-415 Available from:https://www.sralab.org/rehabilitation-measures/neck-disability-index (last accessed 1.5.2020)
3. Vernon H, Mior S. The neck disability index: A study of reliability and validity. Journal of Manipulative and Physiological Therapeutics, 1991, 14:409-15

4. Riddle DL, Stratford PW. Use of generic versus region specific functional status measures on patients with cervical spine disorders. Physical Therapy, 1998;78:951-963
5. Stratford PW, Riddle DL, Binkley JM et al (1999) Using the neck disability index to make decisions concerning individual patients Physiotherapy Canada, 2,107-112
6. Cleland JA, Childs JD, Whitman JM.. Psychometric Properties of the Neck Disability Index and Numeric Pain Rating Scale in patients With Mechanical Neck Pain, Arch Phys Med Rehabil. 2008; 89(1):69-74
7. Young IA, Cleland JA, Michener LA, Brown C. Reliability, Construct Validity, and Responsiveness of the Neck Disability Index, Patient-Specific Functional Scale, and Numeric Pain Rating Scale in Patients with Cervical Radiculopathy, American Journal of Physical Medicine & Rehabilitation, 2010; ;89(10):831-839
8. Jan lucas hoving, Elizabeth F o'leary, ken r niere, sally green, Rachelle buchbinder, Validity of the neck disability index, Northwick park neck pain questionnaire, and problem elicitation technique for measuring disability associated with whiplash-associated disorders, pain,2003;102(3); 273-281
9. Young BA, Walker MJ, Strunce JB, Boyles RE, Whitman JM, Childs JD. Responsiveness of the Neck Disability Index in patients with mechanical neck disorders. Spine, 2009 Jul 24, online article ahead of print.

❑❑❑

133 NIH Stroke Scale

Objective

The National Institutes of Health Stroke Scale (NIHSS) is a systematic assessment tool that provides a quantitative measure of stroke-related neurologic deficit. The NIHSS was originally designed as a research tool to measure baseline data on patients in acute stroke clinical trials. Now, the scale is also widely used as a clinical assessment tool to evaluate acuity of stroke patients, determine appropriate treatment, and predict patient outcome.

The NIHSS can be used as a clinical stroke assessment tool to evaluate and document neurological status in acute stroke patients[1]. The stroke scale is valid for predicting lesion size and can serve as a measure of stroke severity. The NIHSS has been shown to be a predictor of both short and long term outcome of stroke patients[2]. Additionally, the stroke scale serves as a data collection tool for planning patient care and provides a common language for information exchanges among healthcare providers.

The scale is designed to be a simple, valid, and reliable tool that can be administered at the bedside consistently by physicians, nurses or therapists.

Intended Population

Individuals with Stroke

Method of Use

The NIHSS is a 15-item neurologic examination stroke scale used to evaluate the effect of acute cerebral infarction on the levels of consciousness, language, neglect, visual-field loss, extraocular movement, motor strength, ataxia, dysarthria, and sensory loss. A trained observer rates the patent's ability to answer questions and perform activities. Ratings for each item are scored on a 3- to 5-point scale, with 0 as normal, and there is an allowance for untestable items. Scores range from 0 to 42, with higher scores indicating greater severity. A single patient assessment requires less than 10 minutes to complete.

The evaluation of stroke severity depends upon the ability of the observer to accurately and consistently assess the patient. Stroke severity may be stratified on the basis of NIHSS scores as follows:[3]

- Very Severe: >25
- Severe: 15 – 24
- Mild to Moderately Severe: 5 – 14
- Mild: 1 – 5

Evidence

Reliability

Inter-rater reliability for individual elements of the NIHSS has been shown to be generally good[4]. However overall scoring can be inconsistent, proper training is required to use the NIH Stroke Scale accurately[5][6][7].

- A study of 4 patients assessed by 30 physicians and 29 study coordinators, with a space of 3 months between assessments, found that the NIHSS has excellent interrater (ICC = 0.95) and test-retest reliability (ICC = 0.93)
- A study of 20 patients rated by 4 clinicians, with each patient subsequently evaluated by 2 independent observers found Adequate to Excellent interrater agreement for 9 of the 13 items on the NIHSS (Kappa = 0.32 to 0.79); lowest levels of agreement were found for the Facial palsy (Kappa = 0.22) and limb ataxia (Kappa = -0.16) items.

- 4 items have poorly reliability or are redundant (level of consciousness, facial weakness, ataxia, and dysarthria[8]

Validity[9][10]

Outcomes related to NIHSS scores at admission:

- Scores of <5; 80% of stroke survivors will be discharged to home
- Score between 6 and 13 typically require acute inpatient rehabilitation
- Scores of >14 frequently require long-term skilled care

Responsiveness[3]

NIHSS scores were compared to infarction size (measured by computed tomography) on 65 patients at 1 week post stroke. 10 items demonstrated an average of 25% change over 7 days. However, changes in limb ataxia and best gaze may have been overstated.

References

1. Spilker J1, Kongable G, Barch C, Braimah J, Brattina P, Daley S, Donnarumma R, Rapp K, Sailor S. Using the NIH Stroke Scale to assess stroke patients. The NINDS rt-PA Stroke Study Group. J Neurosci Nurs. 1997 Dec;29(6):384-92.
2. H.P. Adams Jr., P.H. Davis, E.C. Leira, K.-C. Chang, B.H. Bendixen, W.R. Clarke, R.F. Woolson, Hansen, MS. Baseline NIH Stroke Scale score strongly predicts outcome after stroke: A report of the Trial of Org 10172 in Acute Stroke Treatment (TOAST). Neurology July 1, 1999 vol. 53 no. 1 126
3. Brott, T., Adams, H. P., Jr., et al. (1989). "Measurements of acute cerebral infarction: a clinical examination scale." Stroke 20(7): 864-870.
4. Josephson SA1, Hills NK, Johnston SC.. NIH Stroke Scale reliability in ratings from a large sample of clinicians. Cerebrovasc Dis. 2006;22(5-6):389-95.
5. André C. The NIH Stroke Scale is unreliable in untrained hands. J Stroke Cerebrovasc Dis. 2002 Jan-Feb;11(1):43-6.
6. Lyden P1, Raman R, Liu L, Emr M, Warren M, Marler J. National Institutes of Health Stroke Scale certification is reliable across multiple venues. Stroke. 2009 Jul;40(7):2507-11.
7. Lyden P, Raman R, Liu L, Grotta J, Broderick J, Olson S, Shaw S, Spilker J, Meyer B, Emr M, Warren M, Marler J. NIHSS training and certification using a new digital video disk is reliable. Stroke. 2005 Nov;36(11):2446-9.
8. Kasner, S. E. (2006). "Clinical interpretation and use of stroke scales." Lancet Neurol 5(7): 603-612.
9. Schlegel, D., Kolb, S. J., et al. (2003). "Utility of the NIH Stroke Scale as a predictor of hospital disposition." Stroke 34: 134-137.
10. Rundek, T., Mast, H., et al. (2000). "Predictors of resource use after acute hospitalization: the Northern Manhattan Stroke Study." Neurology 55: 1180-1187.

NIH Stroke Scale

Patient Identification. ___ ___-___ ___ ___-___ ___

Pt. Date of Birth ___ ___/___ ___/___ ___

Hospital ___________________(___ ___-___ ___)

Date of Exam ___ ___/___ ___/___ ___

Interval: [ ] Baseline [ ] 2 hours post treatment [ ] 24 hours post onset of symptoms ±20 minutes [ ] 7-10 days [ ] 3 months [ ] Other ____________________ (___ ___)

Time: ___ ___:___ ___ [ ]am [ ]pm

Person Administering Scale ________________

Administer stroke scale items in the order listed. Record performance in each category after each subscale exam. Do not go back and change scores. Follow directions provided for each exam technique. Scores should reflect what the patient does, not what the clinician thinks the patient can do. The clinician should record answers while administering the exam and work quickly. Except where indicated, the patient should not be coached (i.e., repeated requests to patient to make a special effort).

Instructions	Scale Definition	Score
1a. Level of Consciousness: The investigator must choose a response if a full evaluation is prevented by such obstacles as an endotracheal tube, language barrier, orotracheal trauma/bandages. A 3 is scored only if the patient makes no movement (other than reflexive posturing) in response to noxious stimulation.	0 = Alert; keenly responsive. 1 = Not alert; but arousable by minor stimulation to obey, answer, or respond. 2 = Not alert; requires repeated stimulation to attend, or is obtunded and requires strong or painful stimulation to make movements (not stereotyped). 3 = Responds only with reflex motor or autonomic effects or totally unresponsive, flaccid, and areflexic	
1b. LOC Questions: The patient is asked the month and his/her age. The answer must be correct - there is no partial credit for being close. Aphasic and stuporous patients who do not comprehend the questions will score 2. Patients unable to speak because of endotracheal intubation, orotracheal trauma, severe dysarthria from any cause, language barrier, or any other problem not secondary to aphasia are given a 1. It is important that only the initial answer be graded and that the examiner not "help" the patient with verbal or non-verbal cues.	0 = Answers both questions correctly. 1 = Answers one question correctly. 2 = Answers neither question correctly.	
1c. LOC Commands: The patient is asked to open and close the eyes and then to grip and release the non-paretic hand. Substitute another one step command if the hands cannot be used. Credit is given if an unequivocal attempt is made but not completed due to weakness. If the patient does not respond to command, the task should be demonstrated to him or her (pantomime), and the result scored (i.e., follows none, one or two commands). Patients with trauma, amputation, or other physical impediments should be given suitable one-step commands. Only the first attempt is scored.	0 = Performs both tasks correctly. 1 = Performs one task correctly. 2 = Performs neither task correctly.	
2. Best Gaze: Only horizontal eye movements will be tested. Voluntary or reflexive (oculocephalic) eye movements will be scored, but caloric testing is not done. If the patient has a conjugate deviation of the eyes that can be overcome by voluntary or reflexive activity, the score will be 1. If a patient has an isolated peripheral nerve paresis (CN III, IV or VI), score a 1. Gaze is testable in all aphasic patients. Patients with ocular trauma, bandages, pre-existing blindness, or other disorder of visual acuity or fields should be tested with reflexive movements, and a choice made by the investigator. Establishing eye contact and then moving about the patient from side to side will occasionally clarify the presence of a partial gaze palsy.	0 = Normal. 1=Partial gaze palsy; gaze is abnormal in one or both eyes, but forced deviation or total gaze paresis is not present. 2 = Forced deviation, or total gaze paresis not overcome by the oculocephalic maneuver.	

3. Visual: Visual fields (upper and lower quadrants) are tested by confrontation, using finger counting or visual threat, as appropriate. Patients may be encouraged, but if they look at the side of the moving fingers appropriately, this can be scored as normal. If there is unilateral blindness or enucleation, visual fields in the remaining eye are scored. Score 1 only if a clear-cut asymmetry, including quadrantanopia, is found. If patient is blind from any cause, score 3. Double simultaneous stimulation is performed at this point. If there is extinction, patient receives a 1, and the results are used to respond to item 11.	0 = No visual loss. 1 = Partial hemianopia. 2 = Complete hemianopia. 3 = Bilateral hemianopia (blind including cortical blindness).	
4. Facial Palsy: Ask – or use pantomime to encourage – the patient to show teeth or raise eyebrows and close eyes. Score symmetry of grimace in response to noxious stimuli in the poorly responsive or non-comprehending patient. If facial trauma/bandages, orotracheal tube, tape or other physical barriers obscure the face, these should be removed to the extent possible	0 = Normal symmetrical movements. 1 = Minor paralysis (flattened nasolabial fold, asymmetry on smiling). 2 = Partial paralysis (total or near-total paralysis of lower face). 3 = Complete paralysis of one or both sides (absence of facial movement in the upper and lower face)	
5. Motor Arm: The limb is placed in the appropriate position: extend the arms (palms down) 90 degrees (if sitting) or 45 degrees (if supine). Drift is scored if the arm falls before 10 seconds. The aphasic patient is encouraged using urgency in the voice and pantomime, but not noxious stimulation. Each limb is tested in turn, beginning with the non-paretic arm. Only in the case of amputation or joint fusion at the shoulder, the examiner should record the score as untestable (UN), and clearly write the explanation for this choice.	0 = No drift; limb holds 90 (or 45) degrees for full 10 seconds. 1 = Drift; limb holds 90 (or 45) degrees, but drifts down before full 10 seconds; does not hit bed or other support. 2 = Some effort against gravity; limb cannot get to or maintain (if cued) 90 (or 45) degrees, drifts down to bed, but has some effort against gravity. 3 = No effort against gravity; limb falls. 4 = No movement. UN = Amputation or joint fusion, explain: ______________ 5a. Left Arm 5b. Right Arm	
6. Motor Leg: The limb is placed in the appropriate position: hold the leg at 30 degrees (always tested supine). Drift is scored if the leg falls before 5 seconds. The aphasic patient is encouraged using urgency in the voice and pantomime, but not noxious stimulation. Each limb is tested in turn, beginning with the non-paretic leg. Only in the case of amputation or joint fusion at the hip, the examiner should record the score as untestable (UN), and clearly write the explanation for this choice.	0 = No drift; leg holds 30-degree position for full 5 seconds. 1 = Drift; leg falls by the end of the 5-second period but does not hit bed. 2 = Some effort against gravity; leg falls to bed by 5 seconds, but has some effort against gravity. 3 = No effort against gravity; leg falls to bed immediately. 4 = No movement. UN = Amputation or joint fusion, explain: ______________ 6a. Left Leg 6b. Right Leg	

7. Limb Ataxia: This item is aimed at finding evidence of a unilateral cerebellar lesion. Test with eyes open. In case of visual defect, ensure testing is done in intact visual field. The finger-nose-finger and heel-shin tests are performed on both sides, and ataxia is scored only if present out of proportion to weakness. Ataxia is absent in the patient who cannot understand or is paralyzed. Only in the case of amputation or joint fusion, the examiner should record the score as untestable (UN), and clearly write the explanation for this choice. In case of blindness, test by having the patient touch nose from extended arm position.	0 = Absent. 1 = Present in one limb. 2 = Present in two limbs. UN = Amputation or joint fusion, explain: ________________	
8. Sensory: Sensation or grimace to pinprick when tested, or withdrawal from noxious stimulus in the obtunded or aphasic patient. Only sensory loss attributed to stroke is scored as abnormal and the examiner should test as many body areas (arms [not hands], legs, trunk, face) as needed to accurately check for hemisensory loss. A score of 2, "severe or total sensory loss," should only be given when a severe or total loss of sensation can be clearly demonstrated. Stuporous and aphasic patients will, therefore, probably score 1 or 0. The patient with brainstem stroke who has bilateral loss of sensation is scored 2. If the patient does not respond and is quadriplegic, score 2. Patients in a coma (item 1a=3) are automatically given a 2 on this item.	0 = Normal; no sensory loss. 1 = Mild-to-moderate sensory loss; patient feels pinprick is less sharp or is dull on the affected side; or there is a loss of superficial pain with pinprick, but patient is aware of being touched. 2 = Severe to total sensory loss; patient is not aware of being touched in the face, arm, and leg.	
9. Best Language: A great deal of information about comprehension will be obtained during the preceding sections of the examination. For this scale item, the patient is asked to describe what is happening in the attached picture, to name the items on the attached naming sheet and to read from the attached list of sentences. Comprehension is judged from responses here, as well as to all of the commands in the preceding general neurological exam. If visual loss interferes with the tests, ask the patient to identify objects placed in the hand, repeat, and produce speech. The intubated patient should be asked to write. The patient in a coma (item 1a=3) will automatically score 3 on this item. The examiner must choose a score for the patient with stupor or limited cooperation, but a score of 3 should be used only if the patient is mute and follows no one-step commands.	0 = No aphasia; normal. 1 = Mild-to-moderate aphasia; some obvious loss of fluency or facility of comprehension, without significant limitation on ideas expressed or form of expression. Reduction of speech and/or comprehension, however, makes conversation about provided materials difficult or impossible. For example, in conversation about provided materials, examiner can identify picture or naming card content from patient's response. 2 = Severe aphasia; all communication is through fragmentary expression; great need for inference, questioning, and guessing by the listener. Range of information that can be exchanged is limited; listener carries burden of communication. Examiner cannot identify materials provided from patient response. 3 = Mute, global aphasia; no usable speech or auditory comprehension.	

10. Dysarthria: If patient is thought to be normal, an adequate sample of speech must be obtained by asking patient to read or repeat words from the attached list. If the patient has severe aphasia, the clarity of articulation of spontaneous speech can be rated. Only if the patient is intubated or has other physical barriers to producing speech, the examiner should record the score as untestable (UN), and clearly write an explanation for this choice. Do not tell the patient why he or she is being tested.	0 = Normal. 1 = Mild-to-moderate dysarthria; patient slurs at least some words and, at worst, can be understood with some difficulty. 2 = Severe dysarthria; patient's speech is so slurred as to be unintelligible in the absence of or out of proportion to any dysphasia or is mute/anarthric. UN = Intubated or other physical barrier, expla in:____________	
11. Extinction and Inattention (formerly Neglect): Sufficient information to identify neglect may be obtained during the prior testing. If the patient has a severe visual loss preventing visual double simultaneous stimulation, and the cutaneous stimuli are normal, the score is normal. If the patient has aphasia but does appear to attend to both sides, the score is normal. The presence of visual spatial neglect or anosagnosia may also be taken as evidence of abnormality. Since the abnormality is scored only if present, the item is never untestable.	0 = No abnormality. 1 = Visual, tactile, auditory, spatial, or personal inattention or extinction to bilateral simultaneous stimulation in one of the sensory modalities. 2 = Profound hemi-inattention or extinction to more than one modality; does not recognize own hand or orients to only one side of space	

Reference: www.stroke.nih.gov/documents/NIH_Stroke_Scale_508C.pdf

134 Nine-Hole Peg Test

Objective

The Nine-Hole Peg Test (9HPT) is used to measure finger dexterity in patients with various neurological diagnoses.

Intended Population

Patients with Stroke, Brain Injury, Parkinson's

Method of Use

Description:

- Administered by asking the client to take the pegs from a container, one by one, and place them into the holes on the board, as quickly as possible
- Participants must then remove the pegs from the holes, one by one, and replace them back into the container
- The board should be placed at the client's midline, with the container holding the pegs oriented towards the hand being tested
- Only the hand being evaluated should perform the test
- Hand not being evaluated is permitted to hold the edge of the board in order to provide stability
- Scores are based on the time taken to complete the test activity, recorded in seconds
- Alternative scoring - the number of pegs placed in 50 or 100 seconds can be recorded. In this case, results are expressed as the number of pegs placed per second
- Stopwatch should be started from the moment the participant touches the first peg until the moment the last peg hits the container

Equipment Required:

- Board (wood or plastic): with 9 holes (10 mm diameter, 15 mm depth), placed apart by 32 mm (Mathiowetz et al, 1985[1]; Sommerfeld et al., 2004[2]) or 50 mm (Heller, Wade, Wood, Sunderland, Hewer, & Ward, 1987[3])
- A container for the pegs: square box (100 x 100 x 10 mm) apart from the board or a shallow round dish at the end of the board (Grice et al, 2003[4])
- 9 pegs (7 mm diameter, 32 mm length) (Mathiowetz et al, 1985[5])
- A stopwatch

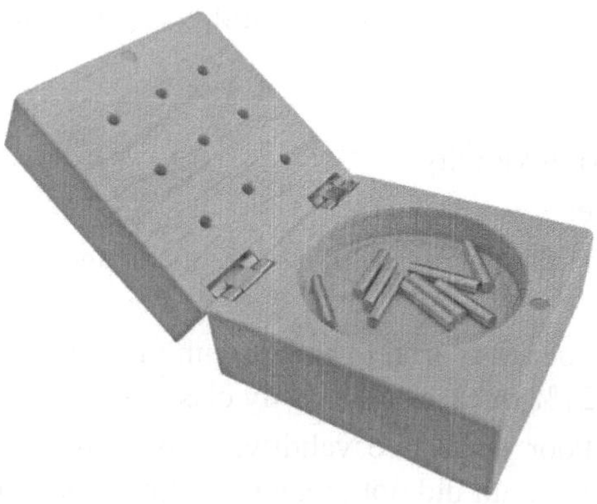

Evidence

Reliability

Test-retest Reliability:

Stroke:

(Chen et al, 2009, Acute and Chronic Stroke) [6]

- Excellent test-retest reliability for entire group (ICC = 0.85)
- Adequate test-retest reliability for individuals with hand spasticity (ICC = 0.64)Excellent test-retest reliability for individuals without hand spasticity (ICC = 0.86)

Parkinson's:

(Earhart et al, 2011) [7]

- Excellent test retest reliability (ICC = 0.88 for dominant hand and ICC = 0.91 for nondominant hand)

Healthy Adults:

(Wang et al 2011; n = 305; mean age = 32 (26); age range = 3 - 85 years) [8]

- Excellent test retest reliability (ICC = 0.95 for right hand, ICC = 0.92 for left hand)

Interrater/Intrarater Reliability:

Healthy Adults:

(Grice et al, 2003, Healthy Adults) [9]

- Excellent interrater reliability for the right hand (r = 0.984)
- Excellent interrater reliability for the left hand (r = 0.993)

Stroke: (Heller et al, 1987; n = 56; mean age = 72 (9.9) years; assessed < 3 months post-stroke, Acute Stroke) [10]

- Adequate to excellent intrarater reliability (r = 0.68 to 0.99)
- Excellent interrater reliability (r = 0.75 to 0.99)

Validity

Criterion Validity:

Stroke:

(Sunderland et al, 1989; n = 38; mean age = 67, Acute Stroke) [11]

- Poor concurrent validity with Frenchay Arm Test: 27% of cases incorrectly classified
- Poor predictive validity: NHPT administered at 1 month did not predict functional outcomes at 6 months post stroke

Healthy Adults:

(Wang et al, 2011) [12]

- Adequate correlation with the Purdue Pegboard test (p = -0.74 to -0.75)
- Excellent correlation with the Bruininks-Oseretsky Test of Motor Proficiency (p = -0.87 to -0.89)

Construct Validity:

Stroke:

(Parker et al, 1986; 2 weeks, 3 & 6 months post onset, Acute Stroke) [13]

- Excellent convergent validity with Motricity Index (r = 0.82)

Responsiveness

Stroke:

(Beebe and Lang, 2009, Acute Stroke) [14]

	Responsiveness:	
	1–3 months	1–6 months
Grip	0.50	0.65
Pinch	0.52	0.56
ARAT	0.55	0.63
9HPT	0.52	0.66
SIS-Hand	1.02	0.86

Responsiveness was calculated using the single population effect size method. Values closer to 1.00 = more responsive to change. Low responsiveness < 0.20; moderate responsiveness < 0.50, and high responsiveness < 0.80

References

1. Mathiowetz, V., Kashman, N., et al. "Grip and pinch strength: normative data for adults." Arch Phys Med Rehabil 1985 66(2): 69-74
2. Sommerfeld, D. K., Eek, E. U., et al. "Spasticity after stroke: its occurrence and association with motor impairments and activity limitations." Stroke 2004 35(1): 134-139
3. Heller, A., Wade, D. T., et al. "Arm function after stroke: measurement and recovery over the first three months." Journal of Neurology, Neurosurgery and Psychiatry 1987 50(6): 714-719
4. Grice, K. O., Vogel, K. A., et al. "Adult norms for a commercially available Nine Hole Peg Test for finger dexterity." The American journal of occupational therapy 2003 57(5): 570-573
5. Mathiowetz, V., Kashman, N., et al. "Grip and pinch strength: normative data for adults." Arch Phys Med Rehabil 1985 66(2): 69-74
6. Chen, H. M., Chen, C. C., et al. "Test-retest reproducibility and smallest real difference of 5 hand function tests in patients with stroke." Neurorehabil Neural Repair 2009 23(5): 435-440

7. Earhart, G. M., Cavanaugh, J. T., et al. "The 9-hole PEG test of upper extremity function: average values, test-retest reliability, and factors contributing to performance in people with Parkinson disease." J Neurol Phys Ther 2011 35(4): 157-163
8. Wang, Y. C., Magasi, S. R., et al. "Assessing dexterity function: a comparison of two alternatives for the NIH Toolbox." Journal of Hand Therapy 2011 24(4): 313-320; quiz 321
9. Grice, K. O., Vogel, K. A., et al. "Adult norms for a commercially available Nine Hole Peg Test for finger dexterity." The American journal of occupational therapy 2003 57(5): 570-573
10. Heller, A., Wade, D. T., et al. "Arm function after stroke: measurement and recovery over the first three months." Journal of Neurology, Neurosurgery and Psychiatry 1987 50(6): 714-719
11. Sunderland, A., Tinson, D., et al. "Arm function after stroke. An evaluation of grip strength as a measure of recovery and a prognostic indicator." British Medical Journal 1989 52(11): 1267
12. Wang, Y. C., Magasi, S. R., et al. "Assessing dexterity function: a comparison of two alternatives for the NIH Toolbox." Journal of Hand Therapy 2011 24(4): 313-320; quiz 321
13. Parker, V. M., Wade, D. T., et al. "Loss of arm function after stroke: measurement, frequency, and recovery." Int Rehabil Med 1986 8(2): 69-73
14. Beebe, J. A. and Lang, C. E. "Relationships and responsiveness of six upper extremity function tests during the first six months of recovery after stroke." J Neurol Phys Ther 2009 33(2): 96-103

❑❑❑

135

Nottingham Health Profile

Objective

The Nottingham Health Profile (NHP) was originally created as a standardised tool to survey health problems and measure medical or social interventions[1]. It was created in the 1970s and developed from more than 2000 statements from more than 700 people about the effects of ill-health[1].

Intended Population

Specific patient groups or the general population.

Method of Use

The NHP is a patient-reported questionnaire. Respondents tick yes or no boxes to answer questions about their health and its effects on their daily life.

The questionnaire is divided into two parts. The first parts comprises 38 questions in six categories: sleep, physical mobility, energy, pain, emotional reactions, and social isolation[1]. This first section is weighted to reflect how severe an impact the respondent thinks their health is having on the above areas of life[1]. The second part of the NHP is made up of seven statements about areas of life that are commonly affected by health: paid employment, jobs around the house, social life, personal relationships, sex life, hobbies and interests, and holidays[1]. Scores on the NHP can range from 0 i.e. no distress to 100 i.e severe distress.

Evidence

Reliability

Many studies have assessed the reliability of the NHP. The original study[1] tested reliability in patients with osteoarthrosis and peripheral vascular disease and found the NHP to be reliable.

Validity

Many studies have assessed the validity of the NHP. In particular, the NHP has been found to be valid for the elderly[1][2], pregnant women[1], and those with minor surgery[3], fractured limbs[4], stroke[5], intermittent claudication[6] or lower limb amputation[7]. The NHP is comparable in validity to the SF-36[2].

Responsiveness

The original authors caution that the NHP does not pick up "milder forms of distress" due to more severe nature of the questions in the first part of the NHP, As a result, it may be difficult to compare the general population and detect change[1].

Miscellaneous

The original authors note that the NHP assesses negative aspects of health rather than positive e.g. well-being[1] which means the NHP can be at odds with more recent conceptions of quality of life which focus on well-being, rather than the absence of ill health.

The NHP has been compared to the SF-36 frequently in literature when assessing quality of life. Due to differences in ceiling effect and sensitivity[2][6][8][9], the SF-36 appears to be more robust a measure than the NHP.

References

1. Hunt SM, McEwen J, Mckenna S. Measuring health status: a new tool for clinicians and epidemiologists. Br J Gen Pract. 1985. 35;273: 185–188. Accessed 30 March 2020.

2. Sharples LD, Todd CJ, Caine N, Tait S. Measurement properties of the Nottingham Health Profile and Short Form 36 health status measures in a population sample of elderly people living at home: Results from ELPHS. Br J Health Psychol. 2000. 5; 3: 217-233.
3. Hunt SM, McKenna SP, McEwen J, et al. Subjective health assessments and the perceived outcome of minor surgery. J Psychosom Re.s 1984; 28: 105-114.
4. McKenna SP, McEwen J, Hunt SM, et al. Changes in the perceived health of patients recovering from fractures. Public Health. 1984; 98: 97-102.
5. Ebrahim S, Barer Nouri F. Use of the Nottingham Health Profile with patients after a stroke. J Epidemiol Community Health. 1986. 40; 2: 166–169. Accessed 31 March 2020.
6. Wann-Hansson C, Hallber IR, Risberg B, Klevsgård R. Health Qual Life Outcomes. A comparison of the Nottingham Health Profile and Short Form 36 Health Survey in patients with chronic lower limb ischaemia in a longitudinal perspective. Health Qual Life Outcomes. 2004; 2: 9. Accessed 31 March 2020.
7. Demet, K., Guillemin, F., Martinet, N., & André, J.-M. Nottingham health profile: Reliability in a sample of 542 subjects with major amputation of one or several limbs. 2002. Prosthet Orthot Int. 26; 2: 120–123.
8. Cabral DL, Laurentino GEC, Damascena CG, Faria CDCM, Melo PG, Teixeira-Salmela LF. Comparisons of the Nottingham Health Profile and the SF-36 health survey for the assessment of quality of life in individuals with chronic stroke. Braz J Phys Ther. 2012. 16; 4: 301-308. Accessed 31 March 2020.
9. Rehabilitation Measures Database. Nottingham Health Profile. Available from https://www.sralab.org/rehabilitation-measures/nottingham-health-profile. Accessed 31 March 2020.

Nottingham Health Profile

Overview:

The Nottingham Health Profile is intended for primary health care, to provide a brief indication of a patient's perceived emotional, social and physical health problems.

Breakdown of questionnaire

(1) Part I: 38 questions in 6 subareas, with each question assigned a weighted value; the sum of all weighted values in a given subarea adds up to 100

- energy level (EL): 3
- pain (P): 8
- emotional reaction (ER): 9
- sleep (S): 5
- social isolation (SI): 5
- physical abilities (PA): 8

(2) Part II: 7 life areas affected Completing questionnaire

- each question answered "Yes" or "No"
- important that all questions are answered
- if the patient is not sure whether to say "yes" or "no" to a problem, s/he are instructed to answer the one more true at that time.

Part I

Question	Yes	No	Section	Weight
I'm tired all the time.			EL	39.20
I have pain at night.			P	12.91
Things are getting me down.			ER	10.47
I have unbearable pain.			P	19.74
I take pills to help me sleep.			S	22.37
I've forgotten what it's like to enjoy myself.			ER	9.31
I'm feeling on edge.			ER	7.22
I find it painful to change position.			P	9.99
I feel lonely.			SI	22.01

I can walk about only indoors.			PA	11.54
I find it hard to bend.			PA	10.57
Everything is an effort			. EL	36.80
I'm waking up in the early hours of the morning.			S	12.57
I'm unable to walk at all.			PA	21.30
I'm finding it hard to make contact with people.			SI	19.36
The days seem to drag.			ER	7.08
I have trouble getting up and down stairs and steps.			PA	10.79
I find it hard to reach for things.			PA	9.30
I'm in pain when I walk.			P	11.22
I lose my temper easily these days.			ER	9.76
I feel there is nobody that I am close to.			SI	20.13
I lie awake for most of the night.			S	27.26
I feel as if I'm losing control.			ER	13.99
I'm in pain when I'm standing.			P	8.96
I find it hard to get dressed by myself.			PA	12.61
I soon run out of energy.			EL	24.00
I find it hard to stand for long (e.g., at the kitchen sink, waiting in a line).			PA	11.20
I'm in constant pain			P	20.86
It takes me a long time to get to sleep.			S	16.10
I feel I am a burden to people.			SI	22.53
Worry is keeping me awake at night.			ER	13.95
I feel that life is not worth living.			ER	16.21
I sleep badly at night.			S	21.70
I'm finding it hard to get along with people.			SI	15.97
I need help to walk about outside (e.g., a walking aid or someone to support me).			PA	12.69
I'm in pain when going up or down stairs.			P	5.83
I wake up feeling depressed.			ER	12.01
I'm in pain when I'm sitting.			P	10.49

Part II

Is your present state of health causing problems with your :	Yes	No
Work? (that is, paid employment)		
Looking after the home? (cleaning & cooking, repairs, odd jobs around the home, etc.)		
Social life? (going out, seeing friends, going to the movies, etc.)		
Home life? (that is, relationships with other people in your home)		
Sex life?		
Interests and hobbies? (sports, arts and crafts, do-it-yourself, etc.)		
Vacations? (summer or winter vacations, weekends away, etc.)		

Interpretation

- number of questions in each section affected
- relative level affected, in which the sum of the relative weights are subtracted from 100%, giving values between 0 and 1, with 0 indicating poor and 1 good health

Reference: https://reseauconceptuel.umontreal.ca/rid%3D1J1WXGYDK-CPP19Z-1ZQY/

❑❑❑

136 Occiput to Wall Distance (OWD)

Objective

The Occiput to Wall Distance is a routine clinical test for thoracic kyphosis that has been in use for many years.

- The occiput-wall distance (OWD) cannot substitute highly accurate clinical measures of kyphosis such as Cobb's angle, OWD has been extensively used in epidemiological studies.
- It has been associated with depressed mood, postural instability, muscle weakness and disability in older women, and may account for a large percentage of the dyspnea and restrictive/ obstructive respiratory dysfunction that often remains unexplained in older persons[1]

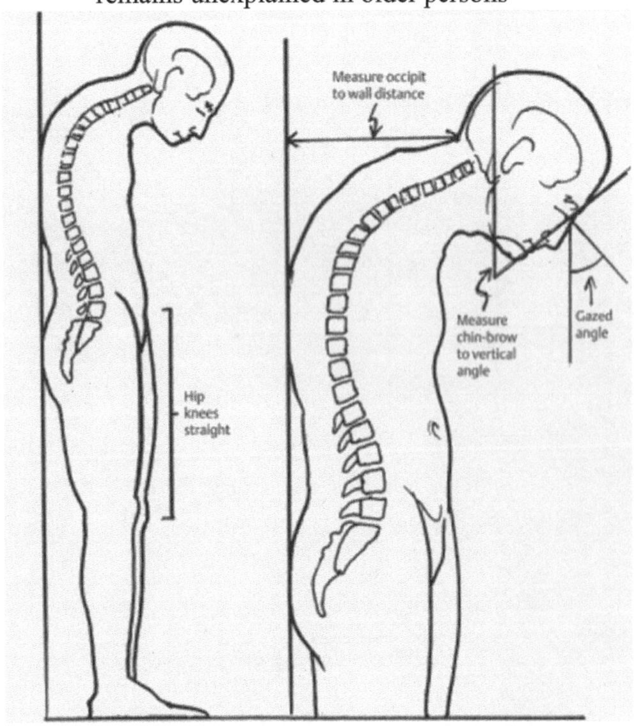

Intended Population

The OWD may be abnormal in kyphosis (forward curvature of the upper thoracic spine) due[3]

- Spondyloarthritis
- Scheuermann's Kyphosis
- Osteoporosis
- Postural instability
- Congenital spinal deformity
- Marked obesity.
- Forward Head Posture
- Upper crossed syndrome

The occiput-wall distance (OWD), has been associated with postural instability, osteoporosis, disability and depression.[1]

OWD is an easily measurable marker of poor physical function in women.

Method of Use

The OWD is measured by having an examinee stand with the back against a wall keeping the posture as straight as possible and with the heels, buttocks and shoulders touching the wall ie standing with both heels and the sacrum against the wall, and with the lower orbital margin and upper margin of the acoustic meatus on the horizontal plane[1].

- While looking forward, the examinee also attempts to have the back of the head (the occiput) touch the wall as well.
- In most normal individuals in this standard position, the occiput will touch the wall and the OWD measurement will be zero.
- If the occiput does not touch the wall, then the OWD is measured with a ruler.

A value greater than 2 cm. is considered to be abnormal[3].

Clinical Significance

In both men and women, walking speed and balance were found to be more severely compromised with higher OWD values.

- This relationship explained by the biomechanical effects of changes in OWD: in particular, the kyphotic posture of the upper dorsal and cervical spine results in anterior displacement of the center of gravity, and is followed by compensatory widening of the base of support and lumbar hyperlordosis.
- This adaptive strategy leads to the balance impairment and involves a consequent increase in the risk of falls.
- Changes in postural control may lead to reduced walking speed, since the cautious reduced step length gait, is an obvious response to postural instability[1]
- Current lifestyles of many people means they spend considerable time in an excessive flexion posture using computers and social media, this can accelerate the development of hyperkyphotic spine in young individuals. The condition can influence general appearance, self-confidence, musculoskeletal problems and work effectiveness of these individuals. Effective early detection (using OWD) and monitoring this condition may prevent or minimize serious consequences and to clearly indicate effectiveness of the treatments.
- OWD can be used to detect the risk of developing hyperkyphosis in many target populations eg school children, office workers and community-dwelling people, OWD > 5 cm had the be

Conclusion

Thoracic kyphosis, assessed using Cobb's angle, has been proved to be associated with poor physical fitness, osteoporosis, and the risk of falls.

Measuring Cobb's angle requires radiologic equipment and therefore this measure is not easily performed.

OWD cannot substitute for Cobb's angle because it does not directly measure the curvature of the spine at a given point, but quantifies the effect of altered curvature.

Thus, OWD is unlikely to reflect kyphotic posture as accurately as Cobb's angle. However, the well-recognized association with several measures of physical limitation confirmed makes OWD a valuable tool for eg treating thoracic kyphosis, epidemiological research[1].

References

1. Antonelli-Incalzi R, Pedone C, Cesari M, Di Iorio A, Bandinelli S, Ferrucci L. Relationship between the occiput-wall distance and physical performance in the elderly: a cross sectional study. Aging clinical and experimental research. 2007 Jun 1;19(3):207-12.Available from:https://www.ncbi.nlm.nih.gov/pmc/articles/PMC2651517/ (last accessed 28.4.2020)
2. University of Ottawa OWD Available from:https://www.youtube.com/watch?v=rOR70O_zTdA (last accessed 28.4.2020)
3. Centers for Disease Control and Prevention. National health and nutrition examination survey. Available from:https://wwwn.cdc.gov/Nchs/Nhanes/2009-2010/ARX_F.htm#Protocol_and_Procedure (last accessed 28.4.2020)
4. Wiyanad, Arpassanan & Thaweewannakij, Thiwabhorn & Wattanapan, Pattra & Sooknuan, Thanat & Mato, Lugkana & Amatachaya, Pipatana & Amatachaya, Sugalya. (2017) Appropriate Occiput-wall Distance to Screen for a Risk of Kyphosis. Available from:https://www.researchgate.net/publication/315773559 Appropriate_Occiput-wall_Distance_to_Screen for_a_Risk_of_Kyphosis/citation/download (last accessed 28.4.2020)

❑❑❑

137 Knee to Wall Test

Purpose

The Weight-bearing lunge test (WBLT) or Dorsiflexion Lunge Test (DFT) is used to assess the dorsiflexion range of movement (DROM) at the ankle joint. [1][2][3]

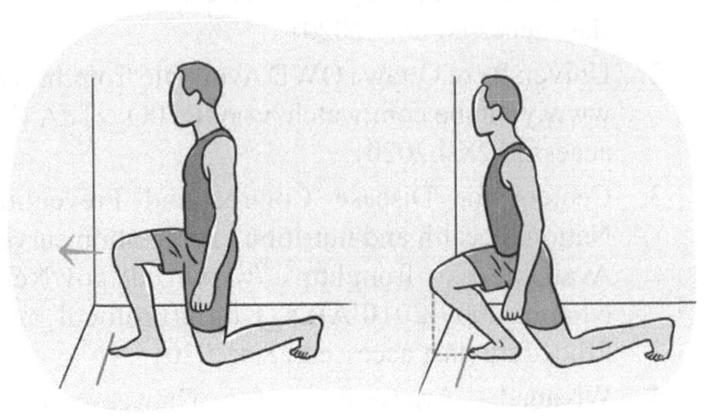

Technique

This test needs to be done against a wall. A standard tape measure (cm) is necessary. Participants are asked to place their foot in such a way that a imaginary line drawn through the heel and big toe are aligned on the tape measure on the floor. Furthermore, a vertical line is drawn on the wall in line with the tape measure. Participants are instructed to lunge forward until their knee touches the wall (vertical line). The heel is required to remain in contact with the floor at all times. The foot is moved away from the wall to the point where the knee can only make slight contact with the wall, while the heel remains in contact with the floor. This puts the ankle joint in maximal dorsiflexion. The leg not being tested can rest on the the floor and participants are allowed to hold onto the wall for support. The maximum distance from the wall to the tip of the big toe is recorded. The distance is measured in centimeters (cm) with each centimeter corresponding to approximately 3.6° of ankle dorsiflexion. [4]

Evidence

The inter-rater reliability for the distance measured for the weight bearing lunge test was R = 0.99 (95% CL: 0.97 - 0.99)[4] The intra-rater reliability for the measurement was also excellent (ICC between 0.98 - 0.99).[3][4] Furthermore, a recent systematic review[1] on the reliability of the of the weight-bearing lunge test reported that there was strong evidence that inter-rater reliability (ICC = 0.80 - 0.99) as well as intra-rater reliability (ICC = 0.65 - 0,99) of the weight-bearing lunge test is good.[1] It was suggested that the weight-bearing lunge test is a reliable method of assessing ankle dorsiflexion range of motion as it provides consistent results and demonstrates reasonable responsiveness.[1]

References

1. Powden CJ, Hoch JM, Hoch MC. Reliability and minimal detectable change of the weight-bearing lunge test: A systematic review.Man Ther. 2015 Aug;20(4):524-32 (last accessed 12 November 2018)
2. Konor MM, Morton S, Eckerson JM, Grindstaff TL. Reliability of three measures of ankle dorsiflexion range of motion. Int J Sports Phys Ther. 2012 Jun; 7(3): 279–287.(last accessed 12 November 2018).
3. Dennis RJ, Finch CF, Elliott BC, Farhart PJ. The reliability of musculoskeletal screening tests used in cricket. Phys Ther Sport. 2008 Feb;9(1):25-33.
4. Bennell KL, Talbot RC, Wajswelner H, Techovanich W, Kelly DH, Hall AJ. Intra-rater and inter-rater reliability of a weight-bearing lunge measure of ankle dorsiflexion.Aust J Physiother. 1998;44(3):175-180. (last accessed 12 November 2018).
5. The Physio Channel. Knee to Wall Test. Available from https://www.youtube.com/watch?v=kbzYML05Vac (last accessed 5 March 2021)

138

Silfverskiold Test

Purpose

The Silfverskiöld test commonly used to identify isolated gastrocnemius contracture associated with several foot and ankle pathologies was first described by Nils Silfverskiöld [1]. The Silfverskiöld test differentiates gastrocnemius tightness from an achilles tendon contracture by evaluating ankle dorsiflexion with the knee extended and then flexed[2].

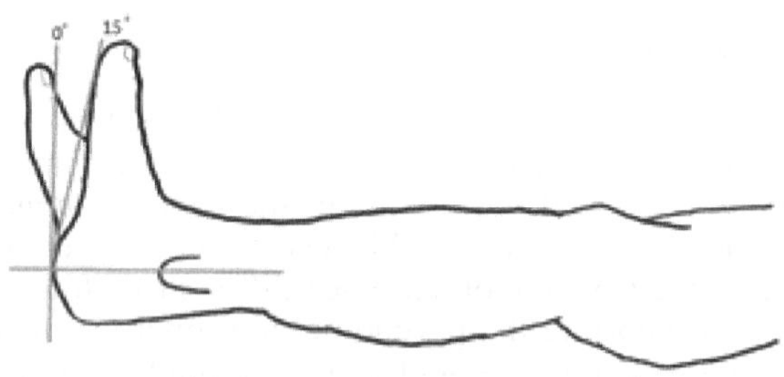

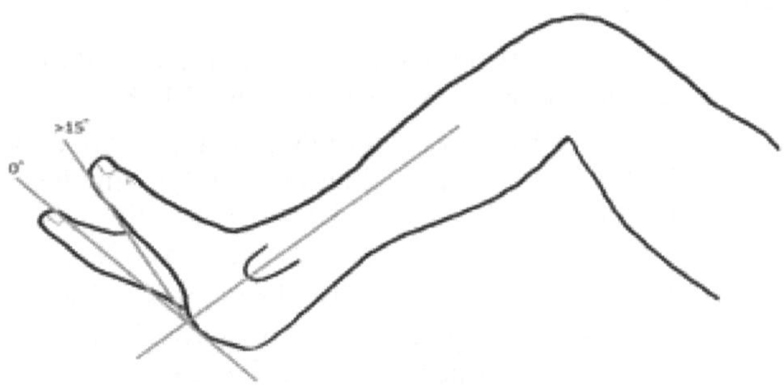

Technique

It measures the dorsiflexion (DF) of the foot at the ankle joint (AJ) with knee extended & flexed to 90 degrees. The test is considered positive when DF at the AJ is greater with knee flexed than extended.

The test is performed with the patient seated or in supine. Two hands are utilized to perform the technique, with one hand neutralizing and locking the subtalar (ST) joint and the other stabilizing the talonavicular (TN) joint and forefoot in order to isolate the ankle joint motion[3]. With the subtalar joint (STJ) in neutral, forefoot is supinated and foot is dorsiflexed with knee in full extension. Measurement is taken of the DF range. Then the test is repeated with knee flexed at 90 degrees.

Less dorsiflexion with a soft and spongy feel when the knee is extended, indicates a gastroc contracture and equally limited DF with the knee flexed and extended, points to either a soleal equinus or an osseous block.

Evidence

Inter- and intrarater reliability testing of the clinical Silfverskiöld test : ICC values of 0.230 to 0.791. poor inter- and intrarater reliability[4].

References

1. SilfverskiöldN.: Reduction of the uncrossed two-joints muscles of the leg to one-joint muscles in spastic conditions. Acta Chir Scand;1924;56:315-30.
2. DiGiovanni CW, Kuo R, Tejwani N, et al: Isolated gastrocnemius tightness. J Bone Joint Surg Am 2002;84(6):962-970.
3. Hansen ST. Functional reconstruction of the foot and ankle. Lippincott Williams & Wilkins; 2000.
4. Molund M, Husebye EE, Nilsen F, Hellesnes J, Berdal G, Hvaal KH. Validation of a New Device for Measuring Isolated Gastrocnemius Contracture and Evaluation of the Reliability of the Silfverskiöld Test. Foot & Ankle International. 2018;39(8):960-965.

❑❑❑

139

Eversion Stress Test

Purpose

The Eversion Stress Test evaluates the integrity of the deltoid ligament and aids in determining the degree of instability after a medial ankle sprain[1][2].

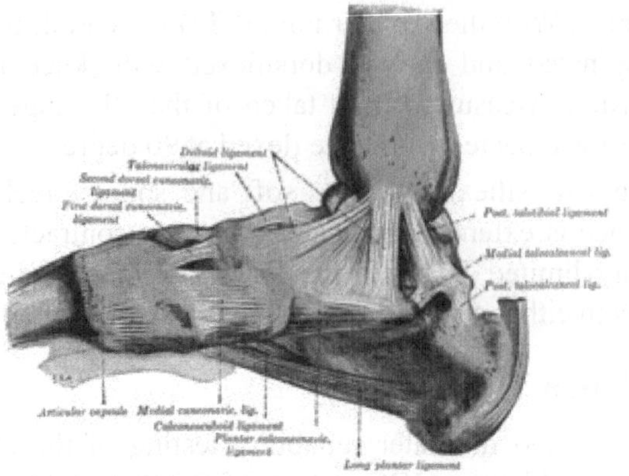

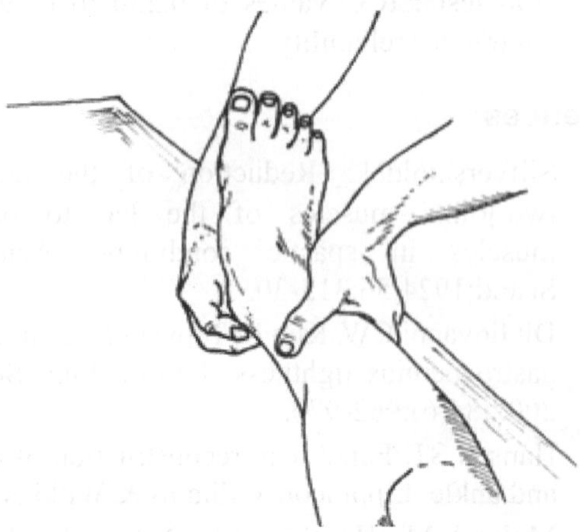

Medial Ankle Ligament

Technique

The patient is supine, side lying, or seated comfortable with the knee bent 90 degrees and gastrocnemius relaxed. The heel is held from below by one hand by the therapist while the other hand holds the lower leg. While maintaining the ankle in a neutral position, the clinician applies an abduction force to the calcaneus to tilt the talus[1]. Increased talar tilt or pain over the deltoid ligament, when compared bilaterally, indicates a positive test. A spongy or indefinite end feel is indicative of a complete tear[3][4]. In the neutral position, a 2-degree or greater tilt during testing when compared bilaterally indicates a high probability of significant injury to the deltoid[5].

Evidence

Studies show that a valgus tilt of the talus occurs when the superficial and deep fibers of the deltoid ligaments are involved. Neutral positioning of the ankle is suggested to test the superficial layer, while testing throughout available ankle range of motion assesses different deltoid fibers[6]. Studies reporting the psychometric properties of this test are scarce and data related to it could not be identified.

References

1. Starkey C, Brown SD. Examination of orthopedic & athletic injuries. FA Davis; 2015 Feb.
2. de Vries JS, Kerkhoffs GM, Blankevoort L, van Dijk CN. Clinical evaluation of a dynamic test for lateral ankle ligament laxity. Knee Surg Sports Traumatol Arthrosc. 2010 May;18(5):628-33.
3. Prentice W, Arnheim D. Principles of athletic training: A competency-based approach. McGraw-Hill Higher Education; 2013 Jan 25.
4. Manganaro D, Alsayouri K. Anatomy, Bony Pelvis and Lower Limb, Ankle Joint. In: StatPearls. StatPearls Publishing, Treasure Island (FL); 2020.
5. Leith JM, McConkey JP, Li D, Masri B. Valgus stress radiography in normal ankles. Foot & ankle international. 1997 Oct;18(10):654-7.
6. Magee DJ. Orthopedic physical assessment 5th ed. St. Louis, Mo, Saunders Elsevier. 2008.

❑❑❑

140 Homan's Sign Test

Purpose

Homan's sign test also called dorsiflexon sign test is a physical examination procedure that is used to test for Deep Vein Thrombosis (DVT). A positive Homan's sign in the presence of other clinical signs may be a quick indicator of DVT. Clinical evaluation alone cannot be relied on for patient management, but when carefully performed, it remains useful in determining the need for additional testing (like D-dimer test, ultrasonography, multidetector helical computed axial tomography (CT), and pulmonary angiography) [1][2].

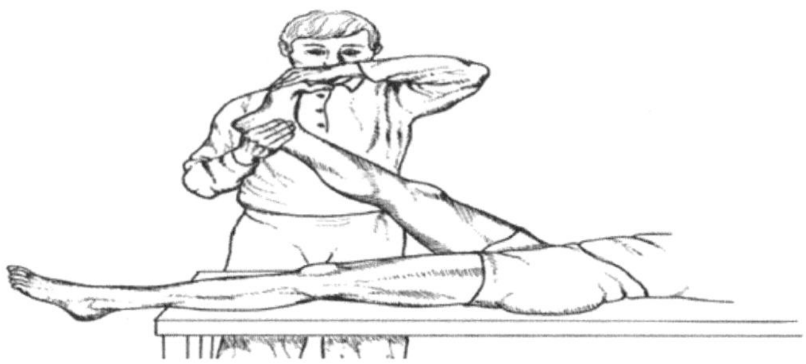

Technique

1. In performing this test the patient will need to actively extend his knee.
2. Once the knee is extended the examiner raises the patient's straight leg to 10 degrees, then passively and abruptly dorsiflexes the foot and squeezes the calf with the other hand.
3. Deep calf pain and tenderness may indicate presence of DVT.

Evidence

Passive, abrupt and forced ankle dorsiflexion with slight knee flexion causes mechanical traction on the posterior tibial vein. This traction stimulates the pain sensitive structures in the lower limb [4] [5].

Differential diagnosis of conditions that demonstrate a positive Homan's sign include intervertebral disc herniation, ruptured Baker's cyst, neurogenic claudication, gastrocnemius spasm, and cellulitis [6].

Accuracy

Homan's sign has low sensitivity and specificity in diagnosing DVT; it can be of value if used in addition to more accurate diagnostic procedures like ultrasonography and venography[7].

Precaution

Vigorous dorsiflexion of the foot is used by surgeons to expel clot from the veins and so this test may have its dangers[8].

Common Errors

A common error that may occur is the examiner not dorsiflexing the patient's foot enough to get a correct interpretation. The knee of the patient must also be in full extension.

Relevance to Physiotherapists

Homan's sign test may serve as a quick and easy way to determine if a patient might be having a DVT and subsequently exercise caution when carrying out certain movements involving the lower limb especially in bedridden and unconscious patients.

References

1. Wheeler HB. Diagnosis of deep vein thrombosis. Review of clinical evaluation and impedance plethysmography. American journal of surgery. 1985 Oct;150(4A):7-13.
2. Patel K, Chun LJ, Deep Venous Thrombosis. Medscape 2017 https://emedicine.medscape.com/article/1911303-workup (Accessed on 3rd July, 2018).
3. Steph Magee. Homan's Sign. Available from https://www.youtube.com/watch?v=R5cevg5Y0Zg [last Accessed on 1/7/2018]
4. Shafer N, Duboff S. Physical signs in the early diagnosis of thrombophlebitis. Angiology. 1971 Jan;22(1):18-30.
5. Mathewson M. A Homan's sign is an effective method of diagnosing thrombophlebitis in bedridden patients. Critical care nurse. 1983 Jul 1;3(4):64-5
6. Hirsh J, Hull RD, Raskob GE. Clinical features and diagnosis of venous thrombosis. Journal of the American College of Cardiology. 1986 Dec 1;8(6 Supplement 2):114B-27B.
7. Ambesh P, Obiagwu C, Shetty V. Homan's sign for deep vein thrombosis: A grain of salt?. Indian Heart Journal. 2017 May;69(3):418.
8. Homans J. Thrombosis of the deep veins of the lower leg, causing pulmonary embolism. New England Journal of Medicine. 1934 Nov 29;211(22):993-7

❑❑❑

141 Thompson Test

Definition/Description

The Thompson test examines the integrity of the Achilles tendon by squeezing the calf. It is performed as a clinical test to identify the presence of a complete Achilles rupture.

Clinically relevant anatomy

The calf musculature of the m. triceps sure group includes:

- m. gastrocnemius, which arises from two heads on the posterior surface of the femur, directly above the two condyles of the femur
- m. soleus, which comes from an inverted U-shaped origin from the posterior aspect of the Tibia, membrane interossei and the head and upper 1/3 of the fibula
- m. plantaris, which arises from the distal lateral portion of the Linea aspera

M. gastrocnemius and m. soleus blend together in the distal portion of the calf and form the tendon of Achilles. The plantaris tendon, when present, lies alongside the heel cord or is somewhat removed from it in its insertion into the medial aspect of the calcaneus.[1]

Tendons are strong, tough bands of inelastic fibrous connective tissue that connect muscle to bone. They consist of elongated cells, minimal ground substance, and collagen fibres. The collagen fibres are packed closely together, parallel to the direction of force. Each collagen fibril is arranged into fascicles, which contain blood vessels and nerve fibres.

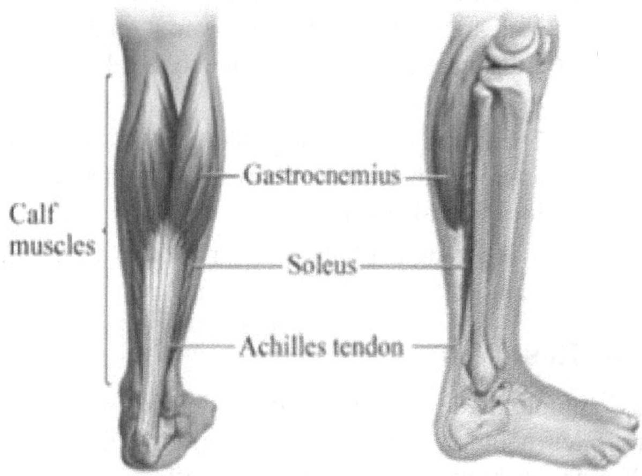

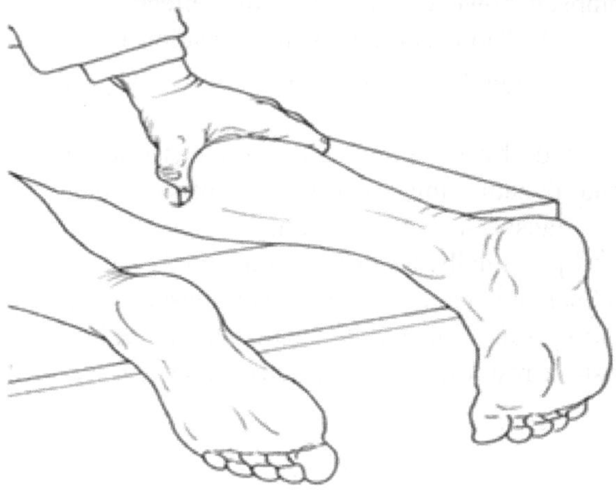

Purpose

The goal of this test is to find out if there is a complete tear present in the Achilles tendon.

Technique

The patient lies prone with his foot over the end of

the table. Alternatively, the patient could lie prone with his knee flexed to 90°. The examiner squeezes the calf muscles, specifically the gastrocnemius - soleus complex, with his hand. Squeezing the calf should cause contraction of the Achilles tendon, resulting in plantar flexion. If the Achilles tendon is completely ruptured, there will not be any apparent plantar flexion.

It is still possible for the m. plantaris and deep toe flexors to also provide plantar flexion even if the Achilles tendon is ruptured & lt; ref & gt; Verhaar JAN, van der Linden AJ. Orthopaedic. Bohn Stafleu van Loghum, 2008, p. 165-166. </ref>. To be sure that the patient has a complete Achilles tendon rupture, there are three additional clinical signs that may be observed to corroborate the diagnosis[2]:

1. On careful inspection, with the patient prone and both ankles fully relaxed, the foot on the ruptured side hangs straight down due to the absence of the tendon tone
2. There may be a palpable gap in the tendon, approximately 3-6cm proximal to the insertion into the calcaneus
3. The strength of the plantar flexion is markedly reduced

Key Research

Simmonds described in 1957 how squeezing the calf muscles could test the rupture of the Achilles tendon. Thompson however had noted this effect in 1955. The Simmonds-Thompson test is an indication for a possible complete rupture, but its mechanism is not completely clear.

A study by Scott and colleagues[3] used an ultrasound to take dynamic images of the calf of two young adults. With transverse compression, the m. gastrocnemius moved proximally, according to the ankle movement. No proximal movement of the m. soleus muscle could be seen. Thompson and Doherty[1]found that the squeezing test gave a positive result when the m. soleus alone was divided. To elucidate these findings, Scott and colleagues separated the m. gastrocnemius tendon from the m. soleus down to 10 cm above the Achilles tendon, the place where the fibres form the tendon. By squeezing a healthy calf, the m. soleus deformed, which made the overlying m. gastrocnemius tendon bow away from the tibia resulting in plantar flexion. The m. soleus did not move in a longitudinal manner, while the m. gastrocnemius muscle moved about 1 cm proximally. These findings confirm the ultrasound findings. When the squeezing test was performed on a divided m. soleus tendon, the m. gastrocnemius did not produce any plantar flexion. Dividing the m. gastrocnemius tendon did not prevent full plantar flexion. We can conclude then that the plantar flexion is caused by bowing the calf tendons and less so by the proximal displacement of the bellies of the m. gastrocnemius.

A study conducted by Douglas and colleagues [4] came up with other findings. The case study consisted of two patients who were diagnosed with a disruption of the m. gastrocnemius tendon and an intact m. soleus tendon after surgical exploration. They could both actively plantar flex their ankles but had a positive Simmonds-Thompson test result. This study indicates that the Thompson test is insufficient as a diagnostic of a complete rupture.

References

1. Thompson TC, Doherty JH. Spontaneous rupture of tendon of Achilles: a new clinical diagnostic test. J Trauma. 1962 Mar;2:126-9.
2. Brukner P, Khan K. Clinical Sports Medicine. 3rd ed. McGraw-Hill Book Company, 2010.
3. Scott BW, Al Chalabi A. How the Simmonds–Thompson test works. J Bone Joint Surg Br. 1992 Mar;74(2):314-5.
4. Douglas J, Kelly M, Blachut P. Clarification of the Simmonds-Thompson test for rupture of an Achilles tendon. Can J Surg. 2009 Jun;52(3):E40-1.

❑❑❑

142 Fingertips to Floor Distance - Special Test

Objective

o assess the total mobility of the lumbo-pelvic region in clients presenting with lumbo-pelvic pain. It is a test that is simple to administer with excellent inter and intra-rater reliability, validity, and responsiveness.

Intended Population

Musculoskeletal conditions of the lumbar-pelvic region eg

- Chronic Low Back Pain
- Ankylosing Spondylitis (Axial Spondylarthritis)
- Radiculopathy Low Back Pain
- Osteoarthritis of the Lumbo-pelvic region

Method of Use

The patient is asked to bend forward and attempt to reach for the floor with their fingertips. The physical therapist then measures the distance between the patient's right long finger and the floor using a standard measuring tape.

Ask the client whether pain, stiffness or both limited the Fingertips to floor (FTF) test. If the FTF test is limited by pain, the location and pain score out of 10 should be documented.

If the FTF test is 0cm or the patient is able to place their palms to the floor with no pain, a different outcome measure should be considered.

As forward bending flexibility is highly variable even in the asymptomatic population no normative values exist. Note- Patients with LBP with or without neural symptoms often present with FTF test measures of greater than 20cm.

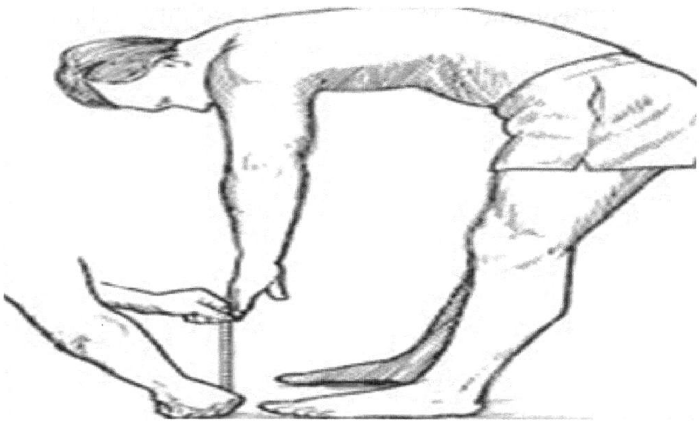

Reliability

The intra- and interobserver reliability were excellent ICC (intraclass correlation coefficient) = .99)[2].

Validity

Spearman's correlation coefficient for trunk flexion assessed by the test and the radiologic measure are excellent (rs =.96).[2]

Responsiveness

.97 for SRM (standardized response mean) and .87 for effect size.

Miscellaneous

FTF test has been criticized for not measuring isolated lumbar flexion ROM, as forward bending range involves pelvic, hip, thoracic spine, Dural and shoulder mobility. However pure lumbar flexion active ROM measures should not be used as an outcome measure to monitor patient progress, as they have been shown to be weakly correlated to the patients' level of disability.[3]

Rainville J et al also found total lumbosacral flexion may be as equally relevant as true lumbar flexion in the measurement of trunk mobility in the clinical examination of patients with chronic low back pain. In regards to their relationship t oa self-reported disability, total flexion seemed to be more relevant to outcome following intensive rehabilitation[4].

References

1. G Gellerman Finger to Floor Test- Lumbo-Pelvic Mobility Available from: https://www.youtube.com/watch?v=8_f9FpyRSsU (last accessed 22 October 2019)
2. Perret C, Poiraudeau S, Fermanian J, Colau MM, Benhamou MA, Revel M. Validity, reliability, and responsiveness of the fingertip-to-floor test. Archives of physical medicine and rehabilitation. 2001;82(11):1566-70.
3. Sullivan MS, Shoaf LD, Riddle DL. The relationship of lumbar flexion to disability in patients with low back pain. Physical therapy. 2000;80(3):240-50.
4. Rainville J, Sobel JB, Hartigan C. Comparison of total lumbosacral flexion and true lumbar flexion measured by a dual inclinometer technique. Spine. 1994 Dec;19(23):2698-701. Available from: https://www.ncbi.nlm.nih.gov/pubmed/7899966 (accessed 22 October 2019)

❑❑❑

143 Oswestry Disability Index

Objective

Patient-completed questionnaire which gives a subjective percentage score of level of function (disability) in activities of daily living in those rehabilitating from low back pain.

Intended Population

Acute or chronic low back pain. Most effective for persistent severe disability while the Roland-Morris is better for mild to moderate disability[1]

Method of Use

Questionnaire examines perceived level of disability in 10 everyday activities of daily living.

The 6 statements are scored from 0 to 5 with the first statement scoring 0 through to the last at 5, e.g.,

Section 1 - Pain intensity

- I have no pain at the moment. Score = 0
- The pain is very mild at the moment. Score = 1
- The pain is moderate at the moment. Score = 2
- The pain is fairly severe at the moment. Score = 3
- The pain is very severe at the moment. Score = 4
- The pain is the worst imaginable at the moment. Score = 5

If more than one box is marked in each section, take the highest score.

The ODI score (index) is calculated as:

For example:

If all 10 sections are completed the score is calculated as follows:

if 16 (total scored) out of 50 (total possible score) x 100 = 32%

If one section is missed (or not applicable) the score is calculated:

If 16 (total scored) / 45 (total possible score) x 100 = 35.5%

Rounding the percentage to a whole number for convenience is suggested.

Interpretation of Scores

0% to 20%: minimal disability:	The patient can cope with most living activities. Usually no treatment is indicated apart from advice on lifting sitting and exercise.
21%-40%: moderate disability:	The patient experiences more pain and difficulty with sitting, lifting and standing. Travel and social life are more difficult and they may be disabled from work. Personal care, sexual activity and sleeping are not grossly affected and the patient can usually be managed by conservative means.
41%-60%: severe disability	Pain remains the main problem in this group but activities of daily living are affected. These patients require a detailed investigation.
61%-80%: crippled:	Back pain impinges on all aspects of the patient's life. Positive intervention is required.
81%-100%:	These patients are either bed-bound or exaggerating their symptoms.

From Paper Based to Electronic Patient Record Systems

Conventionally ODI is applied as paper based forms. By development of internet technologies, online calculator tools for ODI become popular. Electronic patient record (EPR) systems are specialised databases for management on patient's health records. By the integration of EPR and outcome measure databases distance patient assessment can be possible.

In 2007 Irmak and Ergun has developed experimental tool for integration of EPR and online assessment system for ODI and Roland Morris Questionnaire by using different programming languages and databases; PHP-MySQL, C# JavaScript, and MS Access. Currently this system is available for online calculation and assessment for non registered users. For scientists a distance patient assessment interface is also available.

Evidence

Reliability

The ODI addresses a broader concept of disability than that directly related to pain intensity[2].

Validity

Fisher K, Johnston M (1997) Validation of the ODQ, its sensitivity as a measure of change following treatment and its relationship with other aspects of the chronic pain experience Physiotherapy Theory and Practice 13, 67-80

Responsiveness

Bolton JE, Fish RG (1997) Responsiveness of the Revised Oswestry Disability Questionnaire Eur J Chiropractic 45, 1, 9-14

References

1. Davies, Claire C.1; Nitz, Arthur J. Psychometric properties of the Roland-Morris Disability Questionnaire compared to the Oswestry Disability Index: a systematic review. Physical Therapy Reviews, Volume 14, Number 6, December 2009 , pp. 399-408(10)
2. Gronblad M, Hupli M et al (1989) Intercorrelation and test-retest reliability of the pain disability index and the Oswestry disability questionnaire and their correlation with pain intensity in low back pain patients The Clinical Journal of Pain 9, 189-195.
3. Fairbank J, Davies J, Couper J, OBrien J (1980) The Oswestry low back pain disability questionnaire Physiotherapy 66, 8, 271-273
4. Fairbank J, Pynsent P. The Oswestry disablility index. Spine 2000;25:2490-53.
5. Roland M, Fairbank J. The Roland-Morris Disability Questionnaire and the Oswestry Disability Questionnaire. Spine 2000;25:3115-3124
6. Davidson M & Keating J (2001) A comparison of five low back disability questionnaires: reliability and responsiveness. Physical Therapy 2002;82:8-24.

Oswestry Low Back Pain Disability Questionnaire

Fairbank JC, Pynsent PB. The Oswestry Disability Index. Spine 2000 Nov 15;25(22):2940-52; discussion 52.

Instructions

This questionnaire has been designed to give us information as to how your back or leg pain is affecting your ability to manage in everyday life. Please answer by checking ONE box in each section for the statement which best applies to you. We realise you may consider that two or more statements in any one section apply but please just shade out the spot that indicates the statement which most clearly describes your problem.

Section 1 – Pain intensity

I have no pain at the moment

The pain is very mild at the moment

The pain is moderate at the moment

The pain is fairly severe at the moment

The pain is very severe at the moment

The pain is the worst imaginable at the moment

Section 2 – Personal care (washing, dressing etc)

I can look after myself normally without causing extra pain

I can look after myself normally but it causes extra pain

It is painful to look after myself and I am slow and careful

I need some help but manage most of my personal care

I need help every day in most aspects of self-care

I do not get dressed, I wash with difficulty and stay in bed

Section 3 – Lifting

I can lift heavy weights without extra pain

I can lift heavy weights but it gives extra pain

Pain prevents me from lifting heavy weights off the floor, but

I can manage if they are conveniently placed eg. on a table

Pain prevents me from lifting heavy weights, but

I can manage light to medium weights if they are conveniently positioned

I can lift very light weights

I cannot lift or carry anything at all

Section 4 – Walking

Pain does not prevent me walking any distance

Pain prevents me from walking more than 1 mile

Pain prevents me from walking more than 1/2 mile

Pain prevents me from walking more than 100 yards

I can only walk using a stick or crutches

I am in bed most of the time

Section 5 – Sitting

I can sit in any chair as long as

I like can only sit in my favourite chair as long as I like

Pain prevents me sitting more than one hour"

Pain prevents me from sitting more than 30 minutes

Pain prevents me from sitting more than 10 minutes

Pain prevents me from sitting at all

Section 6 – Standing

I can stand as long as I want without extra pain

I can stand as long as I want but it gives me extra pain

Pain prevents me from standing for more than 1 hour

Pain prevents me from standing for more than 30 minutes

Pain prevents me from standing for more than 10 minutes

Pain prevents me from standing at all

Section 7 – Sleeping

My sleep is never disturbed by pain

My sleep is occasionally disturbed by pain

Because of pain I have less than 6 hours sleep

Because of pain I have less than 4 hours sleep

Because of pain I have less than 2 hours sleep

Pain prevents me from sleeping at all

Section 8 – Sex life (if applicable)

My sex life is normal and causes no extra pain

My sex life is normal but causes some extra pain

My sex life is nearly normal but is very painful

My sex life is severely restricted by pain

My sex life is nearly absent because of pain

Pain prevents any sex life at all

Section 9 – Social life

My social life is normal and gives me no extra pain

My social life is normal but increases the degree of pain

Pain has no significant effect on my social life apart from limiting my more energetic interests eg, sport

Pain has restricted my social life and I do not go out as often

Pain has restricted my social life to my home

I have no social life because of pain

Section 10 – Travelling

I can travel anywhere without pain

I can travel anywhere but it gives me extra pain

Pain is bad but I manage journeys over two hours

Pain restricts me to journeys of less than one hour

Pain restricts me to short necessary journeys under 30 minutes

Pain prevents me from travelling except to receive treatment

❑❑❑

144

Pain Catastrophizing Scale

Pain catastrophizing is characterized by the tendency to magnify the threat value of a pain stimulus and to feel helpless in the presence of pain, as well as by a relative inability to prevent or inhibit pain-related thoughts in anticipation of, during, or following a painful event.[1]

Pain catastrophizing affects how individuals experience pain. Sullivan et al 1995 state that people who catastrophize tend to do three things, all of which are measured by this questionnaire.

1. They ruminate about their pain (e.g. "I can´t stop thinking about how much it hurts")
2. They magnify their pain (e.g. "I´m afraid that something serious might happen")
3. They feel helpless to manage their pain (e.g. "There is nothing I can do to reduce the intensity of my pain")

As such, the PCS was developed to help quantify an individual's pain experience, asking about how they feel and what they think about when they are in pain. Compared to other ways of measuring pain-related thoughts, this questionnaire is unique in that the individual does not need to be in pain while completing it.

It is one of the most widely used instruments for measuring catastrophic thinking related to pain, and is used extensively in clinical practice and in research.[2] The Adult Version is available in English and 20 other languages.

Intended Population

For adolescents and adults dealing with pain as the result of various pathology/disease.[3]

Method of Use

People are asked to indicate the degree to which they have the above thoughts and feelings when they are experiencing pain using the 0 (not at all) to 4 (all the time) scale. A total score is yielded (ranging from 0-52), along with three subscale scores assessing rumination, magnification and helplessness.

Evidence

Reliability

The PCS has been shown to have adequate to excellent internal consistency (coefficient alphas stated below):[3][4]

- Total PCS = .87-.93
- Rumination = .85-.91
- Magnification = .66-.75
- Helplessness = .78-.87

Validity

The PCS total and subscales correlated moderately and significantly with the INTRP, the Inventory of Negative Thoughts in Response to Pain, ($p < .01$) providing further evidence of concurrent validity for the PCS. Controlling for general psychological disturbance (MASQGeneral Disturbance) did not substantially change the magnitudes of the correlations between the PCS subscales (.43-.48) or the total PCS (partial $r = .56$, $p < .001$) and the INTRP.[4]

Responsiveness

A total PCS score of 30 represents clinically relevant level of catastrophizing. A total PCS score of 30 corresponds to the 75th percentile of the distribution of PCS scores in clinic samples of chronic pain patients.[3]

Gender Differences

Osman et al found a significant difference between men and women. These authors found that women had higher scores on the Rumination [F(286) = 3.91, $p < .05$] and Helplessness, [F(286) = 5.99, $p < .01$] subscales than did men. Also, women had higher scores on the total PCS score [F(286) = 5.55, $p < .01$] than did men. There was no significant difference between men and women on the Magnification subscale ($p > .05$).[4]

References

1. Quartana PJ, Campbell CM, Edwards RR. Pain Catastrophizing: A Critical Review. Expert Rev Neurother, 2009: 9(5); 745-58.
2. The Development of the Pain Catastrophizing Scale: http://sullivan-painresearch.mcgill.ca/pcs.php
3. Sullivan MJL, Bishop SR, Pivik J. The Pain Catastrophizing Scale: Development and Validation. Psychol Assess, 1995; 7(4): 524-32.
4. Osman A, Barrios FX, Kopper BA, Hauptmann W, Jones J, O'Neill E. Factor structure, Reliability, and Validity of the Pain Catastrophizing Scale. J Behav Med, 1997; 20(6): 589-605.
5. Cano A, Leonard MT, Franz A. The Significant Other Version of the Pain Catastrophizing Scale (PCS-S): Preliminary Validation. Pain, 2005; 119(1-3): 26-37.

Pain Catastrophizing Scale

	Not at all	To a slight degree	To a moderate degree	To a great degree	All the time
I worry all the time about whether the pain will end					
I feel I can't go on					
It's terrible and I think it's never going to get any better					
It's awful and I feel that it overwhelms me					
I feel I can't stand it anymore					
I become afraid that the pain will get worse					
I keep thinking of other painful events					
I anxiously want the pain to go away					
I can't seem to keep it out of my mind					
I keep thinking about how much it hurts					
I keep thinking about how badly I want the pain to stop					
There's nothing I can do to reduce the intensity of the pain					
I wonder whether something serious may happen					

145 Parkinson's Disease Questionnaire (PDQ-8)

Introduction

Parkinson's Disease Questionnaire-8 (PDQ-8)[1] is the brief version of PDQ-39 formulated to reduce the respondent burden and for convenient use in clinical settings in patients of Parkinson Disease, Parkinson's Disease Questionnaire (PDQ-39)[2] consists of 39 questions from 8 dimensions: mobility, activities of daily of living, emotional well-being, stigma, social support, cognition, communication, and bodily discomfort, and therefore can be cumbersome to complete. Parkinson's disease Questionnaire-8 (PDQ-8)[1] is the patient reported outcome measure constructed by taking one question from each of the eight domain of PDQ-39.

Intended Population

It is a quality of life outcome measure used in patient with Parkinson disease.

Method of Use

Equipment Required: Questionnaire based, Pen and paper

Training Required: none

Time Required: 5-10 min

Instrument and Scoring: It is a eight question instrument with a question taken from each domain of: mobility, activities of daily of living, emotional well-being, stigma, social support, cognition, communication, and bodily discomfort.

The question are cored out of 0-4 and the sum is totaled.

The questions are:

1. Had difficulty getting around in public?
2. Had difficulty dressing yourself?
3. Felt depressed?
4. Had problems with your close personal relationships?
5. Had problems with your concentration, e.g. when reading or watching TV?
6. Felt unable to communicate with people properly?
7. Had painful muscle cramps or spasms?
8. Felt embarrassed in public due to having Parkinson's disease?

Psychometric Properties: Inter-rater/ Intra-rater reliability: strong correlation between the summary indices of the PDQ-8 and the PDQ-39 ($r=0.93$, $P<0.001$)[3]

Internal Consistency: acceptable internal consistency(Cronbach's α: 0.80; Item-scale correlation efficient: 0.56–0.72)[3]

Validity: Excellent convergent and concurrent validity[4]

References

1. Peto V, Jenkinson C, Fitzpatrick R. PDQ-39: a review of the development, validation and application of a Parkinson's disease quality of life questionnaire and its associated measures. J Neurol. 1998;245(Suppl 1):S10–S14.
2. Hagell P, Whalley D, McKenna SP, Lindvall O. Health status measurement in Parkinson's disease: validity of the PDQ-39 and Nottingham health profile. Mov Disord. 2003;18:773–783.
3. Chen, K., Yang, YJ., Liu, FT. *et al.* Evaluation of PDQ-8 and its relationship with PDQ-39 in China: a three-year longitudinal study. Health Qual Life Outcomes. 2017. 15, 170. https://doi.org/10.1186/s12955-017-0742-5
4. Huang TT, et al. Quality of life in Parkinson's

disease patients: validation of the Short-Form Eight-item Parkinson's Disease Questionnaire (PDQ-8) in Taiwan. Qual Life Res 2011;20:499-505

Patient Specific Functional Scale

Objective

Patient Specific Functional Scale was developed by Stratford et al 1995 as a self-report outcome measure of function that could be used in patients with varying levels of independence.[1] The aim of PSFS is to provide clinicians with a valid, reliable, responsive and efficient outcome measure that would be easy to use and applicable to a large number of clinical presentations.[2]

Intended Population

The PSFS is a self-reported valid, reliable, and responsive outcome measure for patients with back, neck, knee and upper extremity problems[3][4]. It has also been shown to have a high test-retest reliability in both generic lower back pain and knee dysfunction issues.[5][1] It is also clinically responsive to changes over time with chronic pain patients[6]

Method of Use

1. Patients are asked to identify up to five important activities they are unable to perform or are having difficulty with as a result of their problem eg putting socks on, shopping.
2. Patients are asked to rate (on an 11-point scale) the current level of difficulty associated with each activity.
3. Following the intervention, patients are asked again to rate the activities previously identified (and are given the chance to nominate new problematic activities that might have arisen during that time).
4. "0" represents "unable to perform" and "10" represents "able to perform at prior level"
5. Patients select a value that best describes their current level of ability on each activity assessed.

Advantages

- Gives the patient positive re-enforcement that the intervention is effective[7]
- Keeps therapy goal orientated
- Quick to complete
- Relatively easy for patients to complete
- Helpful to redirect subjective assessment to function as opposed to pain
- Can be used on a wide variety of musculoskeletal and neurological conditions[8]

Disadvantages

- Not obtaining a final PSFS score. For example if a patient cancels their final appointment it is not always possible to ask for the score completion.[7]
- Some patients can find rating their activities on a numerical scale difficult
- Not specific to condition
- May require further outcome measures specific to condition to be completed[4]

Evidence

The PSFS is a valid, reliable, and responsive outcome measure for patients with back, neck, knee and upper extremity problems[3][4]. It has also been shown to have a high test-retest reliability in both generic lower back pain and knee dysfunction issues.[5]

Reliability

A study into cervical radiculopathy found the test-retest reliability of the PSFS to be high (Intraclass correlation coefficient = 0.82; 95% Confidence interval= 0.54–0.93) in comparison with the Neck Disability Index.[9]

Moderate to good reliability for patient with upper extremity musculoskeletal problems ICC = 0,713.[10]

Poor reliability exhibited in patient with cervical radiculopathy.[11]

Validity

PSFS is a valid tool ($p<.001$) in detecting patient with upper extremity problem.[10]

Responsiveness

Adequate responsiveness in patient with cervical radiculopathy (3.3) while the clinically important difference is 2.2.[11]

References

1. Horn KK, Jennings S, Richardson G, Van Vliet D, Hefford C, Abbott JH. The patient-specific functional scale: psychometrics, clinimetrics, and

application as a clinical outcome measure. journal of orthopaedic & sports physical therapy. 2012 Jan;42(1):30-D17.

2. Stratford P, Gill C, Westaway M, Binkley J. Assessing disability and change on individual patients: a report of a patient specific measure. Physiotherapy canada. 1995 Oct;47(4):258-63.
3. Hefford C, Abbott JH, Arnold R, Baxter GD. The patient-specific functional scale: validity, reliability, and responsiveness in patients with upper extremity musculoskeletal problems. journal of orthopaedic & sports physical therapy. 2012 Feb;42(2):56-65.
4. Westaway MD, Stratford PW, Binkley JM. The patient-specific functional scale: validation of its use in persons with neck dysfunction. Journal of Orthopaedic & Sports Physical Therapy. 1998 May;27(5):331-8.
5. Chatman AB, Hyams SP, Neel JM, Binkley JM, Stratford PW, Schomberg A, Stabler M. The Patient-Specific Functional Scale: measurement properties in patients with knee dysfunction. Physical therapy. 1997 Aug 1;77(8):820-9.
6. Maughan EF, Lewis JS. Outcome measures in chronic low back pain. European Spine Journal. 2010 Sep 1;19(9):1484-94.
7. Nicholas P, Hefford C, Tumilty S. The use of the Patient-Specific Functional Scale to measure rehabilitative progress in a physiotherapy setting. Journal of Manual & Manipulative Therapy. 2012 Aug 1;20(3):147-52.
8. Maughan EF, Lewis JS. Outcome measures in chronic low back pain. European Spine Journal. 2010 Sep 1;19(9):1484-94.
9. Cleland JA, Fritz JM, Whitman JM, Palmer JA. The reliability and construct validity of the Neck Disability Index and patient specific functional scale in patients with cervical radiculopathy. Spine. 2006 Mar 1;31(5):598-602.
10. The Patient-Specific Functional Scale: Validity, Reliability, and Responsiveness in Patients With Upper Extremity Musculoskeletal Problems
11. Reliability, Construct Validity, and Responsiveness of the Neck Disability Index, Patient-Specific Functional Scale, and Numeric Pain Rating Scale in Patients with Cervical Radiculopathy.

❑❑❑

146 The Patient-Specific Functional Scale

This useful questionnaire can be used to quantify activity limitation and measure functional outcome for patients with any orthopedic condition.

Clinician to read and fill in below: Complete at the end of the history and prior to physical examination.

Initial Assessment: I am going to ask you to identify up to three important activities that you are unable to do or are having difficulty with as a result of your _________________ problem. Today, are there any activities that you are unable to do or having difficulty with because of your _________________ problem? (Clinician: show scale to patient and have the patient rate each activity).

Follow-up Assessments: When I assessed you on (state previous assessment date), you told me that you had difficulty with (read all activities from list at a time). Today, do you still have difficulty with: (read and have patient score each item in the list)?

Patient-specific activity scoring scheme (Point to one number):

0	1	2	3	4	5	6	7	8	9	10
Unable to perform activity										Able to perform activity at the same level as before injury or problem

(Date and Score)

Activity	Initial					
1						
2						
3						
4						
5						

Total score = sum of the activity scores/number of activities

Minimum detectable change (90%CI) for average score = 2 points

Minimum detectable change (90%CI) for single activity score = 3 points

PSFS developed by: Stratford, P., Gill, C., Westaway, M., & Binkley, J. (1995). Assessing disability and change on individual patients: a report of a patient specific measure. Physiotherapy Canada, 47, 258-263

❑❑❑

147 Pediatric Balance Scale

Objective

The Pediatric Balance Scale is a modified version of the Berg Balance Scale that is used to assess functional balance skills in school-aged children. The scale consists of 14 items that are scored from 0 points (lowest function) to 4 points (highest function) with a maximum score of 56 points.[1]

Intended Population

The Pediatric Balance Scale is intended for use with school-aged children with mild to moderate motor impairments. Pilot testing was performed on children aged 5 to 15 years.[1]

Method of Use

Equipment: The equipment used is[1]:

- Adjustable height bench
- Chair with back support and arm rests
- Stopwatch or watch with a second hand
- Masking tape (1 inch wide)
- Step stool 6 inches in height
- Chalkboard eraser
- Ruler or yardstick
- Small level

Optional equipment that may be helpful includes: 2 child size footprints, blindfold, brightly coloured object at least 2 inches in size, flash cards, 2 inches of adhesive-backed hook Velcro, two 1 foot strips of loop Velcro.

Item Descriptions

1. Sitting to standing
2. Standing to sitting
3. Transfers
4. Standing unsupported
5. Sitting unsupported
6. Standing with eyes closed
7. Standing with feet together
8. Standing with one foot in front
9. Standing on one foot
10. Turning 360 degrees
11. Turning to look behind
12. Retrieving object from floor
13. Placing alternate foot on stool
14. Reaching forward with outstretched arm

Evidence

Reliability

Reliability testing performed with a sample of 20 children ages 5-15 years old with mild to moderate motor impairments showed good test-retest reliability (ICC=0.998) and good interrater reliability (ICC=0.997).[1]

Validity

Validity testing performed with a sample of 30 children ages 4-10 years old with spastic cerebral palsy in GMFCS Levels I-III showed a strong correlation between the Pediatric Balance Scale and the self-care ($r=0.73$, $p<0.001$) and mobility ($r=0.82$, $p<0.001$) dimensions of the Pediatric Disability Evaluation Inventory (PEDI).[2]

Validity testing performed with a sample of 23 children ages 6-15 years old with spastic cerebral palsy (hemiplegia or diplegia) showed a strong correlation ($r=0.797$, $p<0.05$) between the Pediatric Balance Scale and the Selective Control Assessment of Lower Extremity (Scale).[3]

References

1. Franjoine MR, Gunther JS, Taylor MJ. Pediatric balance scale: a modified version of the berg balance scale for the school-age child with mild to moderate motor impairment. Pediatr Phys Ther 2003;15(2):114-28.
2. Duarte Nde A, Grecco LA, Franco RC, Zanon N, Oliveira CS. Correlation between pediatric balance scale and functional test in children with cerebral palsy. J Phys Ther Sci 2014;26(6):849-53.
3. Lim H. Correlation between the selective control assessment of lower extremity and pediatric balance scale scores in children with spastic cerebral palsy. J Phys Ther Sci 2015;27(12):3645-49.

Pediatric Balance Scale

Name Date

Location Examiner

Item Description	Score (0 – 4)	Second (Optional)
1 Sitting to standing		
2. Standing to sitting		
3. Transfers		
4. Standing unsupported		
5. Sitting unsupported		
6. Standing with eyes closed		
7. Standing with feet together		
8. Standing with one foot in front		
9. Standing on one foot		
10. Turning 360 degrees		
11. Turning to look behind		
12. Retrieving object from floor		
13. Placing alternate foot on stool		
14. Reaching forward with outstretched arm		
Total Score		

General instructions

1. Demonstrate each task and give instructions as written A child may receive a practice trial on each item. If the child is unable to complete the task based on their ability to understand the directions, a second practice trial may be given. Verbal and visual directions may be danified through the use of physical prompts.
2. Each item should be scored utilizing the 0 to 4 scale. Multiple trials are allowed on many of the items. The child's performance should be scored based upon the lowest criteria, which describes the child's best performance. If on the first trial a child receives the maximal score of 4, additional trials need not be administered. Several items require the child to maintain a given position for a specific time. Progressively, more points are deducted if the time or distance requirements are not met; if the subject's performance warrants supervision; or if the subject touches an external support or receives assistance from the examiner. Subjects should understand that they must maintain their balance while attempting the tasks. The choice, of which leg stand on or how far to reach, is left to the subject. Poor judgement will adversely influence the performance and the scoring. In addition to scoring items 4,5,6,7,8,9,10, and 13, the examiner may choose to record the exact time in second.

Equipment

The Pediatric Balance Scale was designed to require minimal use of specialized equipment. following is a complete list of items required for administration of this tool adjustable height bench chair with back support and arm rests stopwatch or watch with a second hand masking tape 1inch wide a step stool 6 inches in height chalkboard eraser ruler or yardstick a small level.

The following item are optional and may be helpful during test administration:

2 child-size footprints blindfold a brightly colored object of at least two inches in size flash cards 2 inches of adhesive-backed hook Velcro Two 1foot strips of loop Velcro Two 1foot strip of loop.

1. Sitting to Standing

Special instruction: Items #1 and #2 may be tested simultaneously if, in the determination of the examiner, it will facilitate the best performance of the child.

INSTRUCTIONS: Child is asked to "Hold arms up and stand up." The child is allowed to select the position of his/her arms.

EQUIPMENT: A bench of appropriate height to allow the child's feet to rest supported on the floor with the hips and knees maintained in 90 degrees of flexion.

Best Of Three Trials

4 able to stand without using hands and stabilize independently

3 able to stand independently using hands

2 able to stand using hands after several tries

1 needs minimal assist to stand or to stabilize

0 needs moderate or maximal assist to stand

2. Standing to Sitting

Special instruction: items #1 and #2 may be tested simultaneously if, in the determination of the examiner, it will facilitate the best performance of the child.

INSTRUCTIONS: Child is asked to sit down slowly, without use of hands. The child is allowed to select the position of his/her arms,

EQUIPMENT: A bench of appropriate height to allow the child's feet to rest supported on the floor with the hips and knows maintained in 90 degrees of flexion.

Beat Of Three Trials

4 sits safely with minimal use of hands

3 control descent by using hands

2 uses back of legs against chair to control descent

1 sits independently, but has uncontrolled descent

0 needs assistance to sit

3. Transfers

INSTRUCTIONS: Arrange chair(s) for a stand pivot transfer, touching at a forty-five-degree angle **Ask the child to transfer one way toward a seat with armrests and one way toward a seat without armrests.**

Equipment: Two chairs, or one chair and one bench. One seating surface must have armrests. One chair/bench should be of standard adult se and the other should be of a appropriate height to allow the child to conformably sit with feet supported on the floor and ninety degrees of hip and knee flexion

Best Of Three Trials

4 able to transfer safely with minor use of hands

3 able to transfer safely, definite need of hands

2 able to transfer with verbal cueing and/or supervision (spotting)

1 needs one person to assist

0 needs two people to assist or supervise (close guard) to be safe

4. Standing Unsupported

INSTRUCTIONS: The child is asked to stand for 30 SECONDS without holding on or moving his/her feet. A taped line or footprints may be placed on the floor to help the child maintain a stationary foot position. The child may be engaged in non-stressful conversation to maintain attention span for thirty seconds. Weight shifting and equilibrium responses in feet are acceptable, movement of the foot in space (off the support surface) indicates end of the timed trial.

EQUIPMENT: a stop watch or watch with a second hand a twelve-inch-long masking tape line or two footprints placed shoulder width apart

4 able to stand safely 30 SECONDS

3 able to stand 30 SECONDS with supervision (spotting)

2 able to stand 15 SECONDS unsupported

1 need several tries to stand 10 SECONDS unsupported

0 unable to stand 10 SECONDS unassisted

______**Time in seconds**

5. Sitting with Back Unsupported and Feet Supported on the Floor

INSTRUCTIONS: Please sit with arms folded on your chest for 30 SECONDS. Child may be engaged in non-stressful conversation to maintain attention span for thirty seconds. Time should be stopped if protective reactions are observed in trunk or upper extremities.

EQUIPMENT: a stop watch or watch with a second hand a bench of appropriate height to allow the feet to rest supported on the floor with the hips and knees maintained in ninety degrees of flexion

4 able to stand safely 30 SECONDS

3 able to stand 30 SECONDS with supervision (spotting) or may requires definite use extremities to maintain sitting position

2 able to sit 15 SECONDS

1 able to sit 10 SECONDS

0 unable to sit 10 SECONDS without supported

________**Time in seconds**

6. Standing Unsupported with Eyes Closed

INSTRUCTIONS: The child is asked to stand still with feet shoulder width apart and close his/her eyes for ten seconds. **Direction: "When I say close your eyes, I want you to stand still, close your eyes, and keep them closed until I say open."** If necessary, a blindfold may be used. Weight shifting and equilibrium responses in the feet are acceptable, movement of the foot in space (off the support surface) indicates end of timed trial. A taped line or footprints may be placed on the floor to help the child maintain a stationary fool position.

EQUIPMENT: a stop watch or watch with a second hand a twelve-inch-long masking tape line or two footprints placed shoulder width apart blindfold.

Best Of 3 Trials.

4 able to stand 10 seconds safely

3 able to stand 10 seconds with supervision (spotting)

2 able to stand 3 seconds

1 unable to keep eyes closed 3 seconds but stays steady

0 needs help to keep from falling

_________ **Time in seconds**

7. Standing Unsupported With Feet Together

INSTRUCTIONS: The child is asked to place his/her feet together and stand still without holding on. The child may be engaged in non-stressful conversation to maintain attention span for thirty seconds. Weight shifting and equilibrium responses in feet are acceptable; movement of the foot in space (off the support surface) indicates end of timed trial. A taped line or footprints may be placed on the floor to help the child maintain stationary foot position.

EQUIPMENT: a stop watch or watch with a second hand a twelve-inch-long masking tape line or two footprints placed together

Best Of 3 Trials.

4 able to place feet together independently and stand 30 seconds safely

3 able to place feet together independently and stand for 30 second with supervision (spotting).

2 able to place feet together independently but unable to hold for 30

1 needs help to attain position but able to stand 30 seconds with feet together

0 needs help to attain position and/or unable to hold for 30 seconds

_______ **Time in seconds**

8. Standing Unsupported One Foot in Front

INSTRUCTIONS: The child is asked to stand with one foot in front of the other, heel to toe. If the child cannot place feet in a tandem position (directly in front), they should be asked to step forward far enough to allow the heel of one foot to be placed ahead of the toes of the stationary foot A taped line and/or footprints may be placed on the floor to help the child maintain a stationary foot position. In addition to a visual demonstration, a single physical prompt (assistance with placement) may be given. The child may be engaged in non-stressful conversation to maintain his/her attention span for 30 seconds. Weight shifting and/or equilibrium reactions in the feet are acceptable. Timed trials should be stopped if either foot moves in space (leaves the support surface) and/or upper extremities support is utilized.

EQUIPMENT: a stop watch or watch with a second hand a twelve-inch-long masking tape line or two footprints placed heel to toe

Best of three trials

4 able to place feet tandem independently and hold 30 SECONDS

3 able to place foot ahead of other independently and hold 30 seconds.

Note: the length of the stance should approximate the subject's normal stride width.

2 able to take small step independently and hold 30 SECONDs, or required assistance to place foot in front, but can hold 15 seconds.

1 needs help to step, but can hold 15 seconds

0 loses balance while stepping or standing

______**Time in seconds**

9. Standing on One Leg

INSTRUCTIONS: The child is asked to stand on one leg for as long as he/she is able to without holding on. If necessary, the child can be instructed to maintain his/her arms (hands) on his/her hips (waist). A taped line or footprints may be placed on the floor to help the child maintain a stationary foot position. Weight shifting and/or equilibrium reactions in the feet are acceptable. Timed trials should be stopped if the weight-bearing foot moves in space (leaves the support surface), the up limb touches the opposite leg or the support surface and/or upper extremities are utilized for support

EQUIPMENT: a stop watch or watch with second hand a twelve-inch-long masking tape line or two footprints placed heel to toe

3 Trials Average Score

4 able to lift leg independently and hold 10 seconds

3 able to lift leg independently and hold 5 to 9 seconds

2 able to lift leg independently and hold 3 to 4 seconds

1 tries to lift leg, unable to hold 3 seconds but remains standing

0 unable to try or needs assist to prevent fall

10. Turn 360 Degrees

INSTRUCTIONS: The child is asked to turn completely around in a full circle, STOP, and then turn a full circle in the other direction.

EQUIPMENT: A stop watch or watch with a second hand

4 able to tum 360 degrees safely in 4 seconds or less each way (lotal of less than eight seconds)

3 able to turn 360 degrees safely in one direction only in 4 seconds or less

2 completes turn in other direction requires more than four seconds

1 able to tum 360 degrees safely but slowly needs close supervision (spotting) or constant verbal cueing

0 needs assistance while turning

________**Time in seconds**

11. Turning to Look Behind Left & Right Shoulders While Standing Still

INSTRUCTIONS: The child is asked to stand with his/her feet still, fixed in one place "Follow this object as I move it. Keep watching it as I move it, but don't move your feet."

EQUIPMENT: a brightly colored object of at least two inches in size, or flash card a twelve-inch-long masking tape line or two footprints placed shoulder width apart

4 looks behind/over each should right shifts include trunk rotation

3 looks behind/over one shoulder with trunk rotation, weight shift in the opposite direction is to the level of the shoulder; no trunk rotation

2 turns head to look to level of shoulder, no trunk rotation

1 needs supervision (spotting) when turning: the chin moves greater than half the distance to the shoulder

0 needs assist to keep from losing balance or falling: movement of the chin is less than half the distance to the shoulder the shoulder

12. Pick Up Object from The Floor from A Standing Position

INSTRUCTIONS: The child is asked to pick up a chalkboard eraser placed approximately the length of his/her foot in front of his/her dominant foot. In children, where dominance is not clear, ask the child which hand they want to use and place the object in front of the foot

EQUIPMENT: a chalkboard eraser a taped line or footprint

4 able to pick up an eraser safety and easily

3 able to pick up eraser but needs supervision (spotting)

2 unable to pick up eraser but reaches 1 to 2 inches from eraser and keeps balance independently

1 unable to pick up eraser needs supervision (spotting) while attempting

0 unable to try, needs assist to keep from losing balance or falling

13. Placing Alternate Foot On Step Stool While Standing Unsupported

INSTRUCTIONS: The child is asked to place each foot alternately on the step stool and to continue until each foot has touched the step/stool four times.

EQUIPMENT: a step/stool of four inches in height a stop watch or watch with a second hand

4 stands independently and safely and completes 8 steps in 20 seconds

3 able to stand independently and complete 8 steps >20 seconds

2 able to complete 4 steps without assistance, but requires close supervision (spotting)

1 able to complete 2 steps, needs minimal assistance

0 needs assistance to maintain balance or keep from falling, unable to try

_________**Time in seconds**

14. Reaching Forward with Outstretched Arm While Standing

General Instruction and Set up: A yardstick affixed to a wall via Velcro strips will be used as the measuring tool. A taped line and/or footprints are used to maintain a stationary foot position. The child will be asked to reach as far forward without falling, and without stepping over the line, The MCP joint of the child's fisted hand will be used as the anatomical reference point for measurements. Assistance may be given to initially position the child's arm at 90 degrees. Support may not be provided during the reaching process, if 90 degrees of shoulder flexion cannot be obtained, then this item should be omitted

INSTRUCTIONS: The child is asked to lift his/her arm up like this. "Stretch out your fingers, make a fist, and reach forward as far as you can without moving your feet."

3 Trials Average Results

EQUIPMENT: a yardstick or ruler a taped line or footprints a level

4 can reach forward confidently >10 inches

3 can reach forward >5 inches, safely

2 can reach forward >2 inches, safely

1 reaches forward but needs supervision (spotting)

0 loses balance while trying, requires external support

-Total Test Score

Maximum Score 56

❑❑❑

148 Pelvic Floor Distress Inventory (PFDI - 20)

Objective

The Pelvic Floor Distress Inventory Questionnaire-20 (PFDI-20) is the short-form version of the Pelvic Floor Distress Inventory (PFDI).[1] Similar to the PFIQ-7, it is a health-related quality of life questionnaire for women with pelvic floor conditions to fill out.[1] The PFDI-20 is comprised of 3 scales, which include the Urinary Distress Inventory-6 (UDI-6), Pelvic Organ Prolapse Distress Inventory-6 (POPDI-6), and the Colorectal-Anal Distress Inventory-8 (CRADI-8).[1]

Intended Population

Women over the age of 18 with disorders of the pelvic floor including urinary incontinence, pelvic organ prolapse, and fecal incontinence.[1]

Method of Use

Since it is comprised of the UDI-6, POPDI-6, and the CRADI-8, the PFDI-20 includes 20 questions.[1] Each question begins with a "yes" or "no" response. If "yes," the patient must indicate how much bowl, bladder, or pelvic symptoms have been bothering them in the past 3 months on a 4-point scale that ranges from "not at all" (0) to "quite a bit" (4).[1] The scale scores are found individually by calculating the mean value of their corresponding questions and then multiplying by 25 to obtain a value that ranges from 0 to 100.[1] The sum of the 3 scales are added together to get the PFDI-20 summary score, which ranges from 0 to 300.[1]

Evidence

Correlation

Correlation, represented by r, ranges from -1.0 to +1.0. If the r value is 0 that means there is no correlation. If the r value is close to -1.0 that means that both values will decrease linearly. If the r value is close to +1.0 that means that both values will increase linearly.

Correlation of the short-form versions with the long-form versions:[1]

- UDI-6 r=0.86[1]
- POPDI-6 r=0.92[1]
- CRADI-8 r=0.93[1]

Reliability:

The test-retest reliability, represented by intraclass correlation coefficients (ICC):[1]

- PFDI-20 ICC=0.93[1]
- UDI-6 ICC=0.82[1]
- POPDI-6 ICC=0.91[1]
- CRADI-8 ICC=0.84[1]

Validity:

The PFDI-20 demonstrates construct validity as it demonstrates a significant association with appropriate measures of symptom severity and pelvic floor diagnoses.[1]

Responsiveness

Each of the 3 scales of the PFDI-20 demonstrated moderate to excellent responsiveness with effect size and standardized response mean values ranging from 0.70 to 1.28.[1] The sensitivity of the PFDI-20 as a whole was excellent with an effect size of 1.48 $P < .0001$ and standardized response mean of 1.09 $P < .0001$.[1] The ability of the PFDI-20 to discriminate between subjects who indicated that they were "worse" after surgery from those who indicated they were "better" was excellent with c-statistic of .95.[1]

Clinically Meaningful Change

At the time of creation, the clinically meaningful change in quality of life (MCID)[2] needed to be studied in larger populations.[1] Studies have found minimal importance changes (MIC) ranging from 23 to 45.[1][3][4] For example, in their small sample size, Barber and colleagues (2004)[1] found a change in the summary score of 45 points or more to be meaningful after surgery.[1] However, it is important to consider that patients undergoing surgery also generally have higher scores at baseline.[5]

More recently, Wiegersma and colleagues (2017) [5] aimed to determine the MIC in women undergoing conservative pelvic organ prolapse treatments for mild symptoms.[5] They found that an improvement of 13.5 points to be helpful when evaluating the effects of conservative treatment strategies.[5]

Miscellaneous

The strength of the PFDI-20 is that it is a short form that gives a comprehensive assessment of the effect of pelvic floor disorders on the quality of life of women, rather than assessing just one aspect of pelvic floor function such as urinary incontinence. A more generic quality-of-life form as the SF-36 has demonstrated poor responsiveness in patients undergoing treatment for urinary incontinence. In these patient populations, it may be important to use both a generic quality-of-life instrument and a condition-specific instrument that has demonstrated responsiveness. The PFDI-20 is easy to use in both clinical and research settings.[1]

References

1. Barber MD, Walters MD, Bump RC. Short forms of two condition-specific quality-of-life questionnaires for women with pelvic floor disorders (PFDI-20 adn PFIQ-7). Am J Obstet Gynecol 2005;193:103-113.
2. Crosby RD, Kolotkin RL, Williams GR. Defining clinically meaningful change in health-related quality of life. Journal of clinical epidemiology. 2003 May 1;56(5):395-407.
3. Gelhorn HL, Coyne KS, Sikirica V, Gauld J, Murphy M. Psychometric evaluation of health-related quality-of-life measures after pelvic organ prolapse surgery. Female pelvic medicine & reconstructive surgery. 2012 Jul 1;18(4):221-6.
4. Utomo E, Blok BF, Steensma AB, Korfage IJ. Validation of the pelvic floor distress inventory (PFDI-20) and pelvic floor impact questionnaire (PFIQ-7) in a Dutch population. International urogynecology journal. 2014 Apr 1;25(4):531-44.
5. Wiegersma M, Panman CM, Berger MY, De Vet HC, Kollen BJ, Dekker JH. Minimal important change in the pelvic floor distress inventory-20 among women opting for conservative prolapse treatment. American journal of obstetrics and gynecology. 2017 Apr 1;216(4):397-e1.

Pelvic Floor Distress Inventory (PFDI - 20)

Instructions: Please answer all of the questions in the following survey. These questions will ask you if you have certain bowel, bladder, or pelvic symptoms and, if you do, how much they bother you. Answer these by circling the appropriate number. While answering these questions, please consider your symptoms over the last 3 months. The PFDI-20 has 20 items and 3 scales of your symptoms. All items use the following format with a response scale from 0 to 4.

Symptom scale: 0 = not present 1= not at all
2 = somewhat 3 = moderately 4 = quite a bit

Pelvic Organ prolapse Distress Inventory 6 (POPDI-6)

Do You...	No	Yes
1. Usually experience pressure in the lower abdomen?	0	1 2 3 4 5
2. Usually experience heaviness or dullness in the pelvic area?	0	1 2 3 4 5
3. Usually have a bulge or something falling out that you can see or feel in your vaginal area?	0	1 2 3 4 5
4. Ever have to push on the vagina or around the rectum to have or complete a bowel movement?	0	1 2 3 4 5
5. Usually experience a feeling of incomplete bladder emptying?	0	1 2 3 4 5

6. Ever have to push up on a bulge in the vaginal area with your fingers to start or complete urination?	0	1 2 3 4 5

Colorectal-Anal distress Inventory 8 (CRAD-8)

Do You...	No	Yes
7. Feel you need to strain too hard to have a bowel movement?	0	1 2 3 4 5
8. Feel you have not completely emptied your bowels at the end of a bowel movement?	0	1 2 3 4 5
9. Usually lose stool beyond your control if your stool is well formed?	0	1 2 3 4 5
10. Usually lose stool beyond your control if your stool is loose?	0	1 2 3 4 5
11. Usually lose gas from the rectum beyond your control?	0	1 2 3 4 5
12. Usually have pain when you pass your stool?	0	1 2 3 4 5
13. Experience a strong sense of urgency and have to rush to the bathroom to have a bowel movement?	0	1 2 3 4 5
14. Does part of your bowel ever pass through the rectum and bulge outside during or after a bowel movement?	0	1 2 3 4 5

Urinary distress Inventory 6 (UDI-6)

Do You...	No	Yes
15. Usually experience frequent urination?	0	1 2 3 4 5
16. Usually experience urine leakage associated with a feeling of urgency, that is, a strong sensation of needing to go to the bathroom?	0	1 2 3 4 5
17. Usually experience urine leakage related to coughing, sneezing or laughing?	0	1 2 3 4 5
18. Usually experience small amounts of urine leakage (that is, drops)?	0	1 2 3 4 5
19. Usually experience difficulty emptying your bladder?	0	1 2 3 4 5
20. Usually experience pain or discomfort in the lower abdomen or genital region?	0	1 2 3 4 5

149 Pelvic Floor Impact Questionnaire (PFIQ - 7)

Objective

The Pelvic Floor Impact Questionnaire-7 (PFIQ-7) is a shortened, less comprehensive version of the Pelvic Floor Impact Questionnaire (PFIQ).[1] It was created by Barber and colleagues (2004)[1] to save time, yet remain effective, in clinical and research encounters. It is a health-related quality of life questionnaire for women with pelvic floor conditions to fill out.[1] It includes scales from the Urinary Impact Questionnaire (UIQ-7), Pelvic Organ Prolapse Impact Questionnaire (POPIQ-7), and the Colorectal-Anal Impact Questionnaire-7 (CRAIQ-7),[1] which are short-forms of their the longer versions. It is useful to determine changes in symptom-severity over time and before and after treatments.[1]

Intended Population

Women over the age of 18 with pelvic floor conditions including urinary incontinence, pelvic organ prolapse, and fecal incontinence.[1]

Method of Use

The PFIQ-7 consists of 7 questions that need to be answered 3 times each (corresponds to the scales previously mentioned) considering symptoms related to the bladder or urine, vagina or pelvis, and bowel or rectum and their effect on function, social health, and mental health in the past 3 months.[1] The responses for each question range from "not at all" (0) to "quite a bit" (3).[1] To get scale scores, the mean of each of the 3 scales is individually calculated, which ranges from 0-3, this number is then multiplied by 100 and then divided by 3.[1] The scale scores are then added together to get the total PFIQ-7 score, which ranges from 0-300. A lower score means there is a lesser effect on quality of life.[1]

Evidence

Correlation

Correlation, represented by r, ranges from -1.0 to +1.0. If the r value is 0 that means there is no correlation. If the r value is close to -1.0 that means that both values will decrease linearly. If the r value is close to +1.0 that means that both values will increase linearly.

Correlation of the short-form versions with the long-form versions:[1]

- UIQ-7 r=0.96[1]
- POPIQ-7 r=0.94[1]
- CRAIQ-7 r=0.96[1]

Reliability

The test-retest reliability, represented by intraclass correlation coefficients (ICC):[1]

- PFIQ-7 ICC=0.77[1]
- UIQ-7 ICC=0.81[1]
- POPIQ-7 ICC=0.70[1]
- CRAIQ-7 ICC=0.81[1]

Validity

The PFIQ-7 demonstrates construct validity as it demonstrates a significant association with appropriate measures of symptom severity and pelvic floor diagnoses.[1]

Responsiveness

The PFIQ-7 has shown moderate responsiveness between the pre- and post-operative periods for pelvic and continence surgeries.[1] The standardized response mean (SRM) for all the sub scales fell within the range of 0.5 to

0.7.[1] It showed an effect size of 0.67 and a SRM of 0.63.[1] However, the responsiveness has been shown to be vary amongst different patients.[2] The highest SRMs have been found in the UIQ-7 and the CRAIQ-7 and the lowest SRMs have been found in the POPIQ-7.[2] However, the SRM for the POPIQ-7 increased at 3 and 12 months in patients who underwent surgery for pelvic organ prolapse.[2]

Clinically Meaningful Change

At the time of creation, the clinically meaningful change in quality of life (MCID)[3] needed to be studied in larger populations.[1] However, in their small sample size, Barber and colleagues (2004)[1] found a change in the summary score of 36 points (12%) or more to be meaningful after surgery.

Miscellaneous

The PFIQ-7 demonstrated a statistically significant improvement at 3 to 6 months after surgery, but the responsiveness was somewhat less than the PFDI-20.[1]

References

1. Barber MD, Walters MD, Bump RC. Short forms of two condition-specific quality-of-life questionnaires for women with pelvic floor disorders (PFDI-20 and PFIQ-7). American journal of obstetrics and gynecology. 2005 Jul 1;193(1):103-13.
2. Barber MD, Chen Z, Lukacz E, Markland A, Wai C, Brubaker L, Nygaard I, Weidner A, Janz NK, Spino C. Further validation of the short form versions of the Pelvic Floor Distress Inventory (PFDI) and Pelvic Floor Impact Questionnaire (PFIQ). Neurourology and urodynamics. 2011 Apr;30(4):541-6.
3. Crosby RD, Kolotkin RL, Williams GR. Defining clinically meaningful change in health-related quality of life. Journal of clinical epidemiology. 2003 May 1;56(5):395-407.

Pelvic Floor Impact Questionnaire (PFIQ - 7)

Instructions: Some women find that bladder, bowel, or vaginal symptoms affect their activities, relationships, and feelings. For each question, check the response that best describes how much your activities, relationships, or feelings have been affected by your bladder, bowel, or vaginal symptoms or conditions over the last 3 months. Please make sure you mark an answer in all 3 columns for each question.

How do symptoms or conditions in the following usually affect your	Bladder or urine	Bowel or rectum	Vagina or pelvis
1. Ability to do household chores (cooking, laundry housecleaning)?	Not at all Somewhat Moderately Quite a bit	Not at all Somewhat Moderately Quite a bit	Not at all Somewhat Moderately Quite a bit
2. Ability to do physical activities such as walking, swimming, or other exercise?	Not at all Somewhat Moderately Quite a bit	Not at all Somewhat Moderately Quite a bit	Not at all Somewhat Moderately Quite a bit
3. Entertainment activities such as going to a movie or concert?	Not at all Somewhat Moderately Quite a bit	Not at all Somewhat Moderately Quite a bit	Not at all Somewhat Moderately Quite a bit
4. Ability to travel by car or bus for a distance greater than 30 minutes away from home?	Not at all Somewhat Moderately Quite a bit	Not at all Somewhat Moderately Quite a bit	Not at all Somewhat Moderately Quite a bit
5. Participating in social activities outside your home?	Not at all Somewhat Moderately Quite a bit	Not at all Somewhat Moderately Quite a bit	Not at all Somewhat Moderately Quite a bit

6. Emotional health (nervousness, depression, etc)?	Not at all Somewhat Moderately Quite a bit	Not at all Somewhat Moderately Quite a bit	Not at all Somewhat Moderately Quite a bit
7. Feeling frustrated?	Not at all Somewhat Moderately Quite a bit	Not at all Somewhat Moderately Quite a bit	Not at all Somewhat Moderately Quite a bit

Total × 100 × 100 × 100

Scoring the PFIQ-7: =

All of the items use the following response scale:

0, Not at all; 1, somewhat; 2, moderately; 3, quite a bit PFIQ-7 Score

Scales:

Urinary Impact Questionnaire (UIQ-7): 7 items under column heading "Bladder or urine"

Colorectal-Anal Impact questionnaire (CRAIQ-7): 7 items under column heading "Bowel / rectum"

Pelvic Organ Prolapse Impact Questionnaire (POPIQ-7): Items under column "Pelvis / Vagina"

Scale Scores: Obtain the mean value for all of the answered items within the corresponding scale (possible value 0 – 3) and then multiply by (100/3) to obtain the scale score (range 0-100).

Missing items are dealt with by using the mean from answered items only.

PFIQ-7 Summary Score: Add the scores from the 3 scales together to obtain the summary score (range 0-300)

Reference:

https://www.sralab.org/sites/default/files/201706/Pelvic%20Floor%20Impact%20Questionnaire%20%28PFIQ-7%29.pdf

❑❑❑

150 Pelvic Girdle Questionnaire (PGQ)

Pregnancy-related back and pelvic girdle pain is a common condition varying from self-limiting symptoms of short duration during pregnancy to great pain and disability both during and after pregnancy. Pelvic girdle pain (PGP) generally arises in relation to pregnancy, trauma, arthritis and osteoarthritis. Pain is experienced between the posterior iliac crest and the gluteal fold, particularly in the vicinity of the sacroiliac joints (SIJ). The pain may radiate into the posterior thigh and can also occur in conjunction with/or separately in the pubic symphysis. The endurance capacity for standing, walking, and sitting is diminished. The diagnosis of PGP can be reached after exclusion of lumbar causes. The pain or functional disturbances in relation to PGP must be reproducible by specific clinical tests.[1]

Objective:

The PGQ is a condition-specific instrument that assesses activity limitations and symptoms in patients with pelvic girdle pain. It was developed for patients with pelvic girdle pain during pregnancy as well as postpartum and can be used in research and clinical practice.[1]

Intended Population:

People with Pelvic Girdle Pain during pregnancy and postpartum.[1]

Method of Use:

Self-report questionnaire of 20 activity items and 5 symptom items scored on a 4-point response scale. Each question is scored from 'Not at all' (0) to 'To a large extent' (3). Questions on the activity sub-scale range from difficulty with dressing, climbing stairs, doing housework, rolling in bed to pushing a shopping cart. Item scores are summed and transformed to yield a score of 0 to 100, where 100 is the worst possible score.[1]

Evidence:

There is little evidence for the measurement properties of instruments commonly used for women with pelvic girdle pain. The PGQ is the first condition-specific measure developed for people with PGP. The PGQ had acceptably high reliability and validity in people with PGP both during pregnancy and postpartum, it is simple to administer, and it is feasible for use in clinical practice. [1]

Reliability:

Test-retest reliability showed high intraclass correlation coefficient estimates: .93 (95% confidence interval 0.86–0.96) for the PGQ activity subscale and .91 (95% confidence interval 0.84–0.95) for the PGQ symptom subscale. [1]

Validity:

The PGQ was found to have content and convergent validity [2]

References

1. Stuge, B., Garratt, A., Krogstad Jenssen, H., Grotle, M. The Pelvic Girdle Questionnaire: A Condition-Specific Instrument for Assessing Activity Limitations and Symptoms in People With Pelvic Girdle Pain. Physical Therapy, July 2011 vol. 91 no. 7 1096-1108
2. Rejano-Campo M, Ferrer-Peña R, Urraca-Gesto MA, Gallego-Izquierdo T, Pecos-Martín D, Stuge B, Plaza-Manzano G. Transcultural adaptation and psychometric validation of a Spanish-language

version of the "Pelvic Girdle Questionnaire" Health and Quality of Life Outcomes (2017) 15:30 https://https://hqlo.biomedcentral.com/track/pdf/10.1186/s12955-017-0605-0 [Accessed 13 November 2018]

Pelvic Girdle Questionnaire (PGQ)

Stuge B, Garratt A, Jenssen H, Grotle M. The Pelvic Girdle Questionnaire: A ConditionSpecific Instrument for Assessing Activity Limitations and Symptoms in People with Pelvic Girdle Pain. Physical Therapy. July 2011; 91(7): 10961108.

Name Date

To what extent do you find it problematic to carry out the activities listed below because of pelvic girdle pain? For each activity tick (√) the box that best describes how you are today

How problematic is it for you because of your pelvic girdle pain to:	Not at all (0)	To a small extent (1)	To some extent (2)	To a large extent (3)
1.Dress yourself 2. Stand for less than 10 minutes 3. Stand for more than 60 minutes 4. Bend down 5. Sit for less than 10 minutes 6. Sit for more than 60 minutes 7. Walk for less than 10 minutes 8. Walk for more than 60 minutes 9. Climb stairs 10. Do housework 11. Carry light objects 12. Carry heavy objects 13. Get up/sit down 14. Push a shopping cart 15. Run 16. Carry out sporting activities* 17. Lie down 18. Roll over in bed 19. Have a normal sex life* 20. Push something with one foot				
How much pain do you experience?	**None (0)**	**Some (1)**	**Moderate (2)**	**Considerable (3)**
21. In the morning 22. In the evening				
To what extent because of pelvic girdle pain:	**Not at all (0)**	**To a small extent (1)**	**To some extent (2)**	**To a large extent (3)**
23. Has your leg/have your legs given way? 24. Do you do things more slowly? 25. Is your sleep interrupted?				
Maximum Score 75 **% Disability= (total score/75) x 100**				

❑❑❑

151 Pelvic Organ Prolapse Quantification (POP-Q) System

Objective

The International Continence Society (ICS), the American Urogynecologic Society (AUGS) and the Society of Gynecologic Surgeons came to agreement in 1996, for a graded objective measure to be used in the assessment of female pelvic organ prolapse[1][2]. This system provides characterisation of a woman's prolapse and allows a uniform recording method to be used by clinicians that enables contrast and disclosure of findings[2]. This system was named the 'Pelvic Organ Prolapse Quantification (POP-Q) System' and is generally used in clinical setting [3]. POP-Q is the more routinely used staging system[4] seen in published research[4].

Intended Population

A woman may present in primary care with symptoms of a 'bulge' or 'heaviness' in her vagina with or without incontinence[1][5]. Other symptoms may include urge incontinence, sexual dysfunction, problems with voiding or defecation[1]. On visual inspection a prolapse may be observed but this patient group can also be asymptotic and are identified through other routine procedures, for instance a smear test[5]. A reduction in vaginal or uterine integrity is observed in up to 30-70%[6] of women presenting for usual gynaecology procedures with 3-6% of these women reporting a drop pass the vaginal opening[6].

Method of Use

Pre-examination

Foregoing the procedure ensure the patient has an empty bladder and if feasible an empty rectum[2]. A full bladder during this examination could risk undervaluing the POP-Q score and therefore, miscalculate the staging[7].

The patient is then positioned where the utmost magnitude of the prolapse is shown and can be confirmed by the patient[2]. Positions may include supine, standing or in a birthing chair at 45 degree angle[8]. A Sim's speculum can be used if needed to draw back the anterior and posterior vaginal walls during the examination. All methods and positions utilised during the examination should be documented so that they can be reproduced[2].

Measurement Parameters

The measurement parameters are made up of six distinct locations (Aa, Ba, C, D, Ap, Bp) and three anatomical markers (GH, PB, TVL):

- Point Aa is at the midline of anterior vaginal wall. Where no prolapse is present this location is 3cm up from the hymen (merely interior to the vaginal opening). Parameters from the hymen can be -3cm indicating no anterior vaginal prolapse or +3cm, which is a full prolapse.
- Point Ba refers to the most superior location of the front vaginal wall . This location coexists with Aa (-3cm) in a woman with no anterior prolapse. However, in a woman with full prolapse this location coexists with point C.
- Point C is the lowest edge of the cervix or the vaginal cuff (i.e. hysterectomy scar). This location identifies if the cervix is descending.
- Point D is the topmost point of the posterior vaginal wall. This location can be contrasted with Point C to assess if the entry to the cervix has been extended.
- Point Ap is located midline of posterior vaginal wall 3cm proximal to hymen. The parameters for this point can range from -3cm to +3cm relative to

hymen.

- Point Bp is the uppermost point of the posterior vaginal wall.
- GH is the 'Genital hiatus' that records the length from the urethral opening to the posterior vaginal opening/ hymen. The hiatus refers to the opening in puborectalis muscle, a component of the levator ani muscle group. A larger distance here may indicate laxity in this area.
- PB is the 'perineal body' and is recorded from the posterior aspect of hymen to the mid-anal opening. This will give an insight to the tonicity of superficial pelvic floor. Through vaginal birth the perineal body can be injuried via tears or by an episiotomy.
- TVL refers to 'total vaginal length' measured from hymen to the most distal point[2][9]. Knowing this allows the depth of prolapse to be assessed and reassessed post surgical repair.

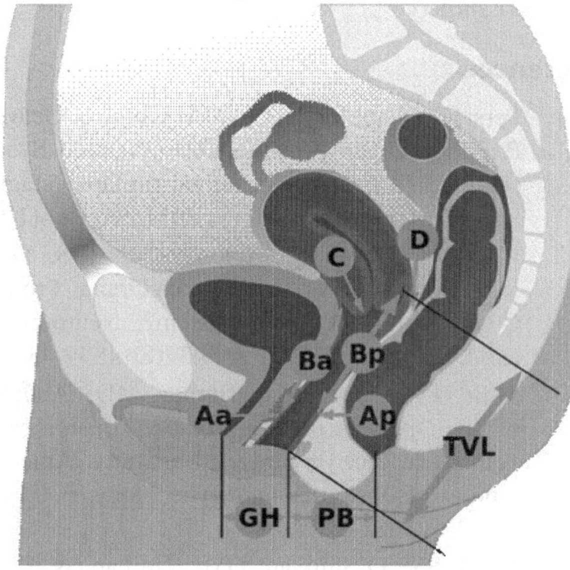

POP-Q System Locations

Recording Measurements

The position of the six distinct locations are measured during a maximum Valsalva or cough with regard to the hymen (that is defined as 0cm). The only exception to this is the measurement of TVL, which is to be recorded at rest when the prolapse is decreased[2].

If a point drops to the hymen it measured as 0cm, if it stays higher than the hymen it is recorded as a negative and if it protrudes past the hymen it is recorded as a positive. All measurements are recorded in centimeters using a ruler or tape measure.

All measurements for each location are recorded on a grid as shown below;

[10]

Anterior Wall (Aa)	Anterior Wall (Ba)	Cervix or cuff (C)
Genital hiatus (gh)	Perineal body (pb)	Total vaginal length (TVL)
Posterior Wall (Ap)	Posterior wall (Bp)	Posterior Fornix (D)

Staging of Prolapse

Once all measurements have been made the stage of the prolapse can be identified in relation to hymen;

- Stage 0: No prolapse is observed (points Aa, Ba, C, D, Ap and Bp are all < / = -3cm).
- Stage 1: The most proximal portion of prolapse is greater than 1 cm above the level of the hymen (points Aa, Ba, C, D, Ap and Bp are all < -1cm).
- Stage 2: The most proximal portion of prolapse is found between 1 cm higher than hymen and 1cm beneath hymen (points Aa, Ba, C, D, Ap and Bp can set at -1cm and +1cm).
- Stage 3: The most distal part of the prolapse extends more than 1cm beneath the hymen but no further than 2 cm, resulting in no measurement larger than TVL (points Aa, Ba, C, D, Ap and Bp can be >/= +2cm and </= TVL -3cm).
- Stage 4: vaginal eversion has taken place or eversion to with 2cm of TVL (points Aa, Ba, C, D, Ap and Bp can be >/= to TVL -2cm)[1][2].

Evidence

Reliability

The POP-Q is a criterion and clearly defined inspection system that is verifiable, uses anatomical landmarks and is reproducible[10][12]. For this reason it is used in clinical research[8]. This system was the initial examination tool in it's field to be comprehensively tested and has attested to show high interobserver and intraobserver reliability[1] in four studies involving 240 participants[12].

Validity

NICE conducted an evidence review for examining pelvic organ prolapse, in which a physical exam and/or POP-Q was compared to index tests;

- Dynamic cystoproctography
- Barium suspension
- Pelvic floor ultrasound
- International Consultation on Incontinence Modular Questionnaire vaginal symptoms (ICIQ-VS)
- Standardised pelvic floor dysfunction questionnaire.

The evidence in this review showed that not any of the index tests attained 'the diagnostic accuracy of the POP-Q reference standard'[5] and recommends that the POP-Q is the examination of preference to assess women suspected of pelvic organ prolapse[5].

Technique Variables

It is important to note that patient position utilised during the POP-Q exam can affect the outcome. For instance a POP-Q exam performed with the patient in a birthing chair at a 45 degree angle will demonstrate a higher stage POP than a patient in supine. Additionally, the full extent of POP is better seen in standing, as a dissimilarity of up to 6cm between a standing and supine exam has been viewed[8].

It has been uncertain whether all the external locations, namely GH and PB, should be recorded at rest or during the patient straining. Testing revealed a marked rise in GH and PB measurements with Valsalva. This is queried to be related to a broadening of levator hiatus, with greater intraabdominal pressure[8]. As a result it is not clear if this broadening with strain is a natural occurrence or due to pelvic floor dysfunction. Therefore, it is advised to record both measurements for GH and PB at rest and with straining, to highlight all aspects of pelvic floor performance[8].

The POP-Q system should be conducted on a patient who has emptied their bladder beforehand. It is found that an empty bladder aids in magnifying a better representation of a prolapse in the six specific locations (Aa, Ba, C, D, Ap, and Bp). However, no influence is seen on GH, PB and TVL with an empty bladder[7].

Despite the POP-Q system being recommended as the reference standard[5], in clinical practice it is found to be time consuming (2-3 minutes in trained professionals) and requires skillfulness in it's application[12]. Associates of ICS and AUGS were surveyed and approximately on one-third of those taking part did not use the POP-Q system routinely in their clinical practice[13]. The main reasons for this is that the POP-Q is considered a complex system and not user friendly. This results in the system not being customary in it's clinical use by specialists globally[13]. A simplified version of the POP-Q has been devised, by The IUGA Standardization of Terminology Committee, to aid in addressing these issues for clinical use[14]. However, for research and urogynecologists, POP-Q will continue to be the benchmark[12].

Clinical Relevance

A pelvic organ prolapse is marked as symptomatic when the foremost border of the prolapse is level or past the level of the hymen (>/= stage 2 POP-Q)[2][15]. This needs to be considered when prescribing a patient's treatment. Physiotherapy aims to manage and maintain a stage 2. However, stage 3 and 4 require further assessment and treatment.

Genital hiatus (GH) measurement of >/= 3.75cm is correlated with and is prognostic of 'apical vaginal support loss'[16]. The GH measurement can check for and identify if further assessment of apical vaginal support is warranted prior planning other treatment such as a hysterectomy or POP repair surgery[16].

References

1. Persu C, Chapple CR, Cauni V, Gutue S, Geavlete P. Pelvic Organ Prolapse Quantification System (POP–Q)–a new era in pelvic prolapse staging. Journal of medicine and life. 2011 Feb 15;4(1):75.
2. Madhu C, Swift S, Moloney-Geany S, Drake MJ. How to use the Pelvic Organ Prolapse Quantification (POP-Q) system?. Neurourology and Urodynamics. 2018 Aug;37(S6):S39-43.
3. Muir TW, Stepp KJ, Barber MD. Adoption of the pelvic organ prolapse quantification system in peer-reviewed literature. American journal of obstetrics and gynecology. 2003 Dec 1;189(6):1632-5.
4. Boyd SS, O'Sullivan DM, Tulikangas P. 29: Implementation of the pelvic organ prolapse quantification system in peer-reviewed journals. American Journal of Obstetrics & Gynecology. 2017 Mar 1;216(3):S591.
5. Guidance NI. Urinary incontinence and pelvic organ prolapse in women: management:© NICE (2019) Urinary incontinence and pelvic organ prolapse in women: Management. BJU Int. 2019;123(5):777-803.
6. Barber MD. Pelvic organ prolapse. Bmj. 2016 Jul 20;354:i3853.
7. Reich A, Kohorst F, Kreienberg R, Flock F.

Influence of bladder volume on pelvic organ prolapse quantification results. Gynecologic and obstetric investigation. 2010;70(2):82-6.

8. Visco AG, Wei JT, McClure LA, Handa VL, Nygaard IE. Effects of examination technique modifications on pelvic organ prolapse quantification (POP-Q) results. International Urogynecology Journal. 2003 Jun 1;14(2):136-40.
9. Haylen BT, De Ridder D, Freeman RM, Swift SE, Berghmans B, Lee J, Monga A, Petri E, Rizk DE, Sand PK, Schaer GN. An International Urogynecological Association (IUGA)/ International Continence Society (ICS) joint report on the terminology for female pelvic floor dysfunction. Neurourology and Urodynamics: Official Journal of the International Continence Society. 2010 Jan;29(1):4-20.
10. Bump RC, Mattiasson A, Bø K, Brubaker LP, DeLancey JO, Klarskov P, Shull BL, Smith AR. The standardization of terminology of female pelvic organ prolapse and pelvic floor dysfunction. American journal of obstetrics and gynecology. 1996 Jul 1;175(1):10-7.
11. Dr Fiona Bach. POP-Q for the MRCOG by ACE Courses. Available from: https://www.youtube.com/watch?v=UyIzjiuUoAs [last accessed 17/09/2020]
12. Raizada N, Mittal P, Suri J, Puri A, Sharma V. Comparative Study to Evaluate the Intersystem Association and Reliability Between Standard Pelvic Organ Prolapse Quantification System and Simplified Pelvic Organ Prolapse Scoring System. The Journal of Obstetrics and Gynecology of India. 2014 Dec 1;64(6):421-4.
13. Auwad W, Freeman RM, Swift S. Is the pelvic organ prolapse quantification system (POPQ) being used? A survey of members of the International Continence Society (ICS) and the American Urogynecologic Society (AUGS). International Urogynecology Journal. 2004 Oct 1;15(5):324-7.
14. Swift S, Morris S, McKinnie V, Freeman R, Petri E, Scotti RJ, Dwyer P. Validation of a simplified technique for using the POPQ pelvic organ prolapse classification system. International Urogynecology Journal. 2006 Nov 1;17(6):615-20.
15. Swift SE, Tate SB, Nicholas J. Correlation of symptoms with degree of pelvic organ support in a general population of women: what is pelvic organ prolapse?. American journal of obstetrics and gynecology. 2003 Aug 1;189(2):372-7.
16. Lowder JL, Oliphant SS, Shepherd JP, Ghetti C, Sutkin G. Genital hiatus size is associated with and predictive of apical vaginal support loss. American journal of obstetrics and gynecology. 2016 Jun 1;214(6):718-e1.

❑❑❑

152 Perme Intensive Care Unit Mobility Score

Objective

- To measure the patient's mobility status. [1]
- The scale scoring starts with the ability of the patient to follow the command and ends in the distance walked in 2 minutes[1]
- The tool is indicative of functional performance especially, patient's walking capacity in the ICU at a specific moment in time. [1]

Intended Population

- Patients with limited independent activities and are in critical illness.[1]

Method of Use

The outcome tool has 15 items and the score ranges from 0 to 32. There are 7 categories (mental status, potential mobility barriers, functional strength, bed mobility, transfers, gait, and endurance). The higher the score, it indicates fewer potential mobility barriers and decreased assistance whereas, the lower the score, it indicates more potential barriers to mobility and more assistance needed for mobility.[1]

The items included in the category mental health are alertness level and ability to follow the command. The alertness level can be scored as unresponsive (0), lethargic(1), and awake and alert(2). The ability to follow command can be scored as no(0) and yes (1). The result from this category helps us to determine the patient's ability to do the mobility. The maximum score of this category is 3.[1]

Potential mobility barriers include items 3 to 6 i.e, use of a mechanical ventilator, pain, use of multiple lines and tubes, use of any drips. The 3rd item is scored as yes(0) or no(1) based on whether the patient is on mechanical ventilation or noninvasive ventilation. Item 4 is pain and if the patient has no pain it is scored as 1 and if the patient has pain or unable to express, it is scored as 0. The 5th item of the scale is related to external appliances or any assistive device and scored as yes(0) and no (1). And if patient has any drip or medication on use, item 6 is scored as yes(0) and no (1).[1]

Functional strength focuses on the capacity of the patient to move the upper and lower limbs. Item 7 assesses the strength of legs whereas item 8 assesses the strength of arms.Each item is again divided into the right and left side and scored as ye(1)s or no(0). The maximum point scored in this category is 4. To achieve the maximal point, the patient must be able to lift both legs against gravity till 20 degrees with knees straight and lift both arms to 45 degrees with the elbow straight. [1]

The 4th category of the scale is bed mobility and it includes items 9 and 10.Patient is asked to do the bed mobility from supine to sit in item 9 and in item 10, the static sitting balance is assessed.the maximum score obtained in this category is 6. [1]

In the category 5, the patient's ability to transfer is assessed. Item 11 addresses the sit to stand, item 12 addresses the standing balance when standing is achieved and item 13 addresses transfer from bed to chair or chair to bed. The scoring of all three items is done based on the assistance required.[1]

The category gait addresses the patient's ability to walk with or without assistance and scored based on the assistance required. The maximum score that can be obtained is 3. [1]

The final category is endurance and it focuses on the patient's capacity to walk in 2 minutes regardless of the level of assistance required including rest periods (sitting or standing), with or without an assistive device. The scoring is done on basis of distance walked and the maximum score obtained is 3. [1]

Evidence

Reliability

Interrater reliability (Cohen κ coefficient) for[2]

- items 2, 3, 5, 6, 7, 8, 13, and 15 was 1.0000
- item 1, 0.8276
- item 4, 0.8000
- item 9, 0.6000
- item 10, 0.7297
- item 11, 0.7260
- item 12, 0.7872
- and item 14, 0.9048

The intraclass correlation coefficient (95% confidence interval) was 0.9880 (0.97743-0.99859)[2]

Validity

- supported by expert concurrence and
- The clinical use of this outcome tool is acceptable.

References

1. Perme C, Nawa RK, Winkelman C, Masud F. A tool to assess mobility status in critically ill patients: the Perme Intensive Care Unit Mobility Score. Methodist DeBakey cardiovascular journal. 2014 Jan;10(1):41.
2. Nawa RK, Lettvin C, Winkelman C, Evora PR, Perme C. Initial interrater reliability for a novel measure of patient mobility in a cardiovascular intensive care unit. Journal of Critical Care. 2014 Jun 1;29(3):475-e1.

Perme Intensive Care Unit Mobility Score

The goal of the Perme Intensive Care Unit Mobility Score is to assess the mobility status of patients in the ICU at a specific moment in time. The authors recommend that (1) the scoring of mobility activities be based on what the patient does and not on what the patient could potentially do, and (2) the score sheet is filled out immediately after the mobility activities are completed.		
Mental Status	1. Alertness upon arrival	The patient alertness is observed upon arrival and initial contact with the rater.
	2. Is the patient able to follow 2 out of 3 commands?	The patient is asked to perform 3 consecutive commands. For patients with obvious and profound weakness of the extremities, we suggest the following commands: blink your eyes, stick your tongue out, move your head up/down.
Potential Mobility Barriers	The evaluator should consider the presence of potential barriers to mobility at any time during the mobility activities.	
	3. Is the patient on mechanical ventilation or noninvasive ventilation?	It includes ventilatory support through an endotracheal tube, tracheostomy, or a mask (noninvasive ventilation).
	4. Pain	The patient experiences or does not experience any pain at any time, during mobility activities.
	5. The patient has 2 or more of the following	The clinician carefully examines the patient and identifies any lines, tubes, catheters, or devices connected to the patient's body, even when not in use. (e.g., central venous catheter not connected to anything, a dialysis catheter when patient is not in dialysis).
	6. Is the patient on any drips?	A drip is considered any kind of continuous intravenous infusion such as: vasopressors, inotropes, insulin, antiarrhythmic, sedation, antibiotics, fluids, electrolyte replacement, blood transfusions, etc.

Bed Mobility	7. Legs	The patient is asked to raise each leg separately, with the knee straight, against gravity. The patient should have approximately 20 degrees of hip flexion and should be supine in semi-recumbent position, otherwise the score is zero
	8. Arms	The patient is asked to raise each arm separately with elbow straight against gravity. The patient should have at least 45 degrees of shoulder flexion, and can be in supine or sitting position.
	9. Supine to sit	The patient is asked to move in bed from supine or semi-recumbent to the sitting position. If the patient is unable to initiate the task, then physical assistance as well as verbal and tactile cues are offered by the clinician in order to complete the task.
	10. Static Sitting balance on side of bed once position is established	The level of assistance should be determined once the patient assumes the sitting position.
Transfers	11. Sit to stand	From the sitting position on the side of bed, chair, wheelchair, or recliner the patient is asked to move into the standing position.
	12. Static standing balance once position was established	The level of assistance should be determined once the patient assumes the standing position.
	13. Transfer from bed to chair OR chair to bed	The patient is asked to move from the bed to a chair, wheelchair, stretcher chair, recliner OR to move from any of those options back to bed. If the patient was already out of bed and did not return to bed, the activity should be scored as "NOT ASSESSED"
Gait	14. Gait	Gait activity is defined as a sequence of foot movements in which the complete gait cycle is completed several times. During the gait activity, the patient can use a walker, cane, any other assistive device, or walk without an assistive device. Steps along the bed or during transfers should not be considered gait.
Endurance	15. Endurance (Distance walked in 2 minutes including sitting or standing rest periods, with or without an assistive device, and regardless of level or assistance required)	The patient is asked to walk as tolerated for 2 minutes. "TWO MINUTES" is defined by having a clinician monitor for a continuous 2-minute period on a watch. The total distance covered in 2 minutes is recorded. When walking, the patient is allowed to take standing or sitting rest breaks as needed. Any resting periods should be included in the 2-minute period.

Perme icu mobility score

Name of evaluator: ICU bed:

	Patient's name or number:	**Date: Time:**
MENTAL STATUS Maximum points = 3	1. Alertness upon arrival Unresponsive = 0 Lethargic = 1 Awake and alert = 2	
	2. Is the patient able to follow 2 out of 3 commands? No = 0 Yes = 1	
POTENTIAL MOBILITY BARRIERS Maximum points = 4 * Upon initial contact with the patient or at any time during the mobility interventions.	3. Is the patient on mechanical ventilation OR noninvasive ventilation? * Yes = 0 No = 1	
	4. Pain * Unable to determine or patient indicates to be in pain = 0 No pain = 1	
	5. The patient has 2 or more of the following: * (circle) Supplemental oxygen device, Foley catheter, ETT, trach, central line, peripheral IV, arterial line, dialysis catheter, PICC, PEG, PEJ, nasogastric tube, chest tube, temporary pacemaker, pulmonary artery catheter, epidural PCA, IABP, LVAD, CRRT, ventriculostomy, lumbar drain, wound VAC, or other. Yes = 0 No = 1	
	6. Is the patient on any drips? * (continuous intravenously infusion: vasopressors, inotropes, insulin, antiarrhythmic, sedation, antibiotics, fluids, electrolyte replacement, blood transfusions, etc.) Yes = 0 No = 1	
FUNCTIONAL STRENGTH Maximum points = 4	7. Legs – Is the patient able to raise the leg against gravity approximately 20 degrees, with knee straight? No = 0 Yes = 1	Left : Right
	8. Arms – Is the patient able to raise arm against gravity approximately 45 degrees, with elbow straight? No = 0 Yes = 1	Left : Right
BED MOBILITY Maximum points = 6	9. Supine to sit Not assessed OR total assistance (< 25%) = 0 Maximum assistance (25% to 50%) = 1 Moderate assistance (50% to 75%) = 2 Minimum assistance (> 75%) OR supervision = 3	
	10. Static sitting balance on side of bed once position is established Not assessed OR total assistance (< 25%) = 0 Maximum assistance (25% to 50%) = 1 Moderate assistance (50% to 75%) = 2 Minimum assistance (> 75%) OR Supervision = 3	
TRANSFERS Maximum points = 9	11. Sit to stand Not assessed OR Total assistance (< 25%) = 0 Maximum assistance (25% to 50%) = 1 Moderate assistance (50% to 75%) = 2 Minimum assistance (> 75%) OR Supervision = 3	
	12. Static standing balance once standing position is established Not assessed OR total assistance (< 25%) = 0 Maximum assistance (25% to 50%) = 1 Moderate assistance (50% to 75%) = 2 Minimum assistance (> 75%) OR supervision = 3	
	13. Transfer from bed to chair OR chair to bed Not assessed OR total assistance (< 25%) = 0 Maximum assistance (25% to 50%) = 1 Moderate assistance (50% to 75%) = 2 Minimum assistance (> 75%) OR supervision = 3	

GAIT Maximum points = 3	14. Gait Not assessed OR total assistance (< 25%) = 0 Maximum assistance (25% to 50%) = 1 Moderate assistance (50% to 75%) = 2 Minimum assistance (> 75%) OR supervision = 3	
ENDURANCE Maximum points = 3	15. Endurance: Distance walked in 2 minutes, regardless of level of assistance required including rest periods (sitting or standing), with or without an assistive device. Unable to walk or not assessed = 0 Distance 5-50 feet = 1 Distance 51-99 feet = 2 Distance ≥ 100 feet = 3	
MAXIMUM POINTS = 32	**TOTAL POINTS**	
Reference : A tool to assess MoBility status in CritiCally ill patients: the perMe intensive Care unit MoBility sCore Christiane Perme, P.T., C.S.S.a; Ricardo Kenji Nawa, P.T., M.Sc.b; Chris Winkelman, Ph.D., R.N.c; Faisal Masud, M.D.d aHouston Methodist Hospital, Houston, Texas; bUniversity of São Paulo, Ribeirão Preto, São Paulo, Brazil; cCase Western Reserve University, Cleveland, Ohio; dHouston Methodist DeBakey Heart & Vascular Center, Houston Methodist Hospital, Houston, Texas		

□□□

153 Physical Activity Scale for the Elderly (PASE)

The awareness regarding improving the physical activity of older adults has been growing among policymakers and healthcare professionals during the past few years. The evidence shows that improving older patients physical ability, lifestyle behaviours and quality of life could promote building resilience and healthy ageing[1].

A physical activity questionnaire is a practical and widely used approach for physical activity assessment in epidemiologic investigations[2].

Activity questionnaires have been used in studies relating physical activity to fall and fracture risk, balance and gait characteristics, bone density, and coronary heart disease in older people[3][4][5][6].

PASE was initially developed in early 90s to provide an instrument to investigate specifically older people with an age-specific physical activity questionnaire, filling what was an important need in epidemiological research at that time[7].

Objective and Intended Population

Physical Activity Scale for the Elderly (PASE) is a brief (5 minutes) and easily scored survey designed specifically to assess physical activity in epidemiological studies of persons age 65 years and older[7].

The **PASE** score combines information on leisure, household and occupational activity[8]. The PASE assesses the types of activities typically chosen by older adults (walking, recreational activities, exercise, housework, yard work, and caring for others. It uses frequency, duration, and intensity level of activity over the previous week to assign a score, ranging from 0 to 793, with higher scores indicating greater physical activity.[9]

Method of Use

Occupational, household and leisure activities are investigated by PASE, over a one-week period[7][10]. The questionnaire can be administered by mail or interview (telephone or in-person)[8]. The observed effect of mode of administration on physical activity estimates is of concern and authors recommend that the telephone version of PASE be the method of first choice, furthermore they suggest that the mail questionnaire be used in a modified form with additional respondent instructions in order to clarify the proper categorisation of activities, thus reducing reporting error in the mail version[7].

The PASE

The questionnaire comprises section on leisure time activity, household activity and work-related activity as follows[10]:

Instruction

Please complete this questionnaire by either circling the correct response or filling in the blank. Here is an example:

During the past 7 days, how often have you seen the sun?

[0.] NEVER

[1.] SELDOM (1-2 DAYS)

[2.] SOMETIMES (3-4 DAYS)

[3.] OFTEN (5-7 DAYS)

Answer all items as accurately as possible. All information is strictly confidential.

Leisure Time Activity

1. Over the past 7 days, how often did you participate in sitting activities such as reading, watching TV, or doing handcrafts?

[0.] NEVER (go to question 2)

[1.] SELDOM (1-2 DAYS) (go to question 1.a and 1.b)

[2.] SOMETIMES (3-4 DAYS) (go to question 1.a and 1.b)

[3.] OFTEN (5-7 DAYS) (go to question 1.a and 1.b)

1.a What were these activities? (open end question)

1.b On average, how many hours did you engage in these sitting activities?

[0.] Less than 1 hour

[1.] 1 but less than 2 hours

[2.] 2 - 4 hours

[3.] more than 4 hours

2. Over the past 7 days, how often did you take a walk outside your home or yard for any reason? For example, for fun or exercise, walking to work, walking the dog, etc

[0.] NEVER (go to question 3)

[1.] SELDOM (1-2 DAYS) (go to question 2.a)

[2.] SOMETIMES (3-4 DAYS) (go to question 2.a)

[3.] OFTEN (5-7 DAYS) (go to question 2.a)

2a. On average, how many hours per day did you spend walking?

[0.] Less than 1 hour

[1.] 1 but less than 2 hours

[2.] 2 - 4 hours

[3.] more than 4 hours

3. Over the past 7 days, how often did you engage in light sport or recreational activities such as bowling, golf with a cart, shuffleboard, fishing from a boat or pier or other similar activities?

[0.] NEVER (go to question 4)

[1.] SELDOM (1-2 DAYS) (go to question 3.a and 3.b)

[2.] SOMETIMES (3-4 DAYS) (go to question 3.a and 3.b)

[3.] OFTEN (5-7 DAYS) (go to question 3.a and 3.b)

3.a What were these activities? (open end question)

3.b On average, how many hours did you engage in these light sport or recreational activities?

[0.] Less than 1 hour

[1.] 1 but less than 2 hours

[2.] 2 - 4 hours

[3.] more than 4 hours

4. Over the past 7 days, how often did you engage in moderate sport and recreational activities such as doubles tennis, ballroom dancing, hunting, ice skating, golf without a cart, softball or other similar activities?

[0.] NEVER (go to question 5)

[1.] SELDOM (1-2 DAYS) (go to question 4.a and 4.b)

[2.] SOMETIMES (3-4 DAYS) (go to question 4.a and 4.b)

[3.] OFTEN (5-7 DAYS) (go to question 4.a and 4.b)

4.a What were these activities? (open end question)

4.b On average, how many hours did you engage in these moderate sport or recreational activities?

[0.] Less than 1 hour

[1.] 1 but less than 2 hours

[2.] 2 - 4 hours

[3.] more than 4 hours

5. Over the past 7 days, how often did you engage in strenuous sport and recreational activities such as jogging, swimming, cycling, singles tennis, aerobic dance, skiing (downhill or cross-country) or other similar activities?

[0.] NEVER (go to question 6)

[1.] SELDOM (1-2 DAYS) (go to question 5.a and 5.b)

[2.] SOMETIMES (3-4 DAYS) (go to question 5.a and 5.b)

[3.] OFTEN (5-7 DAYS) (go to question 5.a and 5.b)

5.a What were these activities? (open end question)

5.b On average, how many hours did you engage in these strenuous sport or recreational activities?

[0.] Less than 1 hour

[1.] 1 but less than 2 hours

[2.] 2 - 4 hours

[3.] more than 4 hours

6. Over the past 7 days, how often did you do any exercisesspecificallytoincreasemusclestrengthand endurance, such as lifting weights or pushups, etc.?

[0.] NEVER (go to question 7)

1.] SELDOM (1-2 DAYS) (go to question 6.a and 6.b)

[2.] SOMETIMES (3-4 DAYS) (go to question 6.a and 6.b)

[3.] OFTEN (5-7 DAYS) (go to question 6.a and 6.b)

6.a What were these activities? (open end question)

6.b On average, how many hours did you engage in these strenuous sport or recreational activities?

[0.] Less than 1 hour

[1.] 1 but less than 2 hours

[2.] 2 - 4 hours

[3.] more than 4 hours

Household Activity

7. During the past 7 days, have you done any light housework, such as dusting or washing dishes?

[1.] NO

[2.] YES

8. During the past 7 days, have you done any heavy housework or chores, such as vacuuming, scrubbing floors, washing windows, or carrying wood?

[1.] NO

[2.] YES

During the past 7 days, did you engage in any of the following activities? Please answer YES or NO for each item.

a. Home repairs like painting, wallpapering, electrical work, etc.

b. Lawn work or yard care, including snow or leaf removal, wood chopping, etc.

c. Outdoor gardening

d. Caring for another person, such as children, dependent spouse, or another adult

Work-related Activity

10. During the past 7 days, did you work for pay or as a volunteer?

[1.] NO

[2.] YES (go to questions 10.a and 10.b)

10a. How many hours per week did you work for pay and or as a volunteer? ____ hours

10b. Which of the following categories best describes the amount of physical activity required on your job and or volunteer work?

1. Mainly sitting with some slight arm movement (Examples: office worker, watchmaker, seated assembly line worker, bus driver, etc.)
2. Sitting or standing with some walking (Examples: cashier, general office worker, light tool and machinery worker)
3. Walking with some handling of materials generally weighing less than 50 pounds (Examples: mailman, waiter/waitress, construction worker, heavy tool and machinery worker)
4. Walking and heavy manual work often requiring handling of materials weighting over 50 pounds (Ex: lumberjack, ston mason, farm or general labourer)

Evidence

PASE shows strong evidences for validity and reliability useful for large epidemiological studies on general population. On more specific conditions this instrument may not be as accurate as required, and further studies on specific conditions are needed.

Validity

Washburn et al. first studied PASE construct validity in early 90s, and it has been established by correlating PASE scores with health status and physiologic measures[7]. PASE scores were positively associated with grip strength (r = 0.37), static balance (r = +0.33), leg strength (r = 0.25) and negatively correlated with resting heart rate (r = - 0.13), age (r = - 0.34) and perceived health status (r = -0.34); and overall Sickness Impact Profile score (r = -0.42)[7], thus showing a strong validity of this instrument.

PASE construct validity has been further studied in 1999. This time it was established by correlating PASE scores with physiologic and performance characteristics: peak oxygen uptake, resting heart rate and blood pressure, percent body fat, and balance[8]. PASE scores were significantly associated ($P<0.05$) with peak oxygen uptake (r = 0.20), systolic blood pressure (r = -0.18) and balance score (r = 0.20); despite this, no significant associations of PASE score and diastolic blood pressure, resting heart rate, or percent body fat were noted[8]. Anyway, these results provided additional evidence for the validity of the PASE as a measure of physical activity suitable for use in epidemiology studies on the association of physical activity, health, and physical function in older individuals[8].

In 2004, PASE stability and convergent validity have been assessed among rural, community dwelling elderly persons using Computer Science and Applications, Inc. Actigraph Monitors (Actigraph) as the direct criterion measure[11]. The study showed there was a statistically significant Spearman correlation coefficient of 0.43 ($p<0.01$) between Actigraph data and total PASE scores[11], thus showing good validity even when compared with digital technologies.

in 2008 Hagiwara et al. evaluated a Japanese translated version of the PASE with three hundred and twenty-five (325) healthy and elderly subjects over 65 years enrolled[12]. Concurrent validity was evaluated by Spearman's rank correlation coefficient between PASE scores and an accelerometer (waking steps and energy expenditure), a physical activity questionnaire for adults in general (the Japan Arteriosclerosis Longitudinal Study Physical Activity Questionnaire, JALSPAQ), grip strength, mid-thigh muscle area per body-weight, static balance and body-fat percentage[12]. The PASE score was significantly correlated with walking steps ($\rho = 0.17$, $P = 0.014$), energy expenditure ($\rho = 0.16$, $P = 0.024$), activity measured with the JALSPAQ ($\rho = 0.48$, $P < 0.001$), mid-thigh muscle area per body-weight ($\rho = 0.15$, $P = 0.006$) and static balance ($\rho = 0.19$, $P = 0.001$)[12]. Therefore, the Japanese version of PASE was shown to have acceptable validity[12].

More recently, PASE validity has been studied for specific conditions. In cancer patients, PASE has shown a low construct validity but a good content validity[13]. In hip osteoarthritis patients, the PASE construct validity was poor revealing that it was unable to assess PA intensity levels. Therefore authors stated that PASE is not recommended as a valid tool to examine PA level for patients with hip OA[14].

Reliability

On Washburn et al. paper from 1993 authors stated that the PASE test-retest reliability coefficient (0.75) exceeded those reported for other physical activity surveys[7]. Back then, test-retest reliability has been assessed over a 3-7 week interval, resulting in a 0.75 (95% CI = 0.69-0.80). Results showed also reliability for mail administration (r = 0.84) was higher than for telephone administration (r = 0.68)[7].

Hagiwara et al. in 2008 evaluated reliability of the PASE Japanese version, by the test–retest method over a period of 3–4 weeks[12]. The proportion of consistency in the response between the first and second surveys was adequately high, with a intraclass correlation coefficient for the PASE score of 0.65, showing this instrument to have acceptable reliability too[12].

Reliability has been evaluated also in specific conditions. In cancer patients, reliability for the PASE scores ranged from good to excellent (ICC = 0.67 to 0.90) [13]; in hip osteoarthritis patients, the test-retest reliability of the total PASE score was moderate, with acceptable ICC, but with large measurement errors[14].

References

1. MacLeod S, Musich S, Hawkins K, Alsgaard K, Wicker ER. The impact of resilience among older adults. Geriatric Nursing. 2016 Jul 1;37(4):266-72.
2. Washburn RA, Montoye HJ. The assessment of physical activity by questionnaire. Am J Epidemiol. 1986 Apr;123(4):563–76.
3. Sorock GS, Bush TL, Golden AL et al. Physical activity and fracture risk in a free-living elderly cohort. J Gerontol 1986; 43: M134-139.
4. Campbell AJ, Borrie MJ, Spears GF. Risk factors for falls in a community-based prospective study of people 70 years and older. J Gerontol 1989; 44: Ml12-117.
5. Dalsky GP, Stocke KS, Ehsani AA et al. Weight-bearing exercise training and lumbar bone mineral content in post-menopausal women. AM Intern Med 1988; 108: 824-828.
6. Marti B, Pekkanen J, Nissinen A et al. Association of physical activity with coronary risk factors and physical ability: twenty year follow-up of a cohort of Finnish men. Age Aging 1989; 18: 103-109.
7. Washburn RA, Smith KW, Jette AM, Janney CA. The physical activity scale for the elderly (PASE): Development and evaluation. Journal of Clinical Epidemiology. 1993 Feb 1;46(2):153–62.
8. Washburn RA, McAuley E, Katula J, Mihalko SL, Boileau RA. The Physical Activity Scale for the Elderly (PASE): Evidence for Validity. Journal of Clinical Epidemiology. 1999 Jul;52(7):643–51.
9. Logan, S.L. et al. (2013). The Physical Activity Scale for the Elderly (PASE) Questionnaire; Does It Predict Physical Health? Int. J. Environ. Res. Public Health: 10, 3967-3986; doi:10.3390/ijerph10093967
10. Physical Activity Scale for the Elderly : Medicine & Science in Sports & Exercise [Internet]. LWW. [cited 2016 Jun 10]. Available from: http://journals.lww.com/acsm-msse/Fulltext/1997/06001/Physical_Activity_Scale_for_the_Elderly.22.aspx
11. Dinger MK, Oman RF, Taylor EL, Vesely SK, Able J. Stability and convergent validity of the Physical Activity Scale for the Elderly (PASE). J Sports Med Phys Fitness. 2004 Jun;44(2):186–92.
12. Hagiwara A, Ito N, Sawai K, Kazuma K. Validity and reliability of the Physical Activity Scale for the Elderly (PASE) in Japanese elderly people. Geriatrics & Gerontology International. 2008 Sep 1;8(3):143–51.
13. Liu RDK, Buffart LM, Kersten MJ, Spiering M, Brug J, van Mechelen W, et al. Psychometric properties of two physical activity questionnaires, the AQuAA and the PASE, in cancer patients. BMC Med Res Methodol. 2011;11:30.
14. Svege I, Kolle E, Risberg MA. Reliability and validity of the Physical Activity Scale for the Elderly (PASE) in patients with hip osteoarthritis. BMC Musculoskelet Disord. 2012;13:26.

❑❑❑

154 International Physical Activity Questionnaire

LONG LAST 7 DAYS SELF-ADMINISTERED FORMAT FOR USE WITH YOUNG AND MIDDLE-AGED ADULTS (15-69 years)

The International Physical Activity Questionnaires (IPAQ) comprises a set of 4 questionnaires. Long (5 activity domains asked independently) and short (4 generic items) versions for use by either telephone or self-administered methods are available. The purpose of the questionnaires is to provide common instruments that can be used to obtain internationally comparable data on health–related physical activity.

Background on IPAQ

The development of an international measure for physical activity commenced in Geneva in 1998 and was followed by extensive reliability and validity testing undertaken across 12 countries (14 sites) during 2000. The final results suggest that these measures have acceptable measurement properties for use in many settings and in different languages, and are suitable for national population-based prevalence studies of participation in physical activity.

Using IPAQ

Use of the IPAQ instruments for monitoring and research purposes is encouraged. It is recommended that no changes be made to the order or wording of the questions as this will affect the psychometric properties of the instruments.

INTERNATIONAL PHYSICAL ACTIVITY QUESTIONNAIRE

We are interested in finding out about the kinds of physical activities that people do as part of their everyday lives. The questions will ask you about the time you spent being physically active in the last 7 days. Please answer each question even if you do not consider yourself to be an active person. Please think about the activities you do at work, as part of your house and yard work, to get from place to place, and in your spare time for recreation, exercise or sport.

Think about all the vigorous and moderate activities that you did in the last 7 days. Vigorous physical activities refer to activities that take hard physical effort and make you breathe much harder than normal. Moderate activities refer to activities that take moderate physical effort and make you breathe somewhat harder than normal.

PART 1: JOB-RELATED PHYSICAL ACTIVITY

The first section is about your work. This includes paid jobs, farming, volunteer work, course work, and any other unpaid work that you did outside your home. Do not include unpaid work you might do around your home, like housework, yard work, general maintenance, and caring for your family. These are asked in Part 3.

1. Do you currently have a job or do any unpaid work outside your home?

Yes No

Skip to PART 2: TRANSPORTATION

The next questions are about all the physical activity you did in the last 7 days as part of your paid or unpaid work. This does not include traveling to and from work.

2. During the last 7 days, on how many days did you do vigorous physical activities like heavy lifting, digging, heavy construction, or climbing up stairs as part of your work? Think about only those physical activities that you did for at least 10 minutes at a time.

_____ days per week

No vigorous job-related physical activity

Skip to question 4

3. How much time did you usually spend on one of those days doing vigorous physical activities as part of your work?

_____ hours per day

_____ minutes per day

4. Again, think about only those physical activities that you did for at least 10 minutes at a time. During the last 7 days, on how many days did you do moderate physical activities like carrying light loads as part of your work? Please do not include walking.

_____ days per week

No moderate job-related physical activity

5. How much time did you usually spend on one of those days doing moderate physical activities as part of your work?

_____ hours per day

_____ minutes per day

6. During the last 7 days, on how many days did you walk for at least 10 minutes at a time as part of your work? Please do not count any walking you did to travel to or from work.

_____ days per week

No job-related walking Skip to PART 2: TRANSPORTATION

7. How much time did you usually spend on one of those days walking as part of your work?

_____ hours per day

_____ minutes per day

PART 2: TRANSPORTATION PHYSICAL ACTIVITY

These questions are about how you traveled from place to place, including to places like work, stores, movies, and so on.
8. During the last 7 days, on how many days did you travel in a motor vehicle like a train, bus, car, or tram?

_____ days per week

No traveling in a motor vehicle Skip to question 10

9. How much time did you usually spend on one of those days traveling in a train, bus, car, tram, or other kind of motor vehicle?

_____ hours per day

_____ minutes per day

Now think only about the bicycling and walking you might have done to travel to and from work, to do errands, or to go from place to place.

10. During the last 7 days, on how many days did you bicycle for at least 10 minutes at a time to go from place to place?

_____ days per week

No bicycling from place to place

11. How much time did you usually spend on one of those days to bicycle from place to place?

_____ hours per day

_____ minutes per day

12. During the last 7 days, on how many days did you walk for at least 10 minutes at a time to go from place to place?

_____ days per week

No walking from place to place Skip to PART 3: HOUSEWORK, HOUSE MAINTENANCE, AND CARING FOR FAMILY

13. How much time did you usually spend on one of those days walking from place to place?

_____ hours per day

_____ minutes per day

PART 3: HOUSEWORK, HOUSE MAINTENANCE, AND CARING FOR FAMILY

This section is about some of the physical activities you might have done in the last 7 days in and around your home, like housework, gardening, yard work, general maintenance work, and caring for your family.

14. Think about only those physical activities that you did for at least 10 minutes at a time. During the last 7 days, on how many days did you do vigorous physical activities like heavy lifting, chopping wood, shoveling snow, or digging in the garden or yard?

_____ days per week

No vigorous activity in garden or yard Skip to question 16

15. How much time did you usually spend on one of those days doing vigorous physical activities in the garden or yard?

_____ hours per day

_____ minutes per day

16. Again, think about only those physical activities that you did for at least 10 minutes at a time. During the last 7 days, on how many days did you do moderate activities like carrying light loads, sweeping, washing windows, and raking in the garden or yard?

_____ days per week

No moderate activity in garden or yard

17. How much time did you usually spend on one of those days doing moderate physical activities in the garden or yard?

_____ hours per day

_____ minutes per day

18. Once again, think about only those physical activities that you did for at least 10 minutes at a time. During the last 7 days, on how many days did you do moderate activities like carrying light loads, washing windows, scrubbing floors and sweeping inside your home?

_____ days per week

No moderate activity inside home Skip to PART

4: RECREATION, SPORT AND LEISURE-TIME PHYSICAL ACTIVITY

19. How much time did you usually spend on one of those days doing moderate physical activities inside your home?

_____ hours per day

_____ minutes per day

PART 4: RECREATION, SPORT, AND LEISURE-TIME PHYSICAL ACTIVITY

This section is about all the physical activities that you did in the last 7 days solely for recreation, sport, exercise or leisure. Please do not include any activities you have already mentioned.

20. Not counting any walking you have already mentioned, during the last 7 days, on how many days did you walk for at least 10 minutes at a time in your leisure time?

_____ days per week

No walking in leisure time Skip to question 22

21. How much time did you usually spend on one of those days walking in your leisure time?

_____ hours per day

_____ minutes per day

22. Think about only those physical activities that you did for at least 10 minutes at a time. During the last 7 days, on how many days did you do vigorous physical activities like aerobics, running, fast bicycling, or fast swimming in your leisure time?

_____ days per week

No vigorous activity in leisure time

23. How much time did you usually spend on one of those days doing vigorous physical activities in your leisure time?

_____ hours per day

_____ minutes per day

24. Again, think about only those physical activities that you did for at least 10 minutes at a time. During the last 7 days, on how many days did you do moderate physical activities like bicycling at a regular pace, swimming at a regular pace, and doubles tennis in your leisure time?

_____ days per week

No moderate activity in leisure time Skip to PART 5: TIME SPENT SITTING

25. How much time did you usually spend on one of those days doing moderate physical activities in your leisure time?

_____ hours per day

_____ minutes per day

PART 5: TIME SPENT SITTING

The last questions are about the time you spend sitting while at work, at home, while doing course work and during leisure time. This may include time spent sitting at a desk, visiting friends, reading or sitting or lying down to watch television. Do not include any time spent sitting in a motor vehicle that you have already told me about.

26. During the last 7 days, how much time did you usually spend sitting on a weekday?

_____ hours per day

_____ minutes per day

27. During the last 7 days, how much time did you usually spend sitting on a weekend day?

_____ hours per day

_____ minutes per day

This is the end of the questionnaire, thank you for participating.

155 Pirani Score

Objective

The Pirani Score is a simple and reliable system to determine severity and monitor progress in the Assessment and Treatment of Clubfoot [1]. This Scoring System uses the different views of the foot to help visualize the issues in the underling soft tissue and bony anatomy. A foot can be assessed in less than a minute and no technical equipment is required.[2]

Developed by Shafique Pirani, a Canadian Orthopaedic Surgeon, who assisted in the development of Clubfoot Services in Uganda and Malawi, it is an easy to use tool, developed to assess the severity of each of the individual components of Clubfoot. It is used both as a means to assess the severity of the Clubfoot at initial presentation and for ongoing monitoring of the patients' progress.

The Pirani Clubfoot Score documents the severity of the deformity and sequential scores are an excellent way to monitor progress. An increase in the Pirani Score between visits may be an indication that a relapse in the Clubfoot Deformity is occurring[3][4].

During Ponseti Management of Clubfoot, the Pirani Score Record shows whether the deformity is correcting normally or whether there is a problem, and the degree of correction of each component of the clubfoot. The Pirani Score is also utilised to assist in determining when to perform the Tenotomy. As highlighted by Dyer et al [2] and others there is significant positive correlation between the initial Pirani score and number of casts required to correct the clubfoot deformity. A Pirani Scoring 4 or more is likely to require at least four casts, and one scoring less than 4 will require three or fewer. A foot with a hindfoot score of 2.5 or 3 has a 72% chance of requiring a tenotomy, which is done when the midfoot score is less than 0.5.

The Pirani Score System is reliable, quick, and easy to use, and provides a good forecast about the likely treatment for an individual foot but a low score does not exclude the possibility that a tenotomy may be required.[2]

Intended Population

The Pirani Score is intended for use as a means to assess the severity of the clubfoot at initial presentation and for ongoing monitoring of the patients' progress.[3]

Methods of Use

The Pirani Scoring System is based on 6 well-described Clinical Signs of Contracture characterizing a severe clubfoot:[3]

- If the sign is severely abnormal it scores 1
- If it is partially abnormal it scores 0.5
- If it is normal it scores 0

Scoring the foot at each visit during treatment enables the health care worker treating the child to document how the foot is responding to manipulation and casting.Many degrees of severity and rigidity of Clubfoot are found at birth. Failures in treatment are related more often to faulty technique of manipulation and casting rather than severity of deformity.

Technique

The examiner is seated. The infant is on the mother's lap. A feeding, relaxed infant allows a more precise examination. The measurements are made while the examiner is gently correcting the foot with minimal effort, and no discomfort.[3]

The Pirani Score key features: [3]

1. Six "Signs" are Assessed
    - Scored depending on Severity - 0, 0.5, or 1
    - 3 Signs in Midfoot
    - 3 Signs in Hindfoot
1. Total Score (TS) varies from 0 to 6 and is the sum of Midfoot and Hindfoot Contracture Scores:

Mid Foot Contracture Score (MFCS)

Varies between 0 and 3 with 3 signs each scored 0, 0.5, or 1

1. **Medial Crease (MC)**
    1.
    - Gently correct the foot, e.g. by lifting the foot holding the second toe
    - Assess the depth of the crease and the presence of other creases
    - The presence of several fine creases is scored 0, two or three moderate creases is scored 0.5, and a single, deep crease where you cannot see the bottom is scored 1. [3]
2. **Curved Lateral Border (CLB)**
    1.
    - Make sure the child's foot is relaxed
    - Observe from the plantar aspect, and use a pen held against the lateral edge of the calcaneum
    - Assess the point on the lateral border of the foot at which it deviates from a straight line
    - If the border of the foot (excluding the phalanges) is straight and without deviation, score 0. If it deviates at the level of the metatarsals, score 0.5. If it deviates at the calcaneo-cuboid joint, score a 1. [3]
3. **Lateral Head of Talus (LHT)**
    1.
    - Palpate the head of the talus with the foot uncorrected (it may be easier to find initially if you move the foot into a more deformed position)
    - Keeping your finger / thumb on the talus, gently correct the foot
    - If the talus completely sinks away under the navicular, score 0. If it moves partially but doesn't completely sink, score 0.5. If it remains fixed and does not sink, score 1. [3]

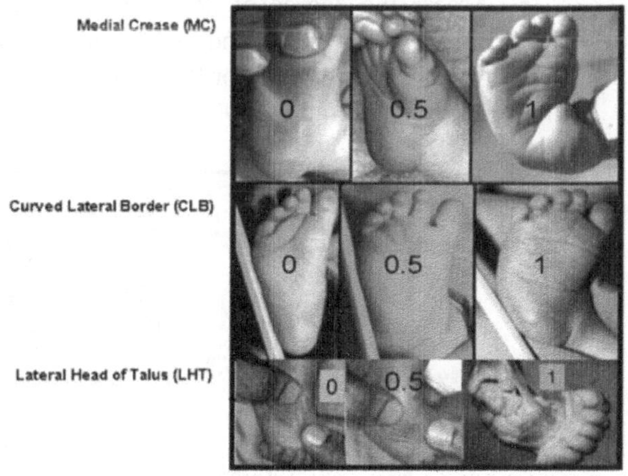

Hindfoot Contracture Score (HFCS)

Varies between 0 and 3

3 signs are each scored 0, 0.5, or 1

1. **Posterior Crease (PC)**
    1.
    - Gently correct the plantarflexion (equinus)
    - Assess the depth of the crease and the presence of other creases
    - The presence of several fine creases is scored 0, two or three moderate creases is scored 0.5, and a single, deep crease where you cannot see the bottom is scored 1. [3]
2. **Empty Heel (EH)**
    1.
    - Hold the foot in mild correction and palpate with a single index finger
    - Ascertain how much flesh there is in the heel between your finger and the calcaneum
    - If it is easy to palpate the calcaneum, which is not far under the skin, score 0. Score 0.5 for a palpable calcaneum which is just felt through a layer of flesh. If the calcaneum is deep under a layer of tissue and very difficult to feel, score 1. (0 is like touching your own chin, 0.5 like touching the tip of your nose, and 1 like touching the soft part of your palm below the base of your thumb). [3]
3. **Rigid Equinus (RE)**
    1.
    - Correct the plantarflexion as much as is comfortable for the child, holding the knee straight

- Assess the degree of dorsiflexion obtained: able to dorsiflex beyond plantigrade = 0, able to reach plantigrade (or 90°) = 0.5, unable to reach plantigrade (or 90°) = 1. [3]

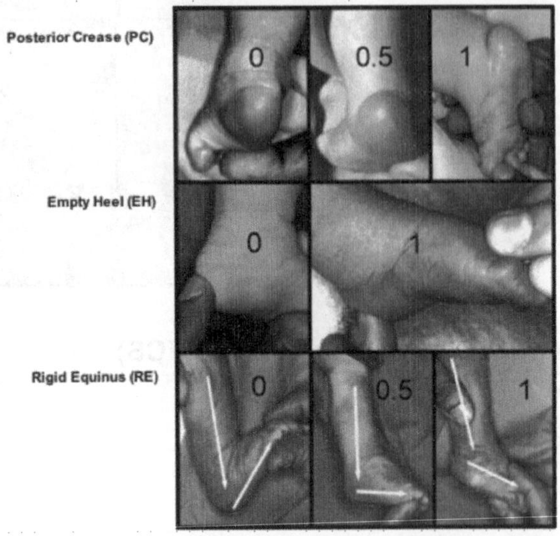

Recording

Pirani Score Record Sheet

The Pirani Score should be recorded at each visit during the correction phase of clubfoot treatment. Most clinics have a paper form to record it. Below is an example of the Global Clubfoot Initiative Pirani Score Form. You will also find two other examples of Clubfoot Assessment Forms including the Global Clubfoot Initiative Pirani Score Form and the CURE Clubfoot Form to record and display the history, physical examination, and treatment in the Resource Section below. [3]

Date										
SIDE	Right	Left	Right	Left	Right	Left	Right	Left	Right	Left	Right	Left
Medial Crease MC												
Curved Lateral Border CLB												
Lateral Head Talus LHT												
MID FOOT CONTRACTURE SCORE (MFCS)												
Posterior Crease PC												
Empty Heel EH												
Rigid Equinus RE												
HIND FOOT CONTRACTURE SCORE (HFCS)												
TOTAL SCORE (TS)												

Pirani Score Graph

Putting the Pirani Score into a Graph:

- If the Midfoot Contracture Score (MFCS), the Hindfoot Contracture Score (HFCS), and the Total Score (TS) are plotted on a simple graph against time, you can follow the improvement of the foot.

Use of Pirani Score to indicate Tenotomy:

- Achilles Tenotomy is the final part of correcting a clubfoot. The Pirani Score can indicate when the foot is ready for a tenotomy. The graph below shows the effects of Ponseti Treatment and Tenotomy on the MFCS, HFCS, and TS. The MFCS drops rapidly with manipulation and casting whereas the HFCS remains high. The tenotomy is done in Week 5 when the MFCS has less than 0.5 but the HFCS remains greater than 1. After the tenotomy, the HFCS improves from 2.5 to 0.5, but does not correct completely.

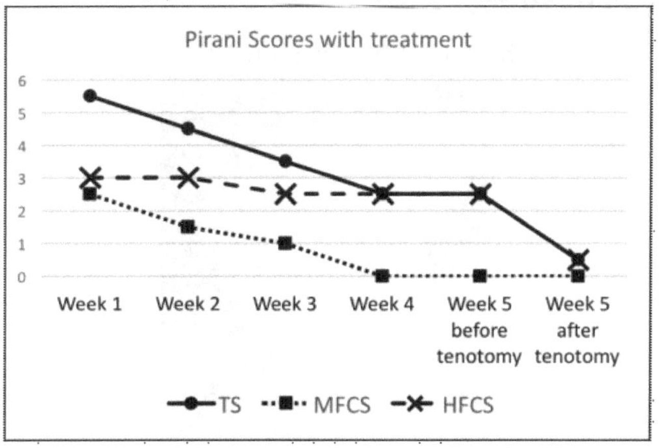

Evidence

The Pirani Scoring system has been found to be both valid and reliable, unlike many other Clubfoot Scoring Systems, which are untested. [5] A higher Pirani Score on presentation may indicate that a higher number of casts will be required, and as such can play a key role as a means for predicting treatment outcomes. [6] In a child with a high initial Hindfoot Contracture Score (HFCS) the likelihood to experience relapse of deformity during the bracing phase is much higher than in those with lower scores and should have close monitoring with special emphasis put on the importance of the use of Foot Abduction Brace when educating parents/carers.[7]

Reliability: Mejabi et al [1] described the Pirani scoring system as a reliable system to determine severity and monitor progress in the treatment of clubfoot. Their study showed significant correlation ($p<0.001$) between the midfoot score, hindfoot score, Pirani score and the number of casts to achieve correction. Also, there was correlation between the Pirani score and the need for tenotomy ($p<0.001$) and the progress of treatment can be monitored with the Pirani score ($p<0.001$). Shaheen et al [8] examined the Interobserver reliability in Pirani Scoring between Paediatric Orthopaedic Surgeons and Physiotherapy Assistants who were trained Nurses with further training to work as Physiotherapy Assistants in Clubfoot management. The mean percentage of agreement of both observers for all Pirani Score Components was 83%. They found moderate to substantial interobserver reliability for the Pirani Score and all its subcomponents. Properly trained physiotherapy assistants are efficient in assessing the degree of severity of clubfoot. [8] Similarly Jillian et al [9] found the Pirani Score to be a reliable measurement tool by plaster technicians for independent assessment of clubfoot. However, they highlight that prior training and supervision in the early phase is necessary. [9]

Validity

Piarani et al [5] demonstrated validity of the Piarni Score with excellent inter-observer reliability by evaluating this clinical scoring system by correlating MRI and clinical scores.

References

1. Mejabi JO, Esan O, Adegbehingbe OO, Orimolade EA, Asuquo J, Badmus HD, Anipole AO. The Pirani Scoring System is Effective in Assessing Severity and Monitoring Treatment of Clubfeet in Children , British Journal of Medicine & Medical Research 17(4): 1-9, 2016
2. Dyer PJ, Davis N. The role of the Pirani scoring system in the management of club foot by the Ponseti method. Bone & Joint Journal. 2006 Aug 1;88(8):1082-4.
3. Africa Clubfoot Training Project. Chapter 4 Africa Clubfoot Training Basic & Advanced Clubfoot Treatment Provider Courses - Participant Manual. University of Oxford: Africa Clubfoot Training Project, 2017.
4. Goriainov V, Judd J, Uglow M. Does the Pirani score predict relapse in clubfoot?. Journal of children's orthopaedics. 2010 Aug 29;4(5):439-44.
5. Pirani S, Hodges D & Sekeramayi F (2003) A reliable and valid method of assessing the amount of deformity in the congenital clubfoot deformity (The Canadian Orthopaedic Research Society and the Canadian Orthopaedic Association conference proceeding) in The Journal of Bone and Joint Surgery 90 (B) SUPP_1, 53
6. Dyer P, Davis N (2006) The role of the Pirani scoring system in the management of clubfoot by the Ponseti method. The Journal of Bone and Joint Surgery 88 (8): 1082-1084
7. Goriainov V, Uglow M (2010) The value of initial Pirani score assessment of clubfoot in predicting recurrence. (British Society for Children's Orthopaedic Surgery conference proceeding) in The Journal of Bone and Joint Surgery 92B, Supp_III, 376.
8. Shaheen S, Jaiballa H, Pirani S. Interobserver reliability in Pirani clubfoot severity scoring between a paediatric orthopaedic surgeon and

a physiotherapy assistant. Journal of Pediatric Orthopaedics B. 2012 Jul 1;21(4):366-8.

9. Jillani SA, Aslam MZ, Chinoy MA, Khan MA, Saleem A, Ahmed SK. A comparison between orthopedic surgeon and allied health worker in Pirani score. J Pak Med Assoc. 2014 Dec;64(12 Suppl 2):S127-30.

Pirani Score Example

Introduction

Scoring the foot at each visit during treatment enables the physiotherapist or health care worker treating the child to document how the foot is responding to the manipulation and casting. It also assists in determining when to perform the Achilles Tenotomy.

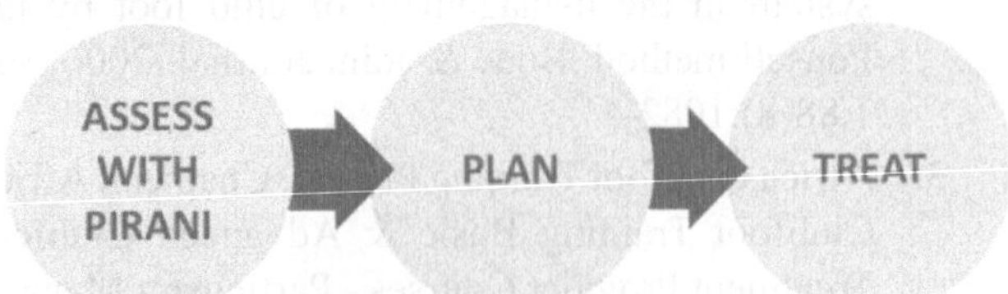

Pirani Score Assessment

Consider the following examples which highlight different elements of the Pirani Score Process.

Example 1 Scoring the Foot

Medial Crease

What is the Medial Crease Score? [1]

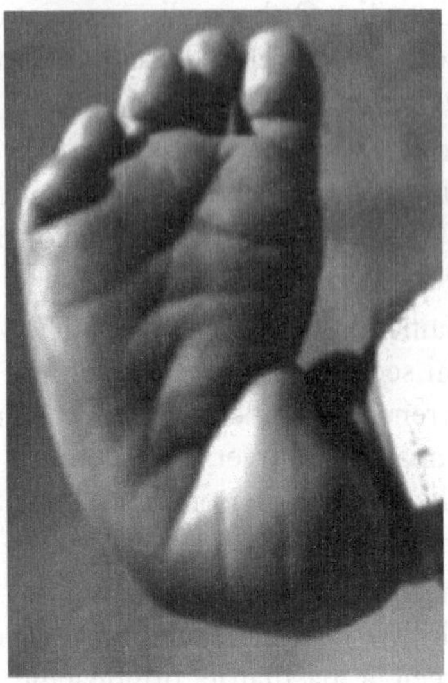

Lateral Border

What is the Lateral Border Score? [1]

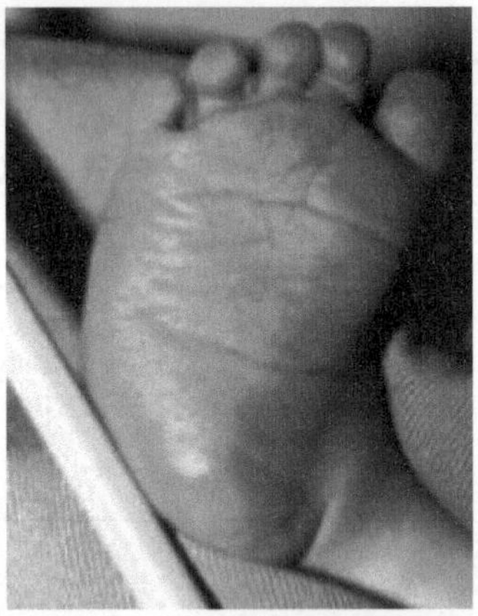

Posterior Crease

What is the Posterior Crease Score? [1]

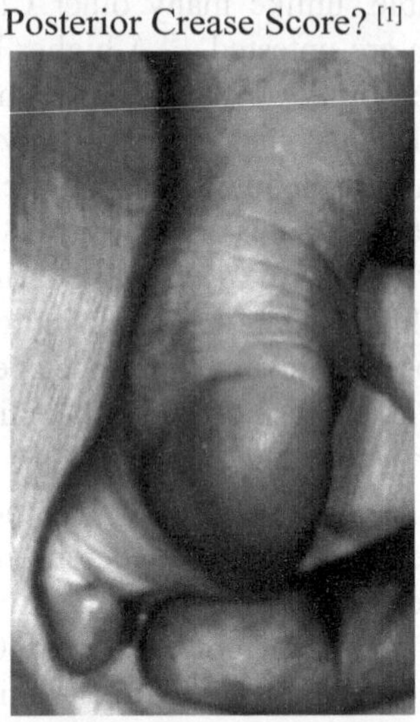

Rigid Equinus Score

If this is the maximum dorsiflexion, what is the Rigid Equinus Score? [1]

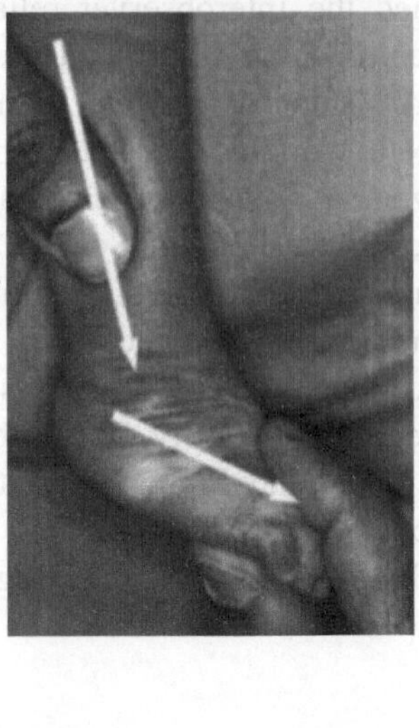

Example 2 Calculating the Pirani Score

After assessment with the Pirani Score, you find: *[1]*

- Medial Crease (MC) = 0
- Curved Lateral Border (CLB) = 0.5
- Lateral Head of Talus (LHT) = 0
- Posterior Crease (PC) = 1
- Empty Heel = 0.5
- Rigid Equinus = 0.5

What is the Total Midfoot Score?

What is the Total Hindfoot Score?

What is the Total Pirani Score?

Is this patient ready to undergo Tenotomy?

Example 3 Determining Readiness for Tenotomy

Based on the following Pirani Scores, which of these patients is ready for Tenotomy? [1]

Patient 1: CLB 0, LHT 0.5, MC 0, PC 0.5, RE 1.0, EH 1.0 Total Score = 3

Patient 2: CLB 0, LHT 0, MC 0, PC 1.0, RE 1.0, EH 1.0 Total Score = 3

Patient 3: *CLB 0, LHT 0, MC 0.5, PC 1.0, RE 1.0, EH 0.5 Total Score = 3*

References

1. Africa Clubfoot Training Project. Chapter 4 How To Assess the Severity of a Clubfoot using the Pirani Score. Africa Clubfoot Training Basic & Advanced Clubfoot Treatment Provider Courses - Participant Manual. University of Oxford: Africa Clubfoot Training Project, 2017.

❑❑❑

156 Postural Assessment Scale for Stroke (PASS)

Objective

PASS is a postural assessment scale specifically designed to assess and monitor postural control after stroke. It contains 12 four-level items of varying difficulty for assessing ability to maintain or change a given lying, sitting, or standing posture.

Intended Population

Stroke patients

Available Versions

The PASS was developed in 1999 by Benaim et al. as an adaptation of the Fugl-Meyer Assessment balance subscale (Benaim et al., 1999). It was originally developed in French and has since been translated into English and Swedish (SwePASS). Short forms of the PASS, with fewer items (5-item SFPASS) and/or smaller scoring scales (PASS-3P), have also been developed.[1]

Modified version of PASS

Method of Use

The PASS consists of 2 sections with a 4-point scale to describe each task. The total score ranges from 0 - 36 and is as follows:[2]

Maintaining Posture

1: **Sitting without support**

0 = cannot sit

1 = can sit with slight support (e.g. by 1 hand)

2 = can sit for more than 10 seconds without support

3 = can sit for 5 minutes without support

2: **Standing with support**

0 = cannot stand, even with support

1 = can stand with strong support of 2 people

2 = can stand with moderate support of 1 person

3 = can stand with support on only 1 hand

3: **Standing without support**

0 = cannot stand without support

1 = can stand without support for

10 seconds or leans heavily on 1 leg

2 = can stand without support for 1 minute or stands slightly asymmetrically

3 = can stand without support for more than 1 minute and at the same time perform arm movements above the shoulder level

4 and **5**: **Standing on the nonparetic / paretic leg**

0 = cannot stand on the leg

1 = can stand on the leg for a few seconds

2 = can stand on the leg for more than 5 seconds

3 = can stand on the leg for more than 10 seconds

Changing a Posture

Scoring of items 6 to 12 is as follows (items 6 to 11 are to be performed with a 50-cm-high examination table, like a Bobath plane; items 10 to 12 are to be performed without any support; no other constraints):

6. **Supine to affected side lateral**
7. **Supine to non-affected side lateral**
8. **Supine to sitting up on the edge of the table**
9. **Sitting on the edge of the table to supine**
10. **Sitting to standing up**
11. **Standing up to sitting down**
12. **Standing, picking up a pencil from the floor**

Items 6 - 12

0 = cannot perform the activity

1 = can perform the activity with much help
2 = can perform the activity with little help
3 = can perform the activity without help

Training requirements

No special training is required, although clinicians should have an understanding of balance impairment and related safety issues following stroke.[1]

Evidence

Reliability

PASS is one of most reliable clinical assessment scale. Mao et al. (2002) examined the inter-rater reliability of the PASS using α-coefficient for individual item reliability and Pearson product moment correlation for total score reliability. Two clinicians assessed patients at 14 days post-stroke on the same day, with a total sample of 112 patients. Inter-rater reliability for individual items was adequate to excellent (median α=0.88, range 0.61-0.96) and inter-rater reliability for the total score was excellent (ICC=0.97, 95% CI 0.95-0.98).

Benaim et al. (1999) measured inter-rater reliability of the PASS using α-coefficient for individual item reliability and Pearson product moment correlation for total score reliability. Two clinicians assessed patients with stroke on the same day, with a total sample of 12 patients. The authors reported adequate to excellent inter-rater reliability for individual items (average α=0.88, range 0.64-1) and excellent inter-rater reliability for the total score (r=0.99, p<0.001). [1]

Validity

PASS is one of the most valid clinical assessments of postural control in stroke patients during the first 3 months after stroke[2]

Mao et al. (2002)[3] examined the predictive validity of the PASS, Berg Balance Scale and the Fugl-Meyer Assessment modified balance scale at 14, 30 and 90 days post-stroke by comparison with the Motor Assessment Scale walking subscale score at 180 days post-stroke, in a sample of 123 patients. The PASS demonstrated excellent predictive validity at all time points (α=0.86-0.90), as measured using Spearman's p correlation coefficient.[2]

Sensitivity

The high sensitivity of the scale during the acute stages of a stroke is excellent and is shown by its' ability to discriminate between patients with right and left brain damage[4]

Miscellaneous

There is strong evidence that a short form of Postural Assessment Scale for Stroke patients, the 5-item PASS-3L, has sound psycho-metric properties in people with stroke[5].

References

1. Heart & Stroke Foundation, Canadian Partnership for Stroke Recovery. Postural Assesment Scale for Stroke Patients (PASS). http://www.strokengine.ca/assess/pass/ (accessed 28 mars 2017)
2. Benaim C, Pérennou DA, Villy J, Rousseaux M, Pelissier JY. Validation of a standardized assessment of postural control in stroke patients: the Postural Assessment Scale for Stroke Patients (PASS). Stroke. 1999 Sep;30:1862-8.
3. Mao HF, Hsueh IP, Tang PF, Sheu CF, Hsieh CL. Analysis and comparison of the psychometric properties of three balance measures for stroke patients. Stroke 2002; 33: 1022-7
4. Poole JL, Whitney SL. Motor assessment scale for stroke patients concurrent validity and interrater reliability. Arch Phys Med Rehabil. 1988;69:195–197.
5. Wang CH, Hsueh IP, Sheu CF, Yao G, Hsieh CL. Psychometric properties of 2 simplified 3-level balance scales used for patients with stroke. Phys Ther 2004;84(5):430-8.

MODIEFIED POSTURAL ASSESMENT SCALE FOR STROKE (PASS)

Only one attempt per item is allowed. Ensure that the patient manages the criteria for the scores below, as well as the criterion for the registered score.A stopwatch is used in items 4 and 7-9 where the patient should maintain a position within a specific time. Item 4 should be performed with the patient´s feet supported on the floor. In items 1-3, 5-6 and 10-12, the patient´s postural balance/control should be scored according to different degrees of support.

1. Supine to affected side lateral

Cannot perform the activity - **0**

Can perform the activity with support from 2 persons-**1**

Can perform the activity with support from 1 person **-2**

Can perform the activity without any hel***p* - 3**

2. Supine to non affected side lateral

Cannot perform the activity-**0**

Can perform the activity with support from 2 persons **-1**

Can perform the activity with support from 1 person-**2**

Can perform the activity without any help **-3**

3. Supine to sitting up on edge of bed

Cannot perform the activity **-0**

Can perform the activity with support from 2 persons-**1**

Can perform the activity with support from 1 person **-2**

Can perform the activity without any help-**3**

4. Sitting without support

Cannot sit-**0**

Can sit with slight support, for example by 1hand-**1**

Can sit for more than 10 seconds without support- **2**

Can sit for 5 minutes without support-**3**

5. Sitting to standing up

Cannot perform the activity **-0**

Can perform the activity with support from 2 persons **-1**

Can perform the activity with support from 1 person **-2**

Can perform the activity without any help **-3**

6. Standing with support

Cannot stand, even with support - **0**

Can stand with strong support from 2 persons **-1**

Can stand with moderate support from 1 person - **2**

Can stand with support of only 1 hand-**3**

7. Standing without support

Cannot stand without support **-0**

Can stand without support for 10 seconds or leans heavily on 1 leg **-1**

Can stand without support for more than 1 minute or stands slightly asymmetrically **-2**

Can stand without support for more than 1 minute and at the same time draw hand/s from forehand to neck (like drawing finger throw the hair) altered with arm/s hanging parallel with the trunk to avoid tiredness-**3**

8. Standing on non paretic leg

Cannot stand on the non paretic leg **-0**

Can stand on the non paretic leg for a few seconds **-1**

Can stand on the non paretic leg for more than 5 seconds - **2**

Can stand on the non paretic leg for more than 10 seconds **-3**

9. Standing on paretic leg

Cannot stand on the non paretic leg **-0**

Can stand on the non paretic leg for a few seconds **-1**

Can stand on the non paretic leg for more than 5 seconds **-2**

Can stand on the non paretic leg for more than 10 seconds-**3**

10. Standing, picking up a shoe from the floor

Cannot perform the activity - **0**

Can perform the activity with support from 2 persons **-1**

Can perform the activity with support from 1 person - **2**

Can perform the activity without any help **-3**

11. Sitting down from standing up

Cannot perform the activity **-0**

Can perform the activity with support from 2 persons **-1**

Can perform the activity with support from 1 person **-2**

Can perform the activity without any help **-3**

12. Sitting on edge of bed to supine

Cannot perform the activity - **0**

Can perform the activity with support from 2 persons **-1**

Can perform the activity with support from 1 person **-2**

Can perform the activity without any help **-3**

❑❑❑

157 Progressive Supranuclear Palsy Rating Scale (PSP-RS)

Introduction

The Progressive Supranuclear Palsy Rating Scale (PSPRS) is a disease specific measure of severity in patients with progressive supranuclear palsy (PSP). It measures disability across 28 items in six domains: daily activities (by history), behaviour, bulbar, ocular motor, limb motor and gait/midline. It was devised by Golbe and Strickland[1]. It is a quantitative measure of disability and attempts to include all of the important areas of clinical impairment in PSP[2].

Intended Population

This scale is targeted toward measuring the severity of clinical impairments in patients with Progressive supranuclear Palsy (PSP).

Method Of Use

Equipment: Scale, Pen, Paper. Cup of water

Training Required:some examination items require prior clinical training

Time Required:10 min[1]

Instrument and Scoring

It is a Clinician reported measuring disability across six domains giving a maximum score of 100[3]. It comprises of 28 items in six areas. Six items are rated on a 3-point scale (0–2) and 22 are rated on a 5-point scale (0–4).

1. The History/Daily Activities area: seven items with a total maximum score of 24,
2. The Mentation area: four items with a maximum score of 16,
3. The Bulbar area: two items with a maximum score of 8,
4. The ocular motor area four items with a maximum score of 16 points,
5. The limb motor area six items with a maximum score of 16.
6. The Gait area: five items with a maximum score of 20.

Item name and score definitions Comments, instructions	
	1.Withdrawal
	0 None
	1 Follows conversation in a group, may respond spontaneously, but rarely if ever initiates exchanges
I. History	2 Rarely or never follows conversation in a group
	2. Irritability
	0 No increase in irritability
	1 Increased, but not interfering with family interactions
	2 Interfering with family interactions
	3. Dysphagia for solids

	0 Normal; no difficulty with full range of food textures
	1 Tough foods must be cut up into small pieces
	2 Requires soft solid diet
	3 Requires pureed or liquid diet
	4 Tube feeding required for some or all feeding
	4.Using knife and fork, buttoning clothes, washing hands and face
	0 Normal
	1 Somewhat slow but no help required
	2 Extremely slow; or occasional help needed
	3 Considerable help needed but can do some things alone
	4 Requires total assistance
	5. Falls
	0 None in the past year
	1 <1 per month; gait may otherwise be normal
	2 1-4 per month
	3 5-30 per month
	4 >30 per month (or chairbound)
	6. Urinary incontinence
	0 None or a few drops less than daily
	1 A few drops staining clothes daily
	2 Large amounts, but only when asleep; no pad required during day
	3 Occasional large amounts in daytime; pad required
	4 Consistent, requiring diaper or catheter awake and asleep
	7. Sleep difficulty
	0 Neither primary nor secondary insomnia
	1 Either primary or secondary insomnia; averages <5 h sleep nightly
	2 Both primary and secondary insomnia; averages <5 h sleep nightly
	3 Either primary or secondary insomnia; averages <5 h sleep nightly
	4 Both primary and secondary insomnia; averages <5 h sleep nightly
	primary insomnia is difficulty falling asleep secondary is difficulty remaining asleep
II. Mentation	
Items 8 -11 use this scale: 0 Clearly absent	8. Disorientation ; Use MMSE items 1^-10 or history to estimate interference in ADLs
1 Equivocal or minimal	9. Bradyphrenia

2 Clearly present, but does not interfere with activities of daily living (ADL)	10. Emotional incontinence
3 Interferes mildly with ADL	11. Grasping/imitative /utilizing behaviour
4 Interferes markedly with ADL	
	12. Dysarthria
	0 None
	1 Minimal; all or nearly all words easily comprehensible
	2 Definite, moderate; most words comprehensible
	3 Severe; may be fluent but most words incomprehensible
III. Bulbar	4 Mute; or a few poorly comprehensible words
	13. Dysphagia
	0 None
	1 Single sips, or fluid pools in mouth or pharynx, but no choking/ coughing
	2 Occasionally coughs to clear fluid; no frank aspiration
	3 Frequently coughs to clear fluid; may aspirate slightly; may expectorate frequently rather than swallow secretions
	4 Requires artificial measures (oral suctioning, tracheostomy or feeding gastrostomy) to avoid aspiration
	14.Voluntary upward command movement
IV. Ocular motor	15.Voluntary downward command movement
Items 14 -16 use this scale:	16.Voluntary left and right command movement
0 Saccades not slow or hypometric; 86 -100% of normal excursion	17. Eyelid dysfunction
	0 None
1 Saccades slow or hypometric; 86 - 100% of normal excursion	1 Blink rate decreased (515/min) but no other abnormality
2 51- 85% of normal excursion	2 Mild inhibition of opening or closing or mild blepharospasm; no visual disability
3 16- 50% of normal excursion	3 Moderate lid-opening inhibition or blepharospasm causing partial visual disability
4 <15% of normal excursion or worse	4 Functional blindness or near-blindness because of involuntary eyelid closure
	18. Limb rigidity
	0 Absent
	1 Slight or detectable only on activation
	2 Definitely abnormal, but full range of motion possible

	3 Only partial range of motion possible
	4 Little or no passive motion possible
V. Limb motor	19. Limb dystonia
	0 Absent
	1 Subtle or present only when activated by other movement
	2 Obvious but not continuous
	3 Continuous but not disabling
	4 Continuous and disabling
	20. Finger tapping
	0 Normal (<14 taps/5 s with maximal amplitude)
	1 Impaired (6 -14 taps/5 s or moderate loss of amplitude
	2 Barely able to perform (0 -5 taps/5 s or severe loss of amplitude)
	21. Toe tapping
	0 Normal (<14 taps/5 s with maximal amplitude)
	1 Impaired (6 -14 taps/5 s or moderate loss of amplitude
	2 Barely able to perform (0 -5 taps/5 s or severe loss of amplitude)
	22. Apraxia of hand movement
	0 Absent
	1 Present, not impairing most functions
	2 Impairing most functions
	23. Tremor in any part
	0 Absent
	1 Present, not impairing most functions
	2 Impairing most functions
	24. Neck rigidity or dystonia
	0 Absent
	1 Slight or detectable only when activated by other movement
	2 Definitely abnormal, but full range of motion possible
	3 Only partial range of motion possible
VI. Gait and midline	19. Limb dystonia
	0 Absent
	1 Subtle or present only when activated by other movement
	2 Obvious but not continuous
	3 Continuous but not disabling
	4 Continuous and disabling
	20. Finger tapping
	0 Normal (<14 taps/5 s with maximal amplitude)

	1 Impaired (6 -14 taps/5 s or moderate loss of amplitude
	2 Barely able to perform (0 -5 taps/5 s or severe loss of amplitude)
	21. Toe tapping
	0 Normal (<14 taps/5 s with maximal amplitude)
	1 Impaired (6 -14 taps/5 s or moderate loss of amplitude
	2 Barely able to perform (0 -5 taps/5 s or severe loss of amplitude)
	22. Apraxia of hand movement
	0 Absent
	1 Present, not impairing most functions
	2 Impairing most functions
	23. Tremor in any part
	0 Absent
	1 Present, not impairing most functions
	2 Impairing most functions
	24. Neck rigidity or dystonia
	0 Absent
	1 Slight or detectable only when activated by other movement
	2 Definitely abnormal, but full range of motion possible
	3 Only partial range of motion possible
VI. Gait and midline	4 Little or no passive motion possible
	25. Arising from chair
	0 Normal
	1 Slow but arises on first attempt
	2 Requires more than one attempt, but arises
	without using hands
	3 Requires use of hands
	4 Unable to arise without assistance
	26. Gait
	0 Normal
	1 Slightly wide-based or irregular or slight pulsion on turns
	2 Must walk slowly or occasionally use walls or helper to avoid falling, especially on turns
	3 Must use assistance all or almost all the time
	4 Unable to walk, even with walker; may be able to transfer
	27. Postural stability
	0 Normal (shifts neither foot or one foot)
	1 Must shift each foot at least once but recovers unaided

	2 Shifts feet and must be caught by examiner
	3 Unable to shift feet; must be caught, but does not require assistance to stand still
	4 Tends to fall without a pull; requires assistance to stand still
	28. Sitting down
	0 Normal
	1 Slightly stiff or awkward
	2 Easily positions self before chair, but descent into chair is uncontrolled
	3 Has difficulty finding chair behind him/her and descent is uncontrolled
	4 Unable to test because of severe postural instability

Psychometric Properties

Reliability: excellent (IRR= 0.86, 95% CI= 0.65–0.98) [1]

Good sensitivity to disease progression[2]

Validity: moderate construct validity[1]

References

1. Golbe LI, Ohman-Strickland PA. A clinical rating scale for progressive supranuclear palsy. Brain. 2007 Jun;130(Pt 6):1552-65.
2. Hewer S, Varley S, Boxer AL, Paul E, Williams DR; AL-108-231 Investigators. Minimal clinically important worsening on the progressive supranuclear Palsy Rating Scale. Mov Disord. 2016 ;31(10):1574-1577.
3. Hall, D.A., Forjaz, M.J., Golbe, L.I., Litvan, I., Payan, C.A.M., Goetz, C.G.,et al. Scales to Assess Clinical Features of Progressive Supranuclear Palsy: MDS Task Force Report. Mov Disord Clin Pract, 2015. 2: 127-134

❑❑❑

158 Patient-Rated Wrist Evaluation Score (PRWE)

Introduction

PRWE is the Patient-Rated Wrist Evaluation.The PRWE is a 15-item questionnaire designed to measure wrist pain and disability in activities of daily living. Developed in 1998 for clinical assessment and is used for specific wrist problems.It is one of the reliable upper extremity outcome instrument.[1]

The PRWE allows patients to rate their levels of wrist pain and disability from 0 to 10, and consists of 2 subscales:

1. Pain subscale: contains 5 items each of which is further rated from 1-10. The maximum score in this section is 50 and minimum 0
2. Function subscale: contains total 10 items which are further divided into 2 sections i.e specific activities (having 6 items) and usual activities (having 4 items). The maximum score in this section is 50 and minimum 0.

Development of PRWE

Scale items were generated using information obtained from patient and expert interviews, biomechanical literature, and other questionnaires.

Items were reduced and refined through expert interviews and pilot testing on small groups of patients. It Surveyed 100 (66 responded) international wrist investigators (IWIW) to generate items particularly. After developing the items PRWE was tested.[2]

Testing the PRWE

A test-retest reliability study was conducted on patients with distal radius (n=64) or scaphoid (n=35) fractures. The total PRWE score's test-retest reliability was excellent over both the short term (2-7 days, ICC > = 0.90) and the long term (1 year, ICC = 0.91). The pain subscale also had excellent short-term and long-term reliability (ICC = 0.90, 0.91, respectively).The function subscale demonstrated excellent short-term reliability (ICC >= 0.88) and moderate long-term disability (ICC = 0.61).[3][4][5]

Objectives

- To determine level of wrist disability
- To set treatment goals
- To determine whether change has occurred
- To communicate in a meaningful way to payers

Scoring

- There are 3 steps to score PRWE

Step 1: Measure the pain score of all 5 items

1. PAIN	
Rate the **average** amount of pain in your wrist over the past week by circling the number that best describes your pain on a scale from 0-10. A zero **(0)** means that you **did not** have any pain and a **ten (10)** means that you had the **worst pain you have ever experienced** or that **you could not do the activity because of pain.**	
RATE YOUR PAIN: Sample Scale ☞	0 1 2 3 4 5 6 7 8 9 10 No Pain Worst Ever
At rest	0 1 2 3 4 5 6 7 8 9 10
When doing a task with a repeated wrist movement	0 1 2 3 4 5 6 7 8 9 10
When lifting a heavy object	0 1 2 3 4 5 6 7 8 9 10
When it is at its worst	0 1 2 3 4 5 6 7 8 9 10
How often do you have pain?	0 1 2 3 4 5 6 7 8 9 10 Never Always

Step 2: Measure the function score of all the 10 items and divide it by 2

2. FUNCTION	
A. SPECIFIC ACTIVITIES	
*Rate the **amount of difficulty** you experienced performing each of the items listed below - over the past week, by circling the number that describes your difficulty on a scale of 0-10. A **zero** (0) means you did not experience any difficulty and a **ten** (10) means it was so difficult you were unable to do it at all.*	
Sample scale →	0 1 2 3 4 5 6 7 8 9 10 No Difficulty Unable To Do
Turn a door knob using my affected hand	0 1 2 3 4 5 6 7 8 9 10
Cut meat using a knife in my affected hand	0 1 2 3 4 5 6 7 8 9 10
Fasten buttons on my shirt	0 1 2 3 4 5 6 7 8 9 10
Use my affected hand to push up from a chair	0 1 2 3 4 5 6 7 8 9 10
Carry a 10lb object in my affected hand	0 1 2 3 4 5 6 7 8 9 10
Use bathroom tissue with my affected hand	0 1 2 3 4 5 6 7 8 9 10
B. USUAL ACTIVITIES	
*Rate the **amount of difficulty** you experienced performing your **usual** activities in each of the areas listed below, over the past week, by circling the number that best describes your difficulty on a scale of 0-10. By "usual activities", we mean the activities you performed **before** you started having a problem with your wrist. A **zero** (0) means that you did not experience any difficulty and a **ten** (10) means it was so difficult you were unable to do any of your usual activities.*	
Personal care activities (dressing, washing)	0 1 2 3 4 5 6 7 8 9 10
Household work (cleaning, maintenance)	0 1 2 3 4 5 6 7 8 9 10
Work (your job or usual everyday work)	0 1 2 3 4 5 6 7 8 9 10
Recreational activities	0 1 2 3 4 5 6 7 8 9 10

Step 3: Add pain and function score.

Total Score = Sum of pain+ function scores (Best Score = 0, Worst Score = 100)

Less score = better outcome

Merits and Demerits

Merits:

- Developed with patient interviews
- Region-specific (wrist) assessment
- Short and quick
- Reliable

Demerits

- Validated / developed from fewer centers
- Region-specific
- No hand dominance

PRWHE

Patient rate wrist/hand evaluation (PRWHE) is the modified version of PRWE. The PRWHE has the same items and scoring system as the PRWE. The PRWHE is preferred in hand/wrist clinics as it is more specific and easier to use and also asses the hand along with wrist.

Changes between the PRWE and PRWHE

1. In the PRWHE, the term "wrist" is replaced with "wrist/hand".
2. The PRWHE has an optional aesthetics question on the form (not part of the scale scoring).

References

1. Angst F, John M, Goldhahn J, et al. Comprehensive assessment of clinical outcome andfckLRquality of life after resection interposition arthroplasty of the thumb saddle joint.fckLRArthritis Rheum 2005;53:205-213
2. MacDermid JC, Turgeon T, Richards RS, etfckLRal. Patient rating of wrisfckLRt pain and disability:fckLRa reliable and valid measurement tool. J Orthop Trauma 1998;12:577-586
3. MacDermid JC, Turgeon T, Richards RS, etfckLRal. Patient rating of wrisfckLRt pain and disability:fckLRa reliable and valid measurement tool. J Orthop Trauma 1998;12:577-586
4. MacDermid JC, Richards RS,Roth JH. DistfckLRal radius fracture:fckLRa prospective outcomefckLRstudy of 275 patients. J Hand Ther 2001;14:154-169
5. MacDermid JC, Roth JH,Richards RS. Pain afckLRnd disability reportedfckLRin the year followingfckLRa distal radius fracture: A cohort stfckLRudy. BMC Musculoskelet Disord 2003;4:24

❑❑❑

159 Quebec Back Pain Disability Scale

Objective

The Quebec back pain disability scale (QBPDS) is a condition-specific questionnaire developed to measure the level of functional disability for patients with low back pain (LBP) that was designed, developed and validated by Kopec et al in 1995. [1] The original purpose of the questionnaire is to take into account the functional limitations related to pain, to monitor the progress of individual patients and to compare the evolution of LBP subjects incorporated in rehabilitation programs. [4] [2] [5]

The Quebec back pain disability scale consists of 20 daily activities that can be categorized into 6 types of activities: [1] [2]

- Bed/rest items 1–3
- Sitting/standing items 4–6
- Ambulation items 7–9
- Movement items 10–12
- Bending/stooping items 13–16
- Handling of large/heavy objects items 17–20.

The various components of the questionnaire were selected from a larger pool of items based on test-retest reliability, item-total correlations, and responsiveness of individual items and by using techniques of factor analysis and item response theory. [1]

The scale exists of one central question: "Do you have trouble today with...?" followed by 20 activities of daily life. Some examples of daily activity: taking something out of the fridge, getting out of bed... In every activity, there are 6 answer categories, measured by using a Likert scale from 0-5 (0 = no effort, 5 = not able to). If the patient suffers a lot that day, he scores that activity with a 5, if it gives no problems a 0. [1] [6] [3] The final outcome is obtained by the sum of the scoring of the degree of difficulty in performing the 20 daily activities. These outcomes score within the range of 0 and 100, determents the level of functional disability, with higher numbers representing greater levels of disability. [1][7]

Intended Population

The Quebec back pain disability scale has been developed for several populations of patients with various disability levels who suffer diseases such as acute LBP, chronic disabling pain, sacroiliac joint dysfunction, lumbar spinal stenosis, disc surgery, and posterior surgical decompression and settings. (level of evidence: 2) [2]

The QBPDS is a useful instrument when someone wants to get an overall impression on the improvement in Pelvic girdle pain. (level of evidence: 2B) [8]

Method of Use

Patients are asked to answer the QBPDS according to the difficulty they have to perform the activities the current day. The QBPDS examines how the lower back pain affects your daily life. It is very important that the patient gives a score for every activity; it is not allowed to skip an activity. (level of evidence: 2A) [2]

The scoring is done by count every digit, circled by the patient. The end score will be between 0 (no limitation) and 100 (totally limited). [4] [2]

It is a very easy questionnaire and takes only five minutes. The QBPDS can be completed by patients by using paper and pen, mail or telephone. [4]

Evidence

The evidence has been extensively examined. (Grade of recommendation: B) [4]

Reliability

The ICC is 0,55 (95% CI = 0,20-0,78) in acute occupational low back pain over a period of four weeks. [1] There is a high internal consistency for the 6-point Likert-scale in other languages (Chronbach's a > 0,90). Davidson and Keating examined the test-retest reliability at patients with low back pain who reported no change during six weeks. They found an ICC of 0,85 ([95% CI] 0,73-0,91). This margin of detection is lower in chronic low back pain patients compared with acute low back pain patients. For patients older than 62 years, who suffer acute low back pain, an ICC of 0,94 and a minimal detectable change of 11,04 over a period of 11 days is established. [2] The English, French and Dutch versions have a good test–retest reliability. (Grade of recommendation: B) [9]

Validity

Construct validity: Construct validity investigates whether the correct variables were measured in relation to the predefined variables. The Quebec back pain disability scale is able to distinguish the difference between patients' disability level and the self-rated health. (Grade of recommendation: B) [2]

The construct validity of the English, French and Dutch version is good. (Grade of recommendation: B) [9]

- Internal construct validity: Kopec, the author of the Quebec back pain disability scale, found an inter-item correlation (r) between 0,24 and 0,87 (a relatively high correlation) and an item-total correlation (r) ranged from 0,59 to 0,86 (a relatively very high correlation). The research, after Kopec's results were published, reported an inter-item correlation lower than 0,80. (Grade of recommendation: B) [2]
  - External construct/convergent validity: There is a moderate to strong correlation between the Quebec back pain disability scale (QBPDS) and other disability questionnaires (Grade of recommendation: B):
  - QBPDS and Roland-Morris disability questionnaire: r = 0,77-0,81
  - QBPDS and Oswestry disability index: r = 0,80- 0,83
  - QBPDS and physical function subscale of SF-36: r =0,67- 0,77 [4]

The correlation between the QBPDS and pain (r=0,54-0,74), psychosocial variables and direct measures of physical function is weak to moderate. (Grade of recommendation: A) [2][4]

Content and face validity: The questionnaire contains various domains of activities which patients and care providers deem important. Because of this and the good measurement properties, the content and face validity is good. (Grade of recommendation: B) [2]

Responsiveness

The responsiveness of the QBPDS is similar to the responsiveness of the Roland-Morris disability questionnaire, modified Oswestry disability questionnaire, Waddell disability index and the physical function subscale of SF-36. (Grade of recommendation: C) [10]

The QBPDS is highly sensitive to change for the score of the individual domains as for the total score (SRM= 0,80 and effect size= 0,62). [11] In addition, the scale is able to recognize small changes in level of disability over time. (Grade of recommendation: B) [2] Davidson and Keating found a minimal detectable change of 19 (95% CI 14-24) at patients with low back pain who reported no change during six weeks. For patients with chronic low back pain is the minimal detectable change 15,8. (Grade of recommendation: B) [2]

The area under the curve (AUC) can be used as a quantitative method to differ patients who improved or deteriorated from the patients who stayed stable. [1] The AUC for the detection of change in patients with chronic low back pain is 0,856. This means that in 85,60 % of the cases the test correctly recognize a change in chronic low back pain. (Grade of recommendation: B) [2]

Miscellaneous

The patients and the clinicians both accept the use of the QBPDS. Researchers (Kopec et al.) declare a low item default (range 0,7-1,8%) [12]. Questionnaires sent by mail had a higher rate of incomplete questionnaires (10.8%). Some patients remarked that a couple of items were not precise enough and the choice between score 0 and 1 and between 4 and 5 wasn't always convenient. The researchers didn't found ceiling or floor effects in the answers. (Grade of recommendation: B) [2]

References

1. J.M. Fritz, J. J Irrgang. A Comparison of a Modified Oswestry Low Back Pain Disability Questionnaire and the Quebec Back Pain Disability Scale. Physical Therapy 2001; 81: 776-788. (level of evidence: 2B)

2. R. Smeets et al. Measures of Function in Low Back Pain/Disorders. Arthritis Care & Research 2011; 63: 158–173 (level of evidence: 2A)
3. L. EM Schoppink et al. Reliability and Validity of the Dutch Adaptation of the Quebec Back Pain Disability Scale. Physical Therapy 1996; 76:268-275. (level of evidence: 2B)
4. P. Calmels et al. Analyse de la littérature: Outils de mesure des paramètres fonctionnels dans la lombalgie (Low back pain disability assessment tools). Annales de réadaptation et de médecine physique 2005; 48: 288–297 (level of evidence: 2A)
5. J.A.Kopec et al. The quebec back pain disability scale: conceptualization and development. Clin Epidemiol 1996; 49(2): 151-161 (level of evidence: 2B)
6. P. Calmels et al. Analyse de la littérature: Outils de mesure des paramètres fonctionnels dans la lombalgie (Low back pain disability assessment tools). Annales de réadaptation et de médecine physique 2005; 48: 288–297 (level of evidence: 2A)
7. L. EM Schoppink et al. Reliability and Validity of the Dutch Adaptation of the Quebec Back Pain Disability Scale. Physical Therapy 1996; 76:268-275. (level of evidence: 2B)
8. A. Vleeming et al. European guidelines for the diagnosis and treatment of pelvic girdle pain. Spine 2008; 17: 794-819 (level of evidence: 2B)
9. M. L. Peters et al. The joint contribution of physical pathology, pain-related fear and catastrophizing to chronic back pain disability. Pain 2005; 113, 45-50 (level of evidence 2B)
10. M. Davidsnon et al. A Comparison of Five Low Back Disability Questionnaires: Reliability and Responsiveness. Physical therapy 2002; 82(1):8-24 (level of evidence: 2B)
11. F. Wilhelm et al. Sensitivity to change of the Quebec Back Pain Disability Scale and the Dallas Pain Questionnaire. Annals of Physical and Rehabilitation Medicine 2010; 53: 15–23 (level of evidence: 2B)
12. J.A.Kopec et al. The quebec back pain disability scale: conceptualization and development. Clin Epidemiol 1996; 49(2): 151-161 (level of evidence: 2B

Quebec Back Pain Disability Scale

This questionnaire is about the way your back pain is affecting your daily life. People with back problems may find it difficult to perform some of their daily activities. We would like to know if you find it difficult to perform any of the activities listed below, because of your back. For each activity there is a scale of 0 to 5. Please choose one response option for each activity (do not skip any activities) and circle the corresponding number. Today, do you find it difficult to perform the following activities because of your back?

		0 Not difficult at all	1 Minimally difficult	2 Somewhat difficult	3 Fairly difficult	4 Very difficult	5 Unable to do
1	Get out of bed	0	1	2	3	4	5
2	Sleep through the night	0	1	2	3	4	5
3	Turn over in bed	0	1	2	3	4	5
4	Ride in a car	0	1	2	3	4	5
5	Stand up for 20-30 minutes	0	1	2	3	4	5
6	Sit in a chair for several hours	0	1	2	3	4	5
7	Climb one flight of stairs	0	1	2	3	4	5
8	Walk a few blocks (300-400 m)	0	1	2	3	4	5
9	Walk several kilometers	0	1	2	3	4	5
10	Reach up to high shelves	0	1	2	3	4	5

11	Throw a ball	0	1	2	3	4	5
12	Run one block (about 100m)	0	1	2	3	4	5
13	Take food out of the refrigerator	0	1	2	3	4	5
14	Make your bed	0	1	2	3	4	5
15	Put on socks	0	1	2	3	4	5
16	Bend over to clean the bathtub	0	1	2	3	4	5
17	Move a chair	0	1	2	3	4	5
18	Pull or push heavy doors	0	1	2	3	4	5
19	Carry two bags of groceries	0	1	2	3	4	5
20	Lift and carry a heavy suitcase	0	1	2	3	4	5

Scoring instructions : The patient is instructed to answer each question on a scale. Add up the selected numbers for a total score.

Interpretation of scores : The minimum score is 20 and the maximum score is 100. Higher scores correlate to greater disability. % of maximal disability = (score) – 20) / 80 * 100% Minimum detectable change (90% confidence) 15 points.

Source: Kopec JA, Esdaile JM, Abrahamowicz M, Abenhaim L, Wood-Dauphinee S, Lamping DL, et al. The Quebec Back Pain Disability Scale. Measurement properties. Spine. 1995 Feb 1;20(3):341-52.

❑❑❑

160 Rancho Los Amigos Level of Cognitive Functioning Scale

Introduction

The Rancho Los Amigos Scale (RLAS), also known as the Ranchos Scale describes the cognitive and behavioral patterns found in brain injury patients as they recover from injury. It was originally developed by the head injury team at the Rancho Los Amigos Hospital in Downey, California to assess patients emerging from a coma. The original scale consisted of eight levels and later on, was revised and is known as the Rancho Los Amigos Revised Scale (RLAS-R). [1] The scale was developed based on assumption that observation of the type, nature, and quality of the patient's behavioral responses can be used to estimate the cognitive level at which the patient is functioning. [2]

The RLAS originally had 8 levels, while the revision added levels 9 and 10 to better reflect the highest levels of recovery. The original levels and the revised levels of the RLAS-R levels were dichotomized into two categories:

- Inferior functioning (RLAS-R 1–8) and
- Superior functioning (RLAS-R 9-10) [3]

Objective

- Used to understand a brain injury patient's abilities, impairments, and prognosis better, as they move through the stages of recovery.
- Facilitates communication among treating healthcare professionals and aids in treatment planning [2][3]

Intended Population

- Brain Injury [2]

Method of Use [1][2]

In the Ranchos Los Amigos Scale, each level is presented as a behavioral description in narrative form and the rater must decide which level best describes the patient's present behaviors. Different levels are given below:

Level I: No Response: Total Assistance

- No response to external stimuli

Level II: Generalized Response: Total Assistance

- Responds inconsistently and non-purposefully to external stimuli
- Responses are often the same regardless of the stimulus

Level III: Localized Response: Total Assistance

- Responds inconsistently and specifically to external stimuli
- Responses are directly related to the stimulus, for example, patient withdraws or vocalizes to painful stimuli
- Responds more to familiar people (friends and family) versus strangers

Level IV: Confused/Agitated: Maximal Assistance

- The individual is in a hyperactive state with bizarre and non-purposeful behavior
- Demonstrates agitated behavior that originates more from internal confusion than the external environment
- Absent short-term memory

Level V: Confused, Inappropriate Non-Agitated: Maximal Assistance

- Shows increase in consistency with following and responding to simple commands
- Responses are non-purposeful and random to more complex commands
- Behavior and verbalization is often inappropriate, and individual appears confused and often confabulates
- If action or tasks is demonstrated individual can perform but does not initiate tasks on own
- Memory is severely impaired and learning new information is difficult
- Different from level IV in that individual does not demonstrate agitation to internal stimuli. However, they can show agitation to unpleasant external stimuli.

Level VI: Confused, Appropriate: Moderate Assistance

- Able to follow simple commands consistently
- Able to retain learning for familiar tasks they performed pre-injury (brushing teeth, washing face) however unable to retain learning for new tasks
- Demonstrates increased awareness of self, situation, and environment but unaware of specific impairments and safety concerns
- Responses may be incorrect secondary to memory impairments but appropriate to the situation

Level VII: Automatic, Appropriate: Minimal Assistance for Daily Living Skills

- Oriented in familiar settings
- Able to perform
- Daily routine automatically with minimal to absent confusion
- Demonstrates carry over for new tasks and learning in addition to familiar tasks
- Superficially aware of one's diagnosis but unaware of specific impairments
- Continues to demonstrate lack of insight, decreased judgment and safety awareness
- Beginning to show interest in social and recreational activities in structured settings
- Requires at least minimal supervision for learning and safety purposes.

Level VIII: Purposeful, Appropriate: Stand By Assistance

- Consistently oriented to person, place and time
- Independently carries out familiar tasks in a non-distracting environment
- Beginning to show awareness of specific impairments and how they interfere with tasks, however, requires standing by assistance to compensate
- Able to use assistive memory devices to recall daily schedule
- Acknowledges other's emotional states and requires only minimal assistance to respond appropriately
- Demonstrates improvement of memory and ability to consolidate the past and future events
- Often depressed, irritable and with low frustration threshold

Level IX: Purposeful, Appropriate: Stand By Assistance on Request

- Able to shift between different tasks and complete them independently
- Aware of and acknowledges impairments when they interfere with tasks and able to use compensatory strategies to cope
- Unable to independently anticipate obstacles that may arise secondary to impairment
- With assistance able to think about consequences of actions and decisions
- Acknowledges the emotional needs of others with stand by-assistance.
- Continues to demonstrate depression and low frustration threshold

Level X: Purposeful, Appropriate: Modified Independent

- Able to multitask in many different environments with extra time or devices to assist
- Able to create own methods and tools for memory retention
- Independently anticipates obstacles that may occur as a result of impairments and take corrective actions

- Able to independently make decisions and act appropriately but may require more time or compensatory strategies
- Demonstrate intermittent periods of depression and low frustration threshold when under stress
- Able to appropriately interact with others in social situations

Psychometric Properties

- Interrater reliabilities ranging from 0.87 to 0.94 and test re-test reliability of 0.82.[2]
- Concurrent validity with the Stover Zeiger scale was 0.92[2]
- Predictive validity from admission to discharge 0.57 to 0.68[2]

References

1. Lin K, Dulebohn SC. Ranchos Los Amigos. Available from : https://www.ncbi.nlm.nih.gov/books/NBK448151/
2. Flannery J, Abraham I. Psychometric properties of a cognitive functioning scale for patients with traumatic brain injury. Western journal of nursing research. 1993 Aug;15(4):465-82. available from: https://journals.sagepub.com/doi/10.1177/019394599301500406
3. Stenberg M, Godbolt AK, Nygren De Boussard C, Levi R, Stålnacke BM. Cognitive impairment after severe traumatic brain injury, clinical course and impact on outcome: a Swedish-Icelandic study. Behavioural neurology. 2015;2015.

❑❑❑

161 Revised Hammersmith Scale (RHS) for Spinal Muscular Atrophy

Objective

The Revised Hammersmith Scale (RHS) is specifically designed outcome measure for people affected by Spinal Muscular Atrophy (SMA)[1] . The Hammersmith Functional Motor Scale (HFMS), was the first outcome measure designed to capture physical abilities in patients with SMA type 2 and 3[2]. An expanded version of the scale was published to be used for patients who were ambulant and it was named the Hammersmith Functional Motor Scale Expanded (HFMSE)[3]. In recent years specialist from all over the world who are working with patients with SMA collaborated together to develop a much better scale by using Rasch analysis. The new scale was called RHS and it provides a more sensitive description of SMA phenotype and progression of the disease.

Intended Population

The RHS was developed to evaluate the broad spectrum of motor functions in patients with SMA. It detects changes for very weak SMA type 2 to very strong SMA type 3. With some of the new pharmaceutical approaches which show great improvements in the weaker end of the spectrum, now there are even children with type 1 who show enough skills in order to pick up points on the scale.

Method of Use

The RHS is an ordinal scale which consists of 33 items with grades of 0,1 and 2. For individuals who can achieve the task without any compensation, it is given a score of 2. For those who only attempt the movement or finish it with some form of compensation is scored 1 and sore of 0 are given when patients are unable to perform any part of the item.

Evidence

The Revised Hammersmith Scale has been performed on 138 subjects before and it showed a very good fit for all of the items[1]. However, it should be noted that the scale is designed to capture a population with a broad spectrum of physical abilities including both ambulant and non-ambulant patients with SMA.

Reliability

The reliability is reported as good with a high Person Separation Index (PSI) of 0.98 and a minimum ceiling effect.

Validity

The RHS has been correlated with the WHO motor milestones showing that the scale captures progressively more difficult motor abilities. Thus, the scale is deemed to possess an established concurrent validity. The RHS also demonstrated discriminative groups validity by distinguishing between SMA type, ambulant status and current WHO functional score.

References

1. Ramsey D, Scoto M, Mayhew A, Main M, Mazzone ES, Montes J, et al. (2017) Revised Hammersmith Scale for spinal muscular atrophy: A SMA specific clinical outcome assessment tool. PLoS ONE 12(2): e0172346. doi:10.1371/journal.pone.0172346
2. Main M, Kairon H, Mercuri E, Muntoni F. The Hammersmith Functional Motor Scale for Children with Spinal Muscular Atrophy: a Scale to Test Ability and Monitor Progress in Children with Limited Ambulation. European Journal of Paediatric Neurology. 2003;7(4):155–9. pmid:12865054

3. O'Hagen JM, Glanzman AM, McDermott MP, Ryan PA, Flickinger J, Quigley J, et al. An expanded version of the Hammersmith Functional Motor Scale for SMA II and III patients. Neuromuscular disorders: NMD. 2007;17(9–10):693–7. Epub 2007/07/31. pmid:1765825

Revised Hammersmith Scale (RHS) for Spinal Muscular Atrophy

Name SMA Type DOB Assessor

Date of assessment Albuterol/Salbutamol Y / N Date of spinal surgery

Please circle highest current level of independent mobility:

None Rolls Bottom shuffles Crawls Walks with KAFO's / AFO's Walks with crutches / frame Independent walking

Comment...

LBC = Limited by contracture *WHO separate scoring at end of RHS

	Test	Instruction	2	1	0	LBC	Comments	RHS Score
SIT-TING	**1* Sitting Using plinth / floor. (Back / feet unsupported)**	Can you sit on the plinth/ chair without using your hands for support for a count of 3?	Sitting unsupported: Ring or 90/90	Maintains seated position via propping with hand/s: Ring or 90/90	Unable to sit		WHO 1* Long sitting	
	2 Hands to head in sitting	Can you show me how you get your hand/ hands to your head? (hands touch head above level of ears/ eyebrows)	Able to bring both hands to head at same time – arms free from side without flexing head or trunk	Able to bring one hand to head – arms free from side without flexing head or trunk c R c L	c Using compensations – flexing head & trunk or "crawling" hand/s c Unable to bring hand to head		Sitting position described: c 90/90 c Ring c Long	
	3 Sitting to lying	Can you lie down in a controlled/ safe way from sitting?	Able to lie down through side lying or using clothes in a controlled/ safe way	Able to lie down by going forwards and rolling sideways, or through prone in a controlled/safe way	Unable or completes in uncontrolled/ unsafe way			

supine	**4 Adduction from crook (hook) lying – supine hips @ 45°, knees @ 90°, feet hip width apart. Passively abduct leg**	Can you bring your leg back to the middle and hold this position for a count of 3?	Able to adduct to bring 1 leg back to neutral	Holds crook lying position for a count of 3	Unable to maintain/ achieve starting position.		c R c L	
	5 Right hip flexion in supine	Can you bring your right knee to your chest? Try to go as far as you can	Full hip flexion achieved	Initiates right hip and knee flexion (>10% of available range of motion)	Unable		flexion contracture > 15 ° present? Hip Y c N c Knee Y c N χ	
	6 Left hip flexion in supine	Can you bring your left knee to your chest? Try to go as far as you can	Full hip flexion achieved	Initiates left hip and knee flexion (>10% of available range of motion)	Unable		flexion contracture > 15 ° present? Hip Y c N c Knee Y c N χ	
	7 Lifts head from supine	Can you lift your head to look at your toes keeping your arms folded for a count of 3?	Can lift head up through neck flexion and holds for a count of 3	c Can lift head with compensatory movements for a count of 3 c Can lift head up momentarily through neck flexion (< a count of 3)	Unable			

ROLL-ING	**8 Supine to side-lying (end position leading leg ends up on top of other)**	Can you roll onto your side? Note: Onto side = shoulders perpendicular to floor, trunk and hips in line with body		Able to roll onto side	Unable to roll onto side in any direction		c R c L	
	9 Rolls supine to prone	Can you roll from your back to your tummy? Try not to use your arms	Rolls fully into prone without pulling/ pushing on arms	Rolls fully into prone by pulling/pushing on arms	Unable to roll into prone in any direction. Does not initiate or complete		c R c L	
prone	**10 Lifting head from prone**	Can you lift your head up keeping your arms by your side for a count of 3	Lifts straight up, arms down by sides for a count of 3	Lifts straight up arms forward for a count of 3	Unable or lifts less than a count of 3			
	11 Prone; prop on forearms	Can you prop yourself on your fore-arms with your head up (not holding your head) For a count of 3	Achieves position and holds head up independently for a count of 3	Maintains position with head supported on hands for a count of 3	Unable or holds for less than a count of 3			
	12* Four-point kneeling/ crawling	Can you get onto your hands and knees and then crawl?	Crawls moving all 4 limbs at least 2 times in a row	Achieves four-point kneeling	Unable		WHO 2*	
ROLL-ING	**13 Rolls prone to supine**	Can you roll from your tummy to your back? Try not to use your arms	Rolls fully into supine without pulling/ pushing on arms	Rolls fully into supine by pulling/pushing on arms	Unable to roll into supine in any direction. Does not initiate or complete		c R c L	

SIT-TING	**14 Lying to sitting**	Can you get from lying (supine) to sitting?	Able via supine / side lying using: c 1 hand c 2 hands	Able by using strategies: c Turns into prone or towards floor c Utilises momentum/ pulls on both legs	Unable			
	15 Sit to Stand (Starting in a 90/90 position using a Plinth / Bench / Chair)	Can you stand up from the chair / bench keeping your arms folded if you can?	Able to stand up without using arms (keeping arms folded, feet do not move)	Stands by using strategies: (circle relevant) Uses hands on legs/chair Turns Prone / Widens Base	Unable			
Standing	**16* Cruising/ supported stand**	Can you walk holding on around furniture?	Cruise at least 5 steps around furniture c R c L	Stands supported for a count of 3	Unable to stand supported		WHO 3 & 4*	
	17* Standing	Can you stand without holding onto anything for a count of 3?	Stands upright and symmetrically, without compensation for a count of 3	Stands but with some degree of compensation for a count of 3	Cannot stand independently, needs support		WHO 5*	
RUN / WALK	**18* Walking**	Can you walk without using any help or aids? Show me	Takes at least 5 steps unaided	Able to take < 5 steps unaided	Unable		WHO 6	
	19 Runs 10m	Can you go as quickly and safely as you can to......(give 10 m marker) "Ready steady GO"	Can run - both feet off the ground	Speeds up walk but always maintains one foot on the floor	c Walks with no extra speed c Only with aids c Unable		TIME:........ seconds	

STAND-ING	**20 Squat down and up**	Can you squat down and stand up again? Pretend you are going to sit on a very low seat - only go as far down as you are able to get up from on your own	Full squat down (without using hands) and up* (with/ without using hands) At least 90° achieved at knees/ hips *must be able to get up from final range	initiates squat in both knees (10° to <90°) with controlled movement +/- using hands on self c Using hands	Unable			
	21 Stand to sit on floor	Can you sit on the floor in a controlled/ safe way from standing? Try not to use your arms	Can you sit on the floor in a con-trolled/ safe way from standing? Try not to use your arms	Sits on floor using hands on floor/body	c Uses furniture c Unable			
MAT	**22 High kneeling**	Can you kneel like this (high kneeling) for a count of 10?	Maintains high kneeling without holding on for a count of 10	Maintains high kneel with one arm sup-port for a count of 10	Unable			
	23 High Kneeling to Right half kneel	Can you bring your LEFT leg up so that your foot is flat on the ground without using your arms and hold for a count of 10?	Able to achieve and maintain posi-tion without arm support for a count of 10	Maintains half kneel with one arm sup-port for a count of 10 With: c support c no support	Unable			
	24 High Kneeling to Left half kneel	Can you bring your RIGHT leg up so that your foot is flat on the ground without using your arms and hold for a count of 10?	Able to achieve and maintain posi-tion without arm support for a count of 10	Maintains half kneel with one arm sup-port for a count of 10 With: c support c no support	Unable			

MAT / FLOOR	**25 Rise from floor**	Can you get up from the floor using as little support as possible and as fast as you can? Stand up as quickly as possible when the instruction "GO" is given	Achieves rise from floor without hands (any unsup-ported method)	Able to get up from floor using hands on floor and/or body	c Able to get up from floor using furniture/ assistance c Unable to get up from floor using any method		If uses ½ kneel: c R (L foot forwards) c L (R foot forwards) Further detail: TIME:.......... seconds	
SINGLE LEG STAND	**26 Stand on one leg – Right**	Can you stand on your right leg for a count of 3?	Able to stand in a relaxed man-ner (no fixation) for a count of 3	Stands but either momentarily or needs a lot of fixation e.g. by knees tightly adducted or other trick	Unable			
	27 Stand on one leg – Left	Can you stand on your left leg for a count of 3?	Able to stand in a relaxed man-ner (no fixation) for a count of 3	Stands but either momentarily or needs a lot of fixation e.g. by knees tightly adducted or other trick	Unable			
	28 Hops – Right	Can you hop on your right leg?		Distinct hop: clears forefoot and heel off floor	Unable			
	29 Hops – Lef	Can you hop on your left leg?		Distinct hop: clears forefoot and heel off floor	Unable			

STAIRS	**30 Ascend stairs 4 standard stairs**	Can you walk up the steps? If support is needed you may only use one rail (can use two hands to one rail)	indepen-dently (without sup-port/rail) ascends using alternating pattern	c Alternating pattern with one sup-port (one rail/hand on body) c Marking time with/without support	Unable			
	31 Descend stairs 4 standard stairs	Can you walk down the steps? If support is needed you may only use one rail (can use two hands to one rail)	Indepen-dently (without sup-port/rail) descends using alternating pattern	c Alternating pattern with one sup-port (one rail/hand on body) c Marking time with/without support	Unable			
STEP	**32 Climbs box step – Right**	Can you step onto the top of the box using your right leg first?	Faces for-wards, climbs up – no support needed	Goes up side-ways or needs support	Unable			
	33 Descends box step – Right	Can you step down from the box using your right leg first?	Faces for-ward, climbs down controlling weight bearing leg. No support needed	Goes down sideways or skips down or needs support	Unable			
	34 Climbs box step – Left	Can you step onto the top of the box using your left leg first?	Faces for-wards, climbs up – no support needed	Goes up side-ways or needs support	Unable			
	35 Descends box step - Left	Can you step down from the box using your left leg first?	Faces for-ward, climbs down controlling weight bearing leg. No support needed	Goes down sideways or skips down or needs support	Unable			

JUMP	36 Jump forwards 30cm (12"	Can you jump as far as you can, with both feet, from this line all of the way to the other line?	Jumps forward and lands with two feet simultaneously moving forward at least 30cm (12")	c Jumps with two feet simultaneously but lands one at a time moving forward/up travelling < 30cm (12") c Jumps and lands with two feet simultaneously moving forward < 30cm (12")	Unable to initiate jump			
			2's =	1's =	0's =		Total =	/69

*WHO DEVELOPMENTAL MILESTONES	Qualifier met:	
	Yes	**No**
W1. Sitting without support: Child sits upright with head erect for at least 10 seconds. Child does not use arms or hands to balance body or support position.		
W2. Hands and knees crawling: Child alternately moves forward or backward on hands and knees. The stomach does not touch the supporting surface. There are continuous and consecutive movement, at least 3 in a row.		
W3. Standing with Assistance: Child stands in upright position on both feet, holding onto a stable object (e.g. furniture) with both hands without leaning on it. The body does not touch the stable object, and the legs support most of the body weight. Child thus stands with assistance for at least 10 seconds.		
W4. Walking with Assistance: Child is in upright position with the back straight. Child makes sideways or forward steps by holding onto a stable object (e.g. furniture) with one or both hands. One leg moves forward while the other supports part of the body weight. Child takes at least 5 steps in this manner.		
W5. Standing Alone: Child stands in upright position on both feet (not the toes) with the back straight. The legs support 100% of the child's weight. There is no contact with a person or object. Child stands alone for at least 10 seconds.		
W6. Walking Alone: Child takes at least 5 steps independently in upright position with the back straight. One leg moves forward while the other supports most of the body weight. There is no contact with the person or object.		
Total WHO Milestones Achieved:	/ 6	

Revised Hammersmith Scale for SMA (RHS) " **Date**

Is this test a true reflection of the subjects ability Y c N c If no please detail why

Comments on Assessment

162 Richmond Agitation-Sedation Scale (RASS)

Introduction

The Richmond Agitation Sedation Scale (RASS) is an instrument designed to assess the level of alertness and agitated behavior in critically-ill patients.[1]

Purpose

The scale was developed by a team of critical care physicians, nurses, and pharmacists with the aim of achieving the following:[1][2]

1. Establish simple and discrete criteria for assessing arousal and agitation;
2. Guide sedation therapy to better meet patients' titration needs; and
3. Improve communication regarding sedation and agitation among healthcare providers.

Structure

The RASS is a 10-point scale ranging from -5 to +4.[1] Levels -1 to -5 denote 5 levels of sedation, starting with "awakens to voice" and ending with "unarousable." Levels +1 to +4 describe increasing levels of agitation. The lowest level of agitation starts with apprehension and anxiety, and peaks at combative and violent. RASS level 0 is "alert and calm." The full scale can be found below:[1]

Richmond Agitation and Sedation Scale

Rass Score	Description
+4	Combative, violet, danger to staff
+3	Pulls or removes tube(s) or catheters; aggressive
+2	Frequent nonpurposeful movement, fights ventilator
+1	Anxious, apprehensive, but not aggressive
0	Alert and calm
-1	Awakens to voice (eye opening/contact) > 10 seconds
-2	Light sedation; briefly awakens to voice (eye opening/contant) < 10 seconds
-3	Moderate sedation; movement or eye opening. No eye contact
-4	Deep sedation; no response to voice, but movement or eye opening to physical stimulation
-5	Unarousable; no response to voice or physical stimulation

Indications

The RASS is mostly applied in mechanically-ventilated patients, but may be used for any individual who is hospitalized.[3] Regular administration and assessment is particularly useful for patients who are critically-ill, are receiving sedative medications, and/or demonstrate fluctuating levels of consciousness.

Procedure

The RASS can be administered in a little as 30-60 seconds.[1] Scoring is based on observation, and response to auditory and physical stimulation. Sessler et al.[1] describe the testing procedure as follows:

Test Procedure and Scoring Instructions

1. Observe patient. Is the patient alert and calm? (score 0)
   a. Does patient have behavior that is consistent with restlessness or agitation? (score +1 to +4 using level criteria)
2. If patient is not alert, in a loud speaking voice state patient's name and direct patient to open eyes and look at speaker. Repeat once if necessary. Can prompt patient to continue looking at speaker.
   a. Patient has eye opening and eye contact, which is sustained for more than 10 seconds (score −1).
   b. Patient has eye opening and eye contact, but this is not sustained for 10 seconds (score −2).
   c. Patient has any movement in response to voice, excluding eye contact (score −3).
3. If patient does not respond to voice, physically stimulate patient by shaking shoulder and then rubbing sternum if there is no response to shaking shoulder.
   a. Patient has any movement to physical stimulation (score −4). b. Patient has no response to voice or physical stimulation (score −5).

Scoring and Interpretation

RASS scoring and interpretation should be based on the sedation protocol being used. For minimal sedation protocols (RASS -2 to 0), sedation should be modified or decreased for a RASS score of -3 or less.[3] Scores of 2 to 4 may indicate under-sedation. At minimum, the patient should be assessed for pain, delirium, and anxiety. In addition, other underlying causes of agitation should be investigated and treated as appropriate.

In select cases, a deep sedation protocol (RASS -4 and -5) may be used.[3] For scores of -3 or higher, sedation should be modified to achieve the desired range.

Psychometric information

The RASS demonstrates strong validity and reliability across a range of critical care populations.[1][4][5][6][7][8][9] Inter-rater reliability has been found to be good to excellent in adult ICU patients on surgical, medical, coronary, cardiac surgery, and neuroscience ICUs.[1][4][5][6][7][9] This includes patients with and without mechanical ventilation and sedative medications. Although most studies were conducted in the United States, inter-rater reliability remained high in Swedish[7] and Portuguese[6] ICU settings as well.

In adult ICU patients in the U.S., the RASS demonstrates good criterion,[4] construct,[1][4] and face validity.[4] Kerson et al.[10] also found high criterion validity in critically-ill children.

Strengths

The RASS has many advantages compared to other sedation-agitation scales. Aside from strong inter-rater reliability[5][7] and ease of administration, use of the RASS improves discrimination between different levels of mild to moderate sedation (+1 to -4).[1] Moreover, the scale is applicable to multiple disciplines, has been heavily studied, and is referenced as a key assessment tool for clinical guidelines related to pain, agitation, and delirium.[11]

Limitations

In patients with severe auditory and visual deficits, the RASS is not a suitable instrument for assessing arousal and agitation.[1] Although the scale is well-researched in the U.S., studies assessing validity and reliability are limited in other geographical locations and languages other than English.

Physical Therapy Implications

For physical therapy clinicians, the RASS can be used to streamline communication regarding sedation and agitation with other healthcare providers. Resulting scores can guide decision making regarding the appropriateness of physical therapy intervention, and treatment priority. The RASS may also identify patients in need of further assessment and management for pain, agitation, and delirium.

References

1. Sessler CN, Gosnell MS, Grap MJ, Brophy GM, O'Neal PV, Keane KA, Tesoro EP, Elswick RK. The Richmond Agitation–Sedation Scale: validity and reliability in adult intensive care unit patients. American journal of respiratory and critical care medicine. 2002 Nov 15;166(10):1338-44.
2. Khan BA, Guzman O, Campbell NL, Walroth

T, Tricker JL, Hui SL, Perkins A, Zawahiri M, Buckley JD, Farber MO, Ely EW. Comparison and agreement between the Richmond Agitation-Sedation Scale and the Riker Sedation-Agitation Scale in evaluating patients' eligibility for delirium assessment in the ICU. Chest. 2012 Jul 1;142(1):48-54.

3. Richmond Agitation-Sedation Scale. Accessed July 5, 2020: https://www.mdcalc.com/richmond-agitation-sedation-scale-rass
4. Ely EW, Truman B, Shintani A, Thomason JW, Wheeler AP, Gordon S, Francis J, Speroff T, Gautam S, Margolin R, Sessler CN. Monitoring sedation status over time in ICU patients: reliability and validity of the Richmond Agitation-Sedation Scale (RASS). Jama. 2003 Jun 11;289(22):2983-91.
5. Rasheed AM, Amirah MF, Abdallah M, Parameaswari PJ, Issa M, Alharthy A. Ramsay sedation scale and richmond agitation sedation scale: A Cross-sectional study. Dimensions of Critical Care Nursing. 2019 Mar 1;38(2):90-5.
6. Almgren M, Lundmark M, Samuelson K. The Richmond Agitation-Sedation Scale: translation and reliability testing in a Swedish intensive care unit. Acta anaesthesiologica scandinavica. 2010 Jul;54(6):729-35.
7. Nassar Junior AP, Pires Neto RC, Figueiredo WB, Park M. Validity, reliability and applicability of Portuguese versions of sedation-agitation scales among critically ill patients. Sao Paulo Medical Journal. 2008 Jul;126(4):215-9.
8. Benítez-Rosario MA, Castillo-Padrós M, Garrido-Bernet B, González-Guillermo T, Martínez-Castillo LP, González A, Asocación Canaria de Cuidados Paliativos (CANPAL) Research Network. Appropriateness and reliability testing of the modified Richmond Agitation-Sedation Scale in Spanish patients with advanced cancer. Journal of pain and symptom management. 2013 Jun 1;45(6):1112-9.
9. Vasilevskis EE, Morandi A, Boehm L, Pandharipande PP, Girard TD, Jackson JC, Thompson JL, Shintani A, Gordon SM, Pun BT, Wesley Ely E. Delirium and sedation recognition using validated instruments: reliability of bedside intensive care unit nursing assessments from 2007 to 2010. Journal of the American geriatrics society. 2011 Nov;59:S249-55.
10. Kerson AG, DeMaria R, Mauer E, Joyce C, Gerber LM, Greenwald BM, Silver G, Traube C. Validity of the Richmond Agitation-Sedation Scale (RASS) in critically ill children. Journal of Intensive Care. 2016 Dec 1;4(1):65.
11. Devlin JW, Skrobik Y, Gélinas C, Needham DM, Slooter AJ, Pandharipande PP, Watson PL, Weinhouse GL, Nunnally ME, Rochwerg B, Balas MC. Clinical practice guidelines for the prevention and management of pain, agitation/sedation, delirium, immobility, and sleep disruption in adult patients in the ICU. Critical care medicine. 2018 Sep 1;46(9):e825-73.

❑❑❑

163

Rivermead Mobility Inde

Objective

The **Rivermead Mobility Index** assesses functional mobility in gait, balance and transfers after stroke

Intended Population

Those with a diagnosis of Stroke, Spinal Cord Injury, Acquired Brain Injury, Lower Limb Amputees

Method of Use

Description:

- The Rivermead Mobility Index is appropriate for a range of disabilities that include anything from being bedridden to being able to run

15 items:

- 14-self-reported items
- 1 direct observation item
- Items progress in difficulty
- Items are coded as either 0 or 1, depending on whether the patient can complete the task according to specific instructions
- Items receive a score of 0 for a "No" response and 1 for a "Yes" response
- Total scores are determined by summing the points for all items
- A maximum of 15 points is possible; higher scores indicate better mobility performance
- A score of "0" indicates an inability to perform any of the activities on the measure

Evidence

Reliability

Test-retest Reliability:

Chronic Stroke:

(Chen et al, 2007; Green, Foster & Young, 2001; n = 22; 1 year post-stroke, assessed twice, with one week between assessments) [1]

- Excellent overall test-retest reliability (ICC = 0.96)
- Excellent test-retest reliability for the following subcategories:

Kappa for turning in bed = 1.0

Kappa for walking inside without aid = 0.89

Kappa for walking outside on uneven ground = 0.83

Kappa for bathing = 0.81

Kappa for picking objects off the floor = 0.79

- Adequate test-retest reliability for the following subcategories:

Kappa for stairs = 0.68

Kappa for lying to sitting = 0.64

Kappa for sitting balance = 0.64

Kappa for transfers = 0.64

Kappa for walking up and down 4 steps = 0.67

Lower Limb Amputees:

(Ryall et al, 2003; n = 62; mean age = 56.8 (18.8) years; mean time post amputation: 4.9 (14.7) years) [2]

- Excellent test-retest reliability (ICC = 0.99)

Interrater/Intrarater Reliability:

Acute Stroke: (Hsueh et al, 2003; n = 57; mean age of 64.2 (11.5) years; assessed at 14, 30, 90, and 180 days post stroke; Taiwanese sample) [3]

- Excellent interrater reliability for total score (ICC = 0.92)
- Poor to excellent interrater reliability for individual subcategories (Weighted Kappa = 0.37 - 0.94)

Validity

Criterion Validity:

Acute Stroke:

(Hsieh et al, 2000; n = 38 inpatients; Sommerfeld & vo Arbin, 2001; n = 115 inpatients aged > 65; Hsueh et al, 2003) [4]

- Excellent predictive validity with Barthel Index 24 days post stroke (r = 0.77)
- RMI scores of > 4 best predictor of early discharge home

Lower Limb Amputees:

(Ryall et al, 2003) [5]

- Adequate concurrent validity with TWT (r = -0.58)
- Only one value is outside the 95% limits of agreement

Construct Validity:

Acute Stroke: (Hsueh et al, 2003) [6]

- Excellent correlation with BI at 14 days post stroke (r = 0.72)
- Excellent correlation with BI at 30 days post stroke (r = 0.88)
- Excellent correlation with BI at 90 days post stroke (r = 0.86)
- Excellent correlation with BI at 180 days post stroke (r = 0.88)

Lower Limb Amputees: (Franchignoni et al, 2003a, n = 140; mean age = 57 (18) years) [7]

- Excellent5elation with TWT (timed walking test) at end of prosthetic training (r = -0.70)

Content Validity:

Acute Stroke: (Hsieh et al, 2000) [8]

- Critical values for two indices, coefficient of reproducibility (> 0.9) and coefficient of scalability (> 0.7), were all exceeded

Lower limb amputees: (Franchignoni et al, 2003a) [9]

- Coefficient of reproducibility was exceeded and ranged from 0.71-1.0
- Coefficient of scalability was not exceeded and ranged from 0.38-0.62

Lower limb amputees: (Ryall et al, 2003) [10]

- Coefficient of reproducibility was exceeded and ranged from 0.91-0.94

Responsiveness

Acute Stroke: (Hsueh et al, 2003) [11]

Days Post Stoke	n	RMI	MRMI	STREAM	BI
14-30	51	1.14	1.31	1.17	1.51
30-90	43	0.86	0.83	0.95	1.07
90-180	43	0.24	0.20	0.40	0.35
14-90	43	1.67	1.56	1.61	2.09
14-180	43	1.94	1.53	1.65	2.01

Values reported as SRM (Standardized Response Mean)

RMI = Rivermead Mobility Index

MRMI = Modified Rivermead Mobility Index

STREAM = Mobility Subscale of the Stroke Rehabilitation Assessment of Movement

BI = Barthel Index

References

1. Chen, H. M., Hsieh, C. L., et al. "The test-retest reliability of 2 mobility performance tests in patients with chronic stroke." Neurorehabil Neural Repair 2007 21(4): 347-352
2. Ryall, N. H., Eyres, S. B., et al. "Is the Rivermead Mobility Index appropriate to measure mobility in lower limb amputees?" Disabil Rehabil 2003 25(3): 143-153
3. Hsueh, I. P., Wang, C. H., et al. "Comparison of psychometric properties of three mobility

measures for patients with stroke." Stroke 2003 34(7): 1741-1745

4. Hsieh, C. L., Hsueh, I. P., et al. "Validity and responsiveness of the rivermead mobility index in stroke patients." Scandinavian Journal of Rehabilitation Medicine 2000 32(3): 140-142
5. Ryall, N. H., Eyres, S. B., et al. "Is the Rivermead Mobility Index appropriate to measure mobility in lower limb amputees?" Disabil Rehabil 2003 25(3): 143-153
6. Hsueh, I. P., Wang, C. H., et al. "Comparison of psychometric properties of three mobility measures for patients with stroke." Stroke 2003 34(7): 1741-1745
7. Franchignoni, F., Brunelli, S., et al. "Is the Rivermead Mobility Index a suitable outcome measure in lower limb amputees?--A psychometric validation study." J Rehabil Med 2003 35(3): 141-144
8. Hsieh, C. L., Hsueh, I. P., et al. "Validity and responsiveness of the rivermead mobility index in stroke patients." Scandinavian Journal of Rehabilitation Medicine 2000 32(3): 140-142
9. Franchignoni, F., Brunelli, S., et al. "Is the Rivermead Mobility Index a suitable outcome measure in lower limb amputees?--A psychometric validation study." J Rehabil Med 2003 35(3): 141-144
10. Ryall, N. H., Eyres, S. B., et al. "Is the Rivermead Mobility Index appropriate to measure mobility in lower limb amputees?" Disabil Rehabil 2003 25(3): 143-153
11. Hsueh, I. P., Wang, C. H., et al. "Comparison of psychometric properties of three mobility measures for patients with stroke." Stroke 2003 34(7): 1741-1745

Rivermead Mobility Index

Score 0 = No 1 = Yes

1. Do you turn over from your back to your side without help?
2. From lying in bed, are you able to get up to sit on the edge of the bed on your own?
3. Could you sit on the edge of the bed without holding on for 10 seconds?
4. Can you (using hands and an aid if necessary) stand up froma chair in less than 15 seconds, and stand there for 15 seconds,
5. Observe patient standing for 10 seconds without any aid.
6. Are you able to move from bed to chair and back without any help?
7. Can you walk 10 metres with an aid if necessary but with no standby help?
8. Can you manage a flight of steps alone, without help?
9. Do you walk around outside alone, on pavements?
10. Can you walk 10 metres inside with no caliper, splint or aid and no standby help?
11. If you drop something on the floor, can you manage to walk 5 meters to pick it up and walk back?
12. Can you walk over uneven ground (grass, gravel, dirt, snow or ice) without help?
13. Can you get in and out of a shower or bath unsupervised, andwash yourself?
14. Are you able to climb up and down four steps with no rail but using an aid if necessary?
15. Could you run 10 metres in 4 seconds without limping? (A fast walk is acceptable.)

❑❑❑

164 Roland-Morris Disability Questionnaire

Objective

First published in 1983, the Roland-Morris Disability Questionnaire[1] is designed to assess self-rated physical disability caused by low back pain. [2]

Intended Population

The Roland-Morris Disability Questionnaire is most sensitive for patients with mild to moderate disability due to acute, sub-acute or chronic low back pain.

For patients with severe disability the Oswestry Disability Indexis recommended. [3]

Method of Use

There are different questionnaires available, which differ from each other in the number of statements: 24-, 18- and 11-item questionnaire. It has also been adapted across cultures and translated for use in different countries.

There are different questionnaires available, which differ from each other in the number of statements: 24-, 18- and 11-item questionnaire. The patient is asked to tick a statement when it applies to him that specific day, this makes it possible to follow changes in time. The end score is the sum of the ticked boxes. The score ranges from 0 (no disability) to 11, 18 or 24 (max. disability) depending on the questionnaire that is used. [2]

Questions

It can be administered face-to-face, electronically or over the phone. There are questionnaires in different languages, available online for free for clinicians to use via the website of the Roland Morris Disability Questionnaire.

1. I stay at home most of the time because of my back.
2. I change position frequently to try and get my back comfortable.
3. I walk more slowly than usual because of my back.
4. Because of my back I am not doing any of the jobs that I usually do around the house.
5. Because of my back, I use a handrail to get upstairs.
6. Because of my back, I lie down to rest more often.
7. Because of my back, I have to hold on to something to get out of an easy chair.
8. Because of my back, I try to get other people to do things for me.
9. I get dressed more slowly then usual because of my back.
10. I only stand for short periods of time because of my back.
11. Because of my back, I try not to bend or kneel down.
12. I find it difficult to get out of a chair because of my back.
14. My back is painful almost all the time.
15. I find it difficult to turn over in bed because of my back.
16. My appetite is not very good because of my back pain.
17. I have trouble putting on my socks (or stockings) because of the pain in my back.
18. I only walk short distances because of my back.
19. I sleep less well because of my back.
20. Because of my back pain, I get dressed with help from someone else.

21. I sit down for most of the day because of my back.
22. I avoid heavy jobs around the house because of my back.
23. Because of my back pain, I am more irritable and bad tempered with people than usual.
24. Because of my back, I go upstairs more slowly than usual.
25. I stay in bed most of the time because of my back.

Reliability

Macedo et al. (2011) looked at the results from different studies for the reliability for the 24-, 18- and 11-item RMDQ: [4]

- Test-retest reliability 24-item: intraclass correlation (ICC) ranges from 0.42 – 0.91
- Test-retest reliability 18-item Stratford: ICC ranges from 0.68 – 0.75
- Test-retest reliability 11-item: ICC ranges from 0.89

Validity

Content validity:

- The RMDQ is limited as it only covers specific physical problems, and not psychological or social problems. In case these problems should be investigated as well, other measuring of these functions is advised.[2]

Construct validity:[2]

- Construct validity defines the degree to which the test measures the variables it is supposed to measure.

The RMDQ correlates well with other tests which measure physical disability:

- Physical subscales of SF-36
- Physical subscales of Sickness Impact Profile
- Quebec Low Back Scale
- Oswestry Disability Questionnaire
- Pain ratings

Responsiveness

Internal responsiveness:[4]

- Internal responsiveness shows the ability of a test to measure differences in time.
- Using effect sizes:
  - 24-item: ranges from 0.63-0.71
  - 18-item Stratford: ranges from 0.73-0.82
  - 11-item: ranges from 0.61-0.69

External responsiveness:[4]

- External responsiveness gives the relation between the results measured with RMDQ and the results measured with the Global Perceived Effect Scale (GPE scale)
- Pearson correleation with GPE Scale:
  - 24-item: ranges from 0.45-0.54
  - 18-item Stratford: ranges from 0.44-0.53
  - 11-item: ranges from 0.39-0.49

References

1. Roland MO, Morris RW. A study of the natural history of back pain. Part 1: Development of a reliable and sensitive measure of disability in low back pain. Spine 1983; 8: 141-144
2. Roland M, Fairbank J. The Roland-Morris Disability Questionnaire and the Oswestry Disability Questionnaire. Spine 2000;25(24):3115-24
3. Davies CC, Nitz AJ.Psychometric properties of the Roland-Morris Disability Questionnaire compared to the Oswestry Disability Index: a systematic review. Physical Therapy Reviews, Volume 14, Number 6, December 2009 , pp. 399-408(10)
4. Macedo LG, Maher CG, Latimer J. Responsiveness of the 24-, 18- and 11-item versions of the Roland Morris Disability Questionnaire. Eur Spine J. 2011;20(3):458-63

❑❑❑

165 Romberg Test

Introduction

The Romberg test is an appropriate tool to diagnose sensory ataxia, a gait disturbance caused by abnormal proprioception involving information about the location of the joints. It is also proven to be sensitive and accurate means of measuring the degree of disequilibrium caused by central vertigo, peripheral vertigo and head trauma.[1] It has been used in clinic for 150 years [2]

Purpose

The Romberg test is used to demonstrate the effects of posterior column disease upon human upright postural control. Posterior column disease involves selective damaging of the posterior column, known as tabes dorsalis neurosyphilis. The Romberg test is used for the clinical assessment of patients with disequilibrium or ataxia from sensory and motor disorders.

Equilibrium is defined as any condition in which all acting forces are cancelled by each other resulting in a stable balanced system. It is maintained through the sensory information from vestibular, somatosensory and visual systems. A patient who has a problem with Proprioception (Somatosensory) can still maintain balance by compensating with vestibular function and vision. In the Romberg test, the patient stands upright and asked to close his eyes. A loss of balance is interpreted as a positive Romberg sign.

The Romberg test was first described in 1846 and was originally described for the condition tabes dorsalis. Before performing the Romberg test, it is necessary to test other aspects of the patient's balance when potential issues with ataxia or disequilibrium are present. Often, proprioceptive challenges are not the first problems faced by this population. Sometimes, it is more simple. It is important to first assess other aspects of balance impairment in order to rule out confounding factors that could lead to a false positive test[3][4].

Clinically Relevant Anatomy

There are three sensory systems that provide input to the cerebellum to maintain truncal stability when the eyes are open:

1. Vision
2. Proprioception
3. Vestibular sense

Only two of the three systems are needed to maintain balance. When visual input is removed, instability due to lack of vision can be teased apart from other sensory impairments. If there is a more severe proprioceptive or vestibular lesion, or if there is a midline cerebellar lesion causing truncal instability, the patient will be unable to maintain the standing position, even when the eyes are open. Note that instability can also be seen with lesions in other parts of the nervous system, such as the upper or lower motor neurons, or the basal ganglia[5][6].

Technique

The Original Romberg test

The test is performed as follows:

1. The patient is asked to remove his shoes and stand with his two feet together. The arms are held next to the body or crossed in front of the body.
2. The clinician asks the patient to first stand quietly with eyes open, and subsequently with eyes closed. The patient tries to maintain his balance. For safety, it is essential that the observer stand close to the patient to prevent potential injury if the patient were to fall. When the patients closes

his eyes, he should not orient himself by light, sense or sound, as this could influence the test result and cause a false positive outcome.

3. The Romberg test is scored by counting the seconds the patient is able to stand with eyes closed.

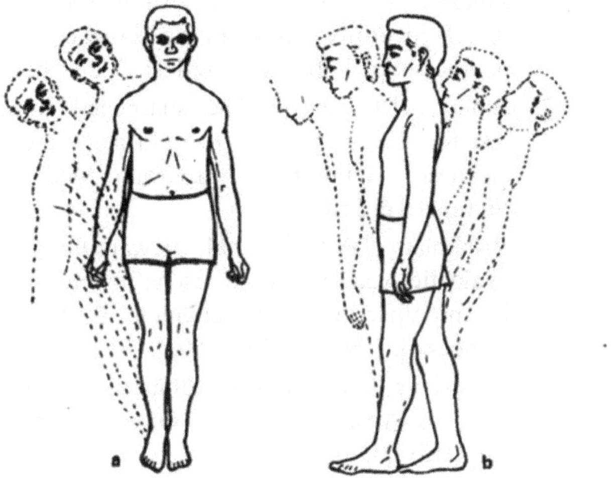

- The literature does not report alternative methods for scoring a Romberg test.
- To make the Romberg test more difficult, the clinician can attempt to disturb the patient's balance with a perturbation. It is important that the clinician does not exaggerate the perturbation.
- A Romberg test can also be used as follow-up assessment for patients with balance and/or proprioception impairments by comparing several different assessments with each other.
- If the clinician observes that the patient is able to stand for longer periods of time with the eyes closed, it is evident that the patient's balance and proprioceptive deficits have decreased[3][7][4][8].
- The Romberg test is positive when the patient is unable to maintain balance with their eyes closed. Losing balance can be defined as increased body sway, placing one foot in the direction of the fall, or even falling.

The Sharpened or Tandem Romberg test

The Sharpened or Tandem Romberg test is a variation of the original test. The implementation is mostly the same. For this second test, the patient has to place his feet in heel-to-toe position, with one foot directly in front of the other. As with the original Romberg test, the assessment is performed first with eyes open and then with eyes closed. The patient crosses his arms over his chest, and the open palm of the hand lies on the opposite shoulder. The patient also distributes his weight over both his feet and holds his chin parallel with the floor[7][4].

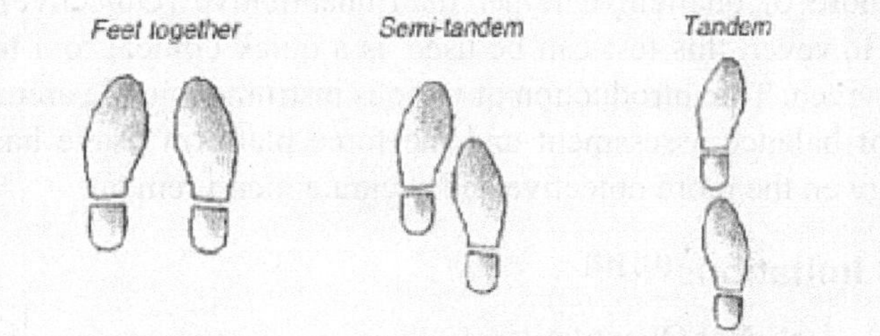

Balance (Sharpened Romberg test). Patient stands with feet together, semi-tandem, and tandem, with eyes open for 10 seconds then closed for 10 seconds in each position.

Obese and older individuals may be unable to stand in this position for prolonged periods of time. For these populations, the Romberg test does not exclusively demonstrate proprioceptive impairments in comparison to other confounding factors[3].

Variables

Although a patient with an acute peripheral vestibular lesion is usually inclined to move towards the side of the problem, it has been shown that chronic vestibular damage (at least partial compensation) does not produce deficits in the standard Romberg test. As well, an individual with proprioceptive problems, accessory to tabes dorsalis, would be unable to stand with the eyes closed and feet together[3].

Many believe that the sharpened Romberg test is a better indicator of vestibular impairment than the original Romberg test. The sharpened Romberg test results give an objective measure of postural stability. This can help to quantify ataxia[3].

Subject, sex, and age do not create a statistically significant difference between normal subjects between the ages of 20 and 49 years; only the Romberg sharpened test with eyes open provided a significant difference ($p < 0.05$) between men and women. Greater instability in subjects less than 20 and more than 50 years of age was also exhibited. When comparing a young and an old cohort, there is a significant difference in performance.

Increasing the difficulty of the tandem Romberg test for patients is not helpful because it also makes the tests more difficult to perform for controls with no symptoms of vestibular disease. This would also make it harder to evaluate the test results. Decreased performance times on the modified Romberg is associated with a concomitant rise in the risk of falling[4][9][10].

Reliability and Validity

There is no consensus in the Reliability (Intra and inter) and validity for Romberg's in the literature as the test is more of qualitative rather than quantitative (Objective). However, this test can be used as a quick clinical tool to screen. The introduction of various instrument in the arena of balance assessment and the force platform usage has given the more objective and accurate measurement.

Limitations[11] [12]

- Not Quantitative
- Low diagnostic sensitivity and specificity
- Low power to determine lesions, predict the risk of falling and reflect the discomfort and ability to perform daily activities.

References

1. Soochan Kim, Mijoo Kim, Nambom Kim, Sungmin Kim, Gyucheol Han.Quantification and Validity of Modified Romberg Tests Using Three-Axis Accelerometers.Green and Smart Technology with Sensor Applications. Communications in Computer and Information Science Volume 338, 2012, pp 254-261.
2. Reicke, N.: The Romberg head-shake test within the scope of equilibrium diagnosis. H.N.O 40, 195–201 (1992)
3. Goebel JA. Practical management of the dizzy patient. Philadelphia: Lippincott Williams & Wilkins, 2008.
4. Black FO, et al. Normal subject postural sway during the Romberg test. Am J Otolaryngol. 1982 Sep-Oct;3(5):309-18.
5. Blumenfeld, H. Neuroexam.com - Romberg test. www.neuroexam.com/neuroexam/content.php?p=37 (accessed 31 Dec 2013).
6. Zelczak TA. Neurologic examination. www.pacificu.edu/optometry/ce/courses/15840/neuroexampg3.cfm (accessed 31 Dec 2013).
7. Johnson BG, et al. The sharpened Romberg test for assessing ataxia in mild acute mountain sickness. Wilderness Environ Med. 2005 Summer;16(2):62-6.
8. Brinkman DMC, et al. Kwantificering en evaluatie van 5 neurologische evenwichtstests bij proefpersonen en patiënten. Ned Tijdschr Geneeskd. 1996;140:2176-80.
9. Longridge NS. Clinical Romberg testing does not detect vestibular disease. Otol Neurotol. 2010 Jul;31(5):803-6.
10. Agrawal Y. The modified Romberg balance test: normative data in US adults. Otol Neurotol, 2011 Oct,32(8):1309–1311.
11. McMichael,K.A., Vander, B.J., Lavery, L., Rodriguez, E., Ganguli, M.: Simple balance and mobility tests can assess falls risk when cognition is impaired. Geriatr. Nurs. 29, 311–323 (2008)
12. O'Neil, D.E., Gill-Body, K.M., Krebs, D.E.: Posturography changes do not predict functional performance changes. Am J. Otol. 19, 797–803 (1998)

❑❑❑

166 Roye Score

Objective

The Roye Score[1] is a 10-item disease-specific instrument to measure outcomes of treatment for clubfoot[2].

Intended Population

This scale is intended for use by mothers of children with idiopathic clubfoot[2] and is used in high income countries[3]. It can be used as an overall measure of clubfoot treatment outcomes with two distinct subscales: function and satisfaction[1].

Method of Use

This disease specific instrument consists of 10 items designed to measure treatment outcomes regarding overall satisfaction, appearance, pain, and physical limitations.

Item	Response Codes			
	1	2	3	4
1. How satisfied are you with the status of your child's foot?	Very Satisfied	Somewhat satisfied	Somewhat dissatisfied	Very dissatisfied
2. How satisfied are you with the appearance of your child's foot?	Very Satisfied	Somewhat satisfied	Somewhat dissatisfied	Very dissatisfied
3. How often is your child teased because of his or her clubfoot?	Never	Sometimes	Usually,	Always
4. How often does your child have problems finding shoes that fit?	Never	Sometimes	Usually,	Always
5. How often does your child have problems finding shoes that he or she likes?	Never	Sometimes	Usually,	Always
6. Does your child ever complain of pain in his or her (affected) foot?	Yes	No, re-coded	No	Yes
7. How limited is your child in his or her ability to walk?	Not at all limited	Somewhat limited	Moderately limited	Very limited
8. How limited is your child in his or her ability to run?	Not at all limited	Somewhat limited	Moderately limited	Very limited
9. How often does your child complain of pain during heavy exercise?	Never	Sometimes	Usually	Always
10. How often does your child complain of pain during moderate exercise?	Never	Sometimes	Usually	Always

Reference:Roye BD, Vitale MG, Gelijns AC, Roye DP Jr. Patient-based outcomes after clubfoot surgery. J Pediatr Orthop. 2001 Jan-Feb; 21(1):42-9.

Evidence

Dietz et al[2] supported the use of the Roye Score as an outcome measure for idiopathic clubfoot in young children by providing evidence of its reliability, validity, and discriminatory power. They also found the Roye score to be sensitive to differences in treatment technique or underlying severity of disease. A more recent study by Smythe et al, in 2018, comparing outcome measures after the Ponsetti method had good inter-observer agreement between the two expert physiotherapists. The study found that Roye Score had a sensitivity of 31.8% (95%CI: 13.9-54.9%) and a specificity of 100% (95%CI: 92-100%) in predicting the need for referral with positive and negative predictive values of 100 and 74.6% respectively[3]

References

1. Roye BD, Vitale MG, Gelijns AC, Roye DP Jr. Patient-based outcomes after clubfoot surgery. J Pediatr Orthop. 2001 Jan-Feb; 21(1):42-9.
2. Dietz FR, Tyler MC, Leary KS, Damiano PC. Evaluation of a disease-specific instrument for idiopathic clubfoot outcome. Clinical orthopaedics and related research. 2009 May 1;467(5):1256-62.
3. Smythe T, Gova M, Muzanuwi R, Foster A, Lavy C. A Comparison of outcome measures used to report clubfoot treatment with the Ponseti method: results from a cohort in Harare, Zimbabwe. BMC Musculoskeletal Disorders (2018) 19:450

❑❑❑

167 SARC-F: A Simple Questionnaire to Rapidly Diagnose Sarcopenia

Introduction

Strength, assistance with walking, rising from a chair, climbing stairs, and falls (SARC-F) questionnaire:

The SARC-F questionnaire is a screening tool that can be rapidly implemented by clinicians to identify probable sarcopenic patients. The questionnaire screens patients for self-reported signs suggestive of sarcopenia, which include deficiencies in strength, walking, rising from a chair, climbing stairs, and experiencing falls. Each of the self-reported parameters receives a minimum and maximum score of 0 and 2, respectively, with the greatest maximum SARC-F score being 10.[1]

Implementation

SARC-F Screen for Sarcopenia: Component Question Scoring

1. Strength: How much difficulty do you have in lifting and carrying 10 pounds?
   None 0 Some 1
   A lot or unable 2
2. Assistance in walking: How much difficulty do you have walking across a room?
   None 0 Some 1
   A lot, use aids, or unable 2
3. Rise from a chair: How much difficulty do you have transferring from a chair or bed?
   None 0 Some 1
   A lot or unable without help 2
4. Climb stairs: How much difficulty do you have climbing a flight of 10 stairs?
   None 0 Some 1
   A lot or unable 2
5. Falls: How many times have you fallen in the past year?
   None 0 less than 3 falls 1
   4 or more falls 2[2]

Data suggests that a SARC-F score of ≥4 best predicts the need for further, more comprehensive evaluation[1]

Validity

The SARC-F proved internally consistent and valid for detecting persons at risk for adverse outcomes from sarcopenia in AAH, BLSA, and NHANES.[3]

References

1. Ardeljan AD, Hurezeanu R. Sarcopenia. StatPearls [Internet]. 2020 Jul 10. Available from:https://www.ncbi.nlm.nih.gov/books/NBK560813/ (accessed 9.3.2021)
2. Malmstrom TK, Morley JE. SARC-F: a simple questionnaire to rapidly diagnose sarcopenia. Journal of the American Medical Directors Association. 2013 Aug 1;14(8):531-2. Available from: https://www.researchgate.net/publication/243966215_SARC-F_A_Simple_Questionnaire_to_Rapidly_Diagnose_Sarcopenia (accessed 10.3.2021)
3. Malmstrom TK, Miller DK, Simonsick EM, Ferrucci L, Morley JE. SARC-F: a symptom score to predict persons with sarcopenia at risk for poor functional outcomes. Journal of cachexia, sarcopenia and muscle. 2016 Mar;7(1):28-36.Available from:https://pubmed.ncbi.nlm.nih gov/27066316/ (accessed 10.3.2021)

❑❑❑

168 Scale for the Assessment and Rating of Ataxia (SARA)

Objective

SARA is a clinical scale developed by Schmitz-Hübsch et al which assesses a range of different impairments in cerebellar ataxia. The scale is made up of 8 items related to gait, stance, sitting, speech, finger-chase test, nose-finger test, fast alternating movements and heel-shin test.[1] Schmitz-Hübsch et al developed the Scale for the Assessment and Rating of Ataxia (SARA) as an alternative to The International Cooperative Ataxia Rating Scale (ICARS). The daily use of ICARS scale in ataxic patients is difficult due to its many assessment items.[2] This new assessment tool has fewer assessment items than the ICARS and therefore has the advantage of easier daily assessment of ataxia. [3]

Intended Population

Currently, the following types of Ataxia have been investigated:

- Spinocerebellar Ataxia[3][4][5]
- Ataxic Stroke [6]
- Friedreich's Ataxia [7] [8]

Method of Use

The SARA is a tool for assessing ataxia. It has eight categories with accumulative score ranging from 0 (no ataxia) to 40 (most severe ataxia). When completing the outcome measure each category is assessed and scored accordingly. Scores for the eight items range as follows:

1. Gait (0-8 points),
2. Stance (0-6 points),
3. Sitting (0-4 points)
4. Speech disturbance (0-6 points)
5. Finger chase (0-4 points)
6. Nose-finger test (0-4 points)
7. Fast alternating hand movement (0-4 points)
8. Heel-shin slide (0-4 points)

Once each of the 8 categories have been assessed, the total is calculated to determine the severity of ataxia.

For motor activities of the four extremities (items 5-8), assessments are performed bilaterally, and the mean values are used to obtain the total score.

Evidence

Spinocerebellar Ataxia

Concurrent validity - Subramony et al found the SARA scale had excellent concurrent validity with the Barthel Index or with Unified Huntington's Disease Rating Scale [10]

Inter/Intra rater reliability - Schmitz-Hübsch et al found the SARA scale to have high inter/intra rater reliability[3]

Ataxia in non Spinocerebellar patients

Freidreichs Ataxia

Construct validity: - Saute et al found the SARA had excellent construct validity with International Cooperative Ataxia Rating Scale (ICARS) and with Friedreich's Ataxia rating Scale [8]

Ataxic Stroke patients

Kim et al found that SARA corresponds well with gait assessments and functional impairments. The scale showed correlation with the Korean Modified Bartel Index and Berg Balance Scale [6]

References

1. Weyer A, Abele M, Schmitz-Hubsch T, Schoch B, Frings M, Timmann D. Reliability And validity of the scale for the assessment and rating of ataxia: a study in 64 Ataxia patients. Movement Disorders 2007;22:1633–7
2. Trouillas P, Takayanagi T, Hallett M, Currier RD, Subramony SH, Wessel K, Bryer A, Diener HC, Massaquoi S, Gomez CM, et al. The Ataxia Neuropharmacology Committee of the World Federation of Neurology. International Cooperative Ataxia Rating Scale for pharmacological assessment of the cerebellar syndrome. J Neurol Sci. 1997;145:205–211.
3. Schmitz-Hübsch T, du Montcel ST, Baliko L, Berciano J, Boesch S, Depondt C, Giunti P, Globas C, Infante J, Kang JS, et al. Scale for the assessment and rating of ataxia: development of a new clinical scale. Neurology. 2006;66:1717–1720.
4. Schmitz-Hübsch T, Fimmers R, Rakowicz M, Rola R, Zdzienicka E, Fancellu R, Mariotti C, Linnemann C, Schöls L, Timmann D, Filla A. Responsiveness of different rating instruments in spinocerebellar ataxia patients. Neurology. 2010 23;74(8):678-84.
5. Ataxia UK. Management of the Ataxias: towards best clinical practice. November 2009 http://www.ataxia.org.uk/Pages/News/Category/clinical-guidlines (accessed 23 Feb 2016)
6. Kim BR, Lim JH, Lee SA, Park S, Koh SE, Lee IS, Jung H, Lee J.Usefulness Of the Scale For the Assessment And Rating Of Ataxia (SARA) In ataxic stroke patients.Ann Rehabil Med 2011;35:772–80
7. Bürk K, Mälzig U, Wolf S, Heck S, Dimitriadis K, Schmitz-Hübsch T, Hering S, Lindig TM, Haug V, Timmann D, Degen I. Comparison of three clinical rating scales in Friedreich ataxia (FRDA). Movement Disorders 2009. 15;24(12):1779-84.
8. Saute JA, Donis KC, Serrano-Munuera C, Genis D, Ramirez LT, Mazzetti P, Pérez LV, Latorre P, Sequeiros J, Matilla-Dueñas A, Jardim LB. Ataxia rating scales—psychometric profiles, natural history and their application in clinical trials. The Cerebellum. 2012 Jun 1;11(2):488-504.
9. Ataxia Study Group. Scale for the Assessment and Rating of Ataxia. http://www.ataxia-study-group.net/html/about/ataxiascales/sara/SARA.pdf (accessed 23 Feb 2016)
10. Subramony SH. SARA—a new clinical scale for the assessment and rating of ataxia. Nature clinical practice Neurology. 2007 Mar 1;3(3):136-7.

Scale for the Assessment and Rating of Ataxia (SARA)

Rater: ________________ date: ____________

patient:____________________

1. Gait

Proband is asked

1. to walk at a safe distance parallel to a wall including a half-turn (turn around to face the opposite direction of gait) and
2. to walk in tandem (heels to toes) without support.

0 Normal, no difficulties in walking, turning and walking tandem (up to one misstep allowed)

1 Slight difficulties, only visible when walking 10 consecutive steps in tandem

2 Clearly abnormal, tandem walking >10 steps not possible

3 Considerable staggering, difficulties in half-turn, but without support

4 Marked staggering, intermittent support of the wall required

5 Severe staggering, permanent support of one stick or light support by one arm required

6 Walking > 10 m only with strong support (two special sticks or stroller or accompanying person)

7 Walking < 10 m only with strong support (two special sticks or stroller or accompanying person)

8 Unable to walk, even supported

Score =

2. Stance

Proband is asked to stand

1. in natural position,

2. with feet together in parallel (big toes touching each other) and

3. in tandem (both feet on one line, no space between heel and toe).

Proband does not wear shoes, eyes are open. For each condition, three trials are allowed.

Best trial is rated.

0 Normal, able to stand in tandem for > 10 s

1 Able to stand with feet together without sway, but not in tandem for > 10s

2 Able to stand with feet together for > 10 s, but only with sway

3 Able to stand for > 10 s without support in natural position, but not with feet together

4 Able to stand for >10 s in natural position only with intermittent support

5 Able to stand >10 s in natural position only with constant support of one arm

6 Unable to stand for >10 s even with constant support of one arm

Score =

3. Sitting

Proband is asked to sit on an examination bed without support of feet, eyes open and arms outstretched to the front.

0 Normal, no difficulties sitting >10 sec

1 Slight difficulties, intermittent sway

2 Constant sway, but able to sit > 10 s without support

3 Able to sit for > 10 s only with intermittent support

4 Unable to sit for >10 s without continuous support

Score =

4. Speech disturbance

Speech is assessed during normal conversation.

0 Normal

1 Suggestion of speech disturbance

2 Impaired speech, but easy to understand

3 Occasional words difficult to understand

4 Many words difficult to understand

5 Only single words understandable

6 Speech unintelligible / anarthria

Score =

5. Finger chase

Rated separately for each side

Proband sits comfortably. If necessary, support of feet and trunk is allowed. Examiner sits in front of proband and performs 5 consecutive sudden and fast pointing movements in unpredictable directions in a frontal plane, at about 50 % of proband´s reach. Movements have an amplitude of 30 cm and a frequency of 1 movement every 2 s. Proband is asked to follow the movements with his index finger, as fast and precisely as possible.

Average performance of last 3 movements is rated.

0 No dysmetria

1 Dysmetria, under/ overshooting target <5 cm

2 Dysmetria, under/ overshooting target < 15 cm

3 Dysmetria, under/ overshooting target > 15 cm

4 Unable to perform 5 pointing movements

Score = Right : Left =

Mean of both sides (Right + Left) / 2 =

6. Nose-finger test

Rated separately for each side

Proband sits comfortably. If necessary, support of feet and trunk is allowed. Proband is asked to point repeatedly with his index finger from his nose to examiner's finger which is in front of the proband at about 90 % of proband's reach. Movements are performed at moderate speed. Average performance of movements is rated according to the amplitude of the kinetic tremor.

0 No tremor

1 Tremor with an amplitude < 2 cm

2 Tremor with an amplitude < 5 cm

3 Tremor with an amplitude > 5 cm

4 Unable to perform 5 pointing movements

Score = Right : Left =

Mean of both sides (Right + Left) / 2 =

7. Fast alternating hand movements

Rated separately for each side

Proband sits comfortably. If necessary, support of feet and trunk is allowed. Proband is asked to perform 10 cycles of repetitive alternation of pro- and supinations of the hand on his/her thigh as fast and as precise as possible. Movement is demonstrated by examiner at a speed of approx. 10 cycles within 7 s. Exact times for movement execution have to be taken.

0 Normal, no irregularities (performs <10s)

1 Slightly irregular (performs <10s)

2 Clearly irregular, single movements difficult to distinguish or relevant interruptions, but performs <10s

3 Very irregular, single movements difficult to distinguish or relevant interruptions, performs >10s

4 Unable to complete 10 cycles

Score = Right : Left =

Mean of both sides (Right + Left) / 2 =

8. Heel-shin slide

Rated separately for each side

Proband lies on examination bed, without sight of his legs. Proband is asked to lift one leg, point with the heel to the opposite knee, slide down along the shin to the ankle, and lay the leg back on the examination bed. The task is performed 3 times. Slide-down movements should be performed within 1 s. If proband slides down without contact to shin in all three trials, rate 4.

0 Normal

1 Slightly abnormal, contact to shin maintained

2 Clearly abnormal, goes off shin up to 3 times during 3 cycles

3 Severely abnormal, goes off shin 4 or more times during 3 cycles

4 Unable to perform the task

Score = Right : Left =

Mean of both sides (Right + Left) / 2 =

❑❑❑

169 Schober Test

Purpose

Schober's test is classically used to determine if there is a decrease in lumbar spine range of motion (flexion), most commonly as a result of ankylosing spondylitis.[1].

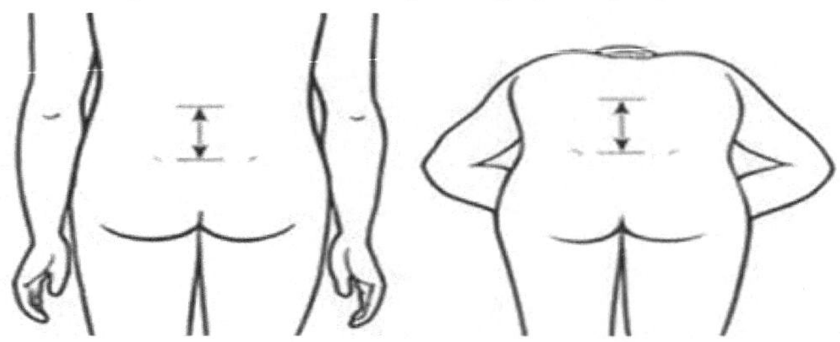

The measurement of this test is useful for

- Screening the status of ankylosing spondylitis disease
- Determination of progression and therapeutic effects of ankylosing spondylitis and other pathologic conditions associated with low back pain[2].

Technique

Schöber Test

- Patient is standing, examiner marks the L5 spinous process by drawing a horizontal line across the patients back.
- A second line is marked 10 cm above the first line.
- Patient is then instructed to flex forward as if attempting to touch his/her toes, examiner remeasures distance between two lines with patient fully flexed.
- The difference between the measurements in erect and flexion positions indicates the outcome of the lumbar flexion [1].

Modified Schober Test (eliminates the errors in identification of lumbosacral junction and makes sure that the entire lumbar spine was included[1][3]

- Patient is standing, examiner marks both posterior superior iliac spine (PSIS) and then draws a horizontal line at the centre of both marks
- A second line is marked 5 cm below the first line.
- A third line is marked 10 cm above the first line.
- Patient is then instructed to flex forward as if attempting to touch his/her toes, examiner remeasures distance between the top and bottom line. [1].

Interpretation

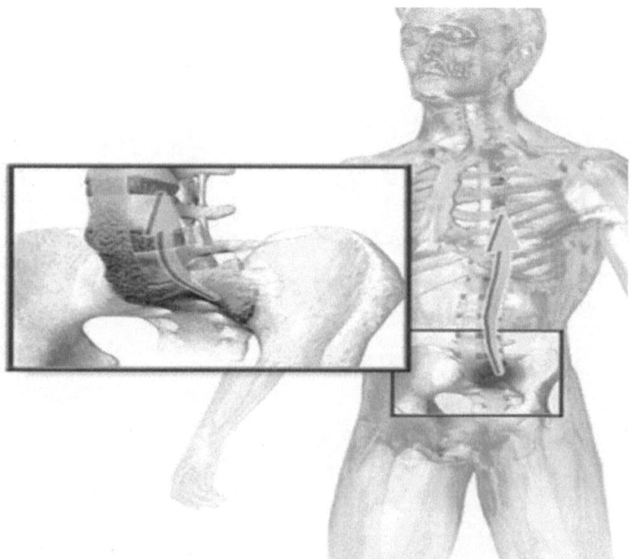

For both versions of the test, an increase of less than 5cm is a positive test and may indicate ankylosing spondylitis (AS). (Image shows region of spine mainly involved in AS)

Positive Schober's Test

Less than 5cm increase in length with forward flexion: Decreased lumbar spine range of motion, ankylosing spondylitis

Clinical Notes

This test is almost exclusively associated with Ankylosing Spondylitis but may also be positive due to a decrease in lumbar range of motion due to pain or congenital anomalies or segmental fusion[4

Evidence

1. Original Schöber Test The validity against radiographs was according to Macrae. strong (r=0.90), according to Rahali-Khachlouf. moderate (r=0.68). The interclass (r=0.90) and intraclass (r=0.96) reliability was found to be excellent[1].
2. Modified Schöber Index The validity against radiographs was according to Macrae. strong (r=0.97), according to Rahali-Khachlouf. moderate (r=0.59). The interclass (r=0.92) and intraclass (r=0.96) reliability were found to be excellent[6].
3. Modified-modified Schöber Test The validity of the modified-modified Schober test is moderate (r=0.67) with an excellent interclass (r=0.91) and intraclass (r=95) reliability[1].

References

1. Rezvani A, Ergin O., Karacan I., Validity and reliability of the Metric Measurements in the Assessment of Lumbar Spine Motion in patients with Ankylosing Spondylitis., 2012, Lippincott Williams & Wilkins, SPINE vol 37, Number 19, pp E1189-E1196 (level of Evidence: 1B)
2. Yen YR, Luo JF, Liu ML, Lu FJ, Wang SR. The anthropometric measurement of schober's test in normal taiwanese population. BioMed research international. 2015;2015.
3. Tousignant M, Poulin L, Marchand S, Viau A, Place C. The Modified–Modified Schober Test for range of motion assessment of lumbar flexion in patients with low back pain: A study of criterion validity, intra-and inter-rater reliability and minimum metrically detectable change. Disability and rehabilitation. 2005 May 20;27(10):553-9.
4. Medisavy Schobers Test Available from:https://medisavvy.com/schobers-test/ (last accessed 30.5.2020)
5. BJC Health Modified Schober's Test for Ankylosing Spondylitis. Available fromhttps://www.youtube.com/watch?v=B9RaFB5BwrQ
6. M Tousignant, Poulin L, Marchand S, , the modified-modified schober test for range of motion assessment of lumbar flexion in patients with low back pain: a study of criterion validity, intra- and inter-rater reliability and minimum metrically detectable change, disability and rehabilitation, 2005, VOL.27, NO.10, Pages 553-559 (Level of evidence: 4)
7. Schober Test for Lumbar Spine Flexion Available from: https://www.youtube.com watch?v=eYOUA9asDu8

❑❑❑

170 Short-form McGill Pain Questionnaire

The publication of the McGill Pain Questionnaire (Melzack, 1975) represented a major (r)evolution in pain research. Pain was mainly described and measured in terms of intensity, but thanks to the MPQ, the qualitative aspect of pain became an important subject in pain research. Pain descriptors were brought together and categorized in three dimensions of pain experience:

- words that described the sensory qualities of the experience in terms of temporal, spatial, pressure, thermal, and other properties
- words that described affective qualities in terms of tension, fear, and autonomic properties that are part of the pain experience
- evaluative words that subjectively described the overall intensity of the total pain experience[1]

The MPQ may be used for a standard registration and evaluation of the complaints of pain in a patient. Furthermore, it can also be used for diagnostics and to control the effects of therapies and/ or pain relief in individual patients.[2]

The short-form McGill Pain Questionnaire (SF-MPQ) is a shorter version of the original MPQ, and was developed later in 1987.

The pain rating index has 2 subscales:

1. Sensory subscale with 11 words, and
2. Affective subscale with 4 words from the original MPQ.

These words or items are rated on an intensity scale as 0 = none, 1 = mild, 2 = moderate and 3 = severe. There's also one item for present pain intensity and one item for a 10 cm visual analogue scale (VAS) for average pain.[3] The SF-MPQ was further revised in 2009 for the use in neuropathic and non-neuropathic pain conditions (SF-MPQ-2). This new version includes 7 additional symptoms related to neuropathic pain, for a total of 22 items with 0-10 numerical response options.[3]

Intended Population

The SF-MPQ has been developed for adults with chronic pain, including pain due to rheumatic conditions,[3] but recent research has also proven usefulness of the SF-MPQ-2 in patients with acute low back pain.[4]

Scoring

The Pain Rating Index can be scored in several ways:

- "Pain Rating Index - rank value": The adjectives are ranked according to increasing intensity so each descriptor can be assigned a higher score.
  - 0 = no pain
  - 1 = mild
  - 2 = discomforting
  - 3 = distressing
  - 4 = horrible
  - 5 = excruciating
- "Pain Rating Index - scale value (VAS)": The pain intensity of each pain descriptor was assessed on a numeric scale in previous research (Melzack and Torgerson in Melzack, 1975). The assigned rating can also be accepted as the score for the pain descriptor.
- "Number of words chosen (NWC)": The number of words chosen by the patient. The higher the total score on the MPQ, the more the pain experience for the patient increases.

Evidence

Reliability

The test-retest reliability of the questionnaire has been evaluated in populations with a variety of conditions, such as osteoarthritis and musculoskeletal pain. For an estimate of the reliability, the intraclass correlation coefficient was used. Since the questionnaire has been translated into 26 languages, the reliability varies depending on the language[3]

When evaluating the test-retest reliability of the SF-MPQ in patients with musculoskeletal pain, the results were adequate (r>70).[3] When examining the same questionnaire in patients with rheumatic pain, the results were significantly higher (r>85). Only the subscale 'current pain' demonstrated a lower intraclass correlation coefficient of 0.75.[5] For the internal consistency reliability, a Cronbach's alpha of r>0.75 has been reported by Melzack et al.[2]

Validity

It was found that the SF-MPQ has more content validity among patients with fibromyalgia than for those with RA. [4] Percentage of use of 15 pain descriptors in 2 groups was significantly different for all words except "throbbing" and "punishing-cruel." The mean intensity score for each word ranged from 1.69 for "sickening" to 2.60 for "tender" in the fibromyalgia group and 1.57 for "fearful" to 2.18 for "aching" in the RA group.[3]

The SF-MPQ has been translated into many different languages. Some studies have demonstrated the validity of the translated versions of the SF-MPQ. The results of the Persian version give a Cronbach's alpha of 0.906, also showing a high internal consistency. There was also a high correlation between the mean VAS and the mean total score (r = 0.926)[6]

Results of the Swedish version indicated that the MPQ 15-item descriptor section was internally consistent (Cronbach's alphas: 0.73-0.89), but lacked content validity in the RA sample. Convergent construct validity was demonstrated by significant correlations between the SF-MPQ and other pain measurements[7]

It this point, one can conclude that the SF-MPQ is a highly valid instrument to evaluate pain in patients with and without neuropathic etiology.[6]

The revised version of the SF-MPQ, the SF-MPQ-2, has been validated for use in chronic pain populations. For example, Lovejoy et al demonstrated an excellent reliability and validity for the use of the SF-MPQ-2 in a group of U.S. veteran patients with chronic neuropathic and non-neuropathic pain.[8][4]

Trudeau et al. conclude that the SF-MPQ-2 is a valid instrument to assess pain qualities in patients with acute low back pain.[4]

Responsiveness

The purpose of the questionnaire is to obtain descriptive values rather than to objectively detect change in time since pain is a subjective concept.[9] Nevertheless, the SF- MPQ has been found to be responsive to change and indicated a clinically valuable difference in a population with musculoskeletal conditions,[3] but the measurement properties vary between groups of patients with pain.[10]

For the osteoarthritis population, however, a prospective observational cohort study demonstrated no significant changes over time. The coefficient was calculated as an estimation of the minimum detectable change.[5]

Another study showed a comparison of the responsiveness of the VAS and the MPQ.

Interpretation of Results

- Clinically important change (CIC): mean improvement in total scores >5 on the 0–45 Norwegian SF-MPQ scale[3]
- Minimum detectable change (MDC) for total, sensory, affective, average, and current pain: 5.2cm, 4.5cm, 2.8cm, 1.4cm, and 1.4cm, respectively[3]

Miscellaneous

Dworkin et al.[11] amended the SF-MPQ to produce a measure (the SF-MPQ-2) that has excellent reliability and validity and provided support for four readily interpretable subscales—continuous pain, intermittent pain, predominantly neuropathic pain, and effective descriptors.

References

1. Melzack R., Ph.D.*: "The McGill Pain Questionnaire", American Society of Anesthesiologists, 2005; 103:199–202. (evidence level = 5)
2. Melzack R, Katz J: "The McGill Pain Questionnaire: Appraisal and current status", Handbook of Pain Measurement, 2nd edition. Edited by Turk DC, Melzack R. New York, Guilford Press, 2001, pp 35–52 (evidence level = 5)
3. Gillian A. Hawker:" Measures of adult pain.", Arthritis Care & Research 2011; 63 (11): 20-252

(Evidence level = 2C)

4. J. Trudeau et al., "Validation of the revised short form McGill Pain Questionnaire (SF-MPQ-2) for self-report of pain qualities in patients with acute low back pain", The Journal of Pain, Volume 13, Issue 4, Supplement, April 2012, Pages S4 (Evidence level = 1B)
5. Grafton KV: "Test-retest reliability of the Short-Form McGill Pain Questionnaire: Rassessment of intraclass correlation coefficients and limits of agreement in patients with osteoarthritis.", Clin J Pain. 2005 Jan-Feb;21(1):73-82 (evidence level= 2B)
6. Farhad Abelmanesh:"Reliability, Validity, and Sensitivity Measures of Expanded and Revised Version of the Short-Form McGill Pain Questionnaire in Iranian Patients with Neuropathic and Non-Neuropathic Pain", Pain Medicine,2012 (evidence level = 1B)
7. C.S. Burckhardt, "A Swedish Version of the Short-Form McGill Pain Questionnaire", 1994, p 77-81, Gothenburg Sweden (evidence level = 1B)
8. T.I. Lovejoy et al., "Evaluation of the Psychometric Properties of the Revised Short-Form McGill Pain Questionnaire", The Journal of Pain, Vol 13, No 12 (December), 2012: pp 1250-1257 (Evidence level = 1B)
9. A. Chauffe et al., "Responsiveness of the VAS and McGill pain questionnaire in measuring changes in musculoskeletal pain", J Sport Rehabil. 2011 May;20(2):250-5. (evidence level= 2C)
10. Strand LI.: "The Short-Form McGill Pain Questionnaire as an outcome measure: test-retest Reliability and responsiveness to change.", Eur J Pain. 2008 Oct;12(7):917-25. (evidence level= 2C)
11. Robert H. Dworkin, Dennis C. Turk, Dennis A. Revicki, Gale Harding, Karin S. Coyne, Sarah Peirce-Sandner, Dileep Bhagwat, Dennis Everton, Laurie B. Burke, Penney Cowan, John T. Farrar, Sharon Hertz, Mitchell B. Max, Bob A. Rappaport and Ronald Melzack. Development and initial validation of an expanded and revised version of the Short-form McGill Pain Questionnaire (SF-MPQ-2). Pain, July 2009, 144(1-2):35-42

Short-form McGill Pain Questionnaire

For this questionnaire, I will provide you a list of words that describe some of the different qualities of pain and related symptoms. Please rate the intensity of each of the pain and related symptoms you felt during the past week on 0 to 10 scale, with 0 being no pain and 10 being the worst pain you can imagine. Use 0 if the word does not describe your pain or related symptoms. Limit yourself to a description of the pain related to your surgery or pelvic pain

Date

Subject Id

1	**Throbbing pain**	none	0	1	2	3	4	5	6	7	8	9	10	worst possible
2	**Shooting pain**	none	0	1	2	3	4	5	6	7	8	9	10	worst possible
3	**Stabbing pain**	none	0	1	2	3	4	5	6	7	8	9	10	worst possible
4	**Sharp pain**	none	0	1	2	3	4	5	6	7	8	9	10	worst possible
5	**Cramping pain**	none	0	1	2	3	4	5	6	7	8	9	10	worst possible
6	**Gnawing pain**	none	0	1	2	3	4	5	6	7	8	9	10	worst possible
7	**Hot-burning pain**	none	0	1	2	3	4	5	6	7	8	9	10	worst possible
8	**Aching pain**	none	0	1	2	3	4	5	6	7	8	9	10	worst possible
9	**Heavy pain**	none	0	1	2	3	4	5	6	7	8	9	10	worst possible
10	**Tender**	none	0	1	2	3	4	5	6	7	8	9	10	worst possible
11	**Splitting pain**	none	0	1	2	3	4	5	6	7	8	9	10	worst possible
12	**Tiring-exhausting**	none	0	1	2	3	4	5	6	7	8	9	10	worst possible
13	**Sickening**	none	0	1	2	3	4	5	6	7	8	9	10	worst possible

14	**Fearful**	none	0	1	2		3	4	5	6	7	8	9	10	worst possible
15	**Punishing-cruel**	none	0	1	2		3	4	5	6	7	8	9	10	worst possible
16	**Electric-shock pain**	none	0	1	2		3	4	5	6	7	8	9	10	worst possible
17	**Cold-freezing pain**	none	0	1	2		3	4	5	6	7	8	9	10	worst possible
18	**Piercing**	none	0	1	2		3	4	5	6	7	8	9	10	worst possible
19	**Pain caused by light touch**	none	0	1	2		3	4	5	6	7	8	9	10	worst possible
20	**Itching**	none	0	1	2		3	4	5	6	7	8	9	10	worst possible
21	**Tingling or 'pins and needles'**	none	0	1	2		3	4	5	6	7	8	9	10	worst possible
22	**Numbness**	none	0	1	2		3	4	5	6	7	8	9	10	worst possible
23	**Present Pain Intensity (PPI)** – Numerical Pain Rating Scale. On a scale from zero to ten, zero indicating no pain and ten indicating worst pain imaginable, rate your pelvic pain														
		none	0	1	2		3	4	5	6	7	8	9	10	worst possible
24	**Evaluative overall intensity of total pain experience. Please check (√) the word that describes the pain in your pelvic area only.**														
No pain	Mild	Discomforting	Distressing	Horrible	Excruciating										

❑❑❑

171 Shoulder Pain and Disability Index (SPADI)

Objective

The Shoulder Pain and Disability Index (SPADI) is a patient completed questionnaire with 13 items assessing pain level and extent of difficulty with ADLs requiring the use of the upper extremities. The pain subscale has 5-items and the Disability subscale has 8-items.

The original version[1] was published in 1991 and has its items scored on the Visual analogue scale while the second version scores its items on the Numerical rating scale(NRS)

SPADI has been translated in many languages including Spanish, Greek, Dutch, Hindi, Thai and Italian each with its own validity and reliability.

Intended Population

SPA DI can be used in the following patient population:

- Shoulder pain[1]
- Rotator cuff disease
- Osteoarthritis
- Rheumatoid arthritis
- Adhesive Capsulitis[2][3]
- Shoulder arthroplasty

Method of Use

The patient is instructed to choose the number that best describes their level of pain and extent of difficulty using the involved shoulder. The pain scale is summed up to a total of 50 while the disability scale sums up to 80. The total SPADI score is expressed as a percentage.

A score of 0 indicates best 100 indicates worst. A higher score shows more disability.

In scoring SPADI, any question missed should be taken out of the total score of each subscale. i.e if 1 question is omitted in the pain section, the total score is divided by 40.

Evidence

Reliability

SPADI was found to have reliability coefficients of ICC ≥ 0.89 in a variety of patient populations.[4] Internal consistency is high with Cronbach α typically exceeding 0.90[4]

Validity

The SPADI demonstrates good construct validity, correlating well with other region-specific shoulder questionnaires.[5][4][6] It has been shown to be responsive to change over time, in a variety of patient populations and is able to discriminate adequately between patients with improving and deteriorating conditions.[7][8][4]

Responsiveness

The minimal clinically important difference has been reported to be 8 points; this represents the smallest detectable change that is important to the patient.[5] However, when SPADI is used repeatedly on the same subject the minimal detectable change is 18 points.[9][10]

References

1. Roach KE, Budiman-Mak E, Songsiridej N, Lertratanakul Y. Development of a Shoulder Pain and Disability Index. Arthritis Care Res 1991; 4: 143–9.
2. Tveitå, E. K., Ekeberg, O. M., Juel, N. G., & Bautz-Holter, E. Responsiveness of the Shoulder Pain and Disability Index in patients with adhesive capsulitis. BMC Musculoskeletal Disorders.

2008: 9(161)

3. Staples MP, Forbes A, Green S, Buchbinder R. Shoulder-specific disability measures showed acceptable construct validity and responsiveness. J Clin Epidemiol 2010; 63: 163–70.
4. Roy JS, MacDermid JC, Woodhouse LJ: Measuring shoulder function: a systematic review of four questionnaires. Arthritis Rheum. 2009, 61 (5): 623-632.
5. Paul A, Lewis M, Shadforth MF, Croft PR, Van Der Windt DA, Hay EM: A comparison of four shoulder-specific questionnaires in primary care. Ann Rheum Dis. 2004, 63 (10): 1293-1299.
6. Bot SD, Terwee CB, van der Windt DA, Bouter LM, Dekker J, de Vet HC: Clinimetric evaluation of shoulder disability questionnaires: a systematic review of the literature. Ann Rheum Dis. 2004, 63 (4): 335-341.
7. Williams JW, Holleman DR, Simel DL: Measuring shoulder function with the Shoulder Pain and Disability Index. J Rheumatol. 1995, 22 (4): 727-732.
8. Beaton DE, Richards RR: Measuring function of the shoulder. A cross-sectional comparison of five questionnaires. J Bone Joint Surg Am. 1996, 78 (6): 882-890.
9. Angst F, Goldhahn J, Drerup S, Aeschlimann A, Schwyzer HK, Simmen BR: Responsiveness of six outcome assessment instruments in total shoulder arthroplasty. Arthritis Rheum. 2008, 59 (3): 391-398.
10. Schmitt JS, Di Fabio RP: Reliable change and minimum important difference (MID) proportions facilitated group responsiveness comparisons using individual threshold criteria. J Clin Epidemiol. 2004, 57 (10): 1008-1018.

Shoulder Pain and Disability Index (SPADI)

Source: Roach KE, Budiman-Mak E, Songsiridej N, Lertratanakul Y. Development of a shoulder pain and disability index. Arthritis Care Res. 1991 Dec;4(4):143-9.

The Shoulder Pain and Disability Index (SPADI) is a self-administered questionnaire that consists of two dimensions, one for pain and the other for functional activities. The pain dimension consists of five questions regarding the severity of an individual's pain. Functional activities are assessed with eight questions designed to measure the degree of difficulty an individual has with various activities of daily living that require upper-extremity use. The SPADI takes 5 to 10 minutes for a patient to complete and is the only reliable and valid region-specific measure for the shoulder.

Scoring instructions

To answer the questions, patients place a mark on a 10cm visual analogue scale for each question. Verbal anchors for the pain dimension are 'no pain at all' and 'worst pain imaginable', and those for the functional activities are 'no difficulty' and 'so difficult it required help'. The scores from both dimensions are averaged to derive a total score.

Interpretation of scores

Total pain score: / 50 x 100 = %

(Note: If a person does not answer all questions divide by the total possible score, eg. if 1 question missed divide by 40).

Total disability score: / 80 x 100 = %

(Note: If a person does not answer all questions divide by the total possible score, eg. if 1 question missed divide by 70)

Total Spadi score: / 130 x 100 = %

(Note: If a person does not answer all questions divide by the total possible score, eg. if 1 question missed divide by 120) The means of the two subscales are averaged to produce a total score ranging from 0 (best) to 100 (worst). Minimum Detectable Change (90% confidence) = 13 points (Change less than this may be attributable to measurement error)

Shoulder Pain and Disability Index (SPADI)

Please place a mark on the line that best represents your experience during the last week attributable to your shoulder problem.

Pain scale

How severe is your pain?

Circle the number that best describes your pain where: 0 = no pain and 10 = the worst pain imaginable

At its worst?	0	1	2	3	4	5	6	7	8	9	10
When lying on the involved side?	0	1	2	3	4	5	6	7	8	9	10
Reaching for something on a high shelf?	0	1	2	3	4	5	6	7	8	9	10
Touching the back of your neck?	0	1	2	3	4	5	6	7	8	9	10
Pushing with the involved arm?	0	1	2	3	4	5	6	7	8	9	10

Disability scale

How much difficulty do you have?

Circle the number that best describes your experience where: 0 = no difficulty and 10 = so difficult it requires help.

Washing your hair?	0	1	2	3	4	5	6	7	8	9	10
Washing your back?	0	1	2	3	4	5	6	7	8	9	10
Putting on an undershirt or jumper?	0	1	2	3	4	5	6	7	8	9	10
Putting on a shirt that buttons down the front?	0	1	2	3	4	5	6	7	8	9	10
Putting on your pants?	0	1	2	3	4	5	6	7	8	9	10
Placing an object on a high shelf?	0	1	2	3	4	5	6	7	8	9	10
Carrying a heavy object of 10 pounds (4.5 kilograms)	0	1	2	3	4	5	6	7	8	9	10
Removing something from your back pocket?	0	1	2	3	4	5	6	7	8	9	10

❑❑❑

172 Six Minute Walk Test / 6 Minute Walk Test

Objective

The six minute walking test (6MWT) was developed by the American Thoracic Society and it was officially introduced in 2002, coming along with a comprehensive guideline[1].

The **6 Minute Walk Test** is a sub-maximal exercise test used to assess aerobic capacity and endurance. The distance covered over a time of 6 minutes is used as the outcome by which to compare changes in performance capacity.

Intended Population

The 6MWT can be used in preschool children (2-5 years), children (6-12 years) adults (18-64 years), elderly adults (65+) with a wide range of diagnoses including. The test was initially designed to help in the assessment of patient with cardiopulmonary issues. Gradually, it was introduced in numerous other conditions. It evaluates the functional capacity of the individual and it provides valuable information regarding all the systems during physical activity, including pulmonary and cardiovascular systems, blood circulation, neuromuscular units, body metabolism, and peripheral circulation[1].

Some conditions where 6MWT can be used are listed below:

- Arthritis
- Fibromyalgia
- Geriatrics
- Multiple Sclerosis
- Parkinson's Disease
- Spinal Cord Injury
- Stroke
- Muscle disorders
- Spinal Muscular Atrophy
- Charcot-Marie-Tooth disease

Method of Use

Equipment Required:

- Stopwatch
- Measuring/trundle wheel to measure distance covered
- 30-metre stretch of unimpeded walkway
- Two cones to mark the distance that needs to be covered
- Pulse oximeter for measuring heart rate and SpO2 (optional)
- Borg Breathlessness Scale (optional)

Set-Up:

- Place cones at either end of the 30 metre stretch as turning points
- Have chairs set up either side and halfway along the walking stretch

Patient Instructions:

- "The object of this test is to walk as far as possible for 6 minutes. You will walk back and forth in this hallway. Six minutes is a long time to walk, so you will be exerting yourself. You will probably get out of breath or become exhausted. You are permitted to slow down, to stop, and to rest as necessary. You may lean against the wall while resting, but resume walking as soon as you are able. You will be walking back and forth around the cones. You should pivot briskly around the cones and continue back the other way without hesitation. Now I'm going to show you. Please watch the way I turn without hesitation."

- Read this standardised encouragement during the test:
- After the 1st minute: "You are doing well. You have 5 minutes to go." When the timer shows 4 minutes remaining: "Keep up the good work. You have 4 minutes to go."

  When the timer shows 3 minutes remaining: "You are doing well. You are halfway done. When the timer shows 2 minutes remaining: "Keep up the good work. You have only 2 minutes left.

  When the timer shows 1 minute remaining: "You are doing well. You only have 1 minute to go. With 15 seconds to go: "In a moment I'm going to tell you to stop. When I do, just stop right where you are and I will come to you."

  At 6 minutes: "Stop"
- If the participant stops at any time prior, you can say: "You can lean against the wall if you would like; then continue walking whenever you feel able."
- Do not use other words of encouragement (or body language) to influence the patient's walking speed. Accompany the participant along the walking course, but keep just behind them. Do not lead them.
- If available record the distance at which the oxygen saturation drops < 88%

Interpretation

An increase in the distance walked indicates improvement in basic mobility. Resnik et al (2011 [3] suggested in Amputee rehabilitation, Post training a difference of at least 45m should be observed for the 6 minutes walk test to be sure that a **"real"** change in the patient's condition.

In some neuromuscular conditions such as Duchenne/Becker muscular dystrophy, Spinal Muscular Atrophy, Charcot-Marie-Tooth disease, and Myasthenia Gravis the 6MWT has been implemented in the assessment of those patients and it has been regularly used to capture any changes, which provides valuable information regarding the natural history of these disorders.

Some studies used the six minute walking test to identify patients with neuromuscular junction dysfunction[4]. By splitting the test into six different components where each minute is a different data point, the researches discovered that the 6MWT can identify any malfunctions in the neuromuscular junctions. Also by comparing the distance covered in the first and the last minute suggested how much the fatigue has influenced the individual.

Evidence

Reliability

Test-Retest Reliability

Alzheimer's Disease:

(Ries et al, 2009, Alzheimer's disease)

- Excellent test-retest reliability for all participants (ICC = 0.98) [5]

Geriatrics:

(Harada et al, 1999; n = 86; mean age = 75 (6) years, Geriatrics)

- Excellent test-retest reliability (r = 0.95) [6]
- (Steffen et al, 2002, Geriatrics)
- Excellent test-retest reliability (ICC = 0.95) [7]

Osteoarthritis:

(Kennedy et al, 2005, Osteoarthritis)

- Excellent test-retest reliability (ICC = 0.94) [8]

Stroke:

(Eng et al, 2004; n = 12 community-dwelling individuals who had a stroke with moderate motor deficits; mean time since stroke onset = 3.5 (2.0) years; mean age = 62.5 (8.6) years, Chronic Stroke) [9]

- Excellent test-retest reliability (ICC = 0.99 distance in meters)
- Excellent test-retest reliability for VO2 (ICC = 0.99)

(Flansbjer et al, 2005, Chronic Stroke) [10]

- Excellent Test-retest reliability (ICC = 0.99)

(Fulk et al, 2008; n = 35 patients who are enrolled in inpatient rehabilitation after stroke; mean age = 67.4 (13.8) years; mean time since stroke onset = 34.5 (17.7) days, Acute Stroke) [11]

- Excellent test-retest reliability for all participants (ICC = 0.862)
- Excellent test-retest reliability for those who

require physical assistance to walk (ICC = 0.97)

- Excellent test-retest reliability for those who can walk without assistance (ICC = 0.80)
- Excellent test-retest reliability for those require an assistive device to walk (ICC = 0.914)

(Wevers et al, 2011, Chronic Stroke) [12]

- Excellent test-retest reliability between first and second 6MWTs outdoors (ICC = 0.96 for GPS and 0.98 for measuring wheel)

TBI:

(Mossberg, 2003, n = 23; mean age 35.5 (12.5) years male, 30.5 (12.8) years female; approximately 12 months since injury, TBI) [13]

- Excellent test re-test reliability (ICC = 0.94)

(VanLoo et al, 2004, n = 13; mean age = 32.5 (11.3) years; average time post injury 11.9 (15.7) months; mean initial GCS 5.8 (2.9); mean PTA 43.8 (39.1) days, TBI) [14]

- Excellent test re-test reliability (ICC = 0.96)

Parkinson's:

(Steffen et al, 2008) [15]

- Excellent test retest reliability (ICC = 0.95 - 0.96)
- Interrater/Intrarater Reliability

Alzheimer's Disease:

(Tappen et al. 1997; n = 33; mean age = 84.7 (3.94) years, Alzheimer's Disease) [16]

- Excellent interrater reliability (ICC = 0.97 - 0.99)
- Excellent intrarater reliability (ICC = 0.76 - 0.9)

SCI:

(Scivoletto et al, 2011; n = 37; median age = 58.5 (range 19–77) years; median time from onset = 24 (range 6–109) months; AIS D = 35, C = 2; Median; WISCI = 16, Chronic SCI) [17]

- Excellent Inter-rater reliability (ICC = 0.99)
- Excellent Intra-rater reliability (ICC = 0.99)

(van Hedel et al, 2005; n = 22; AIS-A = 1, B = 0, C = 3, D = 18; mean age = 52 (20) years) [18]

Tested on 3 occasions within 7 days:

- Excellent inter-rater reliability (r = 0.97)

Determined by comparing the 2 measurements performed by a single therapist

- Excellent intra-rater reliability (r = 0.98)
- Bland Altman plot: Inter-rater reliability > intra-rater reliability and may indicate first test influence over second test

Stroke:

(Kosak & Smith, 2005; n = 18; mean age = 77 (11) years; mean time since stroke onset = 28 (34) day; enrolled in inpatient rehabilitation; mean FIM score at time of admission to inpatient rehabilitation = 68 (17), Acute Stroke)

- Adequate Intra-rater reliability (ICC = 0.74)
- Adequate Inter-rater reliability (ICC = 0.78)

Validity

Criterion Validity

COPD:

(Szekely et al, 1997; n = 47, average age 60.5 (7.5) years, individuals undergoing volume reduction surgery, COPD) [19]

- Inability to walk > 200m before the operation and resting PzCO2 > 45 were the best predictors of unacceptable postoperative outcome and mortality (specificity = 84%, sensitivity = 82%)
- Adequate correlation with length of hospital stay:
- Pre-surgical 6MWT (R = 0.32)
- Post-surgical 6MWT (R = 0.40)

Elderly:

(Harada et al, 1999; n = 86 older adults without significant disease; 35 were recruited from retirement homes and 57 from community centers; mean age = 75 (6) years, Elderly) [20]

- Adequate concurrent validity with:
- Chair stands (r = 0.67)
- Standing balance (r = 0.52)
- Gait speed (r = -0.73)
- *Distance walked was greater in active older healthy adults than in inactive older healthy adults (p < 0.0001)

SCI:

(Lam et al, 2008, SCI) [21]

- Excellent concurrent validity with: 10 Meter Walk Test (r = -0.95)
- Adequate concurrent validity with: Timed Up and

Go (r = -0.88)
- Poor concurrent validity with Walking Index for SCI II (r = 0.60)

Stroke:

(Flansbjer et al, 2005, Chronic Stroke) [22]
- Excellent concurrent validity with:
- TUG (r = -0.89)
- 10 meter comfortable gait speed (r = 0.84)
- 10 meter fast gait speed (r = 0.94)
- Stair Climbing Ascend (r = -0.82)
- Stair Climbing Descend (r = -0.80)

Construct Validity

Geriatrics:

(Harada et al, 1999, Geriatrics) [6]
- Adequate correlation with chair stands (r = 0.67), tandem balance (r = 0.52), and gait speed (r = -0.73)
- Adequate correlation with SF 36 physical function subscale (r = 0.55) and general health perceptions subscale (r = 0.39)
- Poor correlation with BMI (r = -0.07)

SCI:

(van Hedel et al, 2007; longitudinal study looking at 6min and 10 MWT at 1, 3, and 6 mo post injury, incomplete SCI who were able to ambulate 10m within 3 months post SCI n = 51, 22 tetraplegic, 29 paraplegic. Cross sectional study n = 18 incomplete SCI, acute and chronic range 2wks to 8 years AIS-C or D, utilized middle 10m of 14m walk, Acute/Subacute SCI) [18]
- Walking speed differed at each time period (1, 3, 6 mo post) but did not differ between the tests
- Regression analysis performed to look at relationship between the tests at preferred and maximum walking speed Preferred walking speed R2 = 0.87 Maximum walking speed R2 = 0.86

Responsiveness

COPD:

(Casanova et al, 2007, COPD) [23]
- Demonstrates significant decline in those individuals with severe airflow limitation (FEV1 < 50%)
- Decline worsened with disease severity

Geriatrics:

(Perera et al, 2006, Geriatrics) [24]
- Small meaningful change 20 m
- Substantial meaningful change 50 m

SCI:

(van Hedel et al, 2006, SCI)
- For individuals with incomplete SCI, the 6MWT was able to detect walking capacity improvements in patients with less ambulatory impairment during the acute and subacute stages of recovery at 3 and 6 months post injury. Similar findings were not demonstrated with the WISCI II or LEMS.
- Statistically significant responsiveness 1-3 months post injury and 3-6 months post injury with larger effect size noted 1-3 months post injury (found in Lam et al, 2008)
- For individuals with incomplete SCI, the 6MWT was not able to detect walking capacity improvements between 6 and 12 months post injury.
- May be a result of this sample having reached normal walking speeds at 6 months post injury (1.39 m/s)

Further study with a larger sample size needs evaluate responsiveness for chronic (> 12 months) injuries

Stroke:

(Kosak & Smith, 2005, Stroke)
- Over a 3.9 (2) week inpatient rehabilitation stay SRM = 1.52

References

1. Laboratories, A. T. S. C. o. P. S. f. C. P. F. (2002). “ATS statement: guidelines for the six-minute walk test.” Am J Respir Crit Care Med 166(1): 111-117.
2. YSUMediaAcademicComp. Six Minute Walk Test 2012. Available from: http://www.youtube.com/watch?v=JHzsgeudQ1I[last accessed 10/10/14]
3. Resnik, L. and Borgia, M., (2011). Reliability of outcome measures for people with lower-limbfckLRamputations: distinguishing true change from statistical error. Physical Therapy, 91(4), pp. 555-565.

4. Pera, M. C., et al. (2017). "6MWT can identify type 3 SMA patients with neuromuscular junction dysfunction." Neuromuscul Disord 27(10): 879-882.
5. Ries, J. D., Echternach, J. L., et al. "Test-retest reliability and minimal detectable change scores for the timed "up & go" test, the six-minute walk test, and gait speed in people with Alzheimer disease." Phys Ther 2009 89(6): 569-579
6. Harada, N., Chiu, V., et al. "Mobility-related function in older adults: assessment with a 6-minute walk test." Archives of physical medicine and rehabilitation 1999 80(7): 837-841
7. Steffen, T. M., Hacker, T. A., et al. "Age- and gender-related test performance in community-dwelling elderly people: Six-Minute Walk Test, Berg Balance Scale, Timed Up & Go Test, and gait speeds." Physical Therapy 2002 82(2): 128-137
8. Kennedy, D. M., Stratford, P. W., et al. "Assessing stability and change of four performance measures: a longitudinal study evaluating outcome following total hip and knee arthroplasty." BMC Musculoskelet Disord 2005 6: 3
9. Eng, J. J., Dawson, A. S., et al. "Submaximal exercise in persons with stroke: test-retest reliability and concurrent validity with maximal oxygen consumption." Arch Phys Med Rehabil 2004 85(1): 113-118
10. Flansbjer, U. B., Holmback, A. M., et al. "Reliability of gait performance tests in men and women with hemiparesis after stroke." J Rehabil Med 2005 37(2): 75-82
11. Fulk, G. D. and Echternach, J. L. "Test-retest reliability and minimal detectable change of gait speed in individuals undergoing rehabilitation after stroke." J Neurol Phys Ther 2008 32(1): 8-13
12. Wevers, L. E., Kwakkel, G., et al. "Is outdoor use of the six-minute walk test with a global positioning system in stroke patients' own neighbourhoods reproducible and valid?" J Rehabil Med 2011 43(11): 1027-1031
13. Mossberg, K. A. "Reliability of a timed walk test in persons with acquired brain injury." Am J Phys Med Rehabil 2003 82(5): 385-390; quiz 391-382
14. van Loo, M. A., Moseley, A. M., et al. "Test-re-test reliability of walking speed, step length and step width measurement after traumatic brain injury: a pilot study." Brain Inj 2004 18(10): 1041-1048
15. Steffen, T. and Seney, M. "Test-retest reliability and minimal detectable change on balance and ambulation tests, the 36-item short-form health survey, and the unified Parkinson disease rating scale in people with parkinsonism." Physical Therapy 2008 88(6): 733-746
16. Tappen, R. M., Roach, K. E., et al. "Reliability of physical performance measures in nursing home residents with Alzheimer's disease." J Gerontol A Biol Sci Med Sci 1997 52(1): M52-55
17. Scivoletto, G., Tamburella, F., et al. "Validity and reliability of the 10-m walk test and the 6-min walk test in spinal cord injury patients." Spinal Cord 2011 49(6): 736-740
18. van Hedel, H. J., Wirz, M., et al. "Assessing walking ability in subjects with spinal cord injury: validity and reliability of 3 walking tests." Archives of Physical Medicine and Rehabilitation 2005 86(2): 190-196
19 Szekely, L., Oelberg, D., et al. "Preoperative predictors of operative morbidity and mortality in COPD patients undergoing bilateral lung volume reduction surgery." Chest 1997 111(3): 550
20. Harada, N., Chiu, V., et al. "Mobility-related function in older adults: assessment with a 6-minute walk test." Archives of physical medicine and rehabilitation 1999 80(7): 837-841
21. Lam, T., Noonan, V., et al. "A systematic review of functional ambulation outcome measures in spinal cord injury." Spinal Cord 2007 46(4): 246-254
22. Flansbjer, U. B., Holmback, A. M., et al. "Reliability of gait performance tests in men and women with hemiparesis after stroke." J Rehabil Med 2005 37(2): 75-82
23. Casanova, C., Cote, C. G., et al. "The 6-min walking distance: long-term follow up in patients with COPD." Eur Respir J 2007 29(3): 535-540
24. Perera, S., Mody, S., et al. "Meaningful change and responsiveness in common physical performance measures in older adults." Journal of the American Geriatrics Society 2006 54(5): 743-749

❑❑❑

173 Spinal Cord Independence Measure (SCIM)

Objective

The SCIM has been developed to address three specific areas of function in patients with spinal cord injuries (SCI). It looks at self-care (feeding, grooming, bathing, and dressing), respiration and sphincter management, and a patient's mobility abilities (bed and transfers and indoors/outdoors). Additionally, the SCIM can also be used to help guide clinicians in determining treatment goals and objectives for patients with a SCI.[1] By helping clinicians determine areas of limitations for their patients with spinal cord injuries, both therapists and patients alike will be benefitting from this functional measurement tool.

Intended Population

The SCIM has been developed, validated, and found to be highly reproducible for patients with spinal cord injuries.[1]

Method of Use

A clinician or member of the clinical staff scores the patient on the items that this outcome measure addresses. Ideally the information obtained for scoring would be through direct observation of the activities listed, however patient report or interview information can be used. [1]

Equipment Needed

Equipment is not needed to perform and utilize this outcome measure.[2]

Completion Time

The SCIM takes approximately 30-45 mins to administer and score.[2]

Scoring

This outcome measure is very user friendly. Its scoring system is self-explanatory; therefore there isn't a manual to instruct the clinician in the scoring process. Scores range from 0-100, where a score of 0 defines total dependence and a score of 100 is indicative of complete independence. Each subscale score is evaluated within the 100-point scale (self-care: 0-20; respiration and sphincter management: 0-40; mobility: 0-40).[2]

Evidence

The newly revised SCIM produced by Catz-Itzkovich is a valid and highly reproducible measure of daily function in patients with spinal cord injuries.[3]

Reliability

Catz et al. found the interrater reliability to be modestly high with Kappa's ranging from 0.696-0.983 across the tasks listed in each subscale. [4]

Validity

Internal consistency: excellent (Cronbach's alpha = 0.9227) [4]

Criterion Validity: difficult to establish due to a lack of 'gold standard' to measure the SCIM against.[4]

Construct Validity: Excellent correlation between the SCIM and the FIM (r =.85) [4]

Excellent correlation between the SCIM and the Walking Index for Spinal Cord Injury (WISCI). (r = .97)[5]

Responsiveness

The SCIM and the SCIM III were found to be more responsive than the FIM.[6]

Miscellaneous

The newest version of the SCIM was preceded by two previous versions. The SCIM I and II were both found to be valid and reliable but did not take into account intercultural differences. Therefore, the SCIM III was developed in 2002 as an international version of the prior forms.[1] Catz et al. designed this version to encompass patients in every walk of life, regardless of their culture.

References

1. Catz A, Itzkovich M. Spinal cord independence measure: comprehensive ability to rating scale for the spinal cord lesion. JRRD. 2007;44(1):65-68.
2. The Spinal Cord Independence Measure (SCIM). Available at: http://www.scireproject.com/book/export/html/152
3. Catz A, Itzkovich M, Steinberg F, Philo O, et al. The Catz-Itzkovich SCIM: a revised version of the spinal cord independence measure. Disability and Rehabilitation. 2001;23(6):263-268.
4. Catz, A., Itzkovich, M., et al. (1997). "SCIM-spinal cord independence measure: a new disability scale for patients with spinal cord lesions." Spinal Cord. 35(12): 850-856.
5. Morganti, B., Scivoletto, G., et al. (2004). "Walking index for spinal cord injury (WISCI): criterion validation." Spinal Cord. 43(1): 27-33.
6. Dawson, J., Shamley, D., et al. (2008). "A structured review of outcome measures used for the assessment of rehabilitation interventions for spinal cord injury." Spinal Cord. 46(12): 768-780.

Spinal Cord Independence Measure (SCIM)

Self-Care.

1. Feeding (cutting, opening containers, pouring, bringing food to mouth, holding cup with fluid)
0. Needs parenteral, gastrostomy, or fully assisted oral feeding
1. Needs partial assistance for eating and/or drinking, or for wearing adaptive devices
2. Eats independently; needs adaptive devices or assistance only for cutting food and/or pouring and/or opening containers
3. Eats and drinks independently; does not require assistance or adaptive devices.

2. Bathing (soaping, washing, drying body and head, manipulating water tap).

A-upper body; B-lower body

A. 0. Requires total assistance
1. Requires partial assistance
2. Washes independently with adaptive devices or in a specific setting (e.g., bars, chair)
3. Washes independently; does not require adaptive devices or specific setting (not customary for healthy people) (adss)

B. 0. Requires total assistance
1. Requires partial assistance
2. Washes independently with adaptive devices or in a specific setting (adss)
3. Washes independently; does not require adaptive devices (adss) or specific setting

3. Dressing (clothes, shoes, permanent orthoses: dressing, wearing, undressing).

A-upper body; B-lower body

A. 0. Requires total assistance
1. Requires partial assistance with clothes without buttons, zippers or laces (cwobzl)
2. Independent with cwobzl; requires adaptive devices and/or specific settings (adss)
3. Independent with cwobzl; does not require adss; needs assistance or adss only for bzl
4. Dresses (any cloth) independently; does not require adaptive devices or specific setting

B. 0. Requires total assistance
1. Requires partial assistancewith clothes without buttons, zipps or laces (cwobzl)
2. Independent with cwobzl; requires adaptive devices and/or specific settings (adss)
3. Independent with cwobzl without adss; needs assistance or adss only for bzl
4. Dresses (any cloth) independently; does not require adaptive devices or specific setting

4. Grooming (washing hands and face, brushing teeth, combing hair, shaving, applying makeup)
0. Requires total assistance
1. Requires partial assistance
2. Grooms independently with adaptive devices
3. Grooms independently without adaptive devices

SUBTOTAL (0-20)

Respiration and Sphincter Management

5. Respiration

0. Requires tracheal tube (TT) and permanent or intermittent assisted ventilation (IAV)
2. Breathes independently with TT; requires oxygen, much assistance in coughing or TT management
4. Breathes independently with TT; requires little assistance in coughing or TT management
6. Breathes independently without TT; requires oxygen, much assistance in coughing, a mask (e.g., peep) or IAV (bipap)
8. Breathes independently without TT; requires little assistance or stimulation for coughing
10. Breathes independently without assistance or device

6. Sphincter Management - Bladder

0. Indwelling catheter
3. Residual urine volume (RUV) > 100cc; no regular catheterization or assisted intermittent catheterization
6. RUV < 100cc or intermittent self-catheterization; needs assistance for applying drainage instrument
9. Intermittent self-catheterization; uses external drainage instrument; does not need assistance for applying
11. Intermittent self-catheterization; continent between catheterizations; does not use external drainage instrument
13. RUV <100cc; needs only external urine drainage; no assistance is required for drainage
15. RUV <100cc; continent; does not use external drainage instrument

7. Sphincter Management - Bowel

0. Irregular timing or very low frequency (less than once in 3 days) of bowel movements
5. Regular timing, but requires assistance (e.g., for applying suppository); rare accidents (less than twice a month)
8. Regular bowel movements, without assistance; rare accidents (less than twice a month)
10. Regular bowel movements, without assistance; no accidents

8. Use of Toilet (perineal hygiene, adjustment of clothes before/after, use of napkins or diapers).

0. Requires total assistance
1. Requires partial assistance; does not clean self
2. Requires partial assistance; cleans self independently
4. Uses toilet independently in all tasks but needs adaptive devices or special setting (e.g., bars)
5. Uses toilet independently; does not require adaptive devices or special setting)

SUBTOTAL (0-40)

Mobility (room and toilet)

9. Mobility in Bed and Action to Prevent Pressure Sores

0. Needs assistance in all activities: turning upper body in bed, turning lower body in bed, sitting up in bed, doing push-ups in wheelchair, with or without adaptive devices, but not with electric aids
2. Performs one of the activities without assistance
4. Performs two or three of the activities without assistance
6. Performs all the bed mobility and pressure release activities independently

10. Transfers: bed-wheelchair (locking wheelchair, lifting footrests, removing and adjusting arm rests, transferring, lifting feet).

0. Requires total assistance
1. Needs partial assistance and/or supervision, and/or adaptive devices (e.g., sliding board)
2. Independent (or does not require wheelchair)

11. Transfers: wheelchair-toilet-tub (if uses toilet wheelchair: transfers to and from; if uses regular wheelchair: locking wheelchair, lifting footrests, removing and adjusting armrests, transferring, lifting feet)

0. Requires total assistance
1. Needs partial assistance and/or supervision, and/or adaptive devices (e.g., grab-bars)
2. Independent (or does not require wheelchair)

Mobility (indoors and outdoors, on even surface)

12. Mobility Indoors

0. Requires total assistance
1. Needs electric wheelchair or partial assistance to operate manual wheelchair
2. Moves independently in manual wheelchair
3. Requires supervision while walking (with or without devices)

4. Walks with a walking frame or crutches (swing)
5. Walks with crutches or two canes (reciprocal walking)
6. Walks with one cane
7. Needs leg orthosis only
8. Walks without walking aids

13. Mobility for Moderate Distances (10-100 meters)

0. Requires total assistance
1. Needs electric wheelchair or partial assistance to operate manual wheelchair
2. Moves independently in manual wheelchair
3. Requires supervision while walking (with or without devices)
4. Walks with a walking frame or crutches (swing)
5. Walks with crutches or two canes (reciprocal walking)
6. Walks with one cane
7. Needs leg orthosis only
8. Walks without walking aids

14. Mobility Outdoors (more than 100 meters)

0. Requires total assistance
1. Needs electric wheelchair or partial assistance to operate manual wheelchair
2. Moves independently in manual wheelchair
3. Requires supervision while walking (with or without devices)
4. Walks with a walking frame or crutches (swing)
5. Walks with crutches or two canes (reciprocal waking)
6. Walks with one cane
7. Needs leg orthosis only
8. Walks without walking aids

15. Stair Management

0. Unable to ascend or descend stairs
1. Ascends and descends at least 3 steps with support or supervision of another person
2. Ascends and descends at least 3 steps with support of handrail and/or crutch or cane
3. Ascends and descends at least 3 steps without any support or supervision

16. Transfers: wheelchair-car (approaching car, locking wheelchair, removing arm- and footrests, transferring to and from car, bringing wheelchair into and out of car)

0. Requires total assistance
1. Needs partial assistance and/or supervision and/or adaptive devices
2. Transfers independent; does not require adaptive devices (or does not require wheelchair)

17. Transfers: ground-wheelchair

0. Requires assistance
1. Transfers independent with or without adaptive devices (or does not require wheelchair

SUBTOTAL (0-40)

TOTAL SCIM SCORE (0-100) =

❑❑❑

174 Spinal Cord Injury Outcome Measures Overview

Introduction

An Outcome Measure is a test used to objectively determine baseline function of an individual at the beginning of treatment. Once treatment has commenced, the same instrument can be used to determine progress and treatment efficacy. With the move towards Evidence-Based Practice (EBP), objective measures of outcome are important to provide credible and reliable justification for treatment. The instrument should also be convenient to apply for the therapist and comfortable for the individual.

Measuring the effectiveness of interventions is accepted as being central to good practice. An integral part of evaluating clinical practice is to objectively assess the intervention and measure it against a set of outcomes to determine its efficacy. For results to be meaningful, it is imperative that any measures used to assess outcomes in any health care context cover domains (for example pain, physical function, perceived independence) that are relatively specific and appropriate to both the particular context and population that you are working with and have acceptable measurement properties, including: reliability, validity, responsiveness, acceptability and feasibility specific to that population. [1][2]

There has been an increased focus on outcome measurement in the field of spinal cord injury, with creation of common definitions and data sets to ensure that information being collected is both valid and accurate with consistent recording of both clinical and research information. Despite increased use of validated outcome and more frequent assessment, there is still a broad range of outcome measures being used that limits the ability to compare findings from centre to centre or client to client, which has an impact on identification and implementation of best practice. This page presents the best available information on how outcome measures for spinal cord injury might be classified and selected for use, based upon their measurement qualities incorporating the most recent consensus recommendations. [3][4]

SCI EDGE Task Force Recommended Outcome Measures

The SCI EDGE Task Force reviewed 63 outcome measures covering the range of body structure and function, activities and participation evaluating each for psychometrics and clinical utility for individuals with a Spinal Cord Injury. Through literature review, analysis, and a modified Delphi Procedure, recommendations were formulated for outcome measures that are highly recommended for use in individuals with Spinal Cord Injury during each phase of treatment and for each type of injury, with a summary for each of these outcome measures updated or added to the Shirley Ryan Ability Lab Rehabilitation Measures Database. [4]

- 20 measures were recommended or highly recommended for both complete and incomplete spinal cord injury
- 14 measures were recommended or highly recommended for at least 2 levels of acuity
- 23 measures were recommended for use in physiotherapy education
- 32 measures were recommended for use in spinal cord injury research

Results also revealed a number of underrepresented areas. In the Body Structure and Function Domain of the International Classification of Functioning, Disability, and Health, none of the measures for tone or cardiovascular function could be recommended secondary to insufficient research specific to the spinal cord injury population to support a stronger recommendation. Similarly in the Activity Domain, balance, upper limb function, and wheelchair skills were also underrepresented with only 1 of 7 balance measures (ie, Berg Balance Scale) and 2 of 9 upper limb function measures (ie, the Capabilities of Upper Extremity Functioning and the Graded and Redefined Assessment of Sensibility, Strength, and Prehension) receiving a "Recommended" rating. Finally in the Participation Domain, all measures that achieved a "Recommended" or "Highly Recommended" rating in at least 3 of the 5 categories were patient- reported outcomes measuring domains of quality of life, community function, health and wellness, and environmental factors, which all displayed extensive psychometric data available in the chronic spinal cord injury population, but only one recommended in the acute spinal cord injury population, (the Needs Assessment Check-list), as such the Participation-level Outcome Measures are most appropriate to be used in the chronic spinal cord injury population. [4]

Phase of Treatment

Overall 14 measures were recommended or highly recommended for at least 2 levels of acuity providing the ability to compare progress over a longer period of time and covering a number of domains of the International Classification of Functioning, Disability, and Health. The acute spinal cord injury category had a total of 6 "Highly Recommended" Outcome Measures and 7 "Recommended" Outcome Measures in comparison with the chronic spinal cord injury category, which had a total of 6 "Highly Recommended" Outcome Measures and 19 "Recommended" Outcome Measures. Limited research in acute spinal cord injury (0 - 3 months) meant fewer measures could be recommended during this phase of injury. In particular in relation to quality of life and upper limb function were areas in which no recommendations could be made, despite the importance of both areas and have been identified as a need for further research and development. [4]

Type of Injury	AIS Level	Highly Recommended	Recommended
Acute	0-3 Months	6 Minute Walk Test (6MWT) 10 Meter Walk Test (10MWT) Hand Held Myometry Timed Up and Go (TUG) Walking Index for Spinal Cord Injury II (WISCI II) ASIA Impairment Scale	Berg Balance Scale (BBS) Functional Independence Measure (FIM) Manual Muscle Test (MMT) Needs Assessment Checklist Numeric Pain Rating Scale Spinal Cord Independence Measure III (SCIM III) Spinal Cord Injury Functional Ambulation Inventory
Subacute	3-6 Months	6 Minute Walk Test (6MWT) 10 Meter Walk Test (10MWT) Handheld Myometry Timed Up and Go (TUG)	Berg Balance Scale (BBS) Functional Independence Measure (FIM) Manual Muscle Test (MMT) Needs Assessment Checklist Numeric Pain Rating Scale Sickness Impact Profile 68 Spinal Cord Injury Functional Ambulation Inventory Spinal Cord Independence Measure III (SCIM III) Walking Index for Spinal Cord Injury II (WISCI II) Berg Balance Scale (BBS)

			Capabilities of Upper Extremity Instrument (CUE)
			Craig Handicap Assessment & Reporting Technique (CHART)
			Craig Hospital Inventory of Environmental Factors
			Functional Independence Measure (FIM
			Graded and Redefined Assessment of Sensibility, Strength and Prehension (GRASSP)
			Life Satisfaction Questionnaire 9
		6 Minute Walk Test (6MWT)	Manual Muscle Test (MMT)
		10 Meter Walk Test (10MWT)	Multidimensional Pain Inventory, SCI Version
		Handheld Myometry	Reintegration to Normal Living Index
Chronic	> 6 Months	umeric Pain Rating Scale (NRS)	Satisfaction With Life Scale
		World Health Organization Quality of Life - BREF (WHOQOL - BREF)	Short Form 36 (SF-36)
		ASIA Impairment Scale	Sickness Impact Profile 68
			Spinal Cord Injury Functional Ambulation Inventory
			Spinal Cord Injury Functional Ambulation Profile
			Spinal Cord Injury Independence Measure III (SCIM III)
			Timed Up and Go (TUG)
			Walking Index for Spinal Cord Injury II (WISCI II)
			Wheelchair Skills Test (WST)
			Wheelchair Users Shoulder Pain Index

ASIA Impairment Scale Level

Overall 20 measures were given a rating of "Recommended" or "Highly Recommended" in both incomplete and complete spinal cord injury categories including measures covering the Body Structure and Function, Activity, Participation and Environment Domains of the International Classification of Functioning, Disability, and Health. [4]

Type of Injury	AIS Level	Highly Recommended	Recommended
			Capabilities of Upper Extremity Instrument (CUE)

			Craig Handicap Assessment and Reporting Technique
			Craig Hospital Inventory of Environmental Factors
			Functional Independence Measure
			Graded and Redefined Assessment of Sensibility Strength and Prehension
			Life Satisfaction Questionnaire 9
		Handheld Myometry	Manual Muscle Test (MMT)
Motor	AIS A	World Health Organization Quality of Life - BREF (WHOQOL - BREF)	Multidimensional Pain Inventory, SCI Version
Complete	AIS B	ASIA Impairment Scale	Needs Assessment Checklist
			Numeric Pain Rating Scale
			Reintegration to Normal Living Index
			Satisfaction With Life Scale
			Short Form 36 (SF-36)
			Sickness Impact Profile 68
			Spinal Cord Injury Independence Measure III (SCIM III)
			Walking Index for Spinal Cord Injury II (WISCI II)
			Wheelchair Users Shoulder Pain Index
		6 Minute Walk Test (6MWT)	Berg Balance Scale (BBS)
Motor	AIS C	10 Meter Walk Test (10MWT)	Capabilities of Upper Extremity Instrument (CUE)
Incomplete	AIS D	Handheld Myometry Timed Up and Go (TUG)	Craig Handicap Assessment & Reporting Technique (CHART)
		Walking Index for Spinal Cord Injury II (WISCI II)	Craig Hospital Inventory of Environmental Factors
		World Health Organization Quality of Life - BREF (WHOQOL - BREF)	Functional Independence Measure (FIM)
		ASIA Impairment Scale	Graded and Redefined Assessment of Sensibility Strength and Prehension (GRASSP)
			Life Satisfaction Questionnaire 9
			Manual Muscle Test (MMT)
			Multidimensional Pain Inventory, SCI Version
			Needs Assessment Checklist

			Numeric Pain Rating Scale
			Reintegration to Normal Living Index
			Spinal Cord Injury Functional Ambulation Inventory
			Spinal Cord Injury Functional Ambulation Profile
			Satisfaction With Life Scale
			Short Form 36 (SF-36)
			Sickness Impact Profile 68
			Spinal Cord Injury Independence Measure III (SCIM III)
			Wheelchair Users Shoulder Pain Index

SCIRE Spinal Cord Injury Outcome Measures Toolkit

Specific and validated outcome measures data is central to understanding the needs of clients, their level of care, and the services that will enhance their rehabilitation. Developed in 2017 specifically for clinicians working in spinal cord injury rehabilitation, the Spinal Cord Injury Research Evidence (SCIRE) Outcome Measures Toolkit aims to further address the need for common measures in spinal cord injury clinical practice, to support practical and clinically applicable research, and ensures up-to-date educational material. [3]

One hundred and forty-eight outcome measures were initially considered for inclusion with consensus reached for 23 out of 30 clinical areas. In the remaining seven clinical areas, more than one outcome measure was recommended. The final toolkit comprises 33 Outcome Measures across 30 Clinical Areas with sufficient measurement properties for use with a spinal cord injury population. It was highlighted that many of the other measures not selected were missing clinically important measurement properties, such as responsiveness, that assist the most in documenting a client's progress in rehabilitation. As such further research is recommended to establish the clinical suitability of the other measures for later inclusion in the toolkit. [3]

International Classification of Functioning, Disability, and Health Component

ICF Area	Clinical Area	Outcome Measure
	Neurological and Autonomic	International Standards for Neurological Classification of Spinal Cord Injury (ISNCSCI)
	Strength	Surface Electromyography
		Hand-Held Myometer
		Ashworth and Modified Ashworth
	Spasticity	Penn Spasm Frequency Scale
		Pendulum Test
Body Structure and Function	Sensory - Pain	Brief Pain Inventory
		Classification System for Chronic Pain in Spinal Cord Injury
	Skin Health	Braden Scale
		Spinal Cord Injury Pressure Ulcer Scale (SCIPUS)
		CAGE Questionnaire

	Mental Health	Depression Anxiety Stress Scale - 21
		Patient Health Questionnaire - 9
		6 Minute Walk Test (6MWT)
		10 Meter Walk Test (10MWT)
	Lower Limb and Walking	Berg Balance Scale (BBS)
		Timed Up and Go Test (TUG)
		Walking Index for Spinal Cord Injury (WISCI)
		Standing and Walking Toolkit
	Wheeled Mobility	Wheelchair Skills Test (WST)
Activities		Capabilities of Upper Extremity Instrument (CUE)
		Graded Redefined Assessment of Strength, Sensibility and Prehension (GRASSP)
	Upper Limb	Jebsen Hand Function Test
		Sollerman Hand Function Test
		Box and Block Test
		Frenchay Activities Index (FAI)
	Self Care	Lawton Instrumental Activities of Daily Living Scale (IADL)
		Spinal Cord Independence Measure (SCIM)
	Community Reintegration	Craig Handicap Assessment & Reporting Technique (CHART)
		Reintegration to Normal Living Index
Participation	Quality of Life	Short Form-36 (SF-36) World Health Organization Quality of Life - BREF (WHOQOL-BREF)
		Assistive Technology Device Predisposition Assessment (ATD-PA)
Environment	Assistive Technology	Quebec User Evaluation of Satisfaction with Assistive Technology (QUEST)

Conclusion

Spinal cord injury is a medically complex and life-disrupting condition with a high likelihood that secondary health complications, such as pressure ulcers, fractures, or circulatory dysfunction, will develop. Clinicians who work with individuals with a spinal cord injury share a commitment toward providing the best interventions to produce successful out- comes for those that they work with. [3]

The most meaningful determinant of treatment efficacy from the perspective of the individual with a spinal cord injury generally relates to improvements in their ability to function in everyday activities and must be forefront in our minds as health care professionals throughout all stages of treatment and rehabilitation. While there will never be a perfect questionnaire or measure of outcome, choosing the right measure to use involves identifying the most appropriate measure for the chosen population group, context and purpose, where evidence exists to show that the questionnaire has exhibited adequate measurement properties pertaining to that group and/or context. [1][3]

Prior to determining any intervention, careful choice of treatment goals and aims is essential in individuals with a spinal cord injury in order to identify and determine the most appropriate outcome measures to use. This means the therapist can ensure they are providing the most appropriate intervention that meets the treatment goals and expectations of the individual with a spinal cord injury. Use of an outcome measures toolkit, specifically validated for spinal cord injury, should lead to improved identification of best practice and enable clinicians to more effectively monitor client progress. [2][3]

References

1. Dawson J, Shamley D, Jamous MA. A Structured Review of Outcome Measures used for the Assessment of Rehabilitation Interventions for Spinal Cord Injury. Spinal Cord. 2008 x. Dec;46(12):768.
2. Lam T, Noonan VK, Eng JJ. A Systematic Review of Functional Ambulation Outcome Measures in Spinal Cord Injury. Spinal Cord. 2008 Apr;46(4):246.
3. Chan CW, Miller WC, Querée M, Noonan VK, Wolfe DL, SCIRE Research Team. The Development of an Outcome Measures Toolkit for Spinal Cord Injury Rehabilitation: Création d'une Trousse de Mesures des Résultats pour la Réadaptation des Personnes ayant subi une lésion de la Moelle épinière. Canadian Journal of Occupational Therapy. 2017 Apr;84(2):119-29.
4. Kahn JH, Tappan R, Newman CP, Palma P, Romney W, Tseng Stultz E, Tefertiller C, Weisbach CL. Outcome Measure Recommendations From the Spinal Cord Injury EDGE Task Force. Physical Therapy. 2016 Nov 1;96(11):1832-42.
5. RickHansenInstitute. Outcome Measures in SCI Interventions - Dr. Sukhvinder Kalsi-Ryan. Available from: https://youtu.be/2C2Owo7y23Q[last accessed 30/10/18

□□□

175 New Freezing of Gait Questionnaire (NFOG-Q)

Objective

The New Freezing of Gait Questionnaire (NFOG-Q) is a self-reported questionnaire consisting of 9 items that measure freezing of gait (FOG). The NFOG-Q is the renewed version of the FOG-Q, which originally consisted of 6 items.

Intended Population

Patients with Parkinson's Disease and other Parkinson-related Symptoms.

The New Freezing of Gait Questionnaire

Did you experience freezing in the last month?

Yes No

During your worst state—Do you walk:

0 Normally

1 Almost normally—somewhat slow

2 Slow but fully independent

3 Need assistance or walking aid

4 Unable to walk

Are your gait difficulties affecting your daily activities and independence?

0 Not at all

1 Mildly

2 Moderately

3 Severely

4 Unable to walk

Do you feel that your feet get glued to the floor while walking, making a turn or when trying to initiate walking (freezing)?

0 Never

1 Very rarely—about once a month

2 Rarely—about once a week

3 Often—about once a day

4 Always—whenever walking

How long is your longest freezing episode?

0 Never happened

1 1–2 s

2 3–10 s

3 11–30 s

4 Unable to walk for more than 30 s

Method of Use

- The NFOG-Q is easy to administer and requires no equipment.

Evidence

Reliability

A study by Hulzinga et al 2020 [1] concluded that the NFOG-Q is not sufficiently reliable nor responsive to detect small effect sizes.

References

1. Hulzinga F, Nieuwboer A, Dijkstra BW, Mancini M, Strouwen C, Bloem BR, Ginis P. The New Freezing of Gait Questionnaire: Unsuitable as an Outcome in Clinical Trials? Mov Disord Clin Pract. 2020 Jan 14;7(2):199-205.

❑❑❑

176 Tampa Scale of Kinesiophobia

Objective

The original Tampa Scale of Kinesiophobiais (TSK) was first developed in 1991 by R. Miller, S. Kopri, and D. Todd. TSK is 17 items a self-reporting questionnaire based on evaluation of fear of movement, fear of physical activity, and fear avoidance. It was first developed to distinguish between non-excessive fear and phobia in patients with chronic musculoskeletal pain, specifically the fear of movement in patients with chronic low back pain then widely used for different parts of the body. The questionnaire using 4 points to assess that are based on; the model of fear-avoidance, fear of work-related activities, fear of movement, and fear of re-injury[1]. There is another valid, and reliable abbreviated version of the scale that consists of 11 items [2].

It consists of **two subscales**,

Activity avoidance (AA): reflection of activity that may result in an increase in pain or cause injury.

Somatic focus (SF): reflection of beliefs and underlying serious conditions.

Intended Population

Tampa scale used in patients with chronic musculoskeletal pain such as low back pain, neck pain, fibromyalgia. TSK-AA was also valid to use after spinal fusion in adolescents with idiopathic scoliosis[3].

Method of Use

TSK composed of 17 items, scoring range from 1: 4 as follows for items from 1, 2, 3-7, 9-11, 13-15, and 17:

1. Strongly disagree
2. Disagree
3. Agree
4. Strongly agree.

For items 4, 8, 12, and 16 it is vice versa:

1. Strongly disagree.
2. Disagree
3. Agree
4. Strongly agree.

The total score of the scale range from 17- 68, where 17 means no kinesiophobia, 68 means severe kinesiophobia, and score ± 37 indicates there is kinesiophobia.

The shortened version TSK-11 maintains items 1, 2, 3, 5, 6, 7, 10, 11, 13, 15, and 17 from the original scale, and its score range from 11-44.

Evidence

Reliability

Internal consistency, TSK shows a high level of internal consistency across all items and is positively associated with related measures of fear-avoidance, pain catastrophizing, pain-related disability[4].

In the Finnish version of TSK, the test-retest reliability (ICC) = 0.887[5].

Validity

Construct validity: moderate correlation coefficient with measures of pain-related fear, pain catastrophising, and disability in patients with CLBP.

Predictive validity: moderate correlation coefficient with physical performance tests[6].

Concurrent validity is moderate, ranging from r(s) =0.33 to 0.59[7].

Responsiveness

For patients with chronic low back pain, TSK was sensitive to detect clinical changes[8], it was also sensitive to detect changes after spinal fusion[9]. Unlike in patients with ACL injury, it isn't the best way to assess psychological factors according to the Japanese version[10].

References

1. Hudes K. The Tampa Scale of Kinesiophobia and neck pain, disability and range of motion: a narrative review of the literature. The Journal of the Canadian Chiropractic Association. 2011 Sep;55(3):222.
2. Tkachuk GA, Harris CA. Psychometric properties of the Tampa Scale for Kinesiophobia-11 (TSK-11). The Journal of Pain. 2012 Oct 1;13(10):970-7.
3. Ye DL, Plante I, Roy M, Ouellet JA, Ferland CE. The Tampa Scale of Kinesiophobia: Structural Validation among Adolescents with Idiopathic Scoliosis Undergoing Spinal Fusion Surgery. Physical & Occupational Therapy In Pediatrics. 2020 Feb 6:1-1.
4. French DJ, France CR, Vigneau F, French JA, Evans RT. Fear of movement/(re) injury in chronic pain: a psychometric assessment of the original English version of the Tampa scale for kinesiophobia (TSK). Pain. 2007 Jan 1;127(1-2):42-51.
5. Koho P, Aho S, Pohjolainen T, Hurri H. Reliability of Tampa Scale for Kinesiophobia Questionnaire and Comparability of Paper and Computer Versions in Chronic Pain Patients. InOrthopaedic Proceedings 2009 May (Vol. 91, No. SUPP_II, pp. 286-286). The British Editorial Society of Bone & Joint Surgery.
6. Roelofs J, Goubert L, Peters ML, Vlaeyen JW, Crombez G. The Tampa Scale for Kinesiophobia: further examination of psychometric properties in patients with chronic low back pain and fibromyalgia. European Journal of Pain. 2004 Oct 1;8(5):495-502.
7. Swinkels-Meewisse EJ, Swinkels RA, Verbeek AL, Vlaeyen JW, Oostendorp RA. Psychometric properties of the Tampa Scale for kinesiophobia and the fear-avoidance beliefs questionnaire in acute low back pain. Manual therapy. 2003 Feb 1;8(1):29-36.
8. Monticone M, Ambrosini E, Rocca B, Foti C, Ferrante S. Responsiveness of the Tampa Scale of Kinesiophobia in Italian subjects with chronic low back pain undergoing motor and cognitive rehabilitation. European Spine Journal. 2016 Sep 1;25(9):2882-8.
9. Monticone M, Ambrosini E, Rocca B, Foti C, Ferrante S. Responsiveness and minimal clinically important changes for the Tampa Scale of Kinesiophobia after lumbar fusion during cognitive behavioral rehabilitation. European Journal of Physical and Rehabilitation Medicine. 2017 Jun;53(3):351-8.
10. Huang H, Nagao M, Arita H, Shiozawa J, Nishio H, Kobayashi Y, Kaneko H, Nagayama M, Saita Y, Ishijima M, Takazawa Y. Reproducibility, responsiveness and validation of the Tampa Scale for Kinesiophobia in patients with ACL injuries. Health and quality of life outcomes. 2019 Dec 1;17(1):150.

Tampa Scale of Kinesiophobia

The original Tampa Scale of Kinesiophobia (TSK) was developed by R. Miller, S. Kopri, andD. Todd, in 1991. This represents a modified version.

Instructions:

In these days of high-tech medicine, one of the most important sources of information about you is often missing from your medical records: your own feeling or intuitions about what is happening with your body. We hope that the following information will help to fill that gap. Please answer the following questions according to your true feelings, not according to what others think you should believe. Score each statement from strongly disagree to strongly agree by tapping the appropriate box.

	Strongly disagree (1)	Somewhat disagree (2)	Somewhat agree (3)	Strongly agree (4)
1. I'm afraid that I might injury myself if I exercise				
2. If I were to try to overcome it, my pain would increase				
3. My body is telling me I have something dangerously wrong				
4. My pain would probably be relieved if I were to exercise				
5. People aren't taking my medical condition seriously enough				
6. My accident has put my body at risk for the rest of my life				
7. Pain always means I have injured my body				
8. Just because something aggravates my pain does not mean it is dangerous				
9. I am afraid that I might injure myself accidentally				
10. Simply being careful that I do not make any unnecessary move ments is the safest thing I can do to prevent my pain from worsening.				
11. I wouldn't have this much pain if there weren't something potentially dangerous going on in my body				
12. Although my condition is painful, I would be better off if I were physically active				
13. Pain lets me know when to stop exercising so that I don't injure				
14. It's really not safe for a person with a condition like mine to be physically active				
15. I can't do all the things normal people do because it's too easy for me to get injured				
16. Even though something is causing me a lot of pain, I don't think it's actually dangerous				
17. No one should have to exercise when he/she is in pain				

❑❑❑

177 The 4-Stage Balance Test

Objective

A tool to assess a client's mobility and risk of falls, based on his or her ability to hold four progressively more challenging positions[1](evaluates static balance).[2]

Intended Population

The test is intended to be performed on older adults.[2]

Method of Use

Directions - There are four standing positions that get progressively harder to maintain.

1. Stand with your feet side-by-side
2. Place the instep of one foot so it is touching the big toe of the other foot.
3. Tandem stance Place one foot in front of the other, heel touching toes
4. Stand on one foot.[3]

- You should describe and demonstrate each position to the patient.
- Then, stand next to the patient, hold their arm, and help them assume the correct position.
- When the patient is steady, let go, and time how long they can maintain the position, but remain ready to assist the patient if they should lose their balance.
- If the patient can hold a position for 10 seconds without moving their feet or needing support, go on to the next position.
- If not, STOP the test. Patients **should not** use an assistive device (cane or walker) and they should keep their eyes open[3] [4]

Outcome

- Not being able to hold the tandem stance (task number 3) for 10 seconds is an indication of increased risk of fall. [2]
- To reduce their risk of falling, consider implementing gait and balance exercises, or refer them to an evidence-based fall prevention program, such as Otago balance program, Tai Chi.

Reliability

Interclass (Pearson) correlations, with time between test and re-test of 3-4 months, 187 subjects from the community) is reported as moderate (0.66) [5]

Validity

A robust correlation has been reported when comparing the scale with other measurements for balance, in the same subjects. [5]

References

1. National center of nutrition and aging 4 stage balance test Available from:https://nutritionandaging.org/4-stage-balance-test/#wbounce-modal (last accessed 16.10.2020)
2. Phelan EA, Mahoney JE, Voit JC, Stevens JA. Assessment and management of fall risk in primary care settings. Medical Clinics. 2015 Mar 1;99(2):281-93.
3. CDC 4 stage balance test Available from: https://www.cdc.gov/steadi/pdf/4-Stage_Balance_Test-print.pdf (last accessed 16.10.2020)
4. Gardner MM, Buchner DM, Robertson MC, Campbell AJ. Practical implementation of an exercise-based falls prevention program. Age and ageing. 2001 Jan 1;30(1):77-83.
5. Rossiter-Fornoff JE, Wolf SL, Wolfson LI, Buchner DM, FICSIT Group. A cross-sectional validation study of the FICSIT common data base static balance measures. The Journals of Gerontology Series A: Biological Sciences and Medical Sciences. 1995 Nov 1;50(6):M291-7.

❑❑❑

178 The Bath Indices

Introduction

The **Bath Indices** is a functional and disease activity indices used to aid diagnosis and monitor disease activity in people with Ankylosing Spondylitis (AS). It is made up of four indices which are the Bath Ankylosing Spondylitis Metrology Index(BASMI), the Bath Ankylosing Spondylitis Functional Index (BASFI), the Bath Ankylosing Spondylitis Disease Activity Index (BASDAI), and the Bath Ankylosing Spondylitis Patient Global Score (BAS-G). All indices produce a score out of 10, giving a clear numerical outcome each time the indices are used. Also, the four indices have been studied for reliability, speed, variability, reproducibility, and sensitivity to change[1].

178. A "The Bath Ankylosing Spondylitis Functional Index (BASFI)"

Objective

The Bath Ankylosing Spondylitis Functional Index (BASFI) is a set of 10 questions designed to determine the degree of functional limitation in patients with Ankylosing Spondylitis (AS). The 10 questions were chosen with a major input from patients with AS. The first 8 questions are about everyday tasks and dependent on functional anatomy (bending, reaching, changing position, standing, turning, and climbing steps with or without rail) while the final 2 questions assess the patients' ability to cope with everyday life. Each item is scored on a scale of 0-10[2].

A 10 cm visual analogue scale (VAS) was used to answer the questions but it is now being replaced by a numerical pain rating scale (NRS) in many centres [1].

Intended Population

It is a patient self-report questionnaire for the patient with Ankylosing Spondylitis.

Method of Use

BASFI is made up of 10 questions that are related to activities of daily living and are scored with a rating scale from 0 (no functional impairments) to 10 (maximal impairment). Each question is answered on a 10 cm horizontal VAS or a numeric response scale (NRS). A score of 0 indicates the activity was easy and a score of 10 indicates the activity was impossible for the person to accomplish[2].

All scores from questions 1-10 are added and then divided by 10. The mean of the individual scores is calculated to give the overall index score. A higher score indicates a higher degree of functional limitations.

The BASFI Items and Scoring[2]

Please indicate your level of ability with each of the following activities during the past week.

1. Putting on your socks or tights without help or aids (e.g sock aid).
   1 2 3 4 5 6 7 8 9 10
2. Bending from the waist to pick up a pen from the floor without aid.
   1 2 3 4 5 6 7 8 9 10
3. Reaching up to a high shelf without help or aids (e.g helping hand).
   1 2 3 4 5 6 7 8 9 10
4. Getting up from an arm less chair without your hands or any other help.
   1 2 3 4 5 6 7 8 9 10
5. Getting up off the floor without help from lying on your back.
   1 2 3 4 5 6 7 8 9 10
6. Standing unsupported for 10 minutes without discomfort.
   1 2 3 4 5 6 7 8 9 10
7. Climbing 12-15 steps without using a handrail or walking aid.
   1 2 3 4 5 6 7 8 9 10
8. Looking over your shoulder without turning your body.
   1 2 3 4 5 6 7 8 9 10
9. Doing physically demanding activities (e.g physiotherapy exercises, gardening or sports).
   1 2 3 4 5 6 7 8 9 10
10. Doing a full days activities whether it be at home or at work.
    1 2 3 4 5 6 7 8 9 10

Evidence

The BASFI satisfies the criteria required of a functional index: it is quick and easy to complete, is reliable and is sensitive to change across the whole spectrum of disease. Furthermore, over the 3 week period of inpatient treatment, the BASFI revealed a significant improvement in function (20%, $p = 0.004$) while there was a less impressive change in the Dougados functional index (6%, $p = 0.03$). This demonstrates the superior sensitivity of the BASFI: Consistency was good for both indices ($p < 0.001$), as was the relationship between patient perception of function and function as assessed by an external observer ($p < 0.001$)[3].

Reliability

When patients were assessed on their actual performance of eight items from the BASFI representing activities of daily life, adequate to excellent test-retest reproducibility was shown[4]. A significant association between the BASMI and BASFI has also been demonstrated indicating the importance of spinal mobility on an individual's functional status[5].

Validity

Calin et al. (1994) compared BASFI with Dougados functional index, it was found that the BASFI demonstrates a significant improvement in function while there was less change in the Dougados score[3].

Internal consistency reliability and construct validity of BASFI was deemed acceptable by the authors, but they also mentioned that the random measurement error of BASFI was not negligible.[6]

Haywood et al. (2005) reported that BASFI is one of three AS assessment instruments with the most extensive evidence for validity through comparison with instruments that measure similar or related constructs, and/or with measures of mobility.[7]

Responsiveness

There was 20% (P = 0.004) improvement in function over 3 weeks versus 6% (P = 0.03) improvement demonstrated by the Dougados functional index during the physiotherapy treatment over the same 3-week period[3].

Miscellaneous

One of the benefits of the scale in the way it is administered resides in the visual analogue scale which is a lot easier and quicker to use for patients, although it requires a bit of interpretation from the clinician.

178. B. "The Bath AS Disease Activity Index (BASDAI)"

Objective

The Bath Ankylosing Spondylitis Disease Activity Index (BASDAI) is the gold standard for measuring and following disease activity and thus functional status in the person with Ankylosing Spondylitis[8].

Like the BASFI, the BASDAI consists of six 10-cm horizontal visual analogue scales to measure the severity of fatigue, spinal and peripheral joint pain, localized tenderness, and morning stiffness (both qualitative and quantitative)[8]. This VAS has now been replaced by a numerical rating scale (NRS) in many centres[1]. The questions are answered on a 10 cm VAS, anchored with the labels "none" and "very severe" at either end of the first five questions, and with "0 hours" and "two hours" at either end of the question on the duration of morning stiffness. The mean of the two scores for morning stiffness counts as one variable. The final score is defined by calculating the mean of the five items. Final scores range from 0 (best) to 10 (worst).

Intended Population

Persons with Ankylosing Spondylitis.

Method of Use

- BASDAI is a quick and simple index taking between 30 secs and 2 mins to complete. It is a self-reported questionnaire that is made up of 6 questions related to 5 major symptoms: fatigue, spinal pain, joint pain/swelling, areas of localized tenderness, morning stiffness. Each question is answered on a ten-centimetre visual analogue scales. A score of 0 = none (no symptoms), and a score of 10 = very severe symptoms.
- To calculate the mean score, the scores for questions 1 – 4 is added together. The mean for questions 5 and 6 is calculated.
- The mean measurement (score) of questions 5 and 6 is added to the scores from questions 1 to 4. This total is then divided by 5 to give the average. This is the BASDAI score. The higher the BASDAI score, the more severe the patient's disability due to their AS.[8][9]

The BASDAI Item and Scoring[8]

Please tick the box which represents your answer.

All questions refer to last week. (i.e.)

1. How would you describe the overall level of fatigue/tiredness you have experienced?

   1 2 3 4 5 6 7 8 9 10

   none very severe

2. How would you describe the overall level of AS neck, back or hip pain you have had

   1 2 3 4 5 6 7 8 9 10

   none very severe

3. How would you describe the overall level of pain/swelling in joints other than the neck, back or hips you have had?

   1 2 3 4 5 6 7 8 9 10

   none very severe

4. How would you describe the overall level of discomfort you have had from any areas tender to touch or pressure?

   1 2 3 4 5 6 7 8 9 10

   none very severe

5. How would you describe the overall level of morning stiffness you have had from the time you wake up?

   1 2 3 4 5 6 7 8 9 10

   none very severe

   0 1 2 or more

   hr hr hrs

6. How long does your morning stiffness last from the time you wake up?

   1 2 3 4 5 6 7 8 9 10

   none very severe

   0 1 2 or more

   hr hr hr

Reliability

BASDAI demonstrated statistically significant ($p<0.001$) reliability.

Test-retest reliability across the scale responses was said to be good (who said that it is good)[8].

Validity

When compared to a previous disease activity index it is felt that BASDAI is superior in terms of symptoms considered and their weighting. This may be due to the input from patients with AS when the index was developed. The BASDAI was also found to be superior in all aspects to the Newcastle Enthesis Index[8].

The validity of BASDAI was further assessed by Calin et al (1999) have further. They concluded that the BASDAI has excellent content validity[10].

Responsiveness

Following a 3-week physiotherapy course, the BASDAI showed a significant (p=0.009) 16.4% score improvement, therefore demonstrating a sensitivity to change. To conclude, the BASDAI is user friendly, highly reliable, reflects the entire spectrum of the disease and is sensitive to clinical changes[8].

178. C. "The Bath Ankyloysing Spondylitis Metrology Index (BASMI)"

Objective

BASMI is a composite index used internationally in research and clinical practice. It is used to assess clinically significant changes in spinal mobility. With this scale in mind, clinicians and patients may have expectations that a score of zero is representative of normal spinal involvement in a healthy population(4). To accurately assess axial status (cervical, dorsal and lumbar spine, hips and pelvic soft tissue) of individuals with AS and from these derive a metrology index to define clinically significant changes in spinal mobility[11].

Intended Population

The BASMI is a scoring system used to assess the spinal mobility of ankylosis spondylitis.

Method of Use

- The BASMI takes only 7 minutes to apply. It is an index composed of five mobility tests; Cervical rotation, Tragus to wall distance, Lumbar side flexion, Modified Schober's, Intermalleolar distance.
- The scale of the BASMI ranges from 0 to 10, where 0 is no mobility limitation and 10 is a very severe limitation.
- To calculate the scores for each measurement i.e cervical rotation, tragus etc. A mean of the left and right measurements is taken. The scores of each measurement are added together, and this will provide a figure out of 50. Divide this by 5 to give the BASMI score. The higher the BASMI score the more severe the patient's limitation of movement due to their AS.

Calculating the score for each of the BASMI measurement[1]

	0	1	2	3	4	5	6	7	8	9	10
Tragus to Wall (cm)	<10	10-12.9	13-15.9	16-18.9	19-21.9	22-24.9	25-27.9	28-30.9	31-33.9	34-36.9	≥37
Lumbar Side Flexion (cm)	≥20	18-19.9	15.9-17.9	13.8-15.8	11.7-13.7	9.6-11.6	7.5-9.5	5.4-7.4	3.3-5.3	1.2-3.2	<1.2
Lumbar Flexion (modified Schober's) (cm)	>7.0	6.4-7.0	5.7-6.3	5.0-5.6	4.3-4.9	3.6-4.2	2.9-3.5	2.2-2.8	1.5-2.1	0.8-1.4	≤0.7
Cervical Rotation (degrees)	≥85	76.6-84.9	68.1-76.5	59.6-68	51.1-59.5	42.6-51	34.1-42.5	25.6-34	17.1-25.5	8.6-17	≤8.5
Intermalleolar Distance (cm)	≥120	110-119.9	100-109.9	90-99.9	80-89.9	70-79.9	60-69.9	50-59.9	40-49.9	30-39.9	<30

A guide to obtaining the BASMI measurement[1]

Below is a guide for clinicians on how to obtain the five BASMI measurements in a standardised fashion. It is recognised that this represents an 'ideal' scenario that may need adapting depending on the patient's individual posture/ circumstances. However, it is recommended that any changes be carefully documented to ensure measurements are accurate each time the measurements are taken. With all measurements, the patient should be comfortable and suitably undressed.

Measure	Starting Position	Method	Notes
Tragus to wall	Standing bare feet; back to the wall; knees straight; scapulae, buttocks, heels against the wall; shoulders level; outer edges of feet 30 cm apart & feet parallel. Ensure the head in a neutral position (anatomical alignment) as possible.	Patient draws chin in as far as possible (retraction). The examiner has both eyes open and side of face against the wall and measures the distance between the tragus of the ear & the wall, using a rigid ruler	Ensure no cervical extension, rotation, flexion or side flexion occurs. Best to use a wall without a skirting board. Ensure retraction is maintained whilst both sides are measured.

Lumbar Side Flexion	Standing bare feet; back to the wall; knees straight; scapulae, buttocks, heels against the wall; shoulders level; outer edges of feet 30 cm apart & feet parallel.	Before any movement occurs, keeping arms, wrist & fingers straight and shoulders depressed measure from the tip of the middle finger to floor. With arms relaxed by the sides, the patient reaches towards the floor by side flexing and maintaining shoulder depression. Re-measure from the tip of the middle finger to the floor. The difference between the 2 measurements represents the amount of side flexion. Repeat on another side.	Ensure patient keeps arms, fingers & knees straight and heels on the floor. Ensure any forward flexion, extension or rotation of the trunk is avoided. Best to use a wall without a skirting board. May need to accommodate a leg length discrepancy with a block underfoot. (NB: Ensure all conditions are recorded for accurate measurements)
Lumbar Flexion (modified Schober's)	Standing with outer edges of bare feet 30 cm apart and feet in line. Examiner marks a first point midway between the Dimples of Venus, a second point is marked 10 cm above this & a third 5 cm below the first to give a 15 cm line.	Patient flexes forward from the waist with knees fully extended. The distance between the upper and lower 2 marks is measured. Any increase beyond 15 cm represents the amount of movement achieved.	At the end of the movement, you may choose to allow slight knee flexion to decrease the influence of hamstrings. This should be documented.
Cervical Rotation	Patient supine on a plinth. Forehead horizontal & head in a neutral position. May need to use a pillow, books or foam block to achieve this. Carefully document to ensure the same set-up on future re-assessments.	Use goniometer/inclinometer as per manufacturer's instructions. The patient rotates his/her head as far as possible, keeping shoulders still. Measure both sides.	Ensure no neck flexion/side flexion occurs. If the good range of movement may need to lie near the edge of the bed to allow movement to occur
Intermalleolar Distance	patient lies supine on the floor or a wide plinth. Knees in extension	Keeping knees straight & legs in contact with the resting surface, the patient is asked to take legs as far apart as possible. Distance between the medial malleoli is measured	Measure quickly as movement can be painful. Be ready to measure before asking the patient to achieve movement.

Reliability

Inter and Intra – rater reliability has been explored and for repeat assessments of the same participant by the same physiotherapist, differences of BASMI of 1.0 or less are within bounds of error; and likewise, differences of 1.0 or less are within bounds of error if different physiotherapists perform the assessments. Only changes above these limits can be confidently interpreted as true clinical change[12].

Validity

At the level of significance ($p<0.001$), the BASMI proved to be accurate and reproducible for both inter-and intra- observer variability[13].

Responsiveness

The sensitivity of the index to change was found to be significant ($p<0.01$) regardless of the disease severity[13]. Five clinical measurements were included in the index:

❑❑❑

178. D. "The Bath Ankylosing Spondylitis Global Score" (BAS-G)

Objective

It is used to assess the effect of AS on the patient's well being. It consists of two questions that ask patients to indicate, on a 10cm VAS, the effect the disease has had on their well being over the last week and last 6 months[14]. The VRS has now been replaced by numerical rating scales (NRS) in many centres[1].

Intended Population

The BASMI is used for persons with AS.

Method of Use

- BAS-G is consistent with the other measures in the core set, utilizing the '**in the last week**' approach to obtaining a snapshot of current patient status but also it also refers to the patient's average well-being over the last 6 months, which can be helpful to describe longer-term disease progression[14].
- The BAS-G consists of two questions that ask patients' to indicate, on a 10cm VAS, the effect the disease has had on their well-being over the last week and last six months.
- The mean of the two scores gives a BAS-G score of 0 – 10. The higher the score, the greater the perceived effect of the disease on the patient's well-being.

The BAS-G Items and Scoring[1]

1. Please use the scale below to indicate the effect your disease has Score out of 10 had on your well being over the last week.

None 1 2 3 4 5 6 7 8 9 10 Very severe Score out of 10

2. Please use the scale below to indicate the effect your disease has had on your well being over the last six months.

None 1 2 3 4 5 6 7 8 9 10 Very severe Score out of 10

Validity

BAS-G has good construct validity and correlated more strongly with each component of BASDAI and BASFI than with BASMI or with gender[14].

Responsiveness

BAS-G demonstrated statistically significant ($p<0.001$) sensitivity to change. Jones et al, acknowledged that BAS-G cannot stand alone, and should be one element of a complete assessment. However, an index of this type provides a numerical value to the patient's sense of well being. This allows for comparison between consultations, especially when patients may not necessarily be seen by the same clinician on each occasion. The authors of the index conclude that they have formalized and validated a simple, frequently asked question[14].

References

1. Irons K, Harrison H, Thomas A, Martindale J. The Bath Indices: An updated synopsis of the Bath Indices – outcome measures for use with Ankylosing Spondylitis patients and their broader application. London. National Ankylosing Spondylitis Society (NASS), Revised Feb, 2016.
2. Calin A et al. A new approach to defining functional ability in ankylosing spondylitis: The development of the Bath Ankylosing Spondylitis Functional Index (BASFI). Journal of Rheumatology. 1994;Vol 21:2281-5
3. Calin A, Garrett S, Whitelock H, Kennedy LG, O'Hea J, Mallorie P, et al A new approach to defining functional ability in ankylosing spondylitis: the development of the Bath Ankylosing Spondylitis Functional Index. J Rheumatol. 1994 Dec;21(12):2281–5.
4. van Weely SF, van Denderen CJ, van der Horst-Bruinsma IE, et al. Reproducibility of performance measures of physical function based on the BASFI, in ankylosing spondylitis. Rheumatology (Oxford). 2009;48(10):1254-1260.
5. Sieper J, Rudwaleit M, Baraliakos X, Brandt J, Braun J, Burgos-Vargas R, Dougados M, Hermann KG, Landewé R, Maksymowych W, van der Heijde D. The Assessment of SpondyloArthritis international Society (ASAS) handbook: a guide to assess spondyloarthritis. Ann Rheum Dis. 2009 Jun;68 Suppl 2:ii1-44.
6. Madsen OR, Rytter A, Hansen LB, Suetta C, Egsmose C. Reproducibility of the Bath Ankylosing Spondylitis Indices of disease activity (BASDAI), functional status. (BASFI) and overall well-being (BAS-G) in anti-tumour necrosis factor-treated spondyloarthropathy patients. Clin Rheumatol. 2010 Aug;29(8):849-54. https://pubmed.ncbi.nlm.nih.gov/20306214/
7. Haywood KL, Garratt AM, Dawes PT. Patient-

assessed health in ankylosing spondylitis: a structured review. Rheumatology (Oxford). 2005 May;44(5):577–86. https://pubmed.ncbi.nlm.nih.gov/15695297/

8. Garret S et al. A new approach to defining disease status in Ankylosing Spondylitis: The Bath Ankylosing Spondylitis Disease Activity Index (BASDAI). Journal of Rheumatology. 1994;2286-91.
9. Sieper J, Rudwaleit M, Baraliakos X, Brandt J, Braun J, Burgos-Vargas R, Dougados M, Hermann K-G, Landewé R, Maksymowych W and Van der Heijde D. (2009) The assessment of SpondyloArthritis international Society (ASAS) handbook: a guide to assess spondyloarthritis. Ann Rheum Dis (2009): 68 (Suppl 11).
10. Calin A, et al. Defining disease activity in ankylosing spondylitis: is a combination of variables (Bath Ankylosing Spondylitis Disease Activity Index) an appropriate instrument? Rheumatology (Oxford).1999;Vol(9),878-82.
11. Chilton-Mitchell L, Martindale J, Hart A, Goodcare L. Normative Values for the Bath Ankylosis Spondylitis Metrology Index in a UK population. Rheumatology (Oxford). 2013; 52(11): 2086-2090. http://doi.org/10.1093 rheumatology/ket272
12. Martindale JH, Sutton CJ, Goodacre L. An exploration of the inter-and intra-rater reliability of the Bath Ankylosing Spondylitis Metrology Index. Clin Rheumatol. 2021;31(11):1627–1631.
13. Jenkinson TR et al. (1994) Defining spinal mobility in ankylosing spondylitis (AS): The Bath AS Metrology Index. Journal of Rheumatology. 1994;Vol (21):1694-8.
14. Jones SD, Steiner A, Garrett SL, Calin A. The Bath Ankylosing Spondylitis Patient Global Score (BAS-G). British Journal of Rheumatology. 1996;Vol 35:66 – 71.

❑❑❑

179 The Rivermead Post-Concussion Symptoms Questionnaire (RPQ)

Introduction

The Rivermead Post-concussion Symptoms Questionnaire (RPQ) is a simple, freely available, and widely used tool for assessment of the presence and severity of various post-concussion symptoms. The questionnaire was first published in 1995 to assess patients' psychosocial functioning post-concussion[1]. It contains 16 questions targeting physical, cognitive and behavioural domains. It was modified by Eyres et al. is 2005 into RPQ Modified Scoring System (RPQ 13/ RPQ-3)[2].

Intended Population

Individuals showing symptoms of Concussion after a head trauma/ brain injury.[3]

Method of Use

Equipment Required:

Questionnaire based: pen and paper

Training Required:

None

Time Required:

5-10 mins

Instrument

The questionnaire is a self-reported questionnaire containing 16 questions[1]. They are asked if after the accident they experienced any:

Sr. No.	Questions	Scoring				
		0	1	2	3	4
1.	Headaches					
2.	Feelings of Dizziness					
3.	Nausea and Vomiting					
4.	Noise Sensitivity Easily upset by loud noise					
5.	Sleep Disturbance					
6.	Fatigue, tiring more easily					
7.	Being Irritable, easily angered					
8.	Feeling Depressed or Tearful					
9.	Feeling frustrated or Impatient					
10.	Forgetfulness, poor memory					
11.	Poor Concentration					
12.	Taking Longer to Think					

13.	Blurred Vision					
14.	Light Sensitivity, *Easily upset by bright light*					
15.	Double Vision					
16.	Restlessness					
	Are you experiencing any other difficulties?					
1.						
2.						

Scoring:

0 = Not experienced at all

1 = 0 No more of a problem

2 = A mild problem

3 = A moderate problem

4 = A severe problem

Lower the Score, better the conditions.

In the modified version[2]:

RPQ-3: Score of first three questions, Scoring is 0-12; if there is a higher score on the RPQ-3, earlier reassessment and closer monitoring is recommended.

RPQ-13: Sore of next 13 questions, Scoring is 0-52; later cluster of symptoms; greater impact on participation, psychosocial functioning and lifestyle.

Psychometric properties

Reliability[4][5]:

For Head Injury: Excellent test re-test reliability, Excellent inter-rater reliability.

For Mild TBI: Adequate test re-test reliability, Adequate inter-rater reliability.

Validity[6]:

Excellent validity with Hospital Anxiety Depression Scale.

Clinical Significance

The questionnaire can be repeated to monitor a patient's progress over time with changes seen in severity of symptoms, or the range of symptoms. Management can be planned likewise[7].

References

1. King, N. S., Crawford, S., Wenden, F.J., Moss, N.E.G. Wade, D.T. The Rivermead Post Concussion Symptoms Questionnaire: a measure of symptoms commonly experienced after head injury and its reliability. Journal of Neurology. 1995. 242, 587-592
2. Eyres, S., Carey, A., Gilworth, G., Neumann, V., Tennant, A. Construct validity and reliability of the Rivermead Post Concussion Symptoms Questionnaire. Clinical Rehabilitation. 2005. 19, 878-887
3. Crawford S, Wenden FJ, Wade DT. The Rivermead head injury follow up questionnaire: a study of a new rating scale and other measures to evaluate outcome after head injury. J Neurol Neurosurg Psychiatry. 1996 May;60(5):510-4. doi: 10.1136/jnnp.60.5.510.
4. King NS, Crawford S, Wenden FJ, Caldwell FE, Wade DT. Early prediction of persisting post-concussion symptoms following mild and moderate head injuries. Br J Clin Psychol. 1999 Mar;38(1):15-25.doi:10.1348/014466599162638.
5. Asselstine J, Kristman VL, Armstrong JJ, Dewan N. The Rivermead Post-Concussion Questionnaire score is associated with disability and self-reported recovery six months after mild traumatic brain injury in older adults. Brain Inj. 2020;34(2):195-202. doi: 10.1080/02699052.2019.1682670
6. de Guise E, Bélanger S, Tinawi S, Anderson K, LeBlanc J, Lamoureux J, Audrit H, Feyz M. Usefulness of the rivermead postconcussion symptoms questionnaire and the trail-making test for outcome prediction in patients with mild traumatic brain injury. Appl Neuropsychol Adult. 2016;23(3):213-22. doi:10.1080/23279095.2015.1038747.
7. Potter, S., Leigh, E., Wade, D., Fleminger, S. The Rivermead Post Concussion Symptoms Questionnaire. Journal of Neurology, October 2006.1-12.

❑❑❑

180 Timed Up and Go Test (TUG)

Objective

To determine fall risk and measure the progress of balance, sit to stand and walking. Simple screening test that is a sensitive and specific measure of probability for falls among older adults[1].

Intended Population

- This test was initially designed for elderly persons, but is used for in other populations eg Parkinson's - This tool is validated for a population with Parkinson's Disease; Multiple Sclerosis; Hip fracture; Alzheimers; CVA; TKR or THR; Huntington Disease
- It is one of the 4 tests used in the The Balance Outcome Measure for Elder Rehabilitation (BOOMER)

Materials Needed

One chair with armrest

Stopwatch

Tape (to mark 3 meters)

Method

1. Patients wear their regular footwear and can use a walking aid, if needed.
2. The patient starts in a seated position
3. The patient stands up upon therapist's command: walks 3 meters, turns around, walks back to the chair and sits down.
4. The time stops when the patient is seated.
5. Be sure to document the assistive device used.

Note: A practice trial should be completed before the timed trial

Observations

Observe the patient's postural stability, gait, stride length, and sway.

- Note all that apply: Slow tentative pace; Loss of balance; Short strides; Little or no arm swing; Steadying self on walls; Shuffling; En bloc turning; Not using assistive device properly.
- These changes may signify neurological problems that require further evaluation[2].

Cut-off time for high risk of falls

An older adult who takes ≥12 seconds to complete the TUG is at risk for falling.[2]

Cut of scores indicating risk of falls by Population (in seconds)

- Community dwelling adults - 13.5
- Older stroke patients - 14
- Frail elderly - 32.6
- LE amputees - 19
- PD - 11.5
- Hip OA - 10 -
- Vestibular disorders - 11.1[3]

Cut-off times to classify subjects as high risk for falling vary based on the study and participants.

Evidence

Reliability

- Intratester and intertester reliability (ICC) have been reported as high, in elderly populations, from .92-.99.[4]
- Reliability in community-dwelling populations

has been found to be moderate (.56).[4]

- In people with Alzheimers disease reliability is high (ICC = .985-.988).[5]
- An ICC of 0.80 for subjects with Parkinson's was found[6] and excellent (0.95) ICC and excellent reliability in another study[7]. Test retest [8]and the interrator reliability are both high, the TUG can be used to assess differences in the Parkinson's and non Parkinson's populations. [9]

Validity

Construct validity has been shown by correlating TUG scores with gait speed (Pearson r = .75), postural sway (Pearson r = -.48), step length (Pearson r = -.74), Barthel Index (Pearson r = -.79), and step frequency (Pearson r = -.59).[4]

Sensitivity and Specificity

- The sensitivity and specificity have been reported to be 87%[10].
- Moderate sensitivity in predicting falls in PD, so in isolation it might not be enough to predict falls in this population [11]

Minimally Detectable Change (MDC)

- MDC is "the smallest amount of difference in individual scores that represents true change (beyond random measurement error)". [8]
- The MDC was 4.09 seconds in patients with Alzheimers.
- In patients with Parkinson's the MDC was 3.5 seconds[8]

Benefits

- Quick to conduct
- Minimal equipment required
- Highly reliable and valid
- Provides useful outcomes related to reduced falls risk

Negatives

- Unable to predict falls in the community[12]
- Test re-test user error can be high
- Turning is only assessed in the patient's preferred direction [7]

TUG Manual and TUG Cognitive

Previous studies have shown that people with Parkinson's can show gait changes like a decrease in walking speed, step length and pattern. These changes are due to a decrease in automaticity and attentional flexibility. People with Parkinson's are at a higher risk for falls because when performing dual tasks they "prioritize concurrent tasks over postural tasks". [11]

- TUG Manual: Carrying a class of water in one hand while completing the TUG. Low sensitivity of 29% and moderate specificity 68%.[11]
- TUG Cognitive: Counting backwards in threes from a random start point while completing the TUG. Sensitivity of 76.5% and specificity (73.7%). It had a moderate accuracy, so it is not recommended as a sole test for fall. The TUG Cognitive was shown to more discriminative than the TUG or TUG Manual. [11]

In a retrospective study of 36 participants with PD, participant who reported falls in the last 6 months were compared to participants who reported no falls. In this study the optimal cut off times to discriminate between fallers and non-fallers with Parkinson's were as follows:[11]

- TUG: 12 seconds
- TUG Cognitive: 14.7 seconds
- TUG Manual: 13.2 seconds

A cross-sectional quantitative study investigating the effects of age-related visual dependence on motor performances (turning cadence; gait speed) under increased attention demands by adding a motor task and visual stimulus to the Timed Up and Go (TUG) test sub-components demonstrated significant performance differences in the TUG test tasks due to age and visual dependence[13].

References

1. Shumway-Cook A, Brauer S, Woollacott M. Predicting the probability for falls in community-dwelling older adults using the Timed Up & Go Test. Physical therapy. 2000 Sep 1;80(9):896-903.Available from:https://academic.oup.com/ptj/article/80/9/896/2842520 (last accessed 16.10.2020)
2. CDC govt. TUG Available from:https://www.cdc.gov/steadi/pdf/TUG_Test-print.pdf (last accessed 16.10.2020)
3. SR ability lab TUG Available from:https://www.sralab.org/rehabilitation-measures/timed-and-go (last accessed 16.10.2020)

4. Steffen T, Hacker T, Mollinger L. Age- and gender-related test performance in community-dwelling elderly people: six-minute walk test, berg balance scale, timed up go test, and gait speeds. Phys Ther. 2002;82(2):128-137.
5. Ries J, Echternach J, Nof L, Blodgett M. Test-retest reliability and minimal detectable change scores for the timed “up go” test, the six-minute walk test, and gait speed in people with alzheimer disease. Phys Ther. 2009;89(6):569-579.
6. Huang S, Hsieh C, Wu R, Tai C, Lin C, Lu W. Minimal detectable change of the timed “up go” test and the dynamic gait index in people with parkinson disease. Phys Ther. 2011;91(1):114-121.
7. Haas B, Clarke E, Elver L, Gowman E, Mortimer E, Byrd E. The reliability and validity of the L-test in people with Parkinson’s disease. Physiotherapy. 2017 Dec 5.https://www.physiotherapyjournal.com/article/S0031-9406(17)30338-3/fulltext
8. Huang SL, Hsieh CL, Wu RM, Tai CH, Lin CH, Lu WS. Minimal detectable change of the timed “up & go” test and the dynamic gait index in people with Parkinson disease. Physical Therapy. 2011 Jan 1;91(1):114-21. https://www.ncbi.nlm.nih.gov/pubmed/20947672
9. Morris S, Morris ME, Iansek R. Reliability of measurements obtained with the Timed “Up & Go” test in people with Parkinson disease. Physical therapy. 2001 Feb 1;81(2):810-8.
10. Shumway-Cook A, Brauer S, Woollacott M. Predicting the probability for falls in community-dwelling older adults using the timed up & go test. Phys Ther. 2000;80(9):896-903.
11. Vance RC, Healy DG, Galvin R, French HP. Dual tasking with the timed “up & go” test improves detection of risk of falls in people with Parkinson disease. Physical therapy. 2015 Jan 1;95(1):95-102. http://citeseerx.ist.psu.edu/viewdoc/download?doi=10.1.1.883.6123&rep=rep1&type=pdf
12. Barry E, Galvin R, Keogh C, Horgan F, Fahey T. Is the Timed Up and Go test a useful predictor of risk of falls in community dwelling older adults: a systematic review and meta-analysis. BMC geriatrics. 2014 Dec;14(1):14.
13. Almajid R, Tucker C, Wright WG, Vasudevan E, Keshner E. Visual dependence affects the motor behavior of older adults during the Timed Up and Go (TUG) test. Archives of gerontology and geriatrics. 2020 Mar 1; 87:104004.

Timed Up and Go Test (TUG)—Scoring sheet

Date: ___________

Time (seconds): ______

Assistive Device Used:

none: ____

cane: ____

walker: ____

other: ____

Other:

stopped to rest: ____

impaired cognition:____

Risk for

Falls: High Risk (>13.5 seconds): ____

None/low/moderate: (<13.5 seconds):____

❑❑❑

181

Tinetti Test

Description

The Tinetti-test[1] was published by Mary Tinetti (Yale University) to assess the gait and balance in older adults[2] and to assess perception of balance and stability during activities of daily living and fear of falling. It is also called Performance-Oriented Mobility Assessment (POMA).[3] It also is a very good indicator of the fall risk of an individual. It has better test-retest, discriminative and predictive validities concerning fall risk than other tests including Timed Up and Go test (TUG), one-leg stand and functional reach test.[4]

Intended Population

It is used in various settings eg those diagnosed with Multiple Sclerosis, Parkinson's Disease, acquired brain injury, spinal cord injury, stroke and the elderly population.

Procedure

The test requires a hard armless chair, a stopwatch and also, a 15 feet even and uniform walkway. It has 2 sections: one assesses balance abilities in a chair and also in standing; the other assesses dynamic balance during gait on a 15 feet even walkway.

The patient is to sit in an armless chair and will be asked to rise up and stay standing. The patient will then turn 360° and then sit back down.[5] This is to test the patients' balance. Testing this, the evaluator will look at several key points including how does the patient rise from and sits down on his/her chair, whether or not the patient stays upright while sitting and standing, what happens when the patients' eyes are closed or when the patient gets a small push against the sternum.[3]

Next, the patient will have to walk a few meters at a normal speed, followed by turning and walking back at a "fast but safe" speed. The patient will then sit back down. As well as in the first part of the test, there are some points the evaluator has to look at. These are the length and height of the steps, the symmetry and continuity of the steps and straightness of the trunk.

During this test, the patient can use any assistive devices (walking stick, crutches, zimmer frame) they would normally use.[3]

Interpretation

The Tinetti test has a gait score and a balance score. It uses a 3-point ordinal scale of 0, 1 and 2. Gait is scored over 12 and balance is scored over 16 totalling 28. The lower the score on the Tinetti test, the higher the risk of falling.

Tinneti tool score	Risk of fall
≤ 18	High
19-23	Moderate
≥ 24	Low

Gait and Balance

If the patient needs to rise in stages, it is possible that there is a problem with proprioception or cerebellar problems. A shuffling gait, abnormal knee extension, high stepping, toe dragging and an inability to stop or turn are all signs of abnormalities during walking. These signs need to be further evaluated because they could indicate several health problems such as partial vision loss, lowered strength in the knee or hip joints, problems with proprioception, frontal lobe dysfunction or even vascular claudication. When the patient falls into his/her chair upon returning it is indicative of poor knee and/or hip flexion. The study by Usayl I et al. showed that the patients who had a higher score in a half squat (HS) and decline squat (DC) also had a higher score in Tinetti Performance Oriented Mobility Assessment (POMA), thus showing a significant correlation between squat and balance assessment in older patients[6]

Clinimetric Properties

The test and retest values for the POMA-T, POMA-B en POMA-G all varied between .72 and .86. The interrater reliability values all varied between .80 and .93.6 People with a score lower than 26 will have a higher chance of falling. This test has a sensitivity of 70% and a specificity of 52%. This means that 70% of the people with a higher fall risk will have a test score lower than 26. It also means that 52% of the people who have a test score lower than 26 have a higher fall risk and will have a fall within a year. The people who have a score of 26 or lower have a two-fold risk of falling.[7]

References

1. Tinetti ME, Williams TF, Mayewski R, Fall Risk Index for elderly patients based on number of chronic disabilities. Am J Med 1986:80:429-434
2. Berg KO, Wood-Dauphinée SL, Williams JI, Maki B. Measuring balance in the elderly: validation of an instrument. Can J Public Health.1992;83(suppl 2) :S7– S11.
3. Shumway-Cook A, Woollacott MH. Motor control: translating research into clinical practice. Philadelphia : Wolters Kluwer, 2016. level of evidence D
4. Lin MR, Hwang HF, Hu MH, Wu HD, Wang YW, Huang FC. Psychometric comparisons of the timed up and go, one-leg stand, functional reach, and Tinetti balance measures in community-dwelling older people.Journal of the American Geriatric Society, 2004; 52(8):1343-8. level of evidence B
5. Reiman MP, Manske RC. Functional testing in human performance. Champaign: Human kinetics, 2009. level of evidence D
6. Uysal I, Korkmaz NC, Cavlak U. Assessment of the musculoskeletal performance with squat tests and performance-oriented measurements in older adults. Journal of Back and Musculoskeletal Rehabilitation. 2019 Nov 22(Preprint):1-7.
7. Raîche M, Hébert R, Prince F, Corriveau H. Screening older adults at risk of falling with the Tinetti balance scale.Lancet, 2000; 356(9234):1001-2.
8. Bob abd Brad Tinetti Balance Test Available from: https://www.youtube.com watch?v=EBHyLQiZcNI (last accessed 13.11.2019)

TASK	DESCRIPTION OF BALANCE	Possible	Score	Date	Score	Date	Score	Date
1. SITTING BALANCE	Leans or slides in chair	0						
	Steady, safe	1						
2. RISES FROM CHAIR	Unable without help	0						
	Able, uses arms to help up	1						
	Able without using arms	2						
3. ATTEMPTS TO RISE FROM CHAIR	Unable without help	0						
	Able, requires > 1 attempt	1						
	Able to rise in 1 attempt	2						
4. IMMEDIATE STANDING BALANCE (first 5 seconds)	Unsteady (swaggers, moves feet, trunk sways)	0						
	Steady but uses walker or other support	1						
	Steady without walker or other support	2						

5. STANDING BALANCE	Unsteady	0						
	Steady but wide stance (heels 4 inches apart) and uses cane or other support	1						
	Narrows stance without support	2						
6. NUDGED (subject at max position with feet as close together as possible, examiner pushes lightly on subject's sternum with palm of hand 3 times)	Begins to fall	0						
	Staggers, grabs, catches self	1						
	Stead Steady	2						
7. EYES CLOSED (at max position – see #6 above)	Unsteady	0						
	Steady	1						
8. TURNING 360 DEGREES	Discontinuous steps	0						
	Continuous steps	1						
	Unsteady (grabs, swaggers)	0						
	Steady	1						
9. SITTING DOWN	Unsafe (misjudged distance, falls into Chair)	0						
	Uses arms or not a smooth motion	1						
	Safe, smooth motion	2						
10. INITIATION OF GAIT (immediately after told to "go)	Any hesitancy or multiple attempts to start	0						
	No hesitancy	1						
11. STEP LENGTH AND HEIGHT	RIGHT swing food does not pass left stance foot with step	0						
	RIGHT foot passes left stance foot	1						
	RIGHT foot does not clear floor completely with step	0						
	RIGHT foot completely clears floor	1						
	LEFT swing foot does not pass right Stance foot with step	0						
	LEFT foot passes right stance foot	1						
	LEFT foot does not clear floor Completely with step	0						
	LEFT foot completely clears floor	1						
12. STEP SYMMETRY	RIGHT AND LEFT step length not equal (estimate)	0						
	RIGHT AND LEFT step appear equal	1						

13. STEP CONTINUITY	Stopping or discontinuity between steps	0						
	Steps appear to continue	1						
14. PATH (estimated in relation to floor tiles, 12-inch diameter. Observe excursion of 1 foot over about 10 feet of the course)	Marked deviation	0						
	Mild/moderate deviation or uses walking aid	1						
	Straight without walking aid	2						
15. TRUNK	Marked sway or uses walking aid	0						
	No sway – but flexion of knees or back, or spreads arms out while walking	1						
	No sway, no flexion, no use of arms, and no use of walking aid	2						
16. WALKING STANCE	Heels apart	0						
	Heels almost touching while walking	1						
Score – GAIT:								
Score – BALANCE								
Score: BALANCE & GAIT:								
			Rate 1		Rate 2		Rate 3	

182

30 sec Chair Stand Test (30sec-CST)

Overview:

The 30 Second Chair Stand Test, in conjunction with other measures such as the 4-Stage Balance Test, Timed Up and Go (TUG) Test and an assessment of postural hypotension can help to indicate if a patient is at risk of falling.

Purpose:

To test leg strength and endurance:

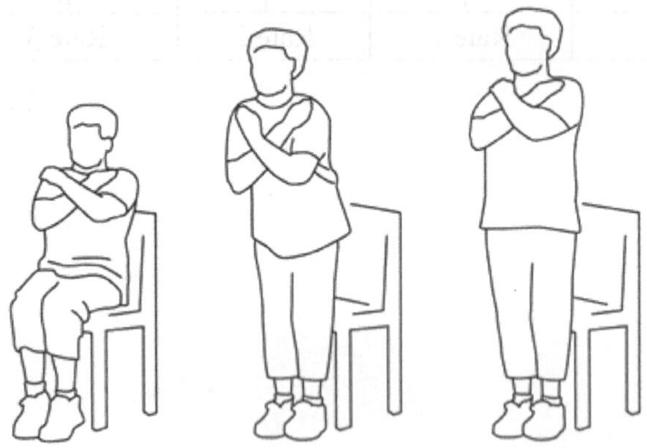

Equipment:

1. A chair with a straight back, without arm rests, placed against a wall to prevent it moving
2. A stopwatch/timer

Instructions to the patient:

1. Sit in the middle of the chair.
2. Place each hand on the opposite shoulder crossed at the wrists.
3. Place your feet flat on the floor.
4. Keep your back straight and keep your arms against your chest.
5. On "Go", rise to a full standing position and then sit back down again.
6. Repeat this for 30 seconds.

On "Go" begin timing.

Do not continue if you feel the patient may fall during the test.

Count the number of times the patient comes to a full standing position in 30 seconds and record it in the box below. If the patient is over halfway to a standing position when 30 seconds have elapsed, count it as a stand. If the patient must use his or her arms to stand then stop the test and record "0" for the number below.

❑❑❑

183 Single Leg Stance Test

Purpose

- The Single leg Stance (SLS) Test is used to assess static postural and balance control.
- Balance assessments (like SLS test) are a valuable clinical tool for monitoring neurological and musculoskeletal status as well as for managing fall risk[1].

Method

- Performed with eyes open and hands on the hips.
- Client must stand unassisted on one leg, timed from the time the other foot leaves the ground till when the foot touches the ground again or the arms leave the hips.
- If unable to stand for 5 seconds or less client at greater risk of injury from fall.[2]

Clinical Implications

Ability to control anticipatory postural adjustments (APAs) prior to lifting one leg while standing in unsupported equilibrium represents a complex motor task that is significantly impaired by eg

- Neurological conditions like multiple sclerosis, Parkinson's disease, Alzheimer's disease, and dementia
- Stroke
- Traumatic brain injury
- General geriatric population
- Lower extremity pathology like knee osteoarthritis (OA), one of the most common chronic health conditions, is associated with significant impairment and disability, and predominantly affects the elderly population[3][1][4].

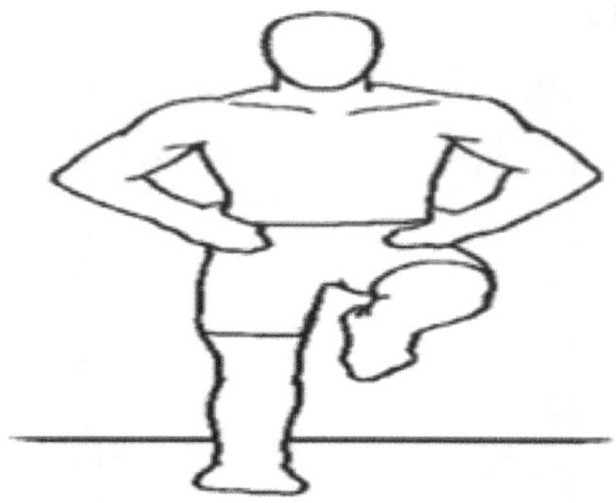

References

1. Zhang C, Talaber A, Truong M, Vargas BB. KD Balance: An objective measure of balance in tandem and double leg stances. Digital Health. 2019 Oct;5:2055207619885573. Available from:https://www.ncbi.nlm.nih.gov/pmc/articles/PMC6831964/ (accessed 13.12.2020)
2. Abilitiy lab SLS Available from:https://www.sralab.org/rehabilitation-measures/single-leg-stance-or-one-legged-stance-test (last accessed 13.12.2020)
3. Hunt MA, McManus FJ, Hinman RS, Bennell KL. Predictors of single-leg standing balance in individuals with medial knee osteoarthritis. Arthritis care & research. 2010 Apr;62(4):496-500. Available from:https://onlinelibrary.wiley.com/doi/full/10.1002/acr.20046 (accessed 13.12.2020)
4. Bonora G, Mancini M, Carpinella I, Chiari L, Ferrarin M, Nutt JG, Horak FB. Investigation of anticipatory postural adjustments during one-leg stance using inertial sensors: evidence from subjects with Parkinsonism. Frontiers in neurology. 2017 Jul 25;8:361 Available from:https://www.frontiersin.org articles/10.3389/fneur.2017.00361/full (accessed 13.12.2020)

❑❑❑

184 Knee Injury and Osteoarthritis Outcome Score

Introduction

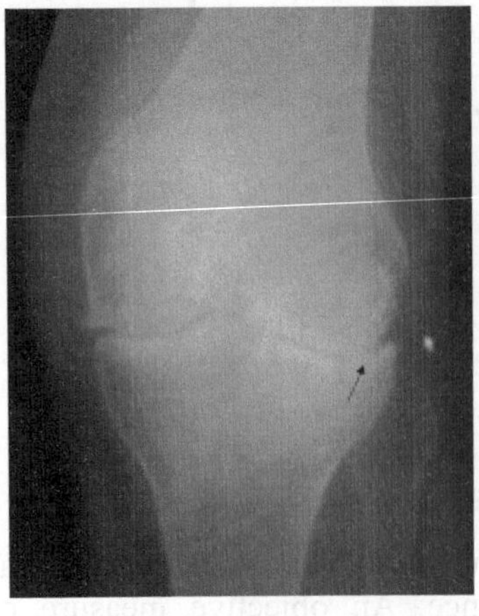

The Knee Injury and Osteoarthritis Outcome Score (KOOS) is a knee-specific instrument, developed to assess the patients' opinion about their knee and associated problems. The KOOS evaluates both short-term and long-term consequences of knee injury. It holds 42 items in 5 separately scored subscales; Pain, other Symptoms, Function in daily living (ADL), Function in Sport and Recreation (Sport/Rec), and knee-related Quality of Life (QOL).It is an extension of the WOMAC Osteoarthritis Index[1].The Knee injury and Osteoarthritis Outcome Score (KOOS) is self-administered.The KOOS proved reliable, responsive to surgery and physical therapy, and valid for patients undergoing anterior cruciate ligament reconstruction. The KOOS meets basic criteria of outcome measures and can be used to evaluate the course of knee injury and treatment outcomes[2].

The questionnaire can be downloaded from here

Development

The KOOS questionnaire was developed in the 1990s as an instrument to assess the patient's opinion about their knee and associated problems. Since the first publication in 1998, the psychometric properties of the KOOS have been assessed in more than twenty individual studies from all over the world. Furthermore, KOOS has been evaluated and compared to other instruments in several reviews[1][3][4][5]

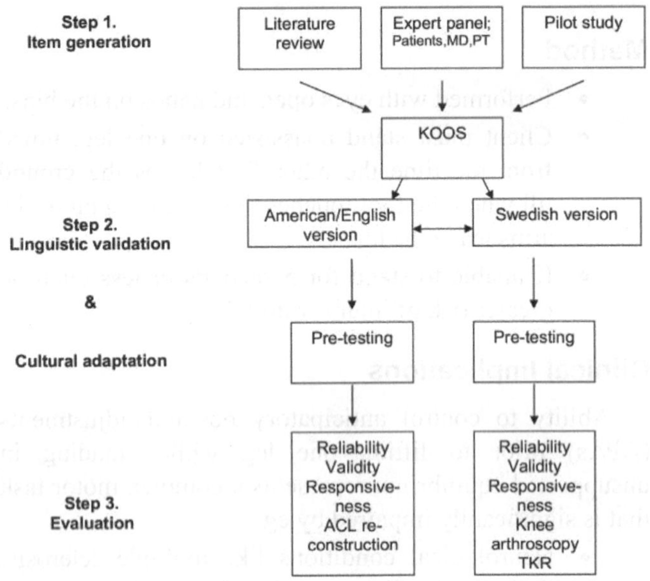

Validation

The KOOS has been validated in several different populations having surgical procedures due to knee complaints. To ensure the instrument being valid for both short-term and long-term consequences, validations have been carried out in different populations with varying diseases and durations and at varying ages and activity levels. Firstly, the American-English version was validated in subjects (age range 18–46) undergoing surgical reconstruction of the ACL[6].Secondly, the Swedish version was validated in subjects (age range 16–79) undergoing knee arthroscopy.[7]. Thirdly, the KOOS was compared to the WOMAC in subjects meniscectomized 16 years previously (age range 38–76) with and without OA[8]. Fourthly, a validation study was carried out in subjects (age range 43–86) treated with total knee replacement for OA[9]. For patients on the waiting-list for total knee replacement for OA, content validity was assessed before surgery by asking the patients to rate the importance of improvement in each of the five KOOS subscales on a 5-point Likert-scale as extremely important, very important, moderately important, somewhat important, or not important at all. For each subscale examples of questions within the subscale were given. Over 90% reported that improvement in the four subscales Pain, Symptoms, Activities of Daily Living, and knee-related Quality of Life was extremely or very important when deciding to have their knee operated on. 51% reported that improvement in functions included in the subscale Sport and Recreation Function such as squatting, kneeling, jumping, turning/twisting and running was extremely or very important when deciding to have their knee operated on. Postoperatively, patients tended to start doing physical functions they did not do prior to the operation.

Convergent and divergent construct validity was determined in comparison to the SF-36[10], and when applicable also to the Lysholm knee scoring scale[11]

Uses

KOOS is intended to be used for:

- knee injury that can result in post traumatic osteoarthritis (OA)
- ACL (anterior cruciate ligament) injury
- Meniscus injury
- Chondral injury
- Ankle and foot problems (FAOS)
- Hip problem (HOOS)
- Rheumatoid arthritis and other inflammatory joint diseases (RAOS)

Advantages of the KOOS

- Inclusion of two different subscales of physical function relating to daily life, and sport and recreation. This enhances the instrument's validity for patients with a wide range of current and expected physical activity levels.
- Short- and long-term time intervals
- Assess changes from week to week induced by treatment (medication, operation, physical therapy) or over years following a primary injury or OA.
- Used in research to assess groups and to monitor individuals.

- Scoring

The five patient-relevant subscales of KOOS are scored separately:

- Pain (nine items)
- Symptoms (seven items)
- ADL Function (17 items)
- Sport and Recreation Function (five items)
- Quality of Life (four items)

A Likert scale is used and all items have five possible answer options scored from 0 (No Problems) to 4 (Extreme Problems) and each of the five scores is calculated as the sum of the items included. Scores are transformed to a 0–100 scale, with zero representing extreme knee problems and 100 representing no knee problems as common in orthopaedic assessment scales and generic measures. Scores between 0 and 100 represent the percentage of total possible score achieved. An aggregate score is not calculated since it is regarded desirable to analyze and interpret the five dimensions separately.

The score is a percentage score from 0 to 100, 0 representing extreme problems and 100 representing no problems. This direction, 100 indicating no problems, is common in orthopaedic instruments and generic measures like the SF-36. In measures developed by rheumatologists, like the WOMAC, 100 usually represents worst possible result.

References

1. Roos EM, Lohmander LS. Knee injury and Osteoarthritis Outcome Score (KOOS): from joint injury to osteoarthritis. Health Qual Life Outcomes 2003;1:64.
2. Roos EM1, Roos HP, Lohmander LS, Ekdahl C, Beynnon BD.Knee Injury and Osteoarthritis Outcome Score (KOOS)--development of a self-administered outcome measure.J Orthop Sports Phys Ther. 1998 Aug;28(2):88-96.
3. Rodriguez-Merchan EC. Knee instruments and rating scales designed to measure outcomes. Journal of orthopaedics and traumatology : official

journal of the Italian Society of Orthopaedics and Traumatology 2012;13:1-6.

4. Collins NJ, Misra D, Felson DT, Crossley KM, Roos EM. Measures of knee function: International Knee Documentation Committee (IKDC) Subjective Knee Evaluation Form, Knee Injury and Osteoarthritis Outcome Score (KOOS), Knee Injury and Osteoarthritis Outcome Score Physical Function Short Form (KOOS-PS), Knee Outcome Survey Activities of Daily Living Scale (KOS-ADL), Lysholm Knee Scoring Scale, Oxford Knee Score (OKS), Western Ontario and McMaster Universities Osteoarthritis Index (WOMAC), Activity Rating Scale (ARS), and Tegner Activity Score (TAS). Arthritis care & research 2011;63 Suppl 11:S208-28.
5. Alviar MJ, Olver J, Brand C, Hale T, Khan F. Do patient-reported outcome measures used in assessing outcomes in rehabilitation after hip and knee arthroplasty capture issues relevant to patients? Results of a systematic review and ICF linking process. Journal of rehabilitation medicine : official journal of the UEMS European Board of Physical and Rehabilitation Medicine 2011;43:374-81.
6. Roos EM, Roos HP, Lohmander LS, Ekdahl C, Beynnon BD: Knee Injury and Osteoarthritis Outcome Score (KOOS)--development of a self-administered outcome measure. J Orthop Sports Phys Ther 1998, 28:88-96.
7. Roos EM, Roos HP, Ekdahl C, Lohmander LS: Knee injury and Osteoarthritis Outcome Score (KOOS)--validation of a Swedish version. Scand J Med Sci Sports 1998, 8:439-448
8. Roos EM, Roos HP, Lohmander LS: WOMAC Osteoarthritis Index--additional dimensions for use in subjects with post-traumatic osteoarthritis of the knee. Western Ontario and MacMaster Universities.Osteoarthritis Cartilage 1999, 7:216-221
9. Roos EM, Toksvig-Larsen S: Knee injury and Osteoarthritis Outcome Score (KOOS) - validation and comparison to the WOMAC in total knee replacement.Health Qual Life Outcomes 2003, 1:17.
10. Ware J. E., Jr., Sherbourne CD: The MOS 36-item short-form health survey (SF-36). I. Conceptual framework and item selection.Med Care 1992, 30:473-483
11. Tegner Y, Lysholm J: Rating systems in the evaluation of knee ligament injuries.Clin Orthop 1985, 43-49.

KOOS KNEE SURVEY

Knee injury and Osteoarthritis Outcome Score (KOOS), English version LK1.0

Today's date: _____/_____/_____

Date of birth: _____/_____/_____

Name:

INSTRUCTIONS: This survey asks for your view about your knee. This information will help us keep track of how you feel about your knee and how well you are able to perform your usual activities. Answer every question by ticking the appropriate box, only one box for each question. If you are unsure about how to answer a question, please give the best answer you can.

Symptoms

These questions should be answered thinking of your knee symptoms during the last week.

S1. Do you have swelling in your knee?

Never Rarely Sometime
Often Always

S2. Do you feel grinding, hear clicking or any other type of noise when your knee moves?

Never Rarely Sometime
Often Always

S3. Does your knee catch or hang up when moving?

Never Rarely Sometime
Often Always

S4. Can you straighten your knee fully?

Always Often Sometimes
Rarely Never

S5. Can you bend your knee fully?

Always Often Sometimes
Rarely Never

Stiffness

The following questions concern the amount of joint stiffness you have experienced during the last week in your knee. Stiffness is a sensation of restriction or slowness in the ease with which you move your knee joint.

S6. How severe is your knee joint stiffness after first wakening in the morning?

None Mild Moderate

Severe Extreme

S7. How severe is your knee stiffness after sitting, lying or resting later in the day?

None Mild Moderate

Severe Extreme

Pain

P1. How often do you experience knee pain?

Never Monthly Weekly

Daily Always

What amount of knee pain have you experienced the last week during the following activities?

P2. Twisting/pivoting on your knee

None Mild Moderate

Sever Extreme

P3. Straightening knee fully

None Mild Moderate

Severe Extreme

P4. Bending knee fully

None Mild Moderate

Severe Extreme

P5. Walking on flat surface

None Mild Moderate

Severe Extreme

P6. Going up or down stairs

None Mild Moderate

Severe Extreme

P7. At night while in bed

None Mild Moderate

Severe Extreme

P8. Sitting or lying

None Mild Moderate

Severe Extreme

P9. Standing upright

None Mild Moderate

Severe Extreme

Function, daily living

The following questions concern your physical function. By this we mean your ability to move around and to look after yourself. For each of the following activities please indicate the degree of difficulty you have experienced in the last week due to your knee.

A1. Descending stairs

None Mild Moderate

Severe Extreme

A2. Ascending stairs

None Mild Moderate

Severe Extreme

For each of the following activities please indicate the degree of difficulty you have experienced in the last week due to your knee

A3. Rising from sitting

None Mild Moderate

Severe Extreme

A4. Standing

None Mild Moderate

Severe Extreme

A5. Bending to floor/pick up an object

None Mild Moderate

Severe Extreme

A6. Walking on flat surface

None Mild Moderate

Severe Extreme

A7. Getting in/out of car

None Mild Moderate

Severe Extreme

A8. Going shopping

None Mild Moderate

Severe Extreme

A9. Putting on socks/stockings

None Mild Moderate

Severe Extreme

A10. Rising from bed

None Mild Moderate

Severe Extreme

A11. Taking off socks/stockings

None Mild Moderate

Severe Extreme

A12. Lying in bed (turning over, maintaining knee position)

None Mild Moderate

Severe Extreme

A13. Getting in/out of bath

None Mild Moderate

Severe Extreme

A14. Sitting

None Mild Moderate

Severe Extreme

A15. Getting on/off toilet

None Mild Moderate

Severe Extreme

For each of the following activities please indicate the degree of difficulty you have experienced in the last week due to your knee.

A16. Heavy domestic duties (moving heavy boxes, scrubbing floors, etc)

None Mild Moderate

Severe Extreme

A17. Light domestic duties (cooking, dusting, etc)

None Mild Moderate

Severe Extreme

Function, sports and recreational activities The following questions concern your physical function when being active on a higher level. The questions should be answered thinking of what degree of difficulty you have experienced during the last week due to your knee.

SP1. Squatting

None Mild Moderate

Severe Extreme

For each of the following activities please indicate the degree of difficulty you have experienced in the last week due to your knee.

A16. Heavy domestic duties (moving heavy boxes, scrubbing floors, etc)

None Mild Moderate

Severe Extreme

A17. Light domestic duties (cooking, dusting, etc

None Mild Moderate

Severe Extreme

Function, sports and recreational activities The following questions concern your physical function when being active on a higher level. The questions should be answered thinking of what degree of difficulty you have experienced during the last week due to your knee.

SP1. Squatting

None Mild Moderate

Severe Extreme

SP2. Running

None Mild Moderate

Severe Extreme

SP3. Jumping

None Mild Moderate

Severe Extreme

SP4. Twisting/pivoting on your injured

None Mild Moderate

Severe Extreme

SP5. Kneeling

None Mild Moderate

Severe Extreme

Quality of Life

Q1. How often are you aware of your knee problem?

Never Monthly Weekly

Daily Constantly

Q2. Have you modified your life style to avoid potentially damaging activities to your knee?

Not at all Mildly Moderately

Severely Totally

Q3. How much are you troubled with lack of confidence in your knee?

Not at all Mildly Moderately

Severely Extremely

Q4. In general, how much difficulty do you have with your knee?

None Mild Moderate

Severe Extreme

Thank you very much for completing all the questions in this questionnaire

185 Hip Disability and Osteoarthritis Outcome Score (HOOS)

Objective

The hip disability and osteoarthritis outcome score (HOOS) is a questionnaire intended to be used to assess the patient's opinion about their hip and associated problems and to evaluate symptoms and functional limitations related to the hip during a therapeutic process [1][2]. Other questionnaires that can be presented are the Western Ontario and McMaster Universities Osteoarthritis Index (WOMAC), the Algo Functional Index (AFI) and the Intermittent and Constant Osteoarthritis Pain Index (ICOAP) [3].

Intended Population

This measuring instrument, judging functions and anatomical qualities combined with activities and participation, is recommended when there is talk of hip disability with or without osteoarthritis (OA). Hip osteoarthritis is a common and chronic musculoskeletal condition and a cause of pain, functional disability and reduced quality of life [4].

The HOOS is meant to be used over short and long-term intervals to assess changes induced by treatment (medication, physical therapy, operation) or over years due to the primary injury or post-traumatic osteoarthritis [2].

Method of Use

The HOOS questionnaire is self-explanatory, user-friendly, patient-administered and takes 7 to 10 minutes to complete.

The outcome score consists of 40 items assessing 5 subscales. The 5 separate patient-relevant dimensions are Pain (P), Symptoms (S), Activity limitations daily living (ADL), Function in sport and recreation (SP) and hip related quality of life (QOL).

Pain (P) includes 10 items with a total score of 40 points, Symptoms (S) includes 5 items with a total score of 20, Activity limitations daily living (ADL) includes 17 items with a total score of 68 and finally Function in sport and recreation (SP) and hip related quality of life both include 4 items with a total score of 16 each.

To answer the questions, standardized answer options are given in 5 Likert-boxes with scores from 0 to 4 (no, mild, moderate, severe and extreme).

To interpret the score, the outcome measure is transformed in a worst to best scale from 0 to 100, with 100 indicating no symptoms and 0 indicating extreme symptoms.

To calculate the total HOOS score the subscales need to be summed up, using following formula for all dimension.

100 – [(patient's score of the subscale x 100)/(total score of the subscale)]

The subscales can be plotted as a HOOS profile, by connecting the mean scores for all 5 dimensions with a line[1][2].

Evidence

Reliability

The Dutch hip disability and osteoarthritis outcome score questionnaire has a good internal consistency and reliability[5]. The HOOS score is entirely based on self-report of functional status and performance. This may be a disadvantage in comparison to instruments that include objective physical examination findings or an assessment of symptoms.

It is recommended to use the HOOS score as a tool to complete additional information [6].

Validity

The construct validity is good with absence of floor and ceiling effects [5].

The hip osteoarthritis outcome score is valid in a sample of subject at a mean of 3 years after hip arthroscopy and for patients with different stadia of hip OA [5][6].

Responsiveness

Thanks to the addition of two subscales, sport and recreation function (SP) and hip related quality of life (QOL), the HOOC shows a higher sensitivity and responsiveness, compared to the Western Ontario and McMaster Universities osteoarthritis index (WOMAC). Patients younger than 66 years report higher responsiveness in all five subscales than patients older than 66 years [1].

Miscellaneous

The hip disability and osteoarthritis outcome score (HOOS) is an extension of the Western Ontario and McMaster Universities Osteoarthritis Index (WOMAC) and Knee Injury and Osteoarthritis Outcome Score (KOOS) [1].

The HOOS questionnaire is also useful compared with the Nonarthritic Hip Score and the modified Harris hip score (MHHS) [6].

References

1. NILSDOTTER A.K., LOHMANDER L.S., KLÄSSBO M., ROOS E.M., Hip disability and osteoarthritis outcome score (HOOS) – validity and responsiveness in total hip replacement, BMC Musculoskeletal Disord., May 2003, level of quality C
2. Pain symptoms ADL, Hip disability and osteoarthritis outcome score (HOOS). www.koos.nu (accessed 23 October)
3. KNGF-guidline, osteoarthritis of the hip and knee. https://www.kngfrichtlijnen.nl/downloads/Osteoarthritis_of_the_hip_and_knee_V06-2010_PRL_ENG.pdf (accessed 23 October)
4. POULSEN E., Conservative treatment of hip osteoarthritis: effect of manual therapy and hip school on pain, function and quality of life – a single-blind randomized controlled trial (abstract), December 2009
5. DE GROOT I.B., REIJMAN M., TERWEE C.B., BEIRMA-ZEINSTRA S.M.A., FAVEJEE M., ROOS E.M., VERHAAR J., Validation of the Dutch version of the hip disability and osteoarthritis outcome score, Osteoarthritis and cartilage, vol. 15 nr. 1, 2007, page. 104-109, level of quality C
6. MARTIN R.L., PHILIPPON M.J., Evidence of validity for the hip outcome score in hip rthroscopy, The journal of arthroscopic and related surgery, vol. 23 nr. 8, August 2007, page. 822-826, level of quality B

Hip Disability and Osteoarthritis Outcome Score (HOOS)

Patient's name (or ref)

Clinician's name (or ref)__________________

INSTRUCTIONS: This survey asks for your view about your hip. This information will help us keep track of how you feel about your hip and how well you are able to do your usual activities. Answer every question by ticking the appropriate box. If you are unsure about how to answer a question, please give the best answer you can.

Symptoms: These questions should be answered thinking of your hip symptoms during the last week.

S1. Do you feel grinding, hear clicking or any other type of noise from you hip?

Never Rarely Sometimes
Often Always

S2. Difficulties spreading legs wide apart

None Mild Moderate
Severe Extreme

S3. Difficulties to stride out when walking

None Mild Moderate
Severe Extreme

Stiffness: The following questions concern the amount of joint stiffness you have experienced during the last week in your hip. Stiffness is a sensation of restriction or slowness in the ease with which you move your hip joint.

S4. How severe is your hip joint stiffness after first wakening in the morning?

None Mild Moderate
Severe Extreme

S5. How severe is your hip stiffness after sitting, lying or resting later in the day?

None Mild Moderate
Severe Extreme

Subtotal: __________________

Pain

P1. How often is your hip painful?

Never Monthly Weekly

Daily Always

What amount of hip pain have you experienced the last week during the following activities?

P2. Straightening your hip fully

None Mild Moderate

Severe Extreme

P3. Bending your hip fully

None Mild Moderate

Severe Extreme

P4. Walking on flat surface

None Mild Moderate

Severe Extreme

P5. Going up or down stairs

None Mild Moderate

Severe Extreme

P6. At night while in bed

None Mild Moderate

Severe Extreme

P7. Sitting or lying

None Mild Moderate

Severe Extreme

P8. Standing upright

None Mild Moderate

Severe Extreme

P9. Walking on a hard surface (asphalt, concrete, etc)

None Mild Moderate

Severe Extreme

P10. Walking on an uneven surface

None Mild Moderate

Severe Extreme

Subtotal: ____________________

Function, daily living: The following questions concern your physical function. By this we mean your ability tomove around and to look after yourself. For each of the following activities please indicate the degree of difficulty you have experienced in the last week due to your hip.

Al. Descending stairs

None Mild Moderate

Severe Extreme

A2. Ascending stairs

None Mild Moderate

Severe Extreme

A3. Rising from sitting

None Mild Moderate

Severe Extreme

A4. Standing

None Mild Moderate

Severe Extreme

A5. Bending to floor/pick up an object

None Mild Moderate

Severe Extreme

A6. Walking on flat surface

None Mild Moderate

Severe Extreme

A7. Getting in/out of car

None Mild Moderate

Severe Extreme

A8. Going shopping

None Mild Moderate

Severe Extreme

A9. Putting on socks/stockings

None Mild Moderate

Severe Extreme

A10. Rising from bed

None Mild Moderate

Severe Extreme

A11. Taking off socks/stockings

None Mild Moderate

Severe Extreme

A12. Lying in bed (turning over, maintaining hip position)

None Mild Moderate

Severe Extreme

A13. Getting in/out of bath

None Mild Moderate

Severe Extreme

A14. Sitting

None Mild Moderate

Severe Extreme

A15. Getting on/off toilet

None Mild Moderate

Severe Extreme

A16. Heavy domestic duties (moving heavy boxes, scrubbing floors, etc)

None Mild Moderate

Severe Extreme

A17. Light domestic duties (cooking, dusting, etc)

None Mild Moderate

Severe Extreme

Subtotal: ____________________

Function, sports and recreational activities: The following questions concern your physical functionwhen being active on a higher level. The questions should be answered thinking of what degree of difficulty you have experienced during the last week due to your hip.

SP1. Squatting

None Mild Moderate

Severe Extreme

SP2. Running

None Mild Moderate

Severe Extreme

SP3. Twisting/pivoting on your injured knee

None Mild Moderate

Severe Extreme

SP4. Walking on uneven surface

None Mild Moderate

Severe Extreme

Subtotal: ____________________

Quality of Life

Q1. How often are you aware of your hip problem?

Never Monthly Weekly

Daily Constantly

Q2. Have you modified your lifestyle to avoid potentially damaging activities to your hip?

Not at all Mildly Moderately

Severely Totally

Q3. How much are you troubled with lack of confidence in your hip?

Not at all Mildly Moderately

Severely Extremely

Q4. In general, how much difficulty do you have with your hip?

None Mild Moderate

Severe Extreme

Subtotal: ____________________

Thank you very much for completing all the questions in this questionnaire

186 Tragus to Wall Test

Objective

To objectively measure the cervical mobility of an individual.

A 2018 review of the Tragus to Wall Test (TWT) noted it is a simple, reliable and valid, clinical indicator of forward flexed posture[1].

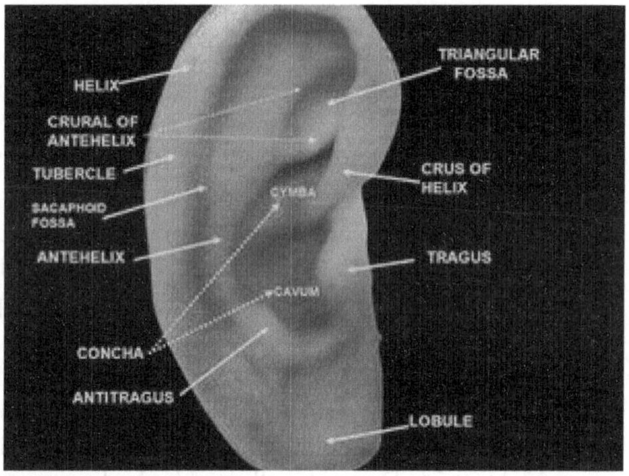

Intended Population

For individuals with a flexed head and neck posture, particularly the elderly and those who have Parkinson's Disease or Ankylosing Spondylitis (Axial Spondyloarthritis) (AS).

Method of Use

Shipe et al (2013) describe the measuring the tragus to wall distance (TWD) as: "the horizontal distance between the tragus, the auricular cartilaginous flap anterior to the external auditory meatus, and a wall."[2] Haywood et al (2004) describe the following: "Horizontal distance between right tragus and wall, standing with heels and buttocks against the wall (to prevent pivoting), knees extended and chin drawn in. Larger distance indicates worse spinal/upper cervical posture. Measured with a retractable steel tape measure."[3]

The TWD can be measured as cued or relaxed, i.e the clinician prompts the individual to assume as close to an anatomical posture as possible e.g "Stand tall.", or the clinician measures the individual in their usual or presenting posture. The measurement can be done standing or sitting and it is worth documenting which position has been used. The TWD can be measured on both the individual's right and left, and then an average can be calculated.

Reference

Haywood et al, 2004: Spinal mobility in ankylosing spondylitis: reliability, validity and responsiveness[3]

Evidence

Reliability

In AS, test-retest correlations have been reported at between 0.93 and 0.95[4]. Inter-tester reliability has also been reported as "excellent" in individuals with PD[5]. However, in individuals aged 18-34 without pathology, Shipe et al [2]observed variable inter-rater reliability results but found that intra-rater reliability was high. The authors subsequently recommended that in clinical practice, the TWT be repeated by the same person.

Validity

In PD, the TWD has shown convergent validity with similar measures (occiput to wall status, C7 to wall distance, photographically derived trunk flexion angle, and inclinometric Thoracic Hyperkyphosis measure)[5].

It has also shown the ability to discriminate between groups (those who could touch occiput to wall when prompted to stand tall) and conditions (cued or relaxed)[5].

Responsiveness

Research reports limited evidence for responsiveness of the TWT[1]. One study[3] reported small to moderate responsiveness to improvement but not deterioration in TWD.

Miscellaneous

Normative Data

The TWT is one measurement in a separate outcome measure, the Bath Ankylosing Spondylitis Metrology Index (BASMI)[6]. As part of a study to produce normative data for the BASMI[7], it was found that TWD did not deteriorate with age[6] . Results from the study showed the TWD was consistent across age groups and gender, which the authors noted was similar to a previous study of normative data using a seated TWT[8]. The authors concluded that TWD is instead disease-specific, in relation to AS.

References

1. Bohannon RW, Tudini F, Constantine D. Tragus-to-wall: A systematic review of procedures, measurements obtained, and clinimetric properties. J Back Musculoskelet Rehabil. 2019;32(1):179-189.
2. Shipe NK, Billek-Sawhney B, Canter TA, Meals DJ, Nestler JM, Stumpff JL. The intra- and inter-rater reliability of the tragus wall distance (TWD) measurement in non-pathological participants ages 18–34. Physiotherapy Theory and Practice. 2013. 29;4: 328-334. Accessed 6 August 2019.
3. Haywood KL, Garratt AM, Jordan K, Dziedzic K, Dawes PT. Spinal mobility in ankylosing spondylitis: reliability, validity and responsiveness. Rheumatology. 2004. 43; 6:750–757. Accessed 6 August 2019.
4. Heuft-Dorenbosch L, Vosse D, Landewé R, Spoorenberg A, Dougados M, Mielants H, van der Tempel H, van der Linden S, van der Heijde D. Measurement of spinal mobility in ankylosing spondylitis: comparison of occiput-to-wall and tragus-to-wall distance. J Rheumatol. 2004. 31; 9:1779-84.
5. Nair P, Bohannon RW, Devaney L, Maloney C, Romano A. Reliability and Validity of Nonradiologic Measures of Forward Flexed Posture in Parkinson Disease. Arch Phys Med Rehabil. 2017. 98; 3:508-516.
6. Chilton-Mitchell L, Martindale J, Hart A, Goodacre L. Normative values for the Bath Ankylosing Spondylitis Metrology Index in a UK population. Rheumatology. 2013. 52; 11: 2086–2090. Accessed 6 August 2019.
7. Jenkinson TR, Mallorie PA, Whitelock HC, Kennedy LG, Garrett SL, Calin A. Defining spinal mobility in ankylosing spondylitis (AS). The Bath AS Metrology Index. J Rheumatol. 1994 Sep;21(9):1694-8.
8. Finnsback C, Mannerkorpi K. Spinal and thoracic mobility—age-related reference values for healthy men and women. Nordisk Fysioterapi. 2005; 9:136-43.
9. Ozaras N, Gulec MG, Celik HK, Demir SE, Guler M. Effect of body shape on tragus-to-wall distance in the normal population. Clin Rheumatol. 2014. 33:1169-71. D may be affected by body mass and weight loss or gain between measurements[9].

❑❑❑

187 Vestibular Oculomotor Motor Screening (VOMS) Assessment

Introduction

Impairments in the vestibulo-ocular system commonly manifest as symptoms of dizziness and visual instability. Nearly 30% of concussed athletes report visual problems during the first week after the injury.[1] Oculomotor impairments and symptoms may manifest as blurred vision, diplopia, impaired eye movements, difficulty in reading, dizziness, headaches, ocular pain, and poor visual-based concentration.[2] Dizziness, which may represent an underlying impairment of the vestibular and/or oculomotor systems, is reported by 50% of concussed athletes[1] and is associated with a 6.4-times greater risk, relative to any other on-field symptom, in predicting protracted (>21 days) recovery.[3]

Concussions can directly impair oculomotor function. Ocular issues (poor eye tracking) after concussion are common. Specifically cranial nerves (CN) III, IV and VI which innervate the eye muscles are susceptible to injury anywhere along the route from brainstem to eye muscles, so this needs to be assessed.

Objective

The Vestibular/Ocular Motor Screening (VOMS) Assessment is used as a brief 5-10 minute concussion screening tool. It has been proposed that it may serve as a single component of a comprehensive approach to the assessment of concussions.[4][5]

Intended population

The test is designed for use with subjects ages 9-40, when used with patients outside this age range, interpretation may vary.

Method of Use

For this test you will need: a tape measure (cm), target with a 14 point font print and a metronome.

The test assesses vestibular and ocular motor impairments via patient-reported symptom provocation after each assessment[4]. The assessment includes a baseline measurement and 5 domains which are recorded in the table provided (see below). Patients verbally rate changes in headache, dizziness, nausea, and fogginess symptoms compared with their immediate pre-assessment state on a scale of 0 (none) to 10 (severe) after each VOMS assessment to determine if each assessment provokes symptoms.

Vestibular/Ocular Motor Test:	Not Tested	Headache 0-10	Dizziness 0-10	Nausea 0-10	Fogginess 0-10	Comments
BASELINE SYMPTOMS:	N/A					
Smooth Pursuits						
Saccades – Horizontal						
Saccades – Vertical						
Convergence (Near Point)						(Near Point in cm): Measure 1: ______ Measure 2: ______ Measure 3: ______
VOR – Horizontal						
VOR – Vertical						
Visual Motion Sensitivity Test						

Baseline Measurement

Prior to performing the 5 domains of the VOMS screen, it is important to establish the patient's baseline symptoms. On a scale of 0-10, ask the patient to score their symptoms at rest for headache, dizziness, nausea & fogginess.

Record: Headache, Dizziness, Nausea & Fogginess ratings at rest.

Domain 1: Smooth Pursuit

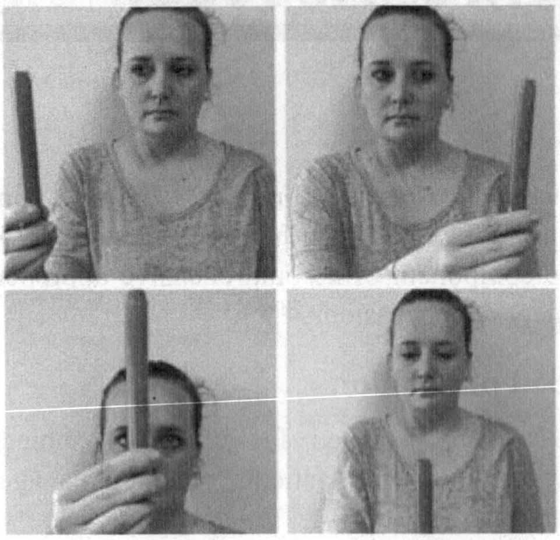

This tests the ability to follow a slowly moving target. The patient and the examiner are seated. The examiner holds a fingertip at a distance of 3 ft. from the patient. The patient is instructed to maintain focus on the target as the examiner moves the target smoothly in the horizontal direction 1.5 ft. to the right and 1.5 ft. to the left of midline. One repetition is complete when the target moves back and forth to the starting position, and 2 repetitions are performed. The target should be moved at a rate requiring approximately 2 seconds to go fully from left to right and 2 seconds to go fully from right to left. The test is repeated with the examiner moving the target smoothly and slowly in the vertical direction 1.5 ft. above and 1.5 ft. below midline for 2 complete repetitions up and down. Again, the target should be moved at a rate requiring approximately 2 seconds to move the eyes fully upward and 2 seconds to move fully downward.

Record: Headache, Dizziness, Nausea & Fogginess ratings after the test.

Domain 2: Saccades

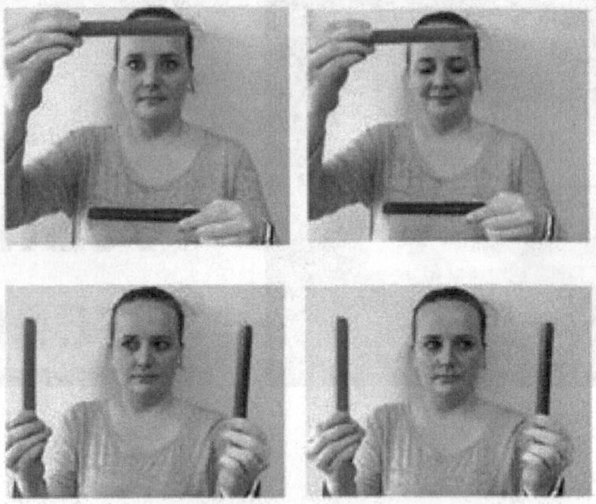

This tests the ability of the eyes to move quickly between targets. The patient and the examiner are seated.

- **Horizontal Saccades**: The examiner holds two single points (fingertips) horizontally at a distance of 3 ft. from the patient, and 1.5 ft. to the right and 1.5 ft. to the left of midline so that the patient must gaze 30 degrees to left and 30 degrees to the right. Instruct the patient to move their eyes as quickly as possible from point to point. One repetition is complete when the eyes move back and forth to the starting position, and 10 repetitions are performed.

Record: Headache, Dizziness, Nausea & Fogginess ratings after the test.

- **Vertical Saccades**: Repeat the test with 2 points held vertically at a distance of 3 ft. from the patient, and 1.5 feet above and 1.5 feet below midline so that the patient must gaze 30 degrees upward and 30 degrees downward. Instruct the patient to move their eyes as quickly as possible from point to point. One repetition is complete when the eyes move up and down to the starting position, and 10 repetitions are performed.

Record: Headache, Dizziness, Nausea & Fogginess ratings after the test.

Domain 3: Convergence

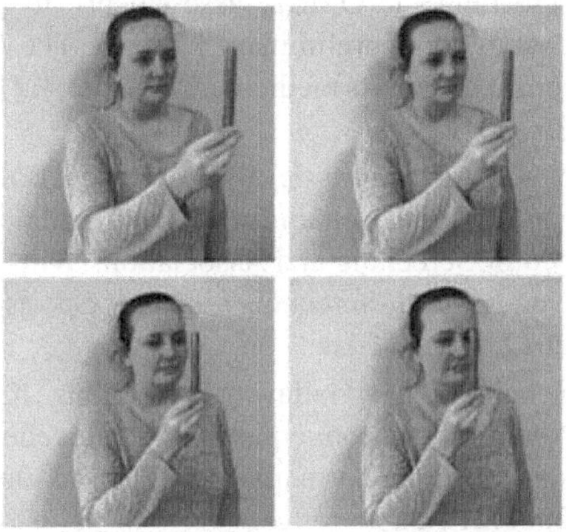

Convergence is assessed by both symptom report and objective measurement of the near point of convergence (NPC).The NPC values are averaged across 3 trials, and normal NPC values are within 5 cm.[6]

Measure the ability to view a near target without double vision. The patient is seated and wearing corrective lenses (if needed). The examiner is seated in front of the patient and observes their eye movement during this test. The patient focuses on a small target (approximately 14 point font size) at arm's length and slowly brings it toward the tip of their nose. The patient is instructed to stop moving the target when they see two distinct images (double vision) or when the examiner observes an outward deviation of one eye. Blurring of the image is ignored. The distance in centimetres between where the target is stopped, and the tip of nose, is measured and recorded using a tape measure. This is repeated a total of 3 times with measures recorded each time.

Record: Headache, Dizziness, Nausea & Fogginess ratings after the test. Abnormal: Near Point of convergence ≥ 6 cm from the tip of the nose.

Domain 4: Vestibular-Ocular Reflex (VOR) Test

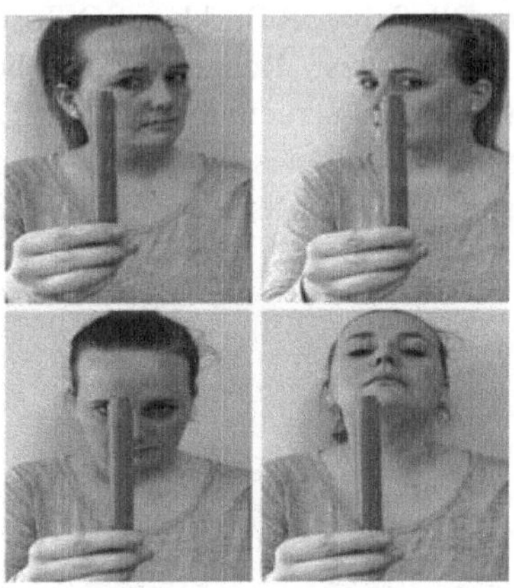

Assess the ability to stabilise vision as the head moves. The patient and the examiner are seated. The examiner holds a target of approximately 14 point font size in front of the patient in the midline at a distance of 3 ft.

- **Horizontal VOR Test**: The patient is asked to rotate their head horizontally while maintaining focus on the target. Using a metronome set at 180 beats per minute (bpm), the head is moved at an amplitude of 20 degrees to each side with the beat. One repetition is complete when the head moves back and forth to the starting position, and 10 repetitions are performed.

Record: Headache, Dizziness, Nausea and Fogginess ratings after the test.

- **Vertical VOR Test**: The test is repeated with the patient moving their head vertically while maintaining focus on the target. Using a metronome set at 180 bpm, the head is moved in an amplitude of 20 degrees up and 20 degrees down with the beat. One repetition is complete when the head moves up and down to the starting position, and 10 repetitions are performed.

Record: Headache, Dizziness, Nausea and Fogginess ratings after the test.

Domain 5: Visual Motion Sensitivity (VMS) Test

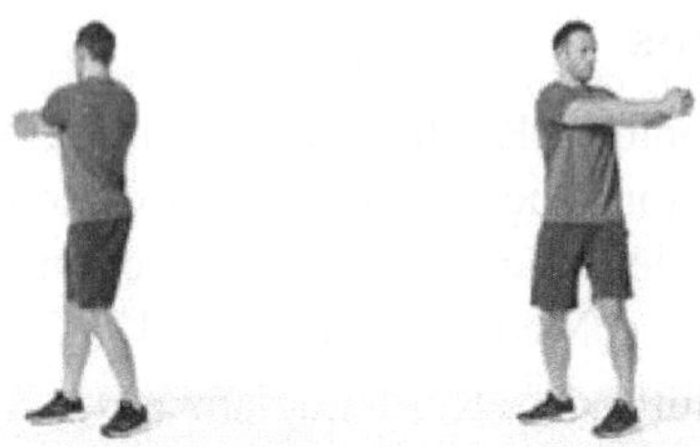

Assess visual motion sensitivity and the ability to inhibit vestibular-induced eye movements using vision.

The patient stands with feet shoulder width apart, facing a busy area of the clinic. The examiner stands next to and slightly behind the patient, so that the patient is guarded but the movement can be performed freely. The patient holds arm outstretched and focuses on their thumb. Set the metronome to 50 bpm. Maintaining focus on their thumb, the patient rotates, together as a unit, their head, eyes and trunk at an amplitude of 80 degrees to the right and 80 degrees to the left, to the beat of the metronome. One repetition is complete when the trunk rotates back and forth to the starting position, and 5 repetitions are performed.

Record: Headache, Dizziness, Nausea & Fogginess ratings after a 10 second pause to allow for latent symptoms after the test[7].

Evidence

The VOMS has demonstrated internal consistency as well as sensitivity in identifying patients with concussions[4][8][9].

Mucha et al[4] found that the test demonstrates internal consistency and basic validity compared with the Post-Concussion Symptom Scale (PCSS). They also suggest that it may "provide preliminary evidence for the use of the VOMS to identify patients with sport-related concussions from healthy controls".

Moran et al[8] supported the implementation of the VOMS baseline assessment into clinical practice, due to a high internal consistency, strong relationships between VOMS items, and a low false-positive rate at baseline in youth athletes.

Anzalon et al[10] suggest that the VOMS can serve as a predictor of recovery time in patients with sports-related concussion.

Worts et al[11] found that the VOMS may be more stable than other screening measures and is less likely to result in false-positives than the King-Devick test in adolescent athletes.

References

1. Kontos AP, Elbin RJ, Schatz P, et al. A revised factor structure for the Post-Concussion Symptom Scale: baseline and postconcussion factors. Am J Sports Med. 2012;40(10):2375-2384.
2. Ciuffreda KJ, Ludlam D, Thiagarajan P. Oculomotor diagnostic protocol for the mTBI population. Optometry. 2011;82(2):61-63.
3. Lau BC, Kontos AP, Collins MW, Mucha A, Lovell MR. Which on-field signs/symptoms predict protracted recovery from sport-related concussion among high school football players? Am J Sports Med. 2011;39(11):2311-2318.
4. Mucha A, Collins MW, Elbin RJ, Furman JM, Troutman-Enseki C, DeWolf RM, Marchetti G, Kontos AP. A brief vestibular/ocular motor screening (VOMS) assessment to evaluate concussions: preliminary findings. The American journal of sports medicine. 2014 Oct;42(10):2479-86.
5. Yorke AM, Smith L, Babcock M, Alsalaheen B. Validity and Reliability of the Vestibular/Ocular Motor Screening and Associations With Common Concussion Screening Tools. Sports Health. 2017;9(2):174-80.
6. Scheiman M, Gallaway M, Frantz KA, et al. Nearpoint of convergence: test procedure, target selection, and normative data. Optom Vis Sci80(3) 2003:214-225
7. Mucha A, Collins MW, Elbin RJ, Furman JM, Troutman-Enseki C, DeWolf RM, Marchetti G, Kontos AP. A brief vestibular/ocular motor screening (VOMS) assessment to evaluate concussions: preliminary findings. The American journal of sports medicine. 2014 Oct;42(10):2479-86.
8. Moran RN, Covassin T, Elbin RJ, Gould D, Nogle S. Reliability and normative reference values for the Vestibular/Ocular Motor Screening (VOMS) tool in youth athletes. The American journal of sports medicine. 2018 May;46(6):1475-80.
9. Moran RN, Covassin T, Elbin RJ. Sex Differences on Vestibular and Ocular Motor Assessment in Youth Athletes. Journal of athletic training. 2019 Apr;54(4):445-8.
10. Anzalone AJ, Blueitt D, Case T, McGuffin T, Pollard K, Garrison JC, Jones MT, Pavur R, Turner S, Oliver JM. A positive vestibular/ocular motor screening (VOMS) is associated with increased recovery time after sports-related concussion in youth and adolescent athletes. The American journal of sports medicine. 2017 Feb;45(2):474-9.
11. Worts PR, Schatz P, Burkhart SO. Test Performance and Test-Retest Reliability of the Vestibular/Ocular Motor Screening and King-Devick Test in Adolescent Athletes During a Competitive Sport Season. Am J Sports Med. 2018;46(8):2004-10.

❑❑❑

188 VISA-A scale

Objective

The VISA-A aims to evaluate the clinical severity for patients with chronic Achilles tendinopathy. It is an easily self-administered questionnaire that evaluates symptoms and their effect on physical activity. It can be used to compare different populations with chronic achilles tendinopathy, and facilitate comparisons between studies. It can be used to determine the patient's clinical severity and provide a guideline for treatments as well as for monitoring the effect of treatment[1] The VISA-A is very user friendly, as it generally takes less than five minutes to complete, even for patients with chronic and severe symptoms. The questionnaire represents a valid, reliable and disease specific questionnaire to measure the condition of the Achilles tendon, but it is not a diagnostic tool. The final version of the questionnaire was named the Victorian Institute of Sport Assessment-Achilles Questionnaire.

Intended Population

- Patients with Achilles tendinopathy.
- Patients who are able to give written informed consent.
- Exclusions: pregnant or nursing women, individuals who have sustained a total rupture of the Achilles tendon.

Method of Use

The questionnaire contains eight questions, covering three necessary domains: 1) pain, 2) functional status, and 3) activity (= three significant domains of dysfunction):

- Questions 1-3 are related to pain. (in this questionnaire, the term "pain" refers specifically to pain in the Achilles tendon region).
- Questions 4-6 are related to function.
- Questions 7-8 are related to activity.
- Question 8 actually contains two questions: a) pain with activity, and b) duration of activity.
- The first seven questions have a score out of 10, and question 8 scores a maximum of 30.
- The first six questions use a VAS so that the patient may report the magnitude of a continuum of subjective symptoms. The final two questions used a categorical rating scale[2]

Answering question 8 is limited to A,B or C and relates to the reality of the patient. The patient automatically loses at least 10 of 20 points if he or she has pain during sports activity.

The maximum score that can be achieved on the question is 100, and would be the score of person who is completely asymptomatic. A lower score indicates more symptoms and greater limitation of physical activity.

A recreational person who has Achilles tendinopathy will not score higher than 70 on the VISA-A scale.

Evidence

Reliability

The VISA-A questionnaire has good test-retest ($r=0.93$), intrarater (thee tests, $r = 0.90$), and interrater ($r=0.90$) reliability as well as good stability when compared one week apart ($R=0.81$).

There are no difference in scores whether the test-retest questionnaires is completed at the first visit or at the second visit ($p=0.58$). Reliability data were analyzed by Pearson 'r, as these data were normally distributed.[2]

It is noted that the VISA-A score does not indicate whether surgery is decided upon, even though it has been shown that there are statistically significant differences between population mean VISA-A scores in non-surgical vs surgical patients.

To internationally compare results, perform multinational studies, or minimize bias originating from subpopulations speaking different languages within one country, a unique protocol of forward and back translations and cultural adaptations as well as "verification of the scaling requirements and validation of and establishing normative values of the new version" are required .

This procedure has been performed and published for the Swedish, Italian, and Turkish versions of the VISA-A questionnaire. Cross-cultural adaptions to Spanish, Portuguese, and Flemish languages have been done but are not reported in journals available in Medline/Pubmed.[1][3][4][5][6]

Validity

The VISA-A score correlates significantly with both Percy and Conochie's grade of severity (Spearman's r =0.58; p<0.01) and that of Curwin and Stanish (Spearman's r=-0.57; p<0.001).[2]

Factor analysis has provided two factors strongly confirming that the questionnaire is valid for evaluating the patient's symptoms and its effect on physical activity. An internal consistency of 0.77 as measured by Cronbach's alpha indicates that no question should be excluded.[2]

The VISA-A questionnaire displays construct validity when used in two populations of patients with Achilles tendinopathy and control subjects. The mean (95% confidence interval) score in non-surgical patients has been shown to be 64 (59-69), in presurgical patients 44 (28-60), and with asymptomatic persons 96 (94-99). VISA-A scores are higher in non-surgical vs presurgical patients (p=0.02) and higher in asymptomatic persons vs presurgical or non-surgical patients (p<0.001).[2]

Responsiveness

The VISA-A questionnaire shows good responsiveness; it is sensitive for clinically important changes over time with treatment, easy for patients to fill out, and the data is easily handled.[7]

Other Languages

The French version of this questionnaire (VISA-AF) is also available. It has been recently shown to have satisfactory levels of construct validity, excellent test–retest reliability, good internal consistency and discriminatory validity, as well as an absence of floor and ceiling effects. [8]

Miscellaneous

Since minimal investigator assistance is required, the VISA-A can be self-administered and risks for potential observer bias are very limited.

The VISA-A questionnaire is not a diagnostic tool, and the score can be reduced or influenced, e.g. lower limb function. Limitations of function limits the subject's ability to score well in question 8, even though the Achilles tendon may be uninjured.

The continuous numerical result of the VISA-A questionnaire is ideal for comparing patients' progress in the clinical setting. Continuous numerical result has the potential to provide utility in both the clinical setting and research. Further studies are needed to determine whether the VISA-A score predicts prognosis[2]

A lower score indicates more symptoms and a larger limitation of physical activity, but there is no evidence that indicates, for example, that a patient with a score of 70 is "cured".

References

1. Silbernagel KG, Thomeé R, Karlsson J. Cross-cultural adaptation of the VISA-A questionnaire, an index of clinical severity for patients with Achilles tendinopathy, with reliability, validity and structure evaluations. BMC Musculoskelet Disord. 2005 Mar 6;6:12.
2. J M Robinson, J L Cook, C Purdam, P J Visentini, J Ross, N Maffulli, J E Taunton, K M Khan, for the Victorian Institute of Sport Tendon Study Group. The VISA-A questionnaire: a valid and reliable index of the clinical severity of Achilles tendinopathy. Br J Sports Med 2001;35:335-341.
3. Lohrer H, Nauck T. Cross-cutrural adaption and validation of the VISA-A questionnaire for German-speaking Achilles tendinopathy patients. BMC Musculoskelet Disord. 2009 Oct 30;10:134.
4. Silbernagel KG, Brorsson A, Lundberg M. The majority of patients with Achilles tendinopathy recover fully when treated with exercise alone: a 5-year follow-up. Am J Sports Med. 2011 Mar;39(3):607-13.
5. Dogramaci Y, Kalaci A, Kücükkübas N, Inandi T, Esen E, Yanat AN. Validation of the VISA-A questionnaire for Turkish language: the VISA-A-Tr study. Br J Sports Med. 2011 Apr;45(5):453-5
6. Maffulli N, Longo UG, Testa V, Oliva F, Capasso G, Denaro V. Italian translation of the VISA-A score for tendinopathy of the main body of the

Achilles tendon. Disabil Rehabil. 2008;30(20-22):1635-9.

7. Karin Grävare Silbernagel, Roland ThomeéfckLRBengt I. Eriksson, and Jon Karlsson. Continued Sports Activity, Using a Pain-Monitoring Model, During Rehabilitation in Patients With Achilles Tendinopathy. Am J Sports Med. 2007 Jun;35(6):897-906.
8. Kaux JF, Delvaux F, Oppong-Kyei J, Dardenne N, Beaudart C, Buckinx F, Croisier JL, Forthomme B, Crielaard JM, Bruyère O. Validity and reliability of the French translation of the VISA-A questionnaire for Achilles tendinopathy. fckLRDisability & Rehabilitation. 2016, 38(26): 2593-9.

The VISA-A questionnaire

An index of the severity of Achilles tendinopathy

In This Questionnaire, The Term Pain Refers Specifically To Pain In The Achilles Tendon Region

1. For how many minutes do you have stiffness in the Achilles region on first getting up?

100 mins 0 1 2 3 4
5 6 7 8 9 10
0 mins

2. Once you are warmed up for the day, do you have pain when stretching the Achilles tendon fully over the edge of a step? (Keeping knee straight)

strong 0 1 2 3 4
severe pain 5 6 7 8
9 10 no pain

3. After walking on flat ground for 30 minutes, do you have pain within the next 2 hours? (If unable to walk on flat ground for 30 minutes because of pain, score 0 for this question).

strong 0 1 2 3 4
severe pain 5 6 7 8
9 10 no pain

4. Do you have pain walking downstairs with a normal gait cycle?

strong 0 1 2 3 4
severe pain 5 6 7 8
9 10 no pain

5. Do you have pain during or immediately after doing 10 (single leg) heel raises from aflat surface?

strong 0 1 2 3 4
severe pain 5 6 7 8
9 10 no pain

6. How many single leg hops can you do without pain?

0 1 2 3 4 5 6
7 8 9 10

7. Are you currently undertaking sport or other physical activity?

0 Not at all

4 Modified training ± modified competition

7 Full training ± competition but not at same level as when symptoms began

10 Competing at the same or higher level as when symptoms began

8. Please complete EITHER A, B or C in this question.

- If you have no pain while undertaking Achilles tendon loading sports please complete Q8a only.
- If you have pain while undertaking Achilles tendon loading sports but it does not stop you from completing the activity, please complete Q8b only.
- If you have pain that stops you from completing Achilles tendon loading sports, please complete Q8c only.

A. If you have no pain while undertaking Achilles tendon loading sports, for how long can you train/practice?

NIL 1-10 mins 11-20 mins
0 7 14
21-30 mins >30 mins
21 30
OR

B. If you have some pain while undertaking Achilles tendon loading sport, but it does not stop you from completing your training/practice for how long can you train/practice?

NIL 1-10 mins 11-20 mins
0 7 14
21-30mins >30 mins
21 30
OR

C. If you have pain that stops you from completing your training/practice in Achilles tendon loading sport, for how long can you train/practice?

NIL 1-10 mins 11-20 mins
0 7 14
21-30mins >30 mins
21 30

Total Score (/ 100) = %

❑❑❑

189 Walking Index for Spinal Cord Injury II (WISCI II)

Objective

The Walking Index for Spinal Cord Injury (WISCI) is a scale that measures the type and amount of assistance (in terms of requirements of assistive devices, or human helpers) required by a person with spinal cord injury (SCI) for walking.[1] It is an ordinal scale which rates people with SCI from being unable to walk to independent walking and designed to indicate the grades of impairment occurring after SCI and their relationship to the function of walking.[2] A year following the release of the 19 level WISCI, it was modified to WISCI II with the inclusion of two levels,[3]

Intended Population

The WISCI/WISCI II was designed as a tool to measure improvement in walking ability specifically for spinal cord injury.[1] It is precisely useful for the following categories of patients:

1. Individuals with SCI that are able to stand and walk with parallel bars are suitable for assessment with the WISCI. Only patients with reciprocal gait should be considered when scoring the WISCI II.[2]
2. A number of individuals with ASIA Impairment Scale grade A below T10 and AIS B, C, D qualify for assessment with the WISCI II.[4]
3. Individuals with tetraplegic presentation require motor strength in their triceps upto a grade of 3 or more to be able to sufficiently support their body weight. [5][6]
4. Individuals presenting with tetrapelgia and arm strength in triceps that is less than grade 3 would not be easily classified by the WISCI.[7]

Method of Use/Scoring

The WISCI assessment is carried out by physical therapist. To score the WISCI/WISCI II the descriptors that relate to the present walking performance of an individual with SCI is observed. Then, appropriate level of highest walking performance is assigned to the patient. The physical therapist selects the level at which the patient is safest as observed, with patient's comfort level described in addition to this. In case other devices apart from those that have been stated in the standard definitions are used during the assessment, they should be documented as descriptors. Also, if there is a discrepancy between two observers, the record with the higher level should be selected. The patient should be observed with the WISCI level documented on using the scale rated from 0 to 20 at baseline (called the Baseline WISCI), the subject is then observed again at the defined interval (called the interval WISCI). The gains in walking can be obtained by simply subtracting the baseline WISCI from the interval WISCI, which is known as the "changed WISCI".[2]

Equipment Needed

The following equipment may be required/recorded during assessment[3]:

1. Walkers (conventional, if rolling walkers are used, they must be identified in the descriptors). A platform walker is considered equivalent to a walker.
2. The use of advanced reciprocating gait orthosis (ARGO) should be excluded.
3. Axillary or Lofstrand (Canadian) crutches may be used.
4. Braces which could mean one or two braces should be identified in the descriptors. For other braces

such as ace wraps or splint should be described under "other".

5. Long leg braces, whether they are locked or unlocked at the ankle must be indicated in the descriptors.
6. Braces must not be covered by clothes to ensure that physical therapist and other professional staff make visual determination that patient has a brace.

Completion Time

The WISCI II may take about 5 to 15 minutes to complete. Especially, during the acute phase, the time required could be longer and shorter during follow-up assessments. [2]

Evidence

Validity

WISCI II has been highly reported to have a high validity in multiple dimensions, which has resulted in it broad acceptance.[2] 24 experts agreed on a hierarchical ranking in SCI walking function in terms of content and face validity for the WISCI.[1][3] A prospective study consisting of 170 subjects in four different countries found that progression through the levels of the scale followed a monotonic pattern, which was observed in over 80% of the subjects.[8] In the study, a 0.91 ($p < 0.001$) correlation between walking capacity from WISCI and impairment (LEMS) was found at the final assessment, which supported construct and content validity. Other studies have also demonstrated the criterion-related, predictive and concurrent validity, and also the convergent and divergent construct validity.[9][8][10][11][12]

Reliability

Marino et al.[13], reported an inter and intra-rater reliability of 1.00 for self-selected WISCI II levels. The inter-rater reliability for maximal level WISCI II was 0.98 and the intra-rater reliability was 1.00.

Reproducibility

In a study[9] carried out on 76 subjects who have chronic SCI, WISCI II demonstrated excellent reproducibility, having an intra-class correlation coefficient of 0.99 for self-selected and maximum WISCI II level. It produced smallest real differences of 0.79 for self-selected level and 0.60 for maximum level which connotes that differences in a WISCI II level can be interpreted as being real in a patient with chronic SCI.

Conclusion

The WISCI has been widely accepted for the assessment of walking function in patients with SCI due to its excellent psychometric properties as well as recommendations by different authorities, It is essential that users carry out the assessment according to the instruction in the testing guide for accurate results.

References

1. Ditunno JF Jr, Ditunno PL, Graziani V, Scivoletto G, Bernardi M, Castellano Vet al. Walking Index for Spinal Cord Injury (WISCI): an international multicenter validity and reliability study. Spinal Cord2000;38,234–243.
2. Ditunno JF, Ditunno PL, Scivoletto G, Patrick M, Dijkers M, Barbeau H, Burns AS, Marino RJ, Schmidt-Read M. The Walking Index for Spinal Cord Injury (WISCI/WISCI II): nature, metric properties, use and misuse. Spinal Cord. 2013 May;51(5):346-55.
3. Ditunno PL, Ditunno JF Jr. Walking Index for Spinal Cord Injury (WISCIII): scale revision. Spinal Cord2001;39,654–656.
4. Ditunno JF. Validation and refinement of the Walking Index for Spinal Cord Injury (WISCI) in a clinical setting. J Spinal Cord Med. 2004;27(2):160.
5. Dobkin BH, Apple D, Barbeau H, Basso M, Behrman A, Deforge D, Ditunno J, Dudley G, Elashoff R, Fugate L, Harkema S. Methods for a randomized trial of weight-supported treadmill training versus conventional training for walking during inpatient rehabilitation after incomplete traumatic spinal cord injury. Neurorehabilitation and Neural Repair. 2003 Sep;17(3):153-67.
6. Morganti B, Scivoletto G, Ditunno P, Ditunno JF, Molinari M. Walking index for spinal cord injury (WISCI): criterion validation. Spinal Cord 2005; 43(1): 27-33.
7. Ditunno JF, Burns AS, Marino RJ. Neurological and functional capacity outcome measures: essential to spinal cord injury clinical trials. Journal of rehabilitation research and development. 2005 May 1;42(3):35.
8. Ditunno JF, Scivoletto G, Patrick M, Biering-Sorensen F, Abel R, Marino R. Validation of the walking index for spinal cord injury in a US and European clinical population. Spinal Cord 2007; 45, 275–291

9. Burns AS, Delparte JJ, Patrick M, Marino RJ, Ditunno JF. The reproducibility and convergent validity of the Walking Index for Spinal Cord Injury (WISCI) in chronic spinal cord injury. Neurorehabil Neural Repair 2011; 25, 149–157
10. Curt A, van Hedel HJ, Klaus D, Dietz V. Recovery from a spinal cord injury: significance of compensation, neural plasticity, and repair. J Neurotrauma 2008; 25, 677–685
11. Morganti B, Scivoletto G, Ditunno P, Ditunno JF, Molinari M. Walking Index for Spinal Cord Injury (WISCI): criterion validation. Spinal Cord 2005; 43, 27–33.
12. van Hedel HJ, Dietz V, Curt A. Assessment of walking speed and distance in subjects with an incomplete spinal cord injury. Neurorehabil Neural Repair 2007; 21, 295–301
13. Marino RJ, Scivoletto G, Patrick M, Tamburella F, Read MS, Burns AS et al. Walking index for spinal cord injury version 2 (WISCI-II) with repeatability of the 10-m walk time: inter- and intrarater reliabilities. Am J Phys Med Rehabil 2010; 89, 7–15
14. Walking Index for SCI II. Emma Marino. Available at https://www.youtube.com watch?v=Fkm6WolhDLw

Instructions for the Use of the Walking Index for Spinal Cord Injury II (WISCI II)

Subject Selection

The purpose of this scale is for use in clinical trials to measure improvements in walking in persons with spinal cord injury. The following outline describes subjects for whom the scale is most commonly utilized.

1. Spinal cord injury subjects who are capable of standing and walking in the parallel bars will be eligible for assessment. Only a reciprocal gait is to be considered in scoring the WISCI scale. Additional inclusion/exclusion criteria may be necessary.
2. Most often ASIA A below T10 and ASIA B, C, and D subjects may qualify3. (Ditunno 2004).
3. Individuals with tetraplegia would require motor strength in triceps of at least grade 3 or be able to support their body weight3,4. (Ditunno 2004, Dobkin 2003).

Standardized Physical Environment and Distance

This is a functional limitation scale, NOT a disability scale. It must be used in a standardized environment with standardized equipment and definitions, which are observed and recorded by professional staff that are trained. The following requirements are necessary:

1. A flat, smooth, non-slippery surface of 10 meters will be utilized.
2. Individuals walk at their own speed and the 10 meters should not be timed.

Standardized Equipment

1. Walkers should be conventional, but if a rolling walker is used, it should be coded as a walker and identified in the descriptors.
2. Use of a platform walker is equivalent to a walker.
3. Crutches can be Lofstrand (Canadian) or axillary.
4. Braces means one or two braces, either long or short, and should be identified in the descriptors. Other devices used for bracing such as ace wraps or splints should be coded as a brace and described under “other”.
5. Whether long leg braces are locked or unlocked at the knees should be identified in the descriptors.
6. Clothing should not cover braces to allow therapists and other professional staff to make a visual determination that the patient has a brace.

Standardized Assistance

1. Any physical contact with the subject, including “contact guard” is considered physical assistance.
2. Supervision should not be regarded as physical assistance.

Scoring

The Walking Index for Spinal Cord Injury Scale (WISCI 2) has demonstrated a response to change in the Spinal Cord Injury Locomotion Trial5 (ISCOS 2004) and in clinical validation studies1,6 (Ditunno 2003, 2004). In scoring the WISCI, check the descriptors that apply to current walking performance, and then assign the highest level of walking performance. In scoring one level, one should choose the level at which the patient is safe as judged by the therapist, with patient’s comfort level described. If devices other than those stated in the standard definitions are used, they should be documented as descriptors. If there is a discrepancy between two observers, the higher level should be chosen.

The subject is observed by the trained personnel and the WISCI level is recorded on the scale of 0 to 20 at baseline (Baseline WISCI). The subject is observed again at the defined interval (Interval WISCI). The change in score is calculated by subtracting the baseline WISCI from the Interval WISCI, which equals the change in WISCI (Changed WISCI). If a group of subjects are enrolled, medians and means may be calculated.

References:

1. Ditunno JF, Ditunno PL, Graziani V, Scivoletto G, Bernardi M, Castellano V, Marchetti M, Brabeau H, Frankel HL, D'Andrea Greve JM, Ko HY, Marshall R, Nance P. Walking Index for spinal cord injury (WISCI): an international multicenter validity and reliability study. Spinal Cord 2000;38:234-243.
2. Ditunno PL, Ditunno JF. Walking index for spinal cord injury (WISCI II): scale revision. Spinal Cord 2001;39:654-656.
3. Morganti B, Scivoletto G, Ditunno P, Ditunno JF, Molinari M. Walking index for spinal cord injury (WISCI): criterion validation. Spinal Cord 2005; 43(1): 27-33.
4. Ditunno JF, West C, Schmidt M, Patrick M. Validation and refinement of the Walking Index for Spinal Cord Injury (WISCI) in a clinical setting. 30th Annual Scientific Meeting of the American Spinal Injury Association, Denver, CO, May 14 – 16, 2004.
5. Doblin BH, Apple D, Barbeau H, Basso M, Behrman A, Deforge D, et el. Methods for a randomized trial of weight-supported treadmill training versus conventional training for walking during inpatient rehabilitation after incomplete traumatic spinal cord injury. Neurorehabil Neural Repair 2003; 17(3):153-167.
6. Ditunno JF, Dobkin BH. Walking index for spinal cord injury (WISCI): response to change in a clinical trial (SCILT) and setting (TJU). Inaugural International Campaign for Cures of spinal cord injury Paralysis (ICCP) Clinical Trials Workshop, Vancouver, Canada, February 20-21, 2004.
7. Ditunno JF, Jr., Burns AS, West C, Patrick M. Clinical validation of the Walking Index in Spinal Cord Injury (WISCI) scale: preliminary report. J Spinal Cord Med 2003;26(Suppl 1):S37.

Walking Index for Spinal Cord Injury (WISCI II) Descriptors

Physical Limitation for walking secondary to impairment is defined at the person level and indicates the ability of a person to walk after spinal cord injury. The development of this assessment index required a rank ordering along a dimension of impairment, from the level of most severe impairment (0) to least severe impairment (20) based on the use of devices, braces and physical assistance of one or more persons. The order of the levels suggests each successive level is a less impaired level than the former. The ranking of severity is based on the severity or the impairment and not on functional independence in the environment. The following definitions standardize the terms used in each item:

Physical assistance: 'Physical assistance of two persons' is moderate to maximum assistance. 'Physical assistance of one person' is minimal to moderate assistance.

Braces: 'Braces' means one or two braces, either short or long leg. (Splinting of lower extremities for standing is considered long leg bracing). 'No braces' means no braces on either leg.

Walker: 'Walker' is a conventional rigid walker without wheels.

Crutches: 'Crutches' can be Lofstrand (Canadian) or axillary.

Cane: 'Cane' is a conventional straight cane.

Level	Description
0	Client is unable to stand and/or participate in assisted walking.
1.	Ambulates in parallel bars, with braces and physical assistance of two persons, less than 10 meters
2.	Ambulates in parallel bars, with braces and physical assistance of two persons, 10 meters.
3.	Ambulates in parallel bars, with braces and physical assistance of one person, 10 meters.
4.	Ambulates in parallel bars, no braces and physical assistance of one person, 10 meters
5.	Ambulates in parallel bars, with no braces and no physical assistance, 10 meters.

6.	Ambulates with walker, with braces and physical assistance of one person, 10 meters.
7.	Ambulates with two crutches, with braces and physical assistance of one person, 10 meters.
8.	Ambulates with walker, no braces and physical assistance of one person, 10 meters.
9.	Ambulates with walker, with braces and no physical assistance, 10 meters.
10.	Ambulates with one cane/crutch, with braces and physical assistance of one person, 10 meters.
11.	Ambulates with two crutches, no braces and physical assistance of one person, 10 meters.
12.	Ambulates with two crutches, with braces and no physical assistance, 10 meters.
13.	Ambulates with walker, no braces and no physical assistance, 10 meters.
14.	Ambulates with one cane/crutch, no braces and physical assistance of one person, 10 meters.
15.	Ambulates with one cane/crutch, with braces and no physical assistance, 10 meters.
16.	Ambulates with two crutches, no braces and no physical assistance, 10 meters.
17.	Ambulates with on devices, no braces and physical assistance of one person, 10 meters.
18.	Ambulates with on devices, with braces and no physical assistance, 10 meters.
19.	Ambulates with one cane/crutch, no braces and no physical assistance, 10 meters.
20.	Ambulates with no devices, no braces and no physical assistance, 10 meters.

Scoring Sheet for the Walking Index for Spinal Cord Injury (WISCI II)

Name________________________________ **Date**________________________

Check descriptors that apply to current walking performance, and then assign the highest level of walking performance. (In scoring a level, one should choose the level at which the patient is safe as judged by the therapist, with patient's comfort level described. If devices other than those stated in the standard definitions are used, they should be documented as descriptors. If there is a discrepancy between two observers, the higher level should be chosen.)

Gait: reciprocal______________________________; swing through___________________________

Devices	Braces	Assistance	Patient reported Comfort level
//bars < 10 meters	Long Leg Braces- Uses 2 Uses 1	Max Assist x 2 people	Very comfortable
//bars < 10 meters	Short Leg Braces- Uses 2 Uses 1	Min/Mod assist x 2 people	Slightly comfortable
Walker- Standard Rolling Platform	Locked at knee ____ Unlocked at knee ____	Min/mod assist x 1 person	Neither comfortable nor uncomfortable
Crutches- Uses 2 Uses 1	Other: __________		Slightly uncomfortable
Canes- Quad Uses 2 Uses 1			Very uncomfortable
No devices	No braces	No assistance	

WISCI Levels

Level	Devices	Braces	Assistance	Distance
0				Unable
1	Parallel bars	Braces	2 persons	Less than 10 meters
2	Parallel bars	Braces	2 persons	10 meters
3	Parallel bars	Braces	1 person	10 meters
4	Parallel bars	No Braces	No assistance	10 meters
5	Parallel bars	Braces	1 person	10 meters
6	Walker	Braces	1 person	10 meters
7	Two crutches	Braces	1 person	10 meters
8	Walker	No Braces	No assistance	10 meters
9	Walker	Braces	No assistance	10 meters
10	One cane/crutch	Braces	1 person	10 meters
11	Two crutches	No Braces	1 person	10 meters
12	Two crutches	Braces	No assistance	10 meters
13	Walker	No Braces	No assistance	10 meters
14	One cane/crutch	No Braces	1 person	10 meters
15	One cane/crutch	Braces	No assistance	10 meters
16	Two crutches	No Braces	No assistance	10 meters
17	No devices	No Braces	1 person	10 meters
18	No devices	Braces	No assistance	10 meters
19	One cane/crutch	No Braces	No assistance	10 meters
20	No devices	No Braces	No assistance	10 meters
Level assigned				

❑❑❑

190 WOMAC Osteoarthritis Index

Objective

The Western Ontario and McMaster Universities Arthritis Index (WOMAC) is widely used in the evaluation of Hip and Knee Osteoarthritis. It is a self-administered questionnaire consisting of 24 items divided into 3 subscales:[1]

1. Pain (5 items): during walking, using stairs, in bed, sitting or lying, and standing upright.
2. Stiffness (2 items): after first waking and later in the day.
3. Physical Function (17 items): using stairs, rising from sitting, standing, bending, walking, getting in / out of a car, shopping, putting on / taking off socks, rising from bed, lying in bed, getting in / out of bath, sitting, getting on / off toilet, heavy domestic duties, light domestic duties WOMAC Index was developed in 1982 at Western Ontario and McMaster Universities. WOMAC is available in over 65 languages and has been linguistically validated.[2][1]

Area of Assessment: Activities of daily living, functional mobility, gait, general health, quality of life.

Intended Population: WOMAC Index was developed for hip and knee osteoarthritis, however it has been used with other rheumatic conditions such as: rheumatoid arthritis, juvenile rheumatoid arthritis, fibromyalgia, systemic lupus erythematosus and low back pain.[1]

Method of Use: The WOMAC takes approximately 12 minutes to complete, and can be taken on paper, over the telephone or computer. Both the computerized and the mobile versions of the test have been found to be comparable to the paper form, with no significant difference.[3][4]

The test questions are scored on a scale of 0-4, which correspond to: None (0), Mild (1), Moderate (2), Severe (3), and Extreme (4).

The scores for each subscale are summed up, with a possible score range of 0-20 for Pain, 0-8 for Stiffness, and 0-68 for Physical Function. Usually a sum of the scores for all three subscales gives a total WOMAC score, however there are other methods that have been used to combine scores.[1]

Higher scores on the WOMAC indicate worse pain, stiffness, and functional limitations.

Evidence

Reliability: The test-retest reliability of the WOMAC varies for the different subscales. The pain subscale has not been consistent across studies, but it generally meets the minimum standard. The physical function subscale is more consistent and has a stronger test-retest reliability. The stiffness subscale has shown low test-retest reliability.[1]

Validity

Responsiveness: The WOMAC Index has been used extensively in clinical trials, and has generally been shown to exhibit greater or comparable responsiveness to change than other tests. This varies, however, for different subscales and types of interventions.[1]

Miscellaneous: Two potential weaknesses of the WOMAC are:

1. The stiffness subscale has low test-retest reliability, and there is little evidence for its measurement properties.
2. Some studies report inadequate factorial validity in the pain and physical function subscales of the WOMAC. Thus, the physical function subscale

might be limited in its ability to detect change if the association between pain and function is weak.[1]

References

1. American College of Rheumatology. Western Ontario and McMaster Universities Osteoarthritis Index (WOMAC). http://www.rheumatology.org/practice/clinical/clinicianresearchers/outcomes-instrumentation/WOMAC.asp. (accessed 12 July 2013).
2. WOMAC Osteoarthritis Index. http://www.womac.org/womac/index.htm. (accessed 12 July 2013).
3. Theiler R, Spielberger J, Bischoff H.A., Bellamy N, Huber J, Kroesen S. Clinical evaluation of the WOMAC 3.0 OA Index in numeric rating scale format using a computerized touch screen version [abstract]. OSTEOARTHR CARTILAGE 2002;10(6):479-481
4. Bellamy N, Wilson C, Hendrikz J, Whitehouse S.L., Patel B, Dennison S, Davis T. Osteoarthritis Index delivered by mobile phone (m-WOMAC) is valid, reliable, and responsive [abstract]. J CLIN EPIDEMIOL 2011;64(2):182-190

WOMAC Osteoarthritis Index

	NONE (0)	SLIGHT (1)	MODERATE (2)	SEVERE (3)	EXTREME (4)
RATE YOUR PAIN WHEN 1.Walking 2. Climbing stairs 3.Sleeping at night 4.Resting Standing					
RATE YOUR STIFFNESS IN THE 1.Morning 2. Evening					
RATE YOUR DIFFICULTY WHEN 1. Descending stairs 2. Ascending stairs 3. Rising from sitting 4. Standing 5. Bending to floor 6. Walking on even floor 7. Getting in/out of car 8. Going shopping 9. Putting on socks 10. Rising from bed 11. Taking off socks 12. Lying in bed 13. Getting in/out of bath 14. Sitting 15. Getting on/off toilet 16. Doing light domestic duties (cooking, dusting) 17. Doing heavy domestic duties (moving furniture)					
Patient Signature				**Date**	
Physical Therapist Signature				**Date**	

❑❑❑

191 Y Balance Test

Purpose

The Y Balance Test (YBT) is a tool used to test a person's risk for injury. It can be used for both the upper quarter and lower quarter. The YBT for the lower quarter (LQYBT) has been thoroughly researched as its protocol is based on research done on the Star Excursion Balance Test. The Star Excursion Balance Test demonstrated reliable results on its ability to predict LE injury in high school basketball players[1], and the LQYBT has identified athletes at increased risk for injury[2].

The YBT for the UQ (UQYBT) has been shown to be a reliable test to assess unilateral UE function in a closed chain position. The UQYBT also has the patient reach in 3 different directions with one UE while in a push-up position [3]. Further research is needed to determine the applicability of the UQYBT.

Reliability

The LQYBT showed good interrater test-retest reliability with an acceptable level of measurement error among multiple raters screening active duty service members, and a second study shows excellent reliability (ICC = 0.88- 0.99) [4] [5]

Resources

The Y-Balance, along with the Functional Movement Screen (FMS), are used in the "Move2Perform Algorithm" software to predict the risk for injury. The components used are:

- Previous injury
- Y-Balance test composite score based on gender, sport and competition level
- Y-Balance Test asymmetry
- Functional Movement Screen (FMS) total score
- Functional Movement Screen Asymmetry
- Pain with testing

Based on the algorithm, patients are then categorized according to risk level (normal, slight increased risk, moderate increased risk, and substantially increased risk).

A. Uses of the Y-balance Test

- A functional movement screening device commonly used to predict the risks of injury in athletes
- Simplified version of the Star Excursion Balance Test (SEBT)
- Also used widely for the measurement of pre- and post-rehabilitation performance, improvement after performance enhancement programs, dynamic balance for fitness programs, and return to-sport-readiness.

B. Types of Tests

1. Y balance test kit includes 3 poles with distance marking in centimeters.
2. It consists of upper quarter test and lower quarter test as seen in the figure below.
3. For upper quarter test: 1 complete trial refers to the 3 reach directions: i.e. Medial, inferolateral, superolateral.
4. For lower quarter test: 1 complete trial refers to the 3 reach directions: i.e. Anterior, posteromedial and posterolateral.

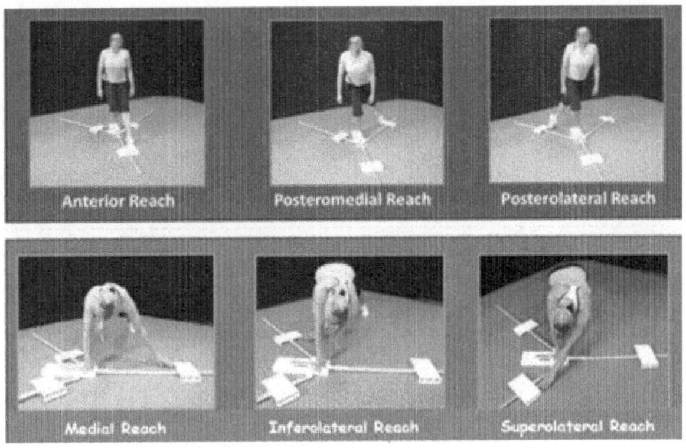

C. **Instructions**

1. Tester should explain the purpose ofYBT and demonstrate to the participant.
2. Participants have to perform 1 complete trial continuously without grounding their foot/hand.
3. Familiarization: Allow two practice trials before recording the actual measurements for each limb.
4. Actual testing: Two successful trials for each limb
5. Perform with barefoot and barehand (No socks and gloves are allowed)

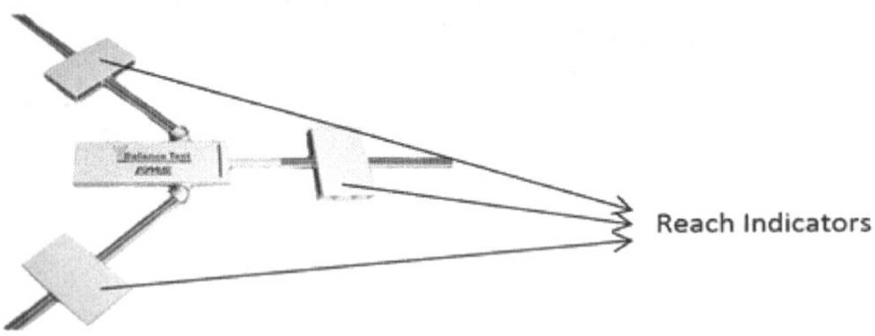

Upper Quarter Testing

1. Push up position; feet shoulder width apart with the shoes off.
2. Stance hand behind the red line and hands underneath the shoulders
3. Push the reach indicator continuously in 3 directions (Medial, Inferior lateral, Superior lateral)
4. Return to the original position under control without touching the ground during the test.
5. Reach foot must always maintain contact with the red target indicator only.
6. Restrict the placement of foot on top of the reach indicator to gain support.
7. The entire trial of three is repeated if there are any faults in the reaches. 8. Repeat the process with the other stance foot.

Lower Quarter Testing

1. Place the longest toe right behind the red line
2. Hands chucked on the hip throughout the entire trial
3. Heels always in contact with the platform
4. Push the reach indicator continuously in three directions (Anterior, Posterior lateral, Posterior medial)
5. Return to the original position under control without touching the ground during the test.
6. Reach foot must always maintain contact with the red target indicator only.
7. Restrict the placement of foot on top of the reach indicator to gain support.
8. The entire trial of three is repeated if there are any faults in the reaches.
9. Repeat the process with the other stance foot. Reach Indicators

D. **What constitute a Successful Trial?**

1. Balance of participant maintained throughout entire trial
2. Participant reaching out maximally to push the reach indicators
3. Do not tilt the foot or the hand on the platform to reach further
4. For lower quarter testing:

a. Arms maintain on hip throughout the entire trial

b. Heels maintain contact on the platform throughout the entire trial

E. **Scoring System**

1. Overall lower quarter: $(Anterior+Posteromedial+Posterolateral)3 \times Limb\ Length \times 100$
2. Overall upper quarter: $(Medial+Inferolateral+Superolateral)3 \times Arm\ Length \times 100$
3. Composite score must be above the risk cut point for that person age gender sports or activity level. If not, they are more likely to get injured.
4. Composite score of the left and right symmetry of each of the reach directions must not be more than 4cm difference.

References

1. Plisky PJ, Rauh MJ, Kaminski TW, Underwood FB. Star excursion balance test as a predictor of lower extremity injury in high school basketball players. J Orthop Sports Phys Ther.

2006;36(12):911-9.
2. Butler RJ, Lehr ME, Fink ML, Kiesel KB, Plisky PJ. Dynamic balance performance and noncontact lower extremity injury in college football players. Sports Health. 2013;5:417-422.
3. Westrick RB, Miller JM, Carow SC, Gerber JP. Exploration of the Y-Balance Test for assessment of upper quarter closed kinetic chain performance. IJSPT. 2012; 7(2): 139-147.
4. Plisky PJ, Gorman PP, Butler RJ, Kiesel KB, Underwood FB, Elkins B. The reliability of an instrumented device for measuring components of the star excursion balance test. N Am J Sports Phys Ther. 2009 May;4(2):92-9.
5. Shaffer SW, Teyhen DS, Lorenson CL, Warren RL, Koreerat CM, Straseske CA, Childs JD. Y-Balance Test: a reliability study involving multiple raters. Mil Med. 2013;178(11):1264-70.

Y-Balance Test – Score Sheet

Right limb length in centimeters: ______________

(Measure from right ASIS to right medial malleolus in supine after performing bilateral bridge)

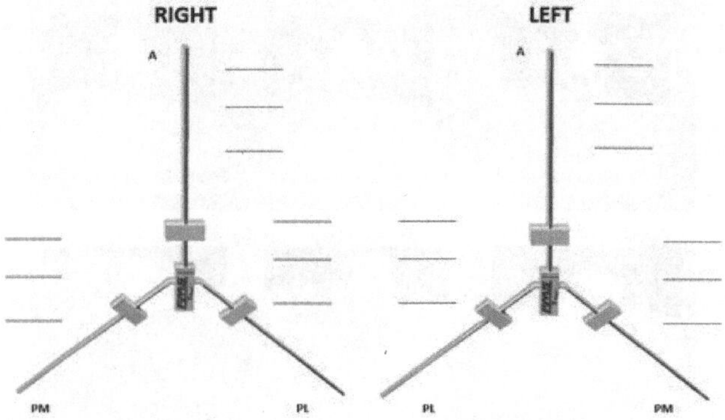

Greatest Successful Reach

	Right	Left	Difference
1. Anterior (A)			
2. Posteromedial (PM)			
3. Posterolateral (PL)			

Composite Score

Right

Left

(Anterior + Posteromedial + Posterolateral) / (3 x Right Limb Length) x 100 =

❑❑❑

192 MODIFIED KUPPUSWAMY SCALE

This is the most commonly used scale for determining the SES of an urban family. Kuppuswamy scale was developed for assessing the SES of an urban individual. It took three parameters into account, namely, education, occupation, and income of the individual

It was modified to enable SES assessment of a family rather than an individual. The parameters were modified as education and occupation of the HOF and the income of. the whole family, pooled from all the sources. These parameters are defined later in this section.

Education of Head of Family	Score	Occupation of Head of Family	Score	Total per Capita Family Income per month (as given originally in 1976)	Score
Professional Degree	7	Professional	10	2000 and Above INR	12
Graduate	6	Semi Profession	6	1000 – 1999 INR	10
Intermediate	5	Clerical / Shop / Farm	5	750- 999 INR	6
High School	4	Skilled Worker	4	500 – 749 INR	4
Middle School	3	Semi-Skilled Worker	3	300 – 499 INR	3
Primary School	2	Unskilled Worker	2	101 – 299 INR	2
Illiterate	1	Unemployed	1	Less than 100 INR	1

The total score is calculated by adding up all the three scores, namely, education, occupation, and total family income. According to the total score thus calculated, the family is placed in the appropriate socioeconomic class as explained in the following Table.

Total Score	Socioeconomic Class
26 – 29	Upper Class
16 – 25	Upper Middle
11 – 15	Lower Middle
5 – 10	Upper Lower
Below 5	Lower

Income of the whole family:

Since the time Kuppuswamy scale has been modified to determine the SES of the family rather than an individual, confusion has prevailed whether the income categories are meant to represent the total family income or per capita income.

The general consensus is that the original modification might have been for the whole family income, even against the argument that this does not consider the family size and may misclassify large families.

We suggest that the student may calculate the socio economic class of the family by applying both i.e. once by using 'total family income' and next by using 'per capita family income'. The resulting categories can be compared, and any difference may be commented upon while presenting the family to the examiner.

Per Capita Family Income:

The income from all the sources should be added up. This is divided by the total number of members of the family, regardless of the age of the individual. For example, even a baby born on the same day is to be counted. The income groups are revised from time to time according to the prevailing All India Consumer Price Index (AICPI). The student should check for the latest cut offs. The last revision before this article has been done using price index of January 2019 (Table below).

Original Income Group	Revised by using AICPI	Score
2000 and Above INR	47348 and above INR	12
1000 – 1999 INR	23674 – 47347 INR	10
750 – 999 INR	17756 – 23673 INR	6
500 – 749 INR	11837 – 17755 INR	4
300 – 499 INR	7102 – 11836 INR	3
101 – 299 INR	2391 – 7101 INR	2
Less than 100 INR	Less than 2390 INR	1

A formula has been developed for future regular updating of the income limits, which uses the latest Consumer Price Index for Industrial Workers (CPI-IW). The latest CPI-IW is available on the web page at http://labourbureaunew.gov.in/LBO_indnum.htm.

Deciding the Occupation Category:

The occupational category of "profession" includes persons who are at a high position and are involved in the decision-making process, laying down policies, and executing them. Most of them have received high education but it is not always the case. To this category belong doctors, senior administrative officers, senior lecturers, college principals, advocates, planters owning large estates, expert musicians, newspaper editors, auditors, architects, managing directors of firms, bank managers, etc.

The "semi-professional" group consists of occupations which involve college education. They may also involve lower grade professional training, but the jobs are essentially of a routine nature. Included in this group are mechanical and electrical engineers, high school teachers, lecturers, junior administrators, junior doctors, insurance inspectors, commission agents, musicians, research assistants, etc.

The third category persons need some training in arithmetic and reading and writing. The work here is also essentially of a repetitive nature. Some typical examples are clerk, typist, and accountant. A shopkeeper as well as a farm owner cannot continue unless they know how to keep accounts and look after the routine management. Many railway occupations such as station master and guard fall under this. Others such as news correspondent, salesman, insurance agents will continue in this category as long as they operate at the routine level. If they show greater initiative, they move into higher categories.

To the "semiskilled" group belong all those persons who need some training to do their routine jobs efficiently, e.g., factory or workshop labourer, laboratory or library attendant, and car cleaner. The petty shopkeeper may also be put into this category because he cannot pursue his occupation without some training regarding where to purchase, how to purchase, and how to sell.

"Unskilled worker": All those who are doing work which involves neither education nor training will come under this category, e.g., watchman, peon, domestic servant, and rickshaw puller.

Unemployed: The lowest category consists of persons who are unemployed irrespective of their general and professional education or training.

References:

- Poornima Tiwari, Shashank Tiwari. Chapter – 13 In: Mastering Practicals in Community Medicine, 2nd ed. Lippincott Williams and Wilkins, New Delhi.
- Aggarwal OP, Bhasin SK, Sharma AK, Chhabra P, Aggarwal K, Rajoura OP. A new instrument (scale) for measuring the socioeconomic status of a family: preliminary study. Indian J Community Med 2005;30(4): 111–4.

- Mishra D, Singh HP. Kuppuswamy's socioeconomic scale—a revision. Ind J Ped 2003;70: 273–4.
- Kuppuswamy B. Manual of Socioeconomic Status (Urban). Delhi: Manasayan; 1981.
- Sharma R, Saini NK. A modification regarding the Kuppuswamy socioeconomic scale. Chron Young Sci 2014;5:84-5
- Sharma R. Kuppuswamy's Socioeconomic Status Scale—Revision for 2011 and Formula for RealTime Updating. Ind J Pediatr 2012 [Epub ahead of print].
- Kuppuswamy's SES Scale for 2019, Online Tool: Available at: http://scaleupdate.weebly.com/real.html ; accessed on 27th March 2019

❑❑❑

193 Kellgren Lawrence Classification for Knee Osteoarthritis

The Kellgren Lawrence grading system is a radiological classification of knee osteoarthritis. It progresses from grade 0 to grade IV and based on x-rays. Knee osteoarthritis is a very common problem prevalent in all sections of society. While most of the changes are related to age, weight is a modifiable factor.

Grading of knee osteoarthritis is needed to gauge the severity of the disease, communication with colleagues and planning for the treatment. There are a number of grading systems devised for knee osteoarthritis, the Kellgren-Lawrence grading scheme is the most widely used and accepted standard for diagnosis of osteoarthritis of the knee.

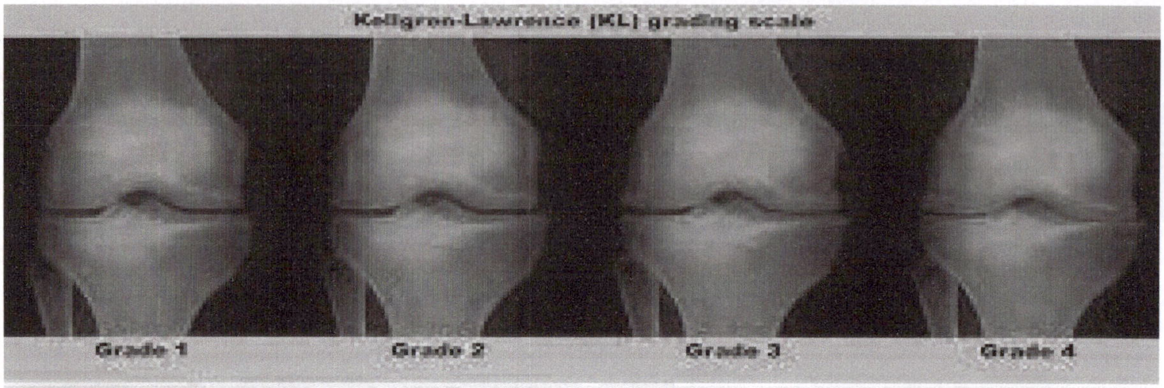

CLASSIFICATION	Normal	Doubtful	Mild	Moderate	Severe
DESCRIPTION	No features of OA	Minute osteophyte: doubtful significance	Definite osteophyte: normal joint space	Moderate joint space reduction	Joint space greatly reduced: subchondral sclerosis

Kellgren Lawrence grading

Grade I = There is a doubtful narrowing of joint space narrowing [A normal joint, therefore, appears to have a space between the bones. Any decrease in space implies a reduction in cartilage cover.] and possible osteophytes [small bony projections that from around joint margins. They are responsible for limiting the range of motion and can cause pain.]

Grade II = There is the presence of osteophytes and possible joint space narrowing on the anteroposterior weight-bearing radiograph. [weight bearing radiographs imply X-rays taken while the person stands on both he feet. A nonweight bearing x-ray is taken when a person is lying down and thus not bearing weight on knees]

Grade III = Grade III Kellgren Lawrence is characterized by multiple osteophytes, definite joint space narrowing, sclerosis [seen as increased white areas in the bone at the joint margin] and possible bony deformity.

Grade IV = It is characterized by large osteophytes, marked joint space narrowing, severe sclerosis, and definitely bony deformity.

❑❑❑